Diagnosis and Treatment of Mitral Valve Disease

A MULTIDISCIPLINARY APPROACH

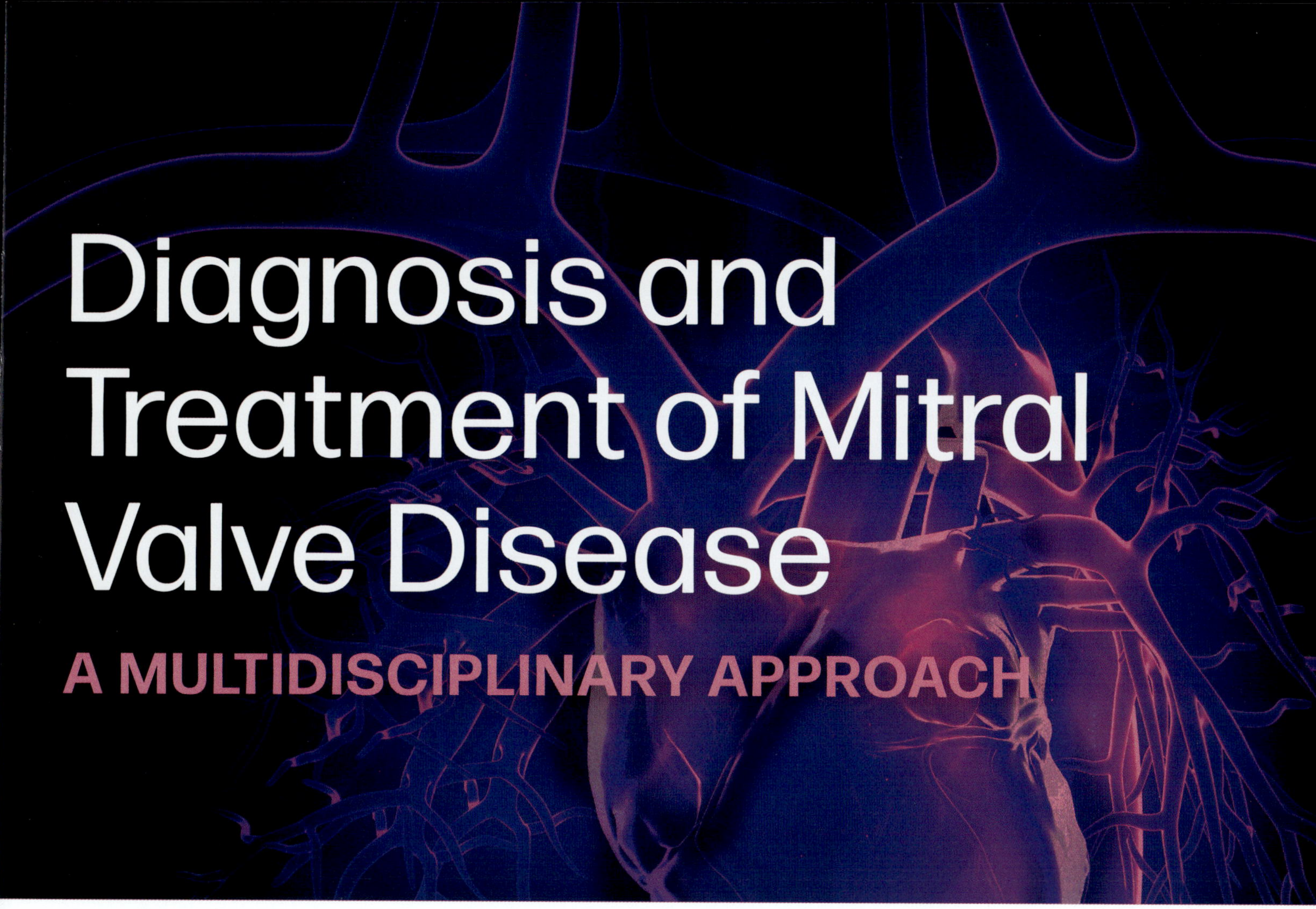

Diagnosis and Treatment of Mitral Valve Disease

A MULTIDISCIPLINARY APPROACH

EDITORS

SCOTT M. GOLDMAN
Director, Structural Heart Program
Lankenau Heart Institute;
Professor of Surgery
Thomas Jefferson University
Wynnewood, Pennsylvania
United States

WILLIAM A. GRAY
Chief of Cardiovascular Division
Lankenau Medical Center and Lankenau Institute of Medical Research
Wynnewood, Pennsylvania
United States

ELSEVIER

Elsevier
1600 John F. Kennedy Blvd.
Ste 1800
Philadelphia, PA 19103-2899

DIAGNOSIS AND TREATMENT OF MITRAL VALVE DISEASE: A MULTIDISCIPLINARY APPROACH ISBN: 978-0-323824781

Notice

Practitioners and researchers must always rely on their own experience and knowledge in evaluating and using any information, methods, compounds or experiments described herein. Because of rapid advances in the medical sciences, in particular, independent verification of diagnoses and drug dosages should be made. To the fullest extent of the law, no responsibility is assumed by Elsevier, authors, editors, or contributors for any injury and/or damage to persons or property as a matter of products liability, negligence or otherwise, or from any use or operation of any methods, products, instructions, or ideas contained in the material herein.

Content Strategist: Jessica L. McCool
Content Development Specialist: Anne E. Snyder
Publishing Services Manager: Shereen Jameel
Project Manager: Gayathri S
Design Direction: Brian Salisbury

Printed in India

Last digit is the print number: 9 8 7 6 5 4 3 2 1

CONTRIBUTORS

Sandra V. Abramson, MD, FACC, FASE
Director
Cardiovascular Imaging Center
Lankenau Medical Center
Wynnewood, Pennsylvania;
Clinical Assistant Professor
Sidney Kimmel Medical College
Philadelphia, Pennsylvania
United States

Michael A. Acker, MD
Chief, Division of Cardiovascular Surgery
Director, Penn Medicine Heart and Vascular Center
Hospital of the University of Pennsylvania
Philadelphia, Pennsylvania
United States

Tariq Ahmad, MD
Interventional Cardiology
Geisinger Wyoming Valley Medical Center
Wilkes-Barre, Pennsylvania
United States

Gorav Ailawadi, MD, MBA
Professor and Chair
Department of Cardiac Surgery
University of Michigan
Ann Arbor, Michigan
United States

Saif Anwaruddin, MD
Director, Interventional Cardiology
St. Vincent's Hospital
Tenet Healthcare
Worcester, Massachusetts
United States

Pavan Atluri, MD
Associate Professor of Surgery
Division of Cardiovascular Surgery
University of Pennsylvania
Philadelphia, Pennsylvania
United States

Shaylyn C. Bennett, MD, MS
Department of Cardiovascular Surgery
Nationwide Children's Hospital
Columbus, Ohio
United States

Philipp Blanke, MD
Department of Radiology
St. Paul's Hospital
Vancouver, British Columbia
Canada

Daniel J.P. Burns, MD, MPhil
Staff Surgeon
Department of Thoracic and Cardiovascular Surgery
Cleveland Clinic
Cleveland, Ohio
United States

Andrew Chatfield, MBChB
Centre for Heart Valve Innovation
St. Paul's Hospital
University of British Columbia
Vancouver, British Columbia
Canada

Chunguang Chen, MD, FACC
Director, Cardiovascular Imaging
Deborah Heart and Lung Center
Browns Mills, New Jersey
United States

Roxanne DeStefano, BS
Structural Heart Therapy Consultant
Philadelphia, Pennsylvania
United States

Steven M. Domsky, MD
Director, Cardiac ICU
Cardiology
Lankenau Medical Center
Wynnewood, Pennsylvania
United States

Amber M. Edwards, MD
Surgeon
Department of Cardiac Surgery
St. Thomas Health
Nashville, Tennessee
United States

Douglas B. Esberg, MD
Director, Cardiac Electrophysiology Lab
Lankenau Medical Center
Wynnewood, Pennsylvania
United States

Clarence M. Findley, MD, PhD
Baylor Scott & White The Heart Hospital
Plano, Texas
United States

A. Marc Gillinov, MD
Department of Thoracic and Cardiovascular Surgery
Heart and Vascular Institute
Cleveland Clinic
Cleveland, Ohio
United States

Eric M. Gnall, DO
Director of ECMO/Acute Mechanical Circulatory Support
Main Line Health
Wynnewood, Pennsylvania
United States

Scott M. Goldman, MD
Director, Structural Heart Program
Lankenau Heart Institute;
Professor of Surgery
Thomas Jefferson University
Wynnewood, Pennsylvania
United States

William A. Gray, MD
Chief of Cardiovascular Division
Lankenau Medical Center and Lankenau Institute of Medical Research
Wynnewood, Pennsylvania
United States

Lee Hafen, MD
Baylor Scott & White The Heart Hospital
Plano, Texas
United States

Rebecca T. Hahn, MD, FACC
Professor of Medicine
Columbia University
Irving Medical Center;
Director, Interventional Echocardiography
New York Presbyterian Hospital
New York, New York
United States

Rim Halaby, MD
Division of Cardiology
Hospital of the University of Pennsylvania
Philadelphia, Pennsylvania
United States

Jason J. Han, MD
Division of Cardiovascular Surgery
University of Pennsylvania
Philadelphia, Pennsylvania
United States

W. Clark Hargrove III, MD
Clinical Professor of Surgery
Division of Cardiovascular Surgery
University of Pennsylvania
Philadelphia, Pennsylvania
United States

Lisa Hathaway Stella, MPH
Executive Director
Interventional Cardiology
Columbia University Irving Medical Center
New York, New York
United States

Katie M. Hawthorne, MD, FACC
Cardiology
Lankenau Medical Center
Lankenau Heart Institute
Wynnewood, Pennsylvania;
Clinical Assistant Professor of Medicine
Sidney Kimmel Medical College
Thomas Jefferson University
Woodbury, New Jersey
United States

Mark R. Helmers, MD
Division of Cardiovascular Surgery
University of Pennsylvania
Philadelphia, Pennsylvania
United States

Howard C. Herrmann, MD
John W. Bryfogle Jr. Professor of Cardiovascular Medicine
Division of Cardiovascular Medicine
Perelman School of Medicine of the University of Pennsylvania
Health System Director for Interventional Cardiology
Hospital of the University of Pennsylvania
Philadelphia, Pennsylvania
United States

Benjamin I. Horn, DO
Fellow, Cardiology
Lankenau Medical Center
Wynnewood, Pennsylvania
United States

Michael Ibrahim, MBBS, PhD
Assistant Professor of Surgery
Associate Director, Penn Mitral Program
Division of Cardiovascular Surgery
University of Pennsylvania
Philadelphia, Pennsylvania
United States

Manju Bengaluru Jayanna, MD, MS
Cardiovascular Diseases Fellow
Lankenau Medical Center
Wynnewood, Pennsylvania
United States

Justin Johannesen, MD
Cardiology Fellow
Cardiology
Rutgers Robert Wood Johnson Medical School
New Brunswick, New Jersey
United States

Samir R. Kapadia, MD, FACC
Chairman, Department of Cardiovascular Medicine
Cleveland Clinic Foundation
Cleveland, Ohio
United States

Elina Khasanova, MD
Clinical Fellow
Radiology
Center for Heart Lung Innovation
St. Paul's Hospital
Vancouver, British Columbia
Canada

Konstantinos P. Koulogiannis, MD
Associate Director, Cardiovascular Core Lab
Department of Cardiovascular Medicine
Morristown Medical Center
Gagnon Cardiovascular Institute
Morristown, New Jersey
United States

Jonathon Leipsic, MD, FRCPC, FSCCT
Vice Chairman
Department of Radiology
University of British Columbia
Vancouver, British Columbia
Canada

Leo Marcoff, MD
Director of Interventional Echocardiography
Department of Cardiovascular Medicine
Morristown Medical Center
Morristown, New Jersey
United States

Gwyneth McNeill, DO
Fellow, Cardiology
Main Line Health
Wynnewood, Pennsylvania
United States

Sehrish Memon, MD
Structural Heart Fellow
Cardiovascular and Structural Heart Disease
Lankenau Medical Center and Lankenau Institute of Medical Research
Wynnewood, Pennsylvania
United States

Ryan A. Moore, MD, MS
Research Fellow
Cleveland Clinic Foundation
Cleveland, Ohio
United States

Vinayak Nagaraja, MBBS, MS, MMed (Clin Epi), FRACP, FCSANZ, FACC
Division of Interventional Cardiology
Department of Cardiovascular Medicine
Cleveland Clinic Foundation
Cleveland, Ohio
United States

Wally Omar, MD
Fellow, Interventional Cardiology
Beth Israel Deaconess Medical Center
Boston, Massachusetts
United States

Yinn Shaung Ooi, MD
Fellow, Cardiology
Lankenau Medical Center
Philadelphia, Pennsylvania
United States

Gosta B. Pettersson, MD, PhD
Vice Chairman and Professor
Department of Thoracic and Cardiovascular Surgery
Cleveland Clinic
Cleveland, Ohio
United States

Duane Pinto, MD, MPH
Associate Professor of Medicine
Harvard Medical School;
Director, Cardiac Catheterization Laboratory
Beth Israel Deaconess Medical Center
Boston, Massachusetts
United States

Michel Pompeu Sá, MD, PhD
Cardiovascular Surgeon
Research Assistant Professor
Lankenau Institute for Medical Research
Wynnewood, Pennsylvania
United States

Nicolas H. Pope, MD
Assistant Professor
Division of Cardiothoracic Surgery
Medical University of South Carolina
Charleston, South Carolina
United States

Basel Ramlawi, MD, FACS, FACC
System Chief
Cardiothoracic Surgery
Lankenau Heart Institute
Wynnewood, Pennsylvania
United States

Carrie Redick, RN, MSN
Director, Interventional Cardiology and Structural Heart
Atlantic Health System
Morristown, New Jersey
United States

Evelio Rodriguez, MD
Chief, Cardiac Surgery
Co-Director of Cardiovascular Service Line
Department of Cardiac Sciences
Ascension Saint Thomas
Nashville, Tennessee
Adjunct Associate Clinical Professor of Medical Education
University of Tennessee Health Science Center
Memphis, Tennessee
United States

K. Marco Rodriguez
Main Line Health Volunteer Research Assistant
Lankenau Medical Center
Wynnewood, Pennsylvania
United States

Roberto Rodriguez, MD, MS
System Surgical Director, Structural Heart Program
Cardiothoracic Surgery
Lankenau Medical Center
Wynnewood, Pennsylvania;
Associate Professor of Surgery
Thomas Jefferson University
Philadelphia, Pennsylvania
United States

Zach Rozenbaum, MD
Department of Cardiology
Lankenau Medical Center
Wynnewood, Pennsylvania
United States;
Faculty of Medicine
Tel Aviv University
Tel Aviv, Israel

Mark J. Russo, MD
Chief
Division of Cardiac Surgery
Director
Structural Heart Disease
Associate Professor of Surgery
Rutgers Robert Wood Johnson Medical School
New Brunswick, New Jersey
United States

Vishal N. Shah, DO
Department of Cardiothoracic Surgery
University of Nebraska Medical Center
Omaha, Nebraska
United States

Serge Sicouri, MD
Director, Cardiac Surgery Research
Lankenau Institute for Medical Research
Wynnewood, Pennsylvania
United States

Robert L. Smith II, MD
Baylor Scott & White The Heart Hospital
Plano, Texas
United States

Benjamin Smood, MD
Resident Physician
Division of Cardiovascular Surgery
University of Pennsylvania
Philadelphia, Pennsylvania
United States

John J. Squiers, MD
Postdoctoral Research Fellow
Department of Cardiothoracic Surgery
Baylor Scott & White The Heart Hospital
Plano, Texas;
Joint Thoracic/General Surgery Resident
Department of Surgery
Baylor University Medical Center
Dallas, Texas
United States

Molly Szerlip, MD
Baylor Scott & White The Heart Hospital
Plano, Texas
United States

Chidinma Tiko-Okoye, MD, MPH
Resident
Department of Surgery
Lankenau Medical Center
Wynnewood, Pennsylvania
United States

Per Wierup, MD, PhD
Staff Surgeon
Heart and Vascular Institute
Cleveland Clinic Foundation
Cleveland, Ohio
United States

PREFACE

The modern era of interventional treatment of mitral valve disease has seen great strides, beginning in 1948. Just think, prior to June 1948, the only accepted treatment for mitral valve disease was medical therapy. But all that would change in Philadelphia, PA, on June 10, 1948, when Charles P. Bailey performed a successful surgical mitral commissurotomy, after which the patient did well for more than 35 years. Also in that same year, Dwight Harken in Boston, MA, began a successful series of that procedure which paved the way for the procedure to be performed safely and effectively. The modern era of interventional treatment of mitral valve disease had arrived! In September of 1960, Albert Starr successfully implanted an artificial heart valve in the mitral position in a patient with mitral stenosis who had undergone two failed attempts at commissurotomy. Percutaneous mitral balloon valvuloplasty (MBV) was introduced in 1984 by Inoue, who developed the procedure as a logical extension of surgical closed commissurotomy.

We believe the time is right to assemble a contributed volume to help guide physicians who seek proficiency in the most modern treatment of mitral valve disease. The volume is not intended as the definitive tome on the subject of mitral valve disease and its treatments, but, rather, a curated volume of those topics that our collective experience has proven most valuable for the success of the physician and the excellence of patient outcomes.

Our aim is that the curated topic areas will help physicians assemble a plan before they undertake any interventional treatment of a patient with mitral valve disease. Not just a plan for which treatment would be the most appropriate for that patient, but a plan for the exact steps in that intervention. This is similar to a "flight plan" in aviation: The pilot does not just plan on when to leave and where to go. The planning involves pre-checking the airplane, planning the route, determining the fuel load required, knowing the weather en route and, alternative airports in case of bad weather, knowing the type of flight (visual or instrument), and planning the proper altitude. Similarly, our experience has shown us that a high degree of preparation prior to arriving in the operating room or catheterization laboratory—a plan—is likely to improve outcomes and procedural efficiency.

The volume includes contributions from a varied team of specialists: surgeons, heart failure specialists, interventional cardiologists, and imaging cardiologists—perhaps the keystone of the team. We are grateful for their contributions and willingness to impart their knowledge so that the next generation of interventional mitral valve specialists can improve their craft and patient outcomes. Key to the efficient functioning of this team is that each member has a depth of knowledge that includes all of these specialties. That is, it is just as important for the imager to understand surgical and transcatheter techniques and capabilities as it is for the surgeon and interventional cardiologist to be able to interpret both diagnostic imaging and imaging required to treat the mitral valve.

We hope this volume helps new mitral valve program teams gain the knowledge needed for a successful start; and, for established programs, to improve, advance, and thrive.

Scott M. Goldman, MD
William A. Gray, MD
Lankenau Heart Institute

FOREWORD

The knowledge necessary to effectively practice clinical medicine is growing exponentially. This is particularly true in the area of valvular heart disease as we are witnessing transformational advancements in the epidemiology, diagnosis, assessment, and management of patients with heart valve disease. The scope of information required to deliver optimal or best clinical practice is demanding a "super-subspecialization" focus on individual heart valves. This is particularly true in mitral valve disease, which is the most common type of valvular heart disease with diverse etiologies and anatomic variants, and with rapidly evolving assessment and management strategies being introduced into clinical practice on a seemingly constant basis. To coalesce the evolving expertise necessary in all areas of clinical care, it is critical that dedicated mitral valve specialists, including general and heart failure cardiologists, imaging experts, structural interventional cardiologists, cardiac surgeons specializing in valvular heart disease, midlevel providers, and researchers be assembled into effective multidisciplinary heart teams. Thus, the multispecialty mitral valve team becomes the vehicle to ensure and render optimal patient care.

The team at the Lankenau Heart Institute headed by Scott Goldman, an expert mitral valve surgeon, and Bill Gray, an equally expert mitral structural interventionalist, embody the quintessential leadership and clinical care structure to deliver optimal mitral valve management in their institution. Fortunately for us, they have assembled their collective experiences and learnings into this work entitled *Diagnosis and Treatment of Mitral Valve Disease*. This comprehensive yet easily readable compendium serves as a "how to do it" resource for any center wishing to embrace best practices in the management of patients with mitral valve disease in the modern era. In addition to sharing their own expertise, Drs. Goldman and Gray have recruited an impressive cadre of world thought leaders to share their knowledge and experience in the 29 chapters arranged in 6 sections. These chapters provide the latest evidence on the pathogenesis, pathophysiology, clinical findings, imaging techniques and medical, surgical, and transcatheter therapy options for patients with mitral valve disease. They also give us practical information as to how to assemble these specialists into a well-functioning multidisciplinary team.

The term "center of excellence" is an oft used term to define centers that provide best-in-class care worthy of a reference center, but not infrequently the actual care delivered falls short of the designation. For centers that truly embrace and desire excellence in mitral valve disease management, this comprehensive resource should serve as the default manual of how to truly achieve the desired lofty status.

As close professional colleagues of Drs. Goldman and Gray, we consider it a privilege to introduce this work to the clinical community caring for patients with mitral valve disease. We are proud of the expert mitral valve care delivered to patients by the Lankenau team and feel fortunate that they have assembled their collective experiences to share with the rest of us in this superb reference manual.

Martin B. Leon, MD
Michael J. Mack, MD

ACKNOWLEDGMENTS

We are fortunate to have begun our medical careers as the modern era of interventional treatment of mitral valve disease had already begun. Learning from those who pioneered new surgical procedures and interventions, we sought to move the field in a direction that would advance the field and improve patient outcomes.

We are hopeful that this contributed volume, *Diagnosis and Treatment of Mitral Valve Disease: A Multidisciplinary Approach*, will help a new generation of surgeons and cardiologists advance the field, establishing their own successful programs, contributing to research in the field, and advancing improved patient outcomes. We have drawn on the expert advice of today's thought leaders, who have made significant contributions to the understanding and betterment of the field. We are certain that these contributions will help those seeking to start new programs or improve existing programs. Our heartfelt thanks to all who have contributed to this volume:

Sandra V. Abramson, Michael A. Acker, Tariq Ahmad, Gorav Ailawadi, Saif Anwaruddin, Pavan Atluri, Manju Bengaluru Jayanna, Shaylyn C. Bennett, Philipp Blanke, Daniel J.P. Burns, Andrew Chatfield, Chunguang Chen, Roxanne DeStefano, Steven M. Domsky, Amber M. Edwards, Douglas B. Esberg, Clarence M. Findley, A. Marc Gillinov, Eric M. Gnall, Lee Hafen, Rebecca T. Hahn, Rim Halaby, Jason J. Han, W. Clark Hargrove III, Lisa Hathaway, Katie M. Hawthorne, Mark R. Helmers, Howard C. Herrmann, Benjamin I. Horn, Michael Ibrahim, Justin Johannesen, Samir R. Kapadia, Elina Khasanova, Konstantinos P. Koulogiannis, Jonathon Leipsic, Leo Marcoff, Gwyneth McNeill, Sehrish Memon, Ryan A. Moore, Vinayak Nagaraja, Wally Omar, Yinn Shaung Ooi, Gosta B. Pettersson, Duane Pinto, Michel Pompeu Sá, Nicolas H. Pope, Basel Ramlawi, Carrie Redick, Evelio Rodriguez, K. Marco Rodriguez, Roberto Rodriguez, Zach Rozenbaum, Mark J. Russo, Vishal N. Shah, Serge Sicouri, Robert L. Smith II, Benjamin Smood, John J. Squiers, Molly Szerlip, Chidinma Tiko-Okoye, and Per Wierup.

We also feel fortunate to be publishing the volume with the world-class science and medical publisher, Elsevier, whose team saw the importance of the work and carried it through to completion. First, we thank Jessica L. McCool, who recognized the importance of contributing to new works in a still-emerging field and signed the volume to the Elsevier portfolio. We thank Anne E. Snyder, who deftly assumed editorial responsibility after the volume was underway and made certain that the volume was developed in a consistent, high-quality manner. Gayathri S, our production project manager, deserves a special thanks for her attention to detail and for ensuring that all contributions were reviewed by contributors and readied for production.

Finally, we thank Main Line Heart Institute, whose focus on providing the best patient care, outcomes, and options has supported our work and research.

Scott M. Goldman, MD
William A. Gray, MD

CONTENTS

VIDEO CONTENTS

22.3. Two-dimensional TEE images of MV in the short-axis view demonstrating MR jet emanating from the A2-P2 segment.

22.4. Three-dimensional TEE images of MV in the short-axis view post MitraClip.

22.5. Two-dimensional TEE images of MV in the 2-chamber view.

23. Transcatheter Valvuloplasty

23.1 Percutaneous transvenous mitral valvuloplasty procedure.

25. Percutaneous Mitral Valve Interventions: Evaluation, Pitfalls, and Complications

25.1. Primary MR: TEE shows ruptured posterior mitral valve leaflet chordae causing severe mitral regurgitation with an eccentric and anterolaterally directed regurgitant jet.

25.2. Primary MR (3D): 3D TEE visualization of the primary MR due to flail P2 scallop.

25.3. MitraClip positioning: Positioning of the MitraClip to grasp A2 and P2.

25.4. Positioning of the second MitraClip.

25.5. Three-dimensional TEE of mitral valve after placement of two MitraClips shows the classic double orifice morphology seen after MitraClip with reduction in the severity of MR.

INTRODUCTION

The past seven decades have seen great advancements in the treatment of mitral valve disease. We have assembled this volume to help individuals and organizations develop successful mitral valve programs. We hope the volume engages, informs, and inspires all who read it to employ key takeaways to start and enhance their own mitral valve programs and improve patient outcomes.

This contributed volume includes chapters from authors who are among the most influential people advancing the treatment of mitral valve disease. Each author has not only contributed their knowledge and expertise to the field but are critical members of a multidisciplinary team at their respective institutions.

We have divided the volume into sections that we believe will facilitate retrieval of key information for the reader. We begin with a Foundations Section that provides a fundamental knowledge base. This includes anatomy of the mitral valve, pathophysiology of the valve, pertinent points of the physical examination, and guidelines for treatment.

Section 2, Diagnostic Tools, includes imaging and diagnostic studies of the mitral valve. The keystone of the diagnosis and therapy of the mitral valve are found in the chapters on transthoracic echo, transesophageal echo, and special imaging considerations. The imaging consideration chapters include MRI, as it is increasing in importance, both quantifying the severity of the disease and limiting pertinent anatomy; CT imaging, because it is key in the planning of transcatheter mitral valve replacement therapy; and cardiac catheterization, because of its importance in the diagnostic evaluation of patients with mitral valve disease. Cardiac catheterization helps define the anatomic and physiologic severity of the disease, can assess the presence of coronary artery disease, and provides an accurate assessment of the state of the pulmonary vasculature and cardiac output.

Section 3, Medical Treatment, includes treatment options for patients with mitral valve disease. This section begins with guideline directed medical therapy of patients with mitral valve disease. Whether as destination treatment for patients with functional mitral valve disease or in preparation for patients who require further intervention, medical therapy remains the first line of treatment.

Surgery remains a mainstay in the treatment of mitral valve disease and is covered in Section 4, Surgical Therapies. Chapters included in this section are based on different surgical approaches and surgical techniques for repair or replacement of the diseased mitral valve. The section begins with a chapter that describes devices and instrumentation that facilitate surgical procedures. The section also includes a chapter that presents the principles of perfusion techniques and myocardial protection necessary to safely conduct these surgical procedures, and chapters presenting different surgical approaches to the mitral valve including the sternotomy approach and the right thoracotomy approach. The addition of endoscopy has allowed for even less invasive surgery and is also included, as is the use of the surgical robot in the surgery of the mitral valve—another reliable, minimally invasive way to treat the mitral valve. Surgical repair of mitral valve regurgitation is presented by a very experienced team in this section, as is replacement of the valve when repair is not feasible. This section concludes with a chapter on evaluation, pitfalls, and complications of surgery.

Section 5 presents transcatheter therapy of the mitral valve. Transcatheter edge-to-edge repair is currently the only FDA-approved transcatheter treatment and is covered here in detail. There are several devices in clinical trial that are also discussed. Another chapter on balloon valvuloplasty, first described in the mid-1980s and an important part of the treatment of rheumatic mitral valve stenosis, is also included. This chapter includes patient selection procedural steps and complications of balloon valvuloplasty. The section concludes with a chapter on the evaluation, pitfalls, and complications of transcatheter therapy.

Chapters in Section 6 provide key takeaways for individuals and organizations seeking to establish successful mitral valve programs. "Establishing the appropriate infrastructure is fundamental to optimizing outcomes and the delivery of care for patients undergoing treatments for mitral valve disease," is a quote from a chapter in this section that discusses the makeup, function, and importance of the multidisciplinary team. Evaluating the structure, processes, and outcomes of a program are key to understanding and maintaining quality. A final chapter discusses the key components necessary to market your program as a comprehensive mitral valve program, how to build a focused outreach plan to optimize internal and external outreach efforts, and how to improve access to care through collaboration with the referral community.

Scott M. Goldman, MD
William A. Gray, MD
Lankenau Heart Institute

1

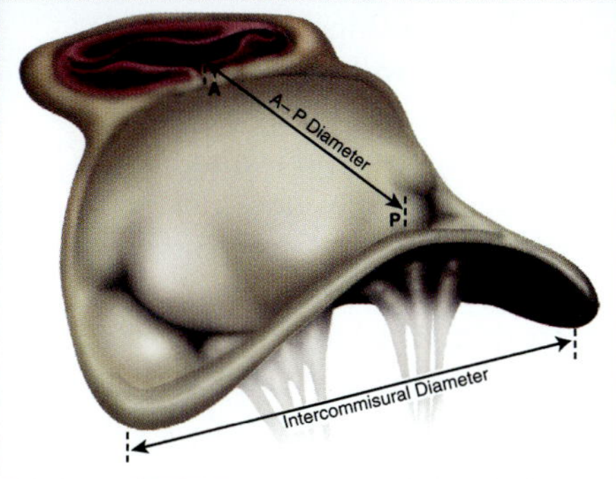

Anatomy of the Mitral Valve

Roberto Rodriguez, Tariq Ahmad

CHAPTER OUTLINE

LEARNING OUTCOMES

- The mitral valve is a complex and highly dynamic structure comprised of various structures that work as a single functional unit.
- The mitral valve annulus is a nonplanar saddle-shaped structure with its highest point at the mid-anterior annulus close to the aortic valve and with a second minor peak at the mid-posterior annulus.
- The fibrous skeleton is concentrated at the base of the ventricular mass and provides electrical insulation at the atrioventricular level and fibrous continuity for the leaflets of the mitral, aortic, and tricuspid valves.
- There are two major types of mitral valve chordae, classified based on their insertion sites to the mitral leaflets. The cords that attach to the leaflet tips are called primary cords, whereas secondary cords are the ones that attach to rough zones of the anterior leaflet and throughout the body of the posterior leaflet.
- The anterior mitral annulus can be divided into three segments (i.e., middle, right, and left). The area of aortic-to-mitral continuity is a dynamic structure that expands during systole and varies in size in response to changes in hemodynamic loading conditions and ventricular contractility.
- The left bundle branch of the cardiac conduction system enters the left ventricular outflow tract (LVOT) posterior to the membranous septum, with the His bundle located at the posteroinferior aspect of the membranous septum and right fibrous trigone.
- With the increasing numbers of mitral valve surgeries, especially reoperations, adequate exposure of the whole mitral valve apparatus through a small left atrium is a key element for successful and expedient intervention.
- A comprehensive knowledge of the mitral valve and its surrounding structure is of utmost importance in order to understand and deal with mitral valve clinical disorders.

INTRODUCTION

Mitral valve is typically 4 to 6 cm^2 in area and is a very dynamic structure. Each of the mitral valve's structural components performs a specific function in order to achieve normal functioning of the valve. In addition to primary mitral valve diseases, the disorders of the left ventricle and left atrium can also lead to abnormal functioning of the mitral valve. In this chapter, we will discuss the normal anatomy of the mitral valve along with the structures that lie around it.

MITRAL VALVE LEAFLETS

The human mitral valve is a highly variable and complex bileaflet structure. Although mitral leaflets are commonly referred to as anterior and posterior but anatomically aortic and mural names, respectively, for these leaflets appear more appropriate. The area where anterior and posterior mitral leaflets come together at their insertion to the mitral annulus is called "commissure." Mitral valve leaflets are noticeably different from each other in many ways but have nearly identical surface areas. The posterior leaflet is narrow but extends two-thirds around the left atrioventricular junction within the inlet portion of the ventricle. The free edge of this leaflet has indentations dividing the leaflet into three scallops. Infrequently these indentations extend deeper into the leaflet but usually not to the annulus, called clefts. Carpentier's nomenclature[1] defines the scallop adjacent to the anterolateral commissure as P1, the central scallop as P2, and the most medial scallop as the P3 segment, which is adjacent to the posteromedial commissure (Fig. 1.1). These scallops can be of variable sizes. The distinguishing feature of the posterior leaflet is the continuity of the left atrial wall myocardium on its atrial surface that can possibly make it prone to displacement in conditions like left atrial enlargement.[2]

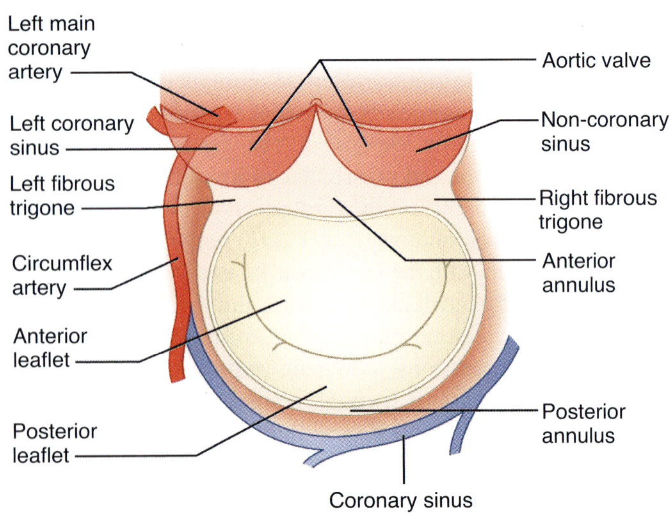

Fig. 1.1 Carpentier's Nomenclature. From (Carpentier AF, Lessana A, Relland JY, et al. The "physio-ring": an advanced concept in mitral valve annuloplasty. *Ann Thorac Surg.* 1995;60[5]:1177–1185; discussion 1185–1186. doi:10.1016/0003-4975(95)00753-8. PMID: 8526596.)

The anterior mitral leaflet is semicircular in shape, extends one-thirds around the annular circumference but is much wider than the posterior leaflet. This leaflet hangs like a curtain left ventricular inlet and outlet. The distinguishing feature of this leaflet is that it is in fibrous continuity with the aortic valve (left and noncoronary cusps), the interleaflet triangle between the aortic cusps that adjoins the interventricular membranous septum and fibrous trigones.[3] Anterior leaflet does not have clear scallops but is divided into A1 through A3 segments corresponding to the adjacent scallops of the posterior leaflet.

Normal mitral valve leaflets are thin, translucent, and pliable. There are three different zones described in these leaflets; (a) the rough zone[4] is nearer to the leaflet tips where the chords are attached. The leaflets are thicker in this area with nodular atrial surfaces and form the coaptation zone; (b) the clear zone (see Fig. 1.5) is next and is devoid of chordal attachments; (c) the basal zone is only present on the posterior leaflet and is the area where basal or tertiary chords are attached.

3D PERSPECTIVE

The four cardiac valvular orifices are not contained within the same plane.[5] In an apical-to-basal direction, the tricuspid valve is the most apical, or most inferior, of the four valves, followed by the mitral valve, aortic valve, and pulmonary valve. The mitral valve is also the most posterior, while the pulmonary valve is the most anterior. The basal planes of the two arterial valves are at right angles to each other.

The plane of the mitral valve is not flat,[6] and it resembles a saddle, just like the origin of its name from "mitra," meaning "bishop's hat" (Fig. 1.2). The highest point is the mid-point of the anterior leaflet. This shape of the mitral valve plays an important role in the distribution of forces during the cardiac cycle as the mitral valve area reduces by 10% to 15% during systole due to annular contraction. The shape of the saddle is further exaggerated by elevation of the highest points in systole when annulus contracts and commissural areas are moved towards the cardiac apex. This function of the mitral valve is affected by left ventricular dilatation leading to mitral annular dilation. The line of coaptation of mitral leaflets is a U-shaped curve. Along the coaptation line, the leaflet tips curl towards the left ventricle leading to an overlap of leaflet's surfaces called coaptation length. This allows persistently adequate leaflet coaptation even in the settings of moderate mitral annular dilation pulling the leaflets apart. In a normal mitral valve, the coaptation line is always below the plane of the mitral annulus, called coaptation depth (Fig. 1.3).

SUB-VALVULAR APPARATUS

Papillary Muscles

There are two papillary muscles classified into anterolateral and posteromedial muscles based on their relationship to the lateral and medial mitral commissures, respectively.[7] The bodies of the papillary muscles originate from the apical third of the left ventricular wall. The anterolateral papillary muscle usually contains a single head and has a dual blood supply from the diagonal

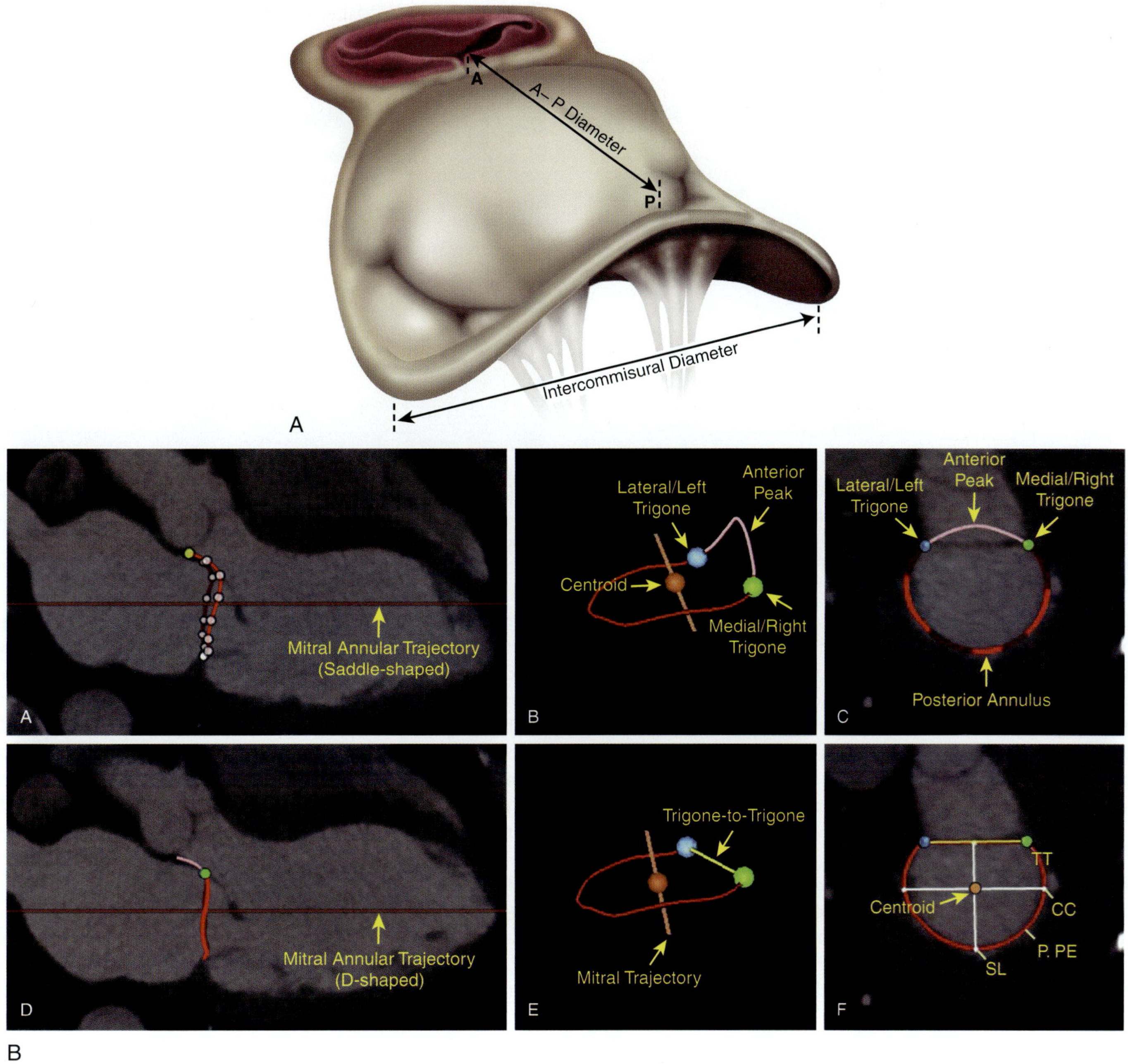

Fig. 1.2 Three-Dimensional Saddle-Shaped Mitral Valve Plane. The plane of the mitral valve is not flat,[6] and it resembles a saddle, just like the origin of its name from "mitra," meaning "bishop's hat". ([A], From Banks T, Razeghi O, Ntalas I, et al. Automated quantification of mitral valve geometry on multi-slice computed tomography in patients with dilated cardiomyopathy—implications for transcatheter mitral valve replacement. *J Cardiovasc Comput Tomogr.* 2018;12(4):329–337. [B], From Blanke P, Naoum C, Webb J, et al. Multimodality imaging in the context of transcatheter mitral valve replacement: establishing consensus among modalities and disciplines. *JACC Cardiovasc Imaging.* 2015;8[10]:1191–1208.)

branch of the left anterior descending artery and the obtuse marginal branch of the left circumflex artery. The posteromedial papillary muscles usually have two heads and receive blood supply from a single vessel, either the right coronary artery or the obtuse marginal branch of the left circumflex artery.

Papillary muscles play an integral role in the proper functioning of the complex mitral valve apparatus (Fig. 1.4). During the first half of the ventricular systole, the entire papillary muscle moves closer to each other and concurrently towards the mitral annulus due to longitudinal contraction of the ventricle base. This coordinated and symmetric movement prevents the distortion of the mitral leaflets when the leaflets move towards the left atrium during the first half of the systole. Additionally, at the same time, annular contraction allows early systolic leaflet

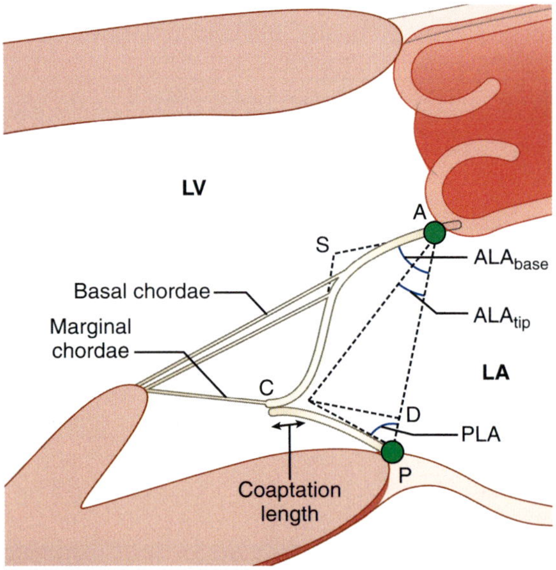

Fig. 1.3 Definition of Mitral Valve Configuration in Parasternal Long-Axis View. *A*, Indicates anterior mitral annulus; *C*, coaptation point; line *AP*, mitral annular diameter; line *CD*, coaptation depth; *LA*, left atrium; *P*, posterior mitral annulus; *S*, basal (or strut) chordae insertion.

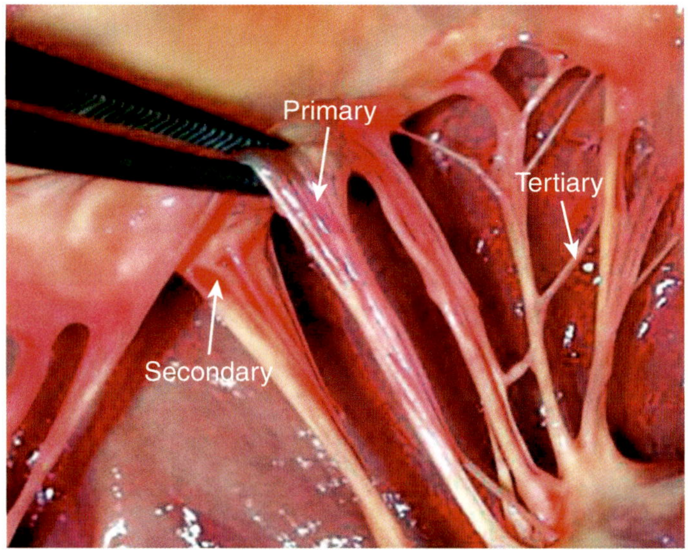

Fig. 1.5 Primary chord attached to the edge of the mitral valve leaflet, and the secondary chord attached to the belly of the mitral valve leaflet. Tertiary chords connect adjacent chords and do not connect to the leaflet.

coaptation by early saddle-shape accentuation. Whereas during late systole, isolated papillary muscle contraction shortens the muscle leading to an increase in distance between papillary muscle tip and the annulus, keeping the mitral leaflets under directed tension and posterior restrain to prevent leaflet prolapse and systolic anterior motion of the anterior leaflet leading to dynamic left ventricular outflow tract obstruction, respectively.

Chordae Tendineae

The chordae tendineae are the fibrous chords that originate from the tips of papillary muscles and attach to the ventricular aspect of the mitral leaflets in a hand held, fan-like pattern. Rarely, the chordae can stem from the basal posterior segment of the left ventricle and attach directly to the basal segments of the posterior mitral leaflet.[8]

There are two major types of the chordae that are classified based on their insertion sites to the mitral leaflets (Fig. 1.5). The chords that attach to the leaflet tips are called primary chords, whereas secondary chords are the ones that attach to rough zones of the anterior leaflet and throughout the body of the posterior leaflet. These chords are formed of tight collagen and elastin network. The primary chords are thinner with limited extensibility to prevent mitral leaflet inversion or flail. Whereas the secondary chords are thick, containing more elastin that makes them more extensible and are less likely to break compared to the primary chords. The anatomy and branching pattern of the chords are highly variable. These chords have the ability to adapt and can lengthen in response to the altering loading conditions.

LEFT ATRIUM

The left atrium is the most posteriorly situated of the cardiac chambers when viewed from the front side of the chest. With the interatrial septum being an oblique structure and mitral orifice higher than the tricuspid, the left atrial chamber is more posteriorly and superiorly situated relative to the right atrial chamber. Accordingly, the pulmonary veins that enter

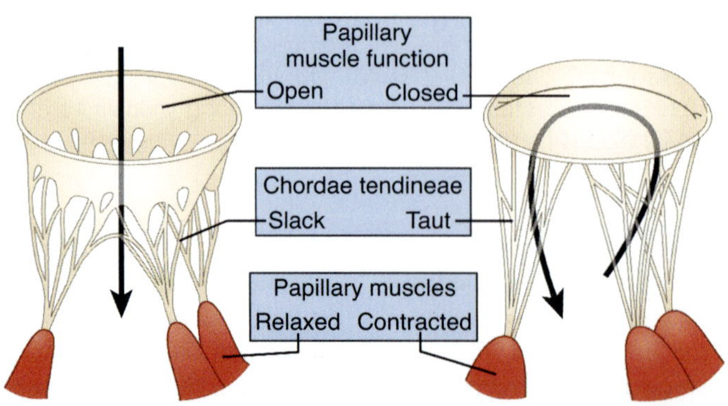

Fig. 1.4 The contraction of these papillary muscles during systole (rhythmic contraction of the ventricles) facilitates blood flow and prevents prolapse.

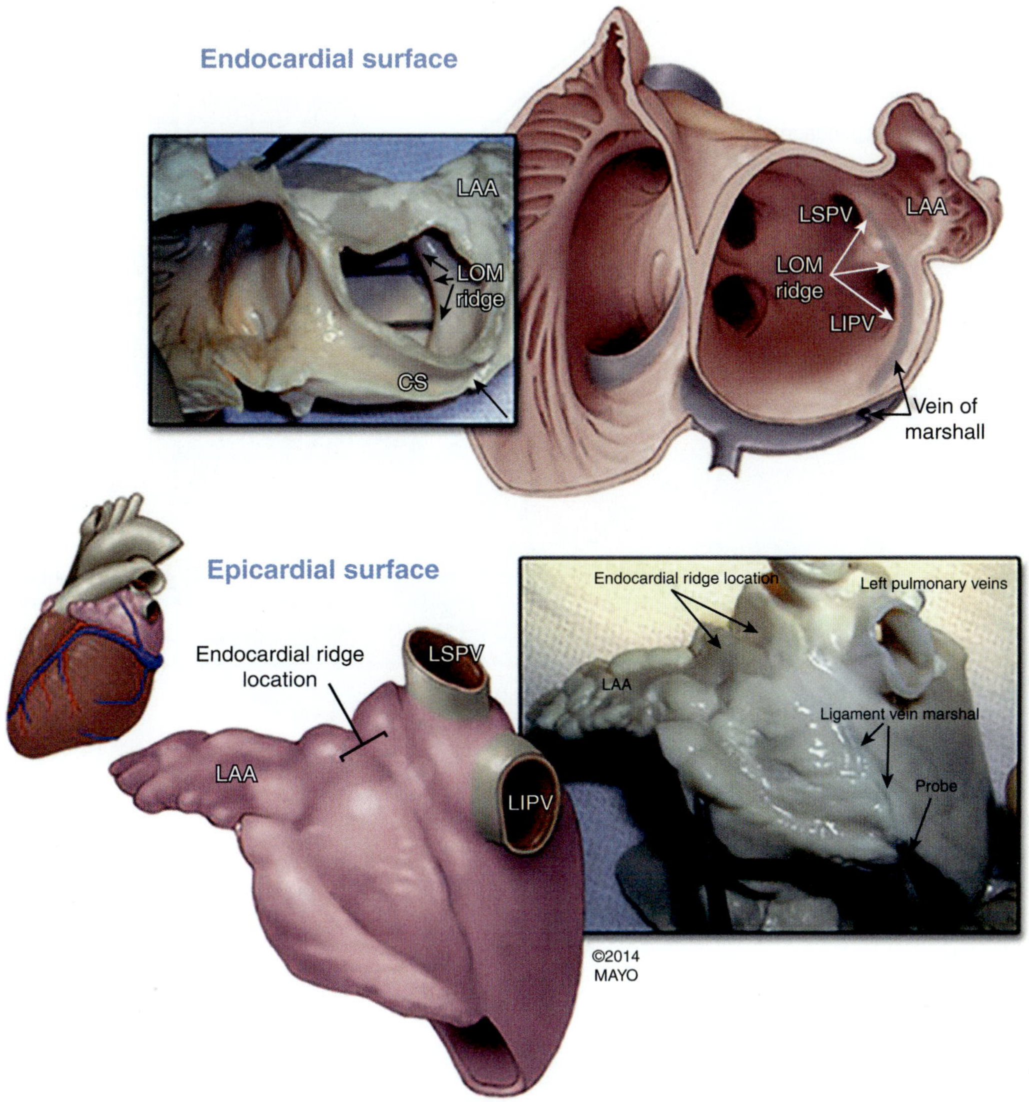

Fig. 1.6 Complexity of Left Atrial Appendage Morphology. Shown are endocardial views of the left atrial appendage from post-mortem specimens of human hearts. Left panel: The left atrial appendage ostia have more of an elliptical rather than a round shape. Middle panel: An endocardial view that shows the relationship of the left atrial appendage ostia, neck, pectinate muscles, and outpouching structure is shown. The smooth left atrium and orifices of pulmonary veins are seen in the figure in relation to the appendage. *CS*, coronary sinus; *LA*, left atrium; *RA*, right atrium; *LIPV*, left inferior pulmonary vein; *LSPV*, left superior pulmonary vein; *LOM*, ligament of Marshall. White arrows point to the outpouching structure of the appendage, where the neck extends outwards to a 3D body. Right panel: An endocardial view of the left atrial appendage showing the complexity of a multi lobed structure, 3D shape, and prominent pectinate ridges. *LAA*, Left atrial appendage. White arrows point towards multiple lobes and pectinate muscles. (From DeSimone CV, Gaba Prakriti Bs, Tri J et al. A review of the relevant embryology, pathohistology, and anatomy of the left atrial appendage for the invasive cardiac electrophysiologist. *J Atr Fibrillation.* 2015;8[2]:1129.)

the posterior part of the left atrium, the left veins located more superior than the right veins (Fig. 1.6). The left atrium has two distinct segments: the main body and the left atrial appendage (LAA). The main body can be further divided into the pulmonary venous segment, the septal segment, and the vestibule, which is the outflow part of the left atrial chamber just above and surrounding the mitral valve. Although the LAA has a well-defined opening called "os," the segments of the left atrial main body do not have any clearly demarcated outlines. Anterior to the left atrium lies the transverse pericardial sinus, and in front of the sinus is the aortic root (Fig. 1.7). Whereas, the tracheal bifurcation, esophagus, and descending thoracic aorta are immediately behind the pericardium overlying the posterior wall of the left atrium.

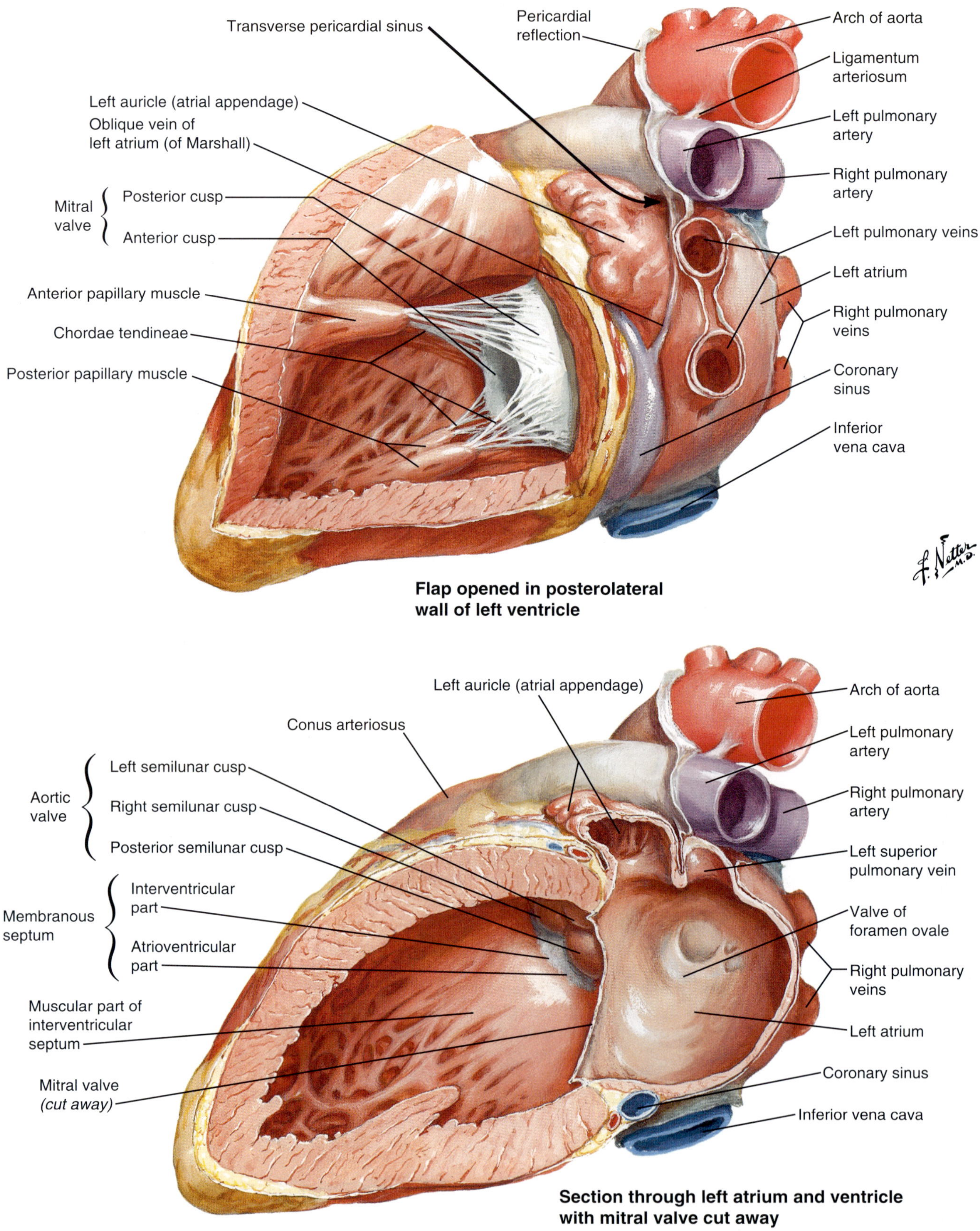

Fig. 1.7 Left Atrium and Left Ventricle Anatomy. (Netter illustration used with permission of Elsevier Inc. All rights reserved. Available from www.netterimages.com.)

The Appendage

The LAA is a pouch-like sac that originates from and lies anterior to the left atrial main body (see Fig. 1.7). The LAA is significantly smaller than the right atrial appendage. The body of the LAA runs parallel to the left upper pulmonary vein. The tip of the appendage points anterior and cephalad in the majority of cases and overlies the base of the pulmonary trunk, the left coronary artery, or the left anterior descending artery. In some cases, the tip can be directed posterior and caudal, or at times into the transverse pericardial sinus. The endocardial surface of LAA is heavily trabeculated with an in-between, paper-thin wall. The LAA has several variations in the size, shape, ostium, and number of lobes.

Septal Segment

Structurally more complex than it appears, the septal segment lies behind the aortic root and transverse pericardial sinus. It is important to appreciate the difference between the true septum (floor of the oval fossa) and atrial wall in-folding as muscle rim in order to obtain safe transseptal access to the mitral valve.

Interatrial groove (Waterston groove)[9] marks the epicardial aspect of the in-folded muscle rim and is not a true septal structure. It can become quite thick, especially in its superior, posterior, and inferior margins. In some patients, the epicardial fat may increase the thickness of the in-folding to 1 to 2 cm in the normal heart. The thickness of more than 2 cm on noninvasive imaging is increasingly reported as indicative of lipomatous hypertrophy.[10]

Pulmonary Venous Segment and Left Lateral Ridge (Coumadin Ridge)

The posterior part of the left atrium receiving the pulmonary veins is its venous segment. In over two-thirds of cases, there are classic four pulmonary vein orifices into the left atrium, whereas in others, common vein orifices are either on the left or right side, or five venous orifices can be seen. In a classic pattern, the right superior pulmonary vein passes behind the junction between the right atrium and the superior caval vein, whereas the inferior pulmonary vein passes behind the inter caval area. The orifices of the right pulmonary veins are directly adjacent to the plane of the atrial septum.

Viewed from within the atrial cavity, the endocardial surface has the appearance of ridges in between the superior and inferior venous orifices. In addition, there is a ridge-like structure between the entrance of the left superior pulmonary vein and the os of the LAA, called the coumadin ridge. Within the fold runs the remnant of the vein of Marshall, abundant autonomic nerve bundles, and a small atrial artery which, in some cases, is the sinus nodal artery. It is recognized as a "Q-tip sign" on echocardiographic imaging and, when prominent, can be mistaken for a thrombus or atrial mass.[11]

During cardiac development, the oblique vein of the left atrium (vein of Marshall) passes from a superior aspect onto the epicardial surface of the left atrium in between the LAA and the left superior pulmonary vein to descend along the posterolateral atrial wall to join the coronary sinus. In some individuals, the lumen of the oblique vein remains patent, forming the persistent left superior cava, draining into the coronary sinus. In the majority of individuals, however, this vein becomes a fibrous strand, the ligament of Marshall.

The Vestibule and the Mitral Isthmus

The smooth outlet zone of the left atrium into the mitral valve is called the vestibule. The myocardium of its distal parts minimally overlaps the atrial surfaces of the mitral leaflets. This can play a role in mitral leaflet stretch leading to functional mitral regurgitation in the settings of atrial cardiopathy due to chronic atrial fibrillation.

The mitral isthmus is a posteroinferior area of the left atrial wall located between the mitral annulus and the left inferior pulmonary vein. Ablation of this area can be important to complete isolation of pulmonary veins.[12] The endocardial surface of the isthmus contains pits and troughs, where some pits are "foramina Lannelongue," draining small cardiac veins. Along the epicardial side of this lies the left circumflex artery and great cardiac vein that continues into the coronary sinus.

FIBROUS SKELETON

The fibrous skeleton is concentrated at the base of the ventricular mass. It provides electrical insulation at the atrioventricular level and fibrous continuity for the leaflets of the mitral, aortic, and tricuspid valves. Its components include the fibrous trigones, the fibrous area of aortic-mitral continuity, the subvalvular collar of the mitral valve, the membranous septum, the interleaflet triangles, the tendon of Todaro, and likely the conus ligament. Most of the mitral annulus is fibrous, but the only true fibrous part of the tricuspid annulus is where the valvar leaflets are attached to the central fibrous body. At the aortic annulus, the fibrous elements support only the noncoronary aortic sinus and parts of the right and left coronary sinuses (Fig. 1.8).

Mitral Annulus

The mitral annulus contains two parts. The anterior part of the annulus is a sheet-like structure made of dense connective tissue that spans the roof of the LV between the fibrous trigones and connects the anterior leaflet of the mitral valve with the interleaflet triangle of the aortic valve. This latter area of aortic-mitral valvar continuity is also known as the aortic-mitral curtain or intervalvular fibrosa. The other part of the annulus is a band-like structure that extends peripherally from the fibrous trigones.[13]

When seen in a short axis, the mitral annulus appears D-shaped with an inter commissural diameter that is longer than the septolateral diameter. During surgical mitral valve repairs, the proportion between these two diameters must be preserved because a mere reduction of the circumference of the mitral orifice alone will not prevent mitral regurgitation.

The complex three-dimensional (3D) geometry of the mitral annulus plays an important physiologic role in the proper and durable function of the mitral valvular complex. In early systole,

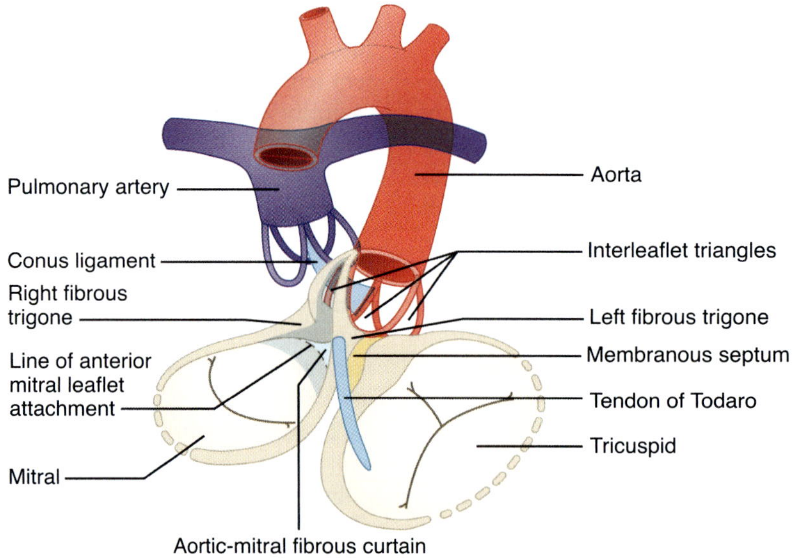

Fig. 1.8 Historic Representation of the Fibrous Skeleton. The majority of the fibrous tissue is concentrated at the fibrous trigones and adjacent connecting structures. There is fibrous tissue in the mitral valvar annulus, but this is hardly ever a continuous ring. The mural tricuspid valvar annulus is exclusively composed of fibroadipose tissue. The hinges of the pulmonary valve are not part of the fibrous skeleton. The conus ligament is an inconsistent structure and is seen in only a small fraction of hearts. *N*, Noncoronary sinus.

the height of the mitral annulus increases along with mild annular contraction along the septolateral dimension, which helps the leaflet coaptation. This annular action can be altered by various conditions[14] such as acute ventricular ischemia, dilated cardiomyopathy, surgical placement of a rigid annuloplasty ring, extensive reduction of the mitral leaflet, or post operative fibrosis, leading to mitral insufficiency.

Epicardial Vessels

The mitral annulus establishes significant anatomic relationships with pericardial vessels. Moving from the left fibrous trigone toward the atrial septum, the left circumflex artery and the great cardiac vein run on the epicardial side of the mitral annulus. The distal left circumflex artery and the coronary sinus run close to the annulus of the anterior mitral leaflet.

Fibrous Trigones and Aorto-Mitral Continuity

The anterior mitral annulus can be divided into three segments (i.e., middle, right, and left). The middle segment is the longest and provides fibrous continuity with the aortic valve (see Fig. 1.8). It extends between the right and left fibrous trigones. The right or left segments of the annulus are attached to the margins of the roof of the left ventricle and extend between the mitral commissures and a fibrous trigone, respectively. This area of aortic-to-mitral continuity is a dynamic structure that expands during systole and varies in size in response to changes in hemodynamic loading conditions and ventricular contractility.[15,16]

The area of fibrous continuity is continuous with the interleaflet triangle between the left and noncoronary sinuses of the aortic valve, with this area forming the posterior wall of the LV outflow tract. Also, this area comes in contact with the left atrial anterior wall. Due to this fibrous area being located at the border between the aortic root, left ventricular outflow tract, and left atrium, it holds an important clinical significance.

Aortic Valve

The aortic valve consists of three structures: the semilunar leaflets, the sinuses of Valsalva, and the interleaflet triangles, which extend from the basal plane forming the ventriculo-aortic junction to the sinotubular junction.

The ventricular musculature supports only around half of the aortic annulus, with the rest being fibrous. Whereas on the mitral side, the fibrous elements (aorto-mitral continuity) support the right side of the right coronary sinus, entire noncoronary sinus, and posterior half of the left coronary sinus. The ventricular musculature is absent or incomplete at the level of the noncoronary sinus due to the fibrous continuity (see Fig. 1.8) between the leaflets of the aortic and mitral valves, along with the presence of the membranous septum.

LEFT VENTRICULAR OUTFLOW TRACT

The left ventricular outflow tract (LVOT) contains muscular and fibrous components. The muscular component is formed by septal and free walls of the left ventricle. The fibrous part of the valvar annulus is formed by the left fibrous trigone, the aortic-mitral curtain, the membranous septum, the right fibrous trigone, and the interleaflet triangle between the noncoronary and right coronary sinuses.[17]

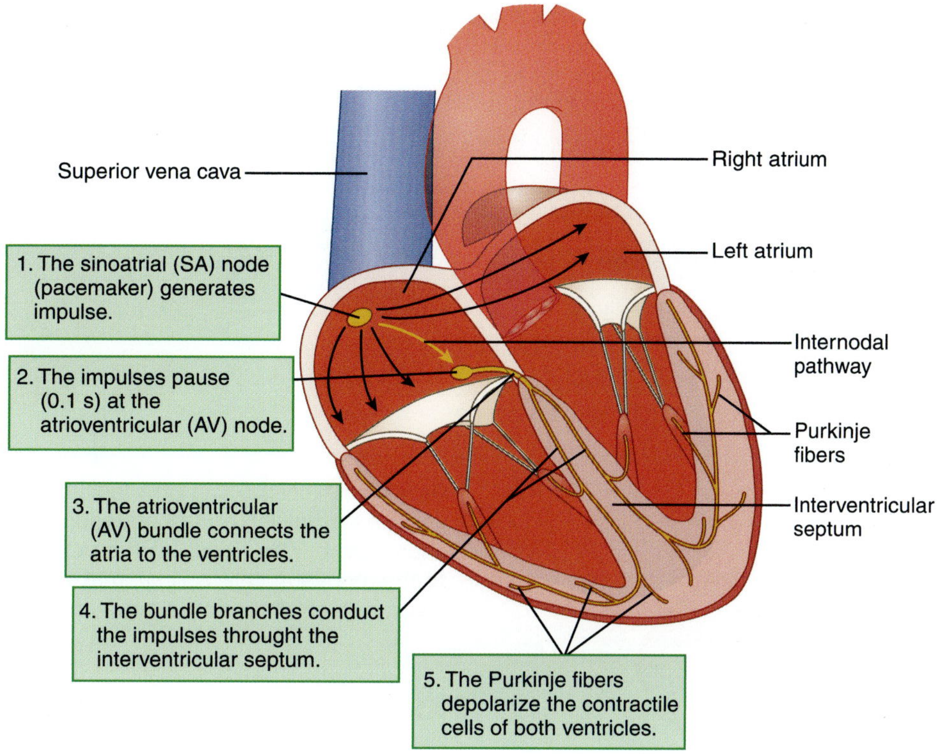

Fig. 1.9 Cardiac Conduction System. Cycle of excitation.

When viewed in a short-axis cross section, the anteromedial wall of the LVOT is formed by the membranous septum, and the interleaflet triangle between the noncoronary and right coronary aortic sinuses, the anterolateral wall of the LVOT is formed by the free wall of the left ventricle and the interleaflet triangle between the left and right coronary sinuses, whereas the posterior wall of the LVOT is formed by the interleaflet triangle between the noncoronary and left coronary sinuses, which is in fibrous continuity with the anterior mitral leaflet. Therefore, the mitral valve contributes to the makeup and function of the LVOT.

Membranous Septum

The membranous septum is located between the top of the muscular ventricular septum and the interleaflet triangle interposed between the no-coronary and right-coronary aortic valvar sinuses. It is divided by the attachment on its right side to the septal leaflet of the tricuspid valve into atrioventricular and interventricular components. The dimensions of the membranous septum and the relative sizes of its two components are variable.[18]

CONDUCTION SYSTEM

The left bundle of the cardiac conduction system (Fig. 1.9)[19] enters the LVOT posterior to the membranous septum, with the His bundle located at the posteroinferior aspect of the membranous septum and right fibrous trigone. In cases of an absent or small membranous septum, the His bundle moves closer to the aortic root. This anatomic variant is associated with a higher risk of conduction injury after percutaneous aortic valve implantation. From the perspective of the left atrium, the atrioventricular node and bundle are related to the vestibular portion that overlies the right fibrous trigonal area of aortic-mitral fibrous continuity. An approximate landmark could be the posteromedial commissure of the mitral valve.

ANATOMICAL APPROACHES TO THE MITRAL VALVE

With the increasing numbers of mitral valve surgeries, especially reoperations, adequate exposure of the whole mitral valve apparatus through a small left atrium is a key element for successful and expedient intervention. This section will briefly describe some of the common surgical approaches for mitral valve operations.

Interatrial Groove (Sondergaard or Waterston Groove)

In this approach, a right thoracotomy incision is made in the anterolateral fourth intercostal space, or a median sternotomy is performed. The right lung is retracted, and the pericardium is divided anterior to the phrenic nerve to expose the lateral wall of the atria in from of the right pulmonary veins. The most common approach to the mitral valve is through an incision starting in front of the right superior pulmonary vein and

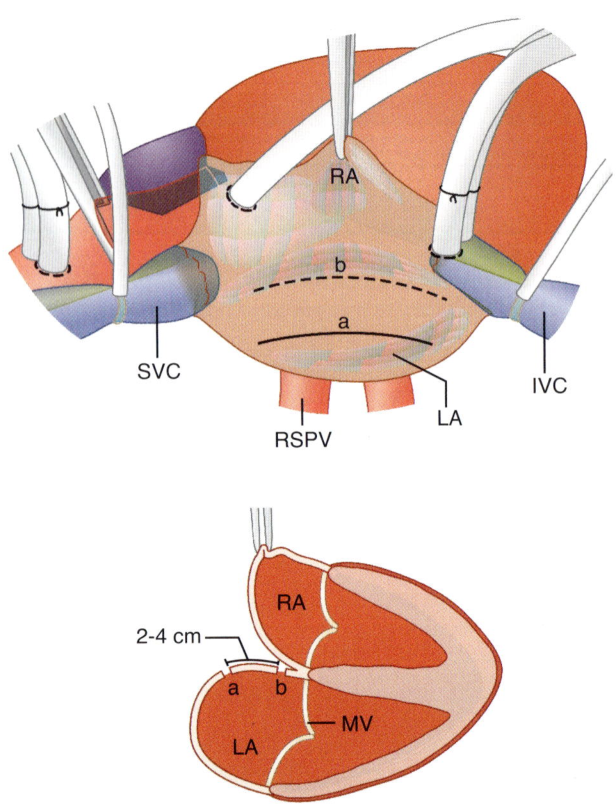

Fig. 1.10 Interatrial Groove Access. (A) At fatty interatrial junction. (B) With dissection into Sondergaard groove and closer to the mitral valve. *IVC*, Inferior vena cava; *LA*, left atrium; *MV*, mitral valve; *RA*, right atrium; *RSPV*, right superior pulmonary vein; *SVC*, superior vena cava.

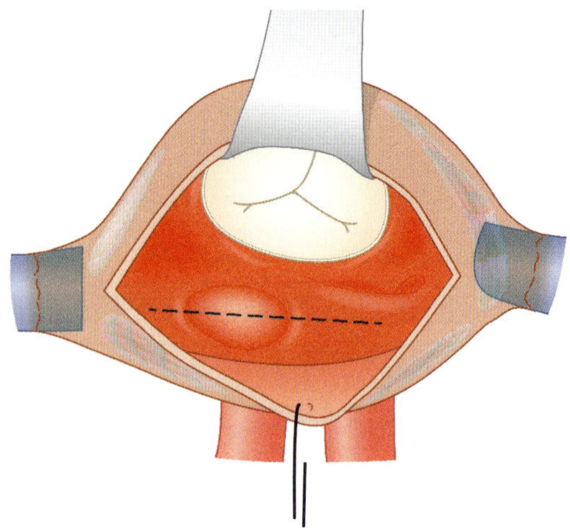

Fig. 1.11 If exposure can be predicted to be difficult, as, in the case of a small left atrium or deep chest, a planned transseptal approach may be used. With a vertical right atriotomy parallel to the atrioventricular sulcus, make a secondary, vertical septal incision through the fossa ovalis, avoiding the coronary sinus.

running parallel to the interatrial groove (Fig. 1.10). But in this area, there are extensive in-foldings of the atrial walls between the right superior pulmonary vein and the venous sinus of the atrium. These enfolded walls form the septum secundum component of the interatrial septum (i.e., the superior limbus of the fossa ovalis). The dissection of this plane was described by Sondergaard and associates in 1955, explaining the repair of atrial septal defects.[20] This groove is filled by a variable amount of fat.[21] Access to this groove is achieved with a combination of sharp and blunt dissection along with reflecting right atrium anteriorly. The incision into the left atrium is then made parallel to the right pulmonary vein but now is approximately 4 to 6 cm closer to the mitral valve compared to the common surgical approach. For more exposure, the incision can be extended superiorly into the roof of the left atrium and inferiorly into the inferior wall of the left atrium in the oblique sinus after mobilization and retraction of the cavae anteriorly.

Various maneuvers can be used to help assist better exposure, such as anterior suspension of the right-sided pericardial flap along with a detachment of the left-sided flap from the back of the sternum, allowing anterior and rightward rotation of the heart. Tilting the operation table head up and rolling it away from the surgeon also aids further exposure. This incision, along with electrical thermocautery (Maze procedure),[22] forms a scar line to treat atrial fibrillation.

Atrial Septal Approach

The above described vertical left atriotomy can be converted into a transseptal approach if mitral valve exposure is inadequate. First, a vertical right atriotomy is performed parallel to the left atrial incision. Then a transverse incision through the fossa ovalis is made perpendicular to the two atriotomies transecting the bridge of tissue between them. Alternatively, a vertical septal incision is made through fossa ovalis parallel to the two atriotomies, avoiding encroaching onto the coronary sinus inferiorly and domes of the left atrium superiorly.

Primary vertical right atriotomy with transseptal approach (Fig. 1.11) can be used in cases of predicted difficult left atrial approach such as deep chest or small left atrium. In the classic Dubost approach,[23] a transverse right atriotomy is performed that extends laterally to the right superior pulmonary vein or into the left atrium between the pulmonary veins. Next interatrial septum is incised at the level of the fossa ovalis perpendicular to the tricuspid valve following a line running 2 cm behind the coronary sinus to avoid conduction pathways, with incision extended to the right pulmonary vein superiorly and ending at the floor of the atrium inferiorly. Excellent exposure to the mitral valve can be obtained with this approach using a single retractor.

Another access can be the superior septal approach,[24] but it can possibly cause atrial dysrhythmias because of potential disruption of the sinoatrial nodal artery (Fig. 1.12). This artery can follow three pathways with half to two-thirds of times courses along the inner anterior border of the right atrium. Less common pathways are either an anterior course, which then goes behind the superior vena cava to reach the sinoatrial node, or its origin from the left circumflex artery with a posterior course on the left atrium and superior vena cava to the sinoatrial node. Due to this reason, a superior septal approach may be considered in patients with underlying permanent atrial fibrillation or complete heart block and not otherwise. In this approach,

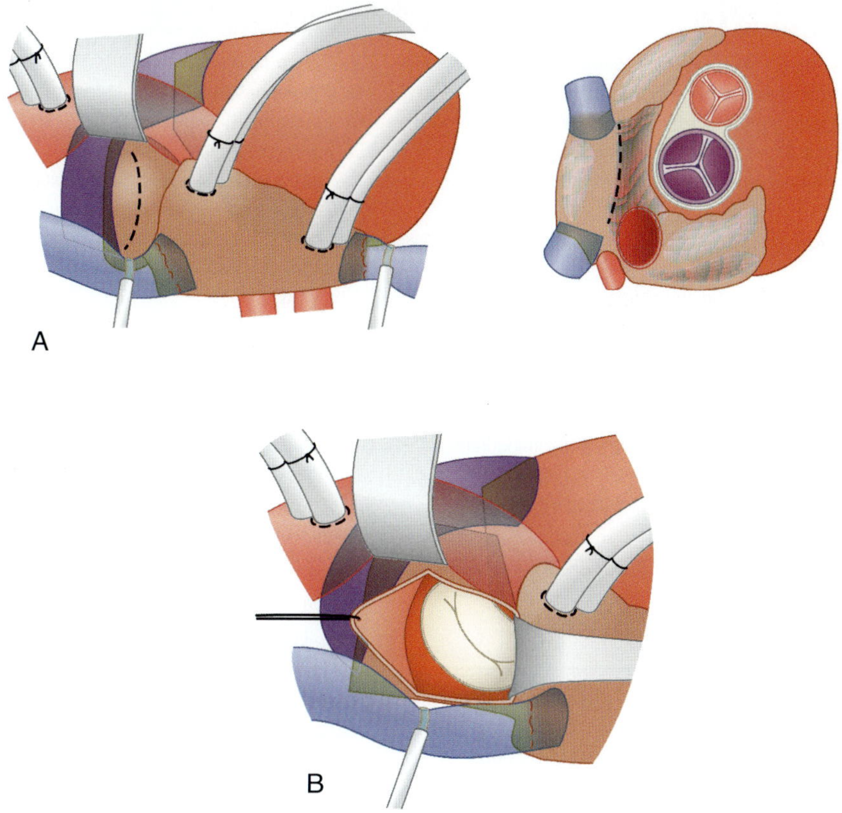

Fig. 1.12 The superior approach to the mitral valve allows adequate exposure of the mitral valve, with minimal to moderate retraction of the aorta and superior vena cava. It also allows a view of the mitral annulus more perpendicular to its plane than do other approaches.

vertical right atriotomy is performed anterior to the sulcus terminalis, extending superiorly to the atrial septum through the appendage. Next, a vertical septal incision is made through the fossa ovalis, extending superiorly to the apex of the right atriotomy, and continues the confluence of these two incisions into the dome of the left atrium.

Left Atrial Dome

This approach[25] provides a view of the mitral annulus more perpendicular to its plane compared to other approaches. First, dissect the aorta and superior vena cava from the right pulmonary artery behind them while avoiding injury to the left coronary artery behind the aorta, and mobilize the superior vena cava from cephalad to the right pulmonary artery inferiorly, to the sulcus terminalis. Next, retract the aorta anteriorly and left, whereas superior vena cava anteriorly and to the right in order to expose the left atrial dome. Then a transverse incision is made to the superior left atrial dome. If an extension of the incision is required, extend it to the right into the right superior pulmonary vein rather than to the left into the thin-walled LAA. If exposure is still not adequate, then the incision may be converted to a modified superior septal approach.

Left Thoracotomy

In some cases of altered anatomy or reoperations, the left thoracotomy approach[26] can be performed by placing an incision in the fourth or fifth anterolateral intercostal space with or without additional fifth rib resection if needed for improved exposure. The pericardium is then opened anterior and parallel to the phrenic nerve. An arterial cannula can be placed in the femoral artery or in descending aorta, in the settings of a competent aortic valve. The left ventricular vent can be placed through the ventricular apex or through the ascending aorta.

The left atrial incision is made parallel to the atrioventricular groove, carried through the thin-walled LAA needing some intricacy with closure techniques.

Percutaneous Transseptal

Percutaneous transseptal access to the left atrium is obtained for a wide array of procedures performed to the mitral valve and structures around it, the list of which is rapidly expanding. Particularly for mitral valve interventions, the access is obtained via the thin segment of the interatrial septum (i.e., fossa ovalis) using specially designed catheters along with needle or wire to burn a controlled hole in the desired location in the fossa using electrocautery, under echocardiographic and fluoroscopic guidance.

In general, these iatrogenic septal defects can be left alone as these pose no significant pathophysiological effects. In some cases, the septal defects can cause hemodynamically significant interatrial shunt needing percutaneous closure.

CASE-BASED ASSESSMENT

1. During surgical mitral valve repair from the right lateral thoracotomy approach, a vertical left atriotomy incision was given anterior to the right superior pulmonary vein at the interatrial sulcus (Sondergaard's groove). Prior to the mitral valve repair, a left-sided Maze procedure and left atrial appendage exclusion were performed. What are the boundaries of the surgical ablation line in this case?
   A. Atriotomy to the mitral valve annulus
   B. Atriotomy to coronary sinus
   C. Pulmonary vein box lesion, which includes the atriotomy
   D. Pulmonary vein box lesion to the base of the appendix
   E. All of the above
2. During transcatheter edge-to-edge mitral valve repair (TEER), the transseptal access was noted to be in an extreme posterior location of the fossa ovalis and possibly in the thick segment of the interatrial septum. An immediate blood collection was noted inside the thick septal wall segment without extension into the pericardial space. What is the space with contained blood called?
   A. Pericardial fatty tissue
   B. Lipomatous hypertrophied atrial septum
   C. Sondergaard groove
   D. Pericardial space
3. The anterolateral papillary muscle usually contains a single head and has a dual blood supply from the diagonal branch of the left anterior descending artery and the obtuse marginal branch of the left circumflex artery. The posteromedial papillary muscle usually has two heads and receives blood supply from?
   A. Single vessel, either the right coronary artery or the obtuse marginal branch of the left circumflex artery
   B. Dual blood supply from right coronary artery and obtuse marginal artery
   C. Single blood supply from the diagonal branch of the left anterior descending artery
   D. Direct blood supply from the left ventricle

See page 315 for the answers.

REFERENCES

1. Carpentier AF, Lessana A, Relland JY, et al. The "physio-ring": an advanced concept in mitral valve annuloplasty. *Ann Thorac Surg.* 1995;60(5):1177–1185; discussion 1185–1186. doi:10.1016/0003-4975(95)00753-8. PMID: 8526596.
2. Kagiyama N, Hayashida A, Toki M, et al. Insufficient leaflet remodeling in patients with atrial fibrillation: association with the severity of mitral regurgitation. *Circ Cardiovasc Imaging.* 2017;10(3):e005451. doi:10.1161/CIRCIMAGING.116.005451 PMID: 28289019.
3. Silver MD, Gotlieb AI, Schoen FJ, et al. *Cardiovascular pathology, Examination of the Heart and of Cardiovascular Specimens in Surgical Pathology.* 3rd ed. New York, Edinburgh: Churchill Livingstone Publishers; 2001.
4. Krawczyk-Ożóg A, Hołda MK, Bolechała F, et al. Anatomy of the mitral subvalvular apparatus. *J Thorac Cardiovasc Surg.* 2018;155(5):2002–2010. doi:10.1016/j.jtcvs.2017.12.061 Epub 2017 PMID: 29397976.
5. Saremi F. *Revisiting Cardiac Anatomy: A Computed-Tomography-Based Atlas and Reference.* Germany: Wiley; 2011.
6. Blanke P, Dvir D, Cheung A, et al. Mitral annular evaluation with CT in the context of transcatheter mitral valve replacement. *JACC Cardiovasc Imaging.* 2015;8(5):612–615.
7. Rusted IE, Scheifley CH, Edwards JE. Studies of the mitral valve. I. Anatomic features of the normal mitral valve and associated structures. *Circulation.* 1952;6(6):825–831. doi:10.1161/01.cir.6.6.825 PMID: 12998105.
8. Lam JH, Ranganathan N, Wigle ED, et al. Morphology of the human mitral valve. I. Chordae tendineae: a new classification. *Circulation.* 1970;41(3):449–458. doi:10.1161/01.cir.41.3.449. PMID: 5415982.
9. Radermecker MA, Limet R. Les différentes voies d'abord de l'oreillette gauche [The different accesses to the left atrium]. *Rev Med Liege.* 2004;59(9):504–508 French. PMID: 15559438.
10. Schwinger ME, Gindea AJ, Freedberg RS, et al. The anatomy of the interatrial septum: a transesophageal echocardiographic study. *Am Heart J.* 1990;119(6):1401–1405. doi:10.1016/s0002-8703(05)80191-7. PMID: 2353623.
11. Piątek-Koziej K, Hołda J, Tyrak K, et al. Anatomy of the left atrial ridge (coumadin ridge) and possible clinical implications for cardiovascular imaging and invasive procedures. *J Cardiovasc Electrophysiol.* 2020;31(1):220–226. doi:10.1111/jce.14307. Epub 2019 Dec 15. PMID: 31808228.
12. Becker AE. Left atrial isthmus: anatomic aspects relevant for linear catheter ablation procedures in humans. *J Cardiovasc Electrophysiol.* 2004;15(7):809–812. doi:10.1046/j.1540-8167.2004.03651.x. PMID: 15250867.
13. Berdajs D, Zünd G, Camenisch C, et al. Annulus fibrosus of the mitral valve: reality or myth. *J Card Surg.* 2007;22(5):406–409. doi:10.1111/j.1540-8191.2007.00449.x. PMID: 17803577.
14. Easley TF, Bloodworth 4th CH, Bhal V, et al. Effects of annular contraction on anterior leaflet strain using an in vitro simulator with a dynamically contracting mitral annulus. *J Biomech.* 2018;66:51–56. doi:10.1016/j.jbiomech.2017.10.045. Epub 2017 Nov 21. PMID: 29169632; PMCID: PMC5767149.
15. Parish LM, Jackson BM, Enomoto Y, et al. The dynamic anterior mitral annulus. *Ann Thorac Surg.* 2004;78(4):1248–1255. doi:10.1016/j.athoracsur.2004.04.055. PMID: 15464480.
16. Timek TA, Green GR, Tibayan FA, et al. Aorto-mitral annular dynamics. *Ann Thorac Surg.* 2003;76(6):1944–1950. doi:10.1016/s0003-4975(03)01078-6. PMID: 14667619.
17. Mori S, Fukuzawa K, Takaya T, et al. Clinical cardiac structural anatomy reconstructed within the cardiac contour using multidetector-row computed tomography: Left ventricular outflow tract. *Clin Anat.* 2016;29(3):353–363. doi:10.1002/ca.22547. Epub 2015 May 14. PMID: 25974872.
18. Saremi F, Hassani C, Sánchez-Quintana D. Septal atrioventricular junction region: comprehensive imaging in adults. *Radiographics.* 2016;36(7):1966–1986. doi:10.1148/rg.2016160010 Epub 2016 Oct 14. PMID: 27740897.
19. Stephenson RS, Atkinson A, Kottas P, et al. High resolution 3-Dimensional imaging of the human cardiac conduction system from microanatomy to mathematical modeling. *Sci Rep.* 2017;7(1):7188. doi:10.1038/s41598-017-07694-8. PMID: 28775383; PMCID: PMC5543124.
20. Sondergaard T, Gotzsche H, Ottosen P, et al. Surgical closure of interatrial septal defects by circumclusion. *Acta Chir Scand.* 1955;109(3–4):188–196 PMID: 13248393.

21. Wilcox BR, Anderson RH. *Surgical Anatomy of the Heart.* New York: Gower Medical; 1985.
22. Kik C, Bogers AJ. Maze procedures for atrial fibrillation, from history to practice. *Cardiol Res.* 2011;2(5):201–207. doi:10.4021/cr79w. Epub 2011 Sep 20. PMID: 28357007; PMCID: PMC5358279.
23. Dubost C, Guilmet D, de Parades B, et al. Nouvelle technique d'ouverture de l'oreillette gauche en chirurgie à coeur ouvert: l'abord bi-auriculaire transseptal [New technique for opening the left atrium in open-heart surgery: the bi-auricular transseptal approach]. *Presse Med.* 1966;74(30):1607–1608 French. PMID: 5932446.
24. Deloche A, Acar C, Jebara V, et al. Biatrial transseptal approach in case of difficult exposure to the mitral valve. *Ann Thorac Surg.* 1990;50(2):318–319. doi:10.1016/0003-4975(90)90765-x. PMID: 2383127.
25. Saksena DS, Tucker BI, Lindesmith GG, et al. The superior approach to the mitral valve. A review of clinical experience. *Ann Thorac Surg.* 1971;12(2):146–153. doi:10.1016/s0003-4975(1065107-7. PMID: 5561368.
26. Clowes Jr GH, Neville WE, Sancetta SM, et al. Results of open surgical correction of mitral valvular insufficiency and description of technique for approach from left side. *Surgery.* 1962;51:138–154 PMID: 13880007.

2

Pathophysiology of Mitral Valve Disease

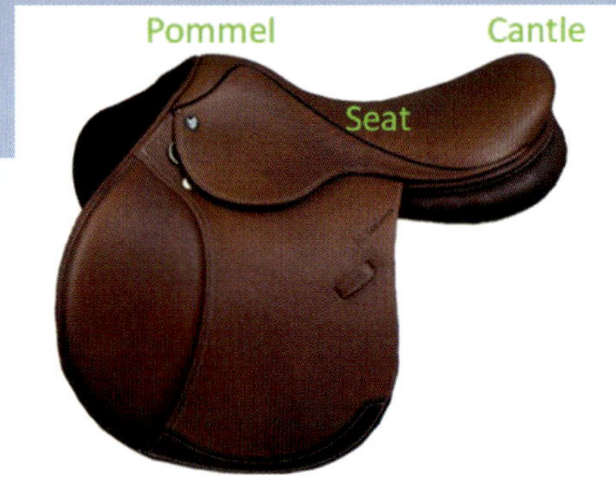

Shaylyn C. Bennett, Scott M. Goldman, Chidinma Tiko-Okoye

CHAPTER OUTLINE

LEARNING OBJECTIVES

- Recognize abnormalities of the mitral valve that lead to a disease state.
- Describe how abnormalities of the mitral valve cause pathology.
- Predict the outcomes of patients with each mitral valve pathology.
- Differentiate functional, primary, and mixed pathology.

INTRODUCTION

Understanding the normal structure and function of the components of the mitral apparatus is key in understanding the resultant pathophysiology when these components, or their interaction with one another, is disrupted. Therefore, we will review the normal physiologic function of the annulus, leaflets, chordae tendineae, and papillary muscles. We will then discuss the two broad categories of mitral valve pathophysiology: Mitral Valve Regurgitation and Mitral Valve Stenosis. Thereafter, we will discuss sequalae of mitral valve disease followed by special populations of mitral valve disease including pregnancy and congenital syndromes.

NORMAL MITRAL VALVE PHYSIOLOGIC FUNCTION

The mitral valve is a dynamic valve whose orifice and shape change during the cardiac cycle.[1] The integrity and synchronized interaction of the components of the mitral valve apparatus: annulus, leaflets, chordae tendinea, and papillary muscles are necessary for normal function.

Annulus

Part of the cardiac skeleton, the *annulus* is a ring of fibrous tissue that anchors the mitral valve at the intersection of the left atrium (LA), left ventricle (LV), and the mitral leaflets. The anterior portion of the annulus, circumscribed by the left and right fibrous trigones, is contiguous with the left coronary and part of the non-coronary cusps of the aortic annulus, and correlates with the pommel in the saddle-shape analogy, making it the highest or most atrial portion of the annulus (Fig. 2.1). This portion of the annulus is more fibrous and is connected to the aortic annulus by the aortic mitral curtain, or a rigid span of fibrous tissue, also known as the intertrigonal region.[2] The anterior portion of the annulus is more fibrous compared to the more muscular posterior portion, making it less prone to dilatation. The lowest point of the annulus, or the seat of the saddle, is located just posterior to the commissures. The posterior portion of the annulus corresponding to the cantle is more loosely attached to the cardiac skeleton and may play a role in the shape-shifting that has been observed in recent studies using the 3D echocardiography.[3]

During diastole, the mitral valve takes on a large, circular shape creating a negligible pressure gradient between the LA and LV facilitating passive left ventricular filling. Advanced imaging in recent studies of healthy subjects has revealed an average mitral annular area of ~10 cm^2, which is significantly larger than the widely accepted "normal" mitral annular area of 4 to 6 cm^2. During systole, the mitral valve must hold the gates against the contractile forces of the LV giving the left ventricular volume only one exit, maintaining forward stroke volume (SV) and cardiac output (CO). Valve closure and leaflet coaptation occurs in early-systole, during iso-volumetric contraction, due to anteroposterior contraction accentuating the saddle-shape.[3]

Leaflets

A continuous sheet of tissue extending from the annulus, the mitral valve leaflets are divided into anterior, posterior, and commissural parts.[1] The anterior and posterior commissures divide the valve into anterior and posterior leaflets. The anterior leaflet is dome-shaped, longer, and thicker than the crescent-shaped posterior leaflet which has a shorter radial length though encompasses a greater circumferential distance of the annulus, approximately 5 cm compared to 3 cm. Some degree of redundant leaflet tissue is necessary for effective coaptation. The normal ratio of the area within the annulus to the area of the leaflet tissue is 1.5 to 2.0.[3] Both anterior and posterior leaflets are described as having three corresponding scallops progressing numerically from anterior to posterior, though only the posterior leaflet has physical demarcations.

As there are variations in tissue characteristics between anterior and posterior leaflets, there are variations in tissue characteristics within each leaflet with the central portion being thinner and parachute-like, the clear zone. The free edges, or coaptation region, are thicker, hydrophilic, protein-rich, and deemed the rough zone and are the primary area of chordae attachment. The area of leaflet attachment to the annulus is termed the basal zone.[1–3] Mitral valve leaflets are composed of four histologic layers: (1) *atrialis*–atrial surface primarily aligned elastic/collagen fibers; (2) *spongiosa*–next layer, predominates in clear zone,

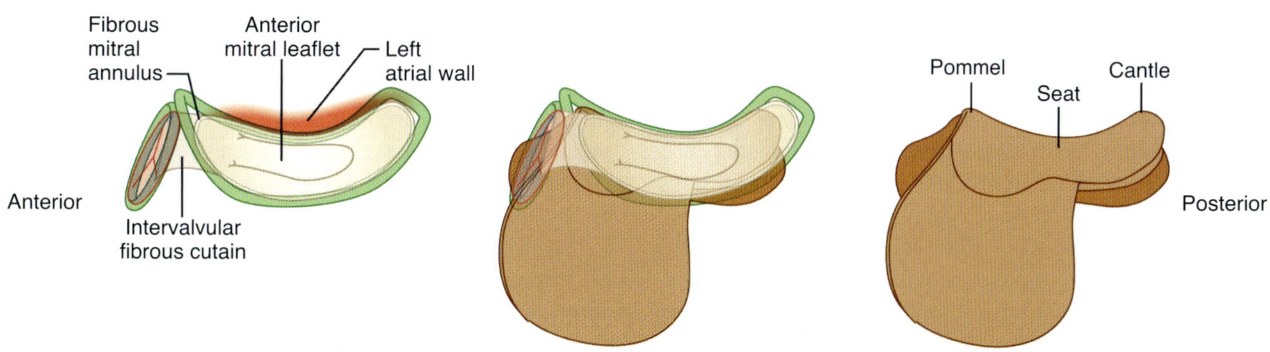

Fig. 2.1 Saddle-Shape of Mitral Valve. In this classic description of mitral valve morphology, the highest anterior portion of the mitral annulus adjacent to the intervalvular fibrous curtain corresponds to the pommel of the saddle. The seat of the saddle corresponds to the lowest portion of the annulus just posterior to the commissures. The posterior portion of the annulus corresponds to the cantle of the saddle.

extracellular matrix of proteoglycans, glycosaminoglycans, and elastic fibers; (3) *fibrosa*–strength layer composed of aligned collagen fibers forming central structural collagenous core; and (4) *ventricularis*–ventricular surface layer of contiguous endothelial cells with elastic and collagen fibers. Both leaflets contain muscle tissue near the annulus which resembles atrial myocardial cells. This tissue is excitable from the atrial side and may contract prior to LV contraction. It has been postulated that this early "leaflet" contraction may be crucial in preventing regurgitation during iso-volumetric contraction of the LV.

Chordae Tendineae

Chordae tendineae arise from the anterolateral (AL) and posteromedial (PM) papillary muscles and insert onto the leaflets.[1,2] They are divided into three types defined by their area of attachment. *Primary* chords attach to the rough zone, or the coaptation region, of both leaflets and are responsible for leaflet apposition. *Secondary* chords attach throughout the body of the leaflet and are said to contribute to normal ventricular geometry. Strut chords are the largest and strongest and attach the tip of each papillary muscle to the body of the anterior leaflet. *Tertiary* chords connect the base of the posterior leaflet directly to the ventricular wall.[2]

The function of the chordae has been controversial.[1] Flail, inversion of the leaflet edge into the atrium, is prevented by the thinner, less elastic, primary chords, also known as marginal chords. Secondary chords, or basal chordae, are larger and more elastic, and serve to transfer loads to the leaflets while protecting the primary chords from this load bearing.[1]

Papillary Muscles

There are typically two large papillary muscles arising from the apical one-third of the LV. The chords attach to these AL or PM papillary muscles. There is, however, considerable variation in papillary muscle anatomy, which explains numerous variations in the number of heads arising from each papillary muscle, as well as the blood supply to each described in the literature.[1,2,4] The AL papillary muscle usually has a single head and a dual blood supply from the left circumflex and left anterior descending coronary arteries. The PM papillary muscle usually has two heads and a single blood supply from either the right or circumflex coronary artery.[3]

Papillary muscles function synchronously with ventricular contraction and leaflet motion to maintain a relatively constant length of the chordae, or distance between the papillary muscles and the leaflets.[3] During early systole, longitudinal ventricular contraction moves the entire papillary muscle closer to the annulus. At this same time, the mitral leaflets are moving atrially. Thus, the distance between the papillary muscles and leaflets remains relatively constant. Later during systole, isolated papillary muscle contraction increases the distance from the tip of the papillary muscle to the annulus and closing leaflets. This creates tension on both leaflets and holds them posteriorly, preventing systolic anterior motion (SAM) and left ventricular outflow tract (LVOT) obstruction.[3] Maintaining the equestrian analogies, one might describe the function of the papillary muscles as that of a skilled rider's arms maintaining the reins (chordae) at a constant length so as not to allow the reins to go slack and taught causing overdue and abrupt impact on the horse's mouth. Using this analogy, one can imagine how discoordination of this complex interaction may result in chordal rupture as the slack chordae suddenly take on the force of LV contraction.

MITRAL REGURGITATION

Let us start by exploring Carpentier's classification which will serve as a guide to describe the structural pathology that results in mitral regurgitation (Fig. 2.2). The French cardiac surgeon, Alain Carpentier so eloquently and humbly described his functional classification at the 1983 meeting of the American Association of Thoracic Surgery (AATS). Per Carpentier, "there are only two functional anomalies: the opening and closing motions of each leaflet are either increased as with *leaflet prolapse* or diminished as with *restricted leaflet motion* (Fig. 2.3).[5]

Carpentier Type I

The Carpentier classification focuses primarily on leaflet position relative to the mitral annular plane. In Carpentier Type I, leaflets have normal opening and closing motion. Primary mitral regurgitation, defined as deriving from the mitral valve apparatus, can occur due to leaflet perforation or cleft.[6] Leaflet perforation can be iatrogenic from interventional procedures. Endocarditis of the mitral valve or direct extension of endocarditis of the aortic valve via their shared fibrous trigone can also result in leaflet perforation.

Leaflet Perforation

Leaflet perforation may be iatrogenic, secondary to trauma, or occur due to infective endocarditis, inflammation of the endocardial lining secondary to infection.[7] Endothelial damage, most commonly affecting the valve leaflets, is followed by thrombotic vegetations which then provide a substrate for bacterial colonization similar to a petri dish. Invasion, usually starting from the coaptive surface, damages leaflet and chordal tissue, and among its many detrimental effects are aneurysm formation and leaflet perforation.

Libman-Sacks endocarditis refers to the sterile fibrin-platelet thrombi vegetations and inflammatory valvular changes which are one of the cardiac manifestations of systemic lupus erythematosus (SLE).[8] It is sometimes also referred to as non-bacterial thrombotic endocarditis (NBTE) or "marantic" endocarditis, and in addition to SLE is associated with malignancy, most commonly adenocarcinoma. The latter term comes from the associated wasting, or cachexia, that can be seen in these patients. Libman-Sacks most commonly affects the mitral valve, followed by the aortic valve. Vegetations differ from the mobile, narrow base of their infectious counterpart in that they are characteristically immobile and sessile. This condition is usually not of hemodynamic significance; however, may manifest as acute or chronic mitral regurgitation (MR). It has also been associated with cerebrovascular and peripheral arterial embolism, cognitive dysfunction, superimposed infective endocarditis, and need for high-risk valvular surgery. Libman-Sacks endocarditis

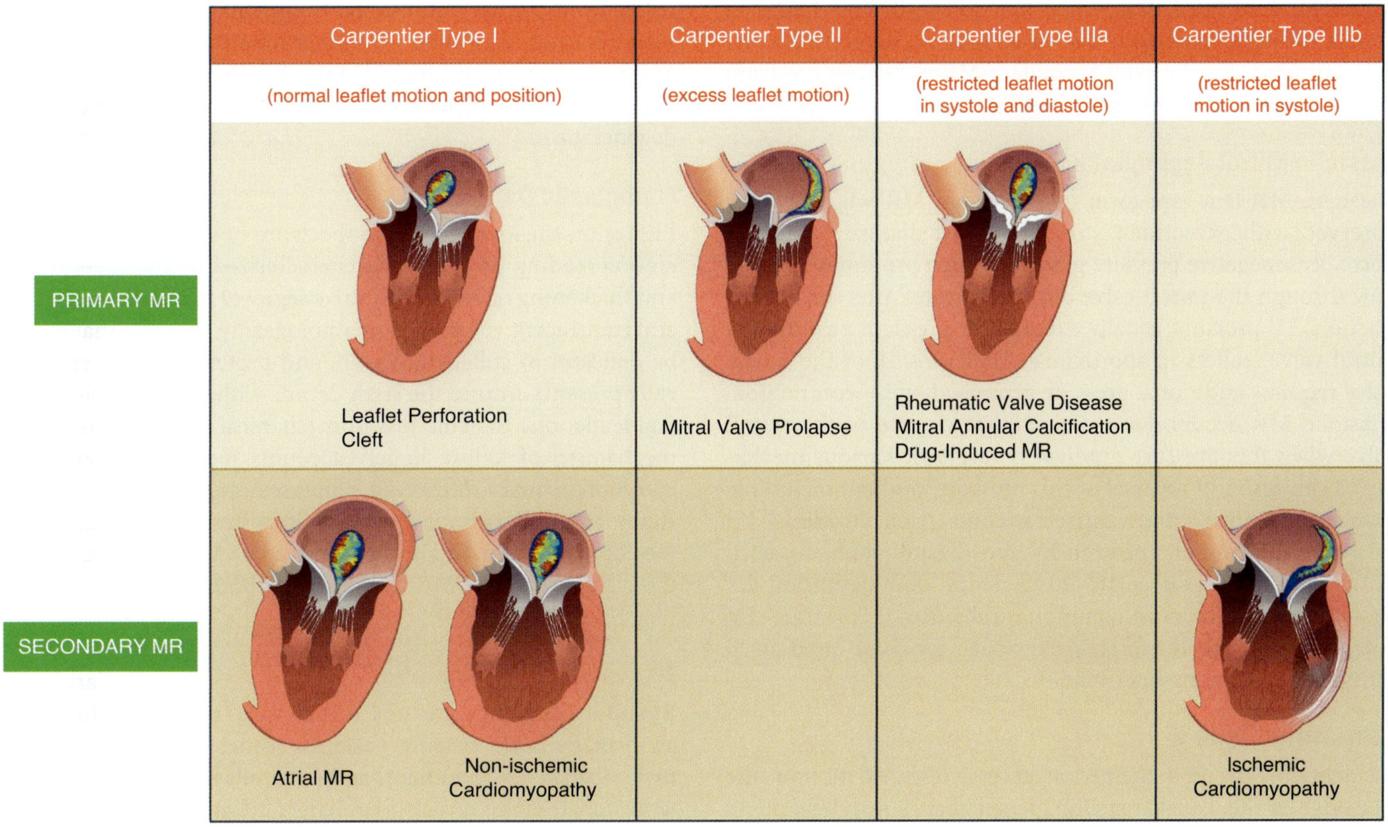

Fig. 2.2 Carpentier Classification. Depicts the classical Carpentier classification based on leaflet motion and divides this into primary and secondary mitral regurgitation *(MR)*. (From El Sabbagh A, Reddy YNV, Nishimura RA. Mitral valve regurgitation in the contemporary era: insights into diagnosis, management, and future directions. *J Am Coll Cardiol Imaging*. 2018;11[4]:628–643.)

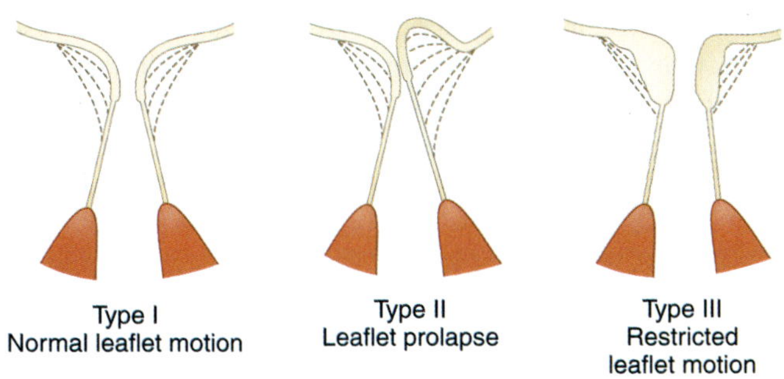

Fig. 2.3 Carpentier's Physiopathological Classification. Diagrammatic representation. Drawings represent a mitral valve apparatus with the posterior leaflet *(left)*, the anterior leaflet *(right)*, two papillary muscles, and the chordae. *Dotted lines* represent the course of the leaflets between opening and closing positions.

is included here as it has been implicated in several reported cases of leaflet perforation.

Mitral Valve Clefts

Mitral valve clefts are deep, congenital indentations in the leaflet extending to the annulus.[6] They are a rare cause of MR which prior to three-dimensional echocardiography (3DE) were almost always found in association with congenital heart disease. The anterior mitral leaflet is formed by the fusion of the superior and inferior atrioventricular (endocardial) cushions. It makes sense then that cleft mitral valves have been most often associated with endocardial cushion defects such as atrioventricular (AV) canals and ostium primum atrial septal defects (ASDs).[2,9] Mitral valve clefts may also occur in the posterior leaflet not associated with other congenital defects.

Annular Dilatation

Secondary mitral regurgitation in Carpentier Type I occurs due to an increased annular area or annular deformation resulting in a larger, flatter annulus, and loss of its saddle-shape configuration. The annulus of the mitral valve is dynamic with left atrial contraction reducing presystolic area, facilitating early leaflet motion and adequate coaptation.[10] When this atriogenic contraction is non-functional, equivalent reduction of annular area is possible via ventricular contraction; however, this is delayed and results in increased MR. Conditions which lead to an increase in mitral annular area include: left atrial dilation and non-ischemic/dilated cardiomyopathy.[6] Atrial fibrillation alone usually results in mild MR due to isolated annular dilation, but can cause more severe MR depending on the degree of left atrial dilation.[10] In patients with atrial fibrillation, severe tricuspid regurgitation is more common than severe MR due to the more robust fibrous skeleton of the mitral annulus better resisting significant dilation. Interestingly, Gertz et al. found that successful ablation led to decreased LA and annular dimensions with associated decrease in MR. However, in patients with recurrent atrial fibrillation, there was no significant change in annular dimensions despite decreased LA size, suggesting a primary annular association.[11] Secondary MR is derived not from the mitral apparatus, but from the LV or LA.

Diastolic Mitral Regurgitation

Diastolic MR is a rare form of functional MR which can be observed with or without structural heart disease.[12] There is normally a negative pressure gradient which promotes forward flow through the mitral valve during diastole. After atrial contraction, LV pressure usually exceeds LA pressure pushing the mitral valve leaflets to approximate. Full closure of the mitral valve requires additional pressure generated by LV contraction. Diastolic MR occurs due to incomplete closure of the mitral valve when this pressure gradient is reversed. Various mechanisms can result in reversal of this pressure gradient including: asynchronous atrial and ventricular contraction, "overdue" LV systole, significant elevation in LV end-diastolic pressure such as occurs with severe aortic insufficiency, and significant LV dysfunction.[2,13] The most common mechanism is "overdue" LV systole commonly due to atrioventricular block or rapid atrial arrhythmia with long intermission.

Carpentier Type II

Carpentier Type II is defined as excessive leaflet motion, the free edge of the leaflet traveling greater than 2 mm beyond its normal coaptation point at the annulus during systole. In his initial article, Carpentier, using Barlow's description, states that this must be clearly delineated from billowing, in which excess leaflet tissue protrudes into the LA during systole while the free edge remains in apposition below the annulus. Fig. 2.4 depicts the difference between prolapse and billowing, and the conglomeration thereof. While the terminology may be confusing and inconsistent in the literature, all mitral valve prolapse (MVP) fails under Carpentier Type II, and is the most frequent cause of MR in developed countries, affecting 2% to 5% of the population. The spectrum of myxomatous degeneration, from fibroelastic deficiency (FED), to myxomatous disease, and finally Barlow's disease (BD; diffuse myxomatous degeneration) encompasses many of the etiologies of MVP. MVP may result from primary autosomal dominant disorder of variable penetrance or associated with other inherited disorders such as Marfan syndrome or Ehlers-Danlos syndrome.[7,14] Table 2.1 provides a more complete list of syndromic causes of myxomatous degeneration.

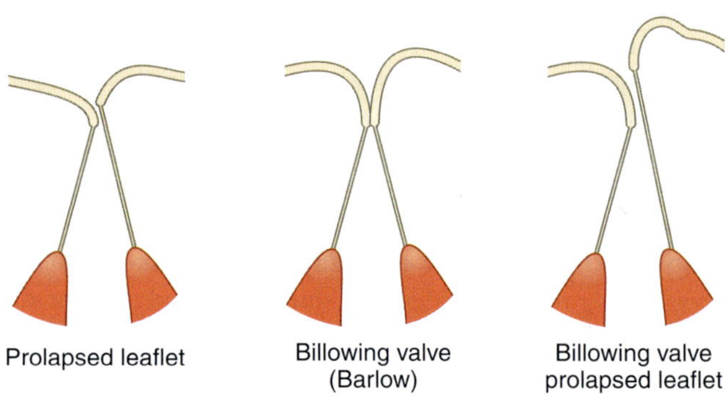

Fig. 2.4 Carpentier's Depiction of Billowing Versus Prolapse. Line drawing depicting leaflets, chordae, and papillary muscles showing prolapsed leaflet with free edge above the normal coaptation plane *(left)*, billowing leaflet with free edges remaining at level of normal coaptation plane and doming of leaflet extending atrially *(middle)*, and finally a combination of both *(right)*.

Fibroelastic Deficiency

FED is on the low end of the spectrum of myxomatous degeneration leading to MVP. It is characterized by the redundancy and thickening of one mitral valve segment in an otherwise thin and translucent valve.[2] Histopathologically, these valves tend to be deficient in collagen, elastin, and proteoglycans. FED typically presents around the sixth decade with ruptured chord and flail leaflet due to acute loss of mechanical integrity. This acute mechanism of failure largely accounts for it being the most common primary mitral valve disease requiring surgical repair. Acute MR and pulmonary edema may result from rupture of the chordae. The pathophysiology of acute MR is described after the classification of MR as there are numerous etiologies that may result in acute MR.

Myxomatous Degeneration

Prolapse from myxomatous mitral valve disease results from abnormally large, usually posterior leaflet comprised of loose myxomatous tissue, rather than dense collagen and elastin. Leaflet histopathology reveals fragmented collagen, increased extracellular proteoglycans, and fibrosis.[7] This results in elongated, stretched out leaflets and attenuated chordae prone to rupture. The valve may have an overall thickened, gelatinous, scalloped appearance. The prolapse caused by myxomatous degeneration is usually asymptomatic and may have resultant MR; however, in more severe cases, annular enlargement and elongated chordae can cause more profound MR. In rare cases, patients may experience symptoms from atrial or ventricular arrhythmias, thromboembolic events, and infective endocarditis.

TABLE 2.1 Syndromic Causes of Myxomatous Degeneration

Syndrome	Associated Genetic Mutation(s)	Estimated Prevalence of MVP
Marfan	FBN1	25%–45%
Ehlers-Danlos	COL5A1, COL5A2	6%
Loeys-Dietz	TGFBR1, TGFBR2	21%
Aneurysms-osteoarthritis	SMAD3	45%
Hypertrophic cardiomyopathy	MYN7, MYBPC3, TNNT2, TNNI3	3%
Osteogenesis imperfecta	COL1A1, COL1A2	Unknown
Pseudoxanthoma elasticum	ABCC6	Unknown

MVP, Mitral valve prolapse.

(Adapted from Fishbein GA, Fishbein MC. Mitral valve pathology. *Curr Cardiol Rep.* 2019;21(7):61.)

Barlow's Disease (Diffuse Myxomatous Degeneration)

Barlow first associated MR with the characteristic midsystolic click and following systolic murmur in the 1960s.[15] As previously mentioned, it was Carpentier who distinguished BD from MVP.[16] Per Carpentier, BD is defined as: bileaflet prolapse greater than 2 mm, a billowing valve with excessively thickened leaflets greater than 3 mm, and severe annular dilation. There are, in fact, pathologic features which differentiate BD from other mitral regurgitant pathologies including significantly thicker leaflets, which are histologically explained by a larger spongiosa layer with infiltration into the fibrosa layer. The larger spongiosa layer is due to accumulation of mucopolysaccharides, which disrupt normal collagen bundles leading to larger billowing leaflet.[17] BD usually results in chronic, rather than acute, MR; however, it is associated with poor outcomes, arrhythmias, and sudden cardiac death.[6]

Malignant Mitral Valve Prolapse

Dating back to the early 1980s, there have been reports of sudden death in young otherwise healthy patients with MVP. These sudden deaths occurred in the absence of severe MR or coexistent coronary artery disease, leading to the notion that there is a malignant form of this usually benign condition. This malignant MVP has also been associated with bileaflet disease (Barlow's), ventricular arrhythmias, and idiopathic LV systolic dysfunction. A recent study by Garbi et al. showed a mean age of 38, a slight male predominance (51.7%), and extensive bileaflet prolapse with annular dilatation.[18] Thickened, elongated chords with thickened ballooning leaflets characteristic of BD were present in all cases. Myocardial fibrosis has also been implicated in cases of sudden cardiac death related to MVP. Recent studies present strong evidence of an associated cardiomyopathy with malignant MVP with myocardial and papillary muscle fibrosis seen on pathology and cardiac MRI, abnormal myocardial contraction pattern, and Pickelhaube Sign on tissue doppler correlating with high strain.[18–21] These findings have also been associated with complex ventricular arrhythmias. Some studies have correlated QT dispersion and sudden cardiac death (SCD) with leaflet thickness and the degree of MVP.[22,23] This makes sense as the larger, billowing leaflet would generate more tension or strain on the associated papillary muscle and myocardium. This may explain the localized abnormal myocardial contraction and hypertrophy compensating for the greater strain created by the enlarged leaflet. However, malignant MVP seems to be unrelated to MR severity. Recent studies have implicated mitral annular disjunction (MAD) in malignant MVP. MAD is defined as detachment of the roots of the mitral annulus from the ventricular myocardium with atrial displacement of the leaflet hinge point, and has been associated with malignant ventricular arrhythmias, MVP, and ventricular fibrosis.[2]

While sudden cardiac death is rare in MVP, the risk is double that in the normal population. This explains the flurry of research in this area as we strive to identify those patients at greatest risk of sudden cardiac death and determine the best management. There is still much that remains controversial, and further study needs to be done in this area.

Traumatic/Iatrogenic Mitral Regurgitation

Traumatic MR is exceedingly rare, but should be considered in blunt cardiac trauma especially with new onset heart failure.[24] MR from blunt cardiac trauma may occur immediately, usually associated with a damaged papillary muscle, or days to months later depending upon the injured component of the valve apparatus. Penetrating cardiac injuries may also result in MR, hopefully with more innate heightened suspicion given the mechanism.

There are various mechanisms by which iatrogenic MR has occurred. These include percutaneous interventions, surgical interventions, and intracardiac left ventricular assist devices. Transcatheter procedures that involve entering the LV, such as transcatheter aortic valve replacement (TAVR), or insertion of an axial flow left ventricular assist device should be very carefully monitored by echocardiography to avoid irreversible damage to the mitral valve. Pigtail catheters and curved guidewires which are used partially to avoid iatrogenic perforation can wrap around chordae becoming stuck and result in significant MR.[25]

Flail

Flail leaflet may result from any of the subtypes of Type II MR and is distinguished from prolapse by loss of normal attachment to the ventricular myocardium to the extent that the leaflet tip points upward toward atrium.[2] Leaflet detachment may affect only one scallop or a smaller portion of a leaflet, in which case, it is deemed a partial flail. The classic flail leaflet refers to the detachment of the majority of the anterior, or posterior, leaflet from its papillary muscle as may occur with chordal rupture or papillary muscle rupture such as in the setting of acute MI.

Carpentier Type IIIa

Type IIIa is defined as restricted leaflet motion during systole and diastole. Most conditions in this category may also be considered "post-inflammatory," with the possible exception of medication-induced MR as its mechanism is mostly unknown.

Rheumatic Heart Disease

Rheumatic heart disease is the most common etiology of Type IIIa disease. Recurrent inflammation leads to thickened, restricted leaflets, commissural fusion, and chordal fusion, a combination which more frequently leads to mitral stenosis, but also causes MR or mixed disease. A more in-depth discussion of rheumatic heart disease is included in the section on mitral stenosis. Echocardiographic findings of rheumatic MR include "hockey stick" appearance of the valve and either centrally or eccentrically directed MR.[2]

Radiation-Induced

Radiation-induced valvular heart disease, again, begins with tissue injury and inflammation leading to diffuse fibrosis and calcification. Radiation-induced valvular disease has a predilection for the aortic-mitral curtain and further distinguishes itself from rheumatic heart disease by lack of commissural fusion.[2] Valvular dysfunction typically occurs many years after radiation exposure and may manifest as MR, mitral stenosis, or mixed disease.

Endocarditis

Treated endocarditis leaves lasting effects on the previously infected valve.[7] In addition to the more acute effects of endocarditis such as leaflet perforation (Type I) and chordal rupture (Type II), chronic effects result in Type III MR. Similar to the pathophysiology of rheumatic heart disease, inflammation results in diffuse fibrosis, which can result in MR due to restricted leaflet motion.

Medication-Induced

Several medications previously on the market have been implicated in causing MR. Two medications used to treat migraines, methysergide and ergotamine, led to valve fibrosis. Pergolide and cabergoline, ergot-derived dopamine receptor agonists used in the treatment of Parkinson's disease caused similar fibrosis. "Fen-phen" fenfluramine and phentermine appetite suppressant, fenfluramine or dexfenfluramine alone were all associated with thick, dense, fibrous tissue covering leaflets and chordae leading to MR.[7] The mechanism has been postulated to involve the central serotoninergic pathways due to its similarities to carcinoid syndrome.

Carpentier Type IIIb

Type IIIb is secondary MR due to leaflet restriction during systole. It is the second most common mechanism requiring mitral valve repair following Type II.

Ischemic

Ischemic leaflet restriction occurs post-myocardial infarction in 20% to 25% of patients, usually due to displacement of the posterior papillary muscle. This occurs partly due to LV remodeling and enlargement with apical and lateral displacement of the papillary muscle, leading to tethered leaflets. Resulting morphology has been described as tenting of the leaflets. If one thinks of the leaflet as tent material, the stakes (papillary muscles) for the free edge have been moved closer to the ventricular wall and the apex, effectively shortening the tie ropes (chordae). As blood fills the tent material, the result is a narrower, more peaked tent in which the free edge cannot reach the level of the annulus. The free edge is unable to reach its coaptation point leading to MR, typically posteriorly-directed. The mitral annulus also plays a significant role with these patients having a larger anterior-posterior diameter with absence of annular folding, saddle-shape accentuation in early systole.[3] Mid- to late-systolic Type IIIb MR occurs due to asymmetric, paradoxical papillary muscle movement.

Non-Ischemic Dilated Cardiomyopathy

Non-ischemic dilated cardiomyopathy results in dilatation of the LV with spherical remodeling.[26] This results in symmetric papillary muscle displacement with simultaneous enlargement of the mitral annulus leading to progressive tethering and leaflet tenting. This typically results in central MR. The pathophysiology of postoperative severe secondary MR with low EF as is frequently seen in non-ischemic dilated cardiomyopathy is worth discussing. Correcting MR results in an increased afterload on the already failing LV due to eliminating this path for exit of blood during systole. This may result in low cardiac output syndrome (LOS) postoperatively.[27] The incidence of LOS seems to be unrelated to LV volume reduction procedures, and may be predicted by a low preoperative total SV, deceleration time of early transmitral flow wave, and the slope of the preload recruitable stroke-work relationship.[27]

Modified or Expanded Carpentier Classification

Due to more advanced imaging, some additional subtypes have been added to the original Carpentier classification as other causes of mitral valve regurgitation have come to light. These will be described in the following sections.

Carpentier Type IVa

Hypertrophic obstructive cardiomyopathy (HOCM), in addition to septal hypertrophy, is associated with numerous abnormalities of the mitral valve apparatus, which result in MR. The most common of these are: elongated leaflet, anterior and basilar displacement of the AL papillary muscle, insertion of the AL papillary muscle into the mid-portion of the anterior leaflet, anterior mitral tenting resulting from papillary muscle displacement and fibrotic, retracted secondary chordae, all of which contribute to systolic anterior motion (SAM).[28] Other factors that contribute to SAM include reduced coaptation-septum distance and the *Venturi effect*–increased flow velocity in the LVOT. MR in HOCM most commonly results when the posterior leaflet is not able to move anteriorly with the anterior leaflet, resulting in malcoaptation and a posterolaterally directed regurgitant jet.[2] This may result from the posterior leaflet being too short or lacking sufficient mobility. A less common cause of MR in SAM occurs due to calcification or fibrosis of the leaflets. Type IVa refers to MR resulting from native SAM.

Carpentier Type IVb

MR may also result from SAM as an iatrogenic outcome of surgical correction of the mitral valve.[28] In this context, SAM results from posterior leaflet resection with resulting anterior displacement of the coaptive surface into the outflow tract. Postoperative SAM may also result from an inappropriately sized annuloplasty ring, which is smaller than the circumference forcing excess tissue of the anterior leaflet into the LVOT.[17] If one thinks of the posterior leaflet as a hammock hanging from the trigones, no matter how one resects part of the leaflet, the hammock will shorten and will move anteriorly.

Carpentier Type IVc

Composes hemodynamic-induced MR.

Hypovolemia

Hypovolemia leads to decreased LV volume. Especially in an acute setting, such as acute blood loss, the ventricle also becomes hyperdynamic. The septum moves toward the anterior leaflet during this period of acutely decreased ventricular volume leading to LV outflow tract obstruction. The anterior leaflet of the mitral valve is pulled into the LVOT. Blood being ejected from the ventricle is essentially baffled by the anterior leaflet back into the LA.

Drug-Induced

Ionotropic or chronotropic agents such as dobutamine, epinephrine, isoproterenol, cocaine, and methamphetamine can cause MR by a similar mechanism as hypovolemia. As the ventricle increases contraction, increasing SV and decreasing ventricular volume, the LVOT is again obstructed and blood is ejected back into the LA along the anterior leaflet of the mitral valve. Similarly, with chronotropic agents, decreased time for ventricular filling decreases ventricular volume.

Carpentier Type V

Type V MR is referred to as a hybrid, and describes a combination of conditions contributing to the MR. For example, a patient with rheumatic valve disease (Type IIIa) with endocarditis-induced perforation (Type I).[2]

Table 2.2 provides a summary of the expanded Carpentier classification covered in this chapter.

Pathophysiology of Acute Mitral Regurgitation

Acute MR can result from leaflet perforation (Carpentier Type I); however, severe acute MR is usually due to papillary muscle rupture or chordal rupture. Chordal rupture can be spontaneous or occur as a result of myxomatous disease, FED, or infective endocarditis.[25] Etiologies of papillary muscle rupture include endocarditis, spontaneous associated with myxomatous mitral valve disease, iatrogenic, and ischemic. Ischemic papillary muscle rupture is most commonly due to an inferior ST-elevation myocardial infarction (STEMI).[29] This is due to posterior location of the papillary muscles, and the typically single vessel blood supply to the PM papillary muscle coming from either the right coronary artery, or obtuse marginal branch of the left circumflex coronary artery.[3,10] MR secondary to papillary muscle rupture is not usually caused by a large area of ischemic myocardium, but a rather small posterior, or inferior infarction or subendocardial infarction affecting the tip of the papillary muscle. Large areas of infarction result in decreased ventricular power and therefore are less likely to result in papillary muscle rupture.

The acute onslaught of blood resulting from rupture of papillary muscle equates to acute volume overload on the LV and LA. This results in rapid increase in LA pressures, pulmonary congestion, and hypoxia, as well as low forward flow from the LV and cardiogenic shock. Unilateral (right-sided) pulmonary congestion may occur from an anteriorly directed jet going into the right pulmomary veins. Due to low LV end-systolic pressure, MR is shifted to early systole; therefore, the murmur may be short and unimpressive. While perhaps counterintuitive, rapidly titratable vasodilators such as sodium nitroprusside and nicardipine can be helpful in the treatment of acute MR, if systemic pressures will tolerate them. They function to decrease the resistance to forward flow, increasing the proportion of blood being ejected via the aorta versus regurgitated into the LA. Intra-aortic balloon counterpulsation (IABP). This can provide the same reduction in LV afterload, thereby decreasing regurgitant volume while supporting systemic pressures, rather than further decreasing them as with vasodilators. Depending upon the amount of hemodynamic instability, additional assist devices may be necessary, such as Impella (Abiomed, Danvers, MA), to maintain systemic perfusion and overall stability while preparing for prompt mitral valve surgery or intervention. While acute MR is a spectrum, severe acute MR with hemodynamic instability will likely require surgical or percutaneous intervention.[29]

Transient SAM in Takotsubo cardiomyopathy is an uncommon cause of acute MR. Severe MR occurs as a result of hyperdynamic contraction of the base of the LV creating SAM. Concomitant LV dysfunction inherent to Takotsubo cardiomyopathy can result in cardiogenic shock.[25] A schematic of the causes of acute MR adapted from this article is included (Fig 2.5).

Stages of Chronic Mitral Regurgitation

The 2020 American College of Cardiology (ACC)/American Heart Association (AHA) Clinical Practice Guidelines break down chronic MR into primary (Table 2.3) and secondary (Table 2.4) categories for the purposes of staging.[29]

TABLE 2.2 Summary Table of Expanded Carpentier Classification Covered in This Chapter

	Type I	Type II	Type IIIa	Type IIIb	Type IVa	Type IVb	Type IVc	Type V
	Normal Leaflet Motion and Position	Excess Leaflet Motion	Restricted Leaflet Motion in Systole and Diastole	Restricted Leaflet Motion in Systole	Native SAM	Iatrogenic SAM	Hemodynamic Induced	Hybrid
1°	Perforation Cleft	MVP FED MD Barlow's Flail	RHD Radiation-induced Endocarditis Medication-induced		SAM 2/2 HOCM	SAM 2/2 Surgery or Procedure		
2°	Atrial Dialation NIDC Diastolic			Ischemic NIDC			Hypovolemia Ionotropes Chronotropes	

1°, Derived from the mitral valve apparatus; *2°, derived from the left atrium or ventricle; FED,* fibroelastic deficiency; *HOCM,* hypertrophic obstructive cardiomyopathy*; MD,* myxomatous degeneration*; MVP,* mitral valve prolapse*; NIDC,* non-ischemic dilated cardiomyopathy; *RHD,* rheumatic heart disease*; SAM,* systolic anterior motion.

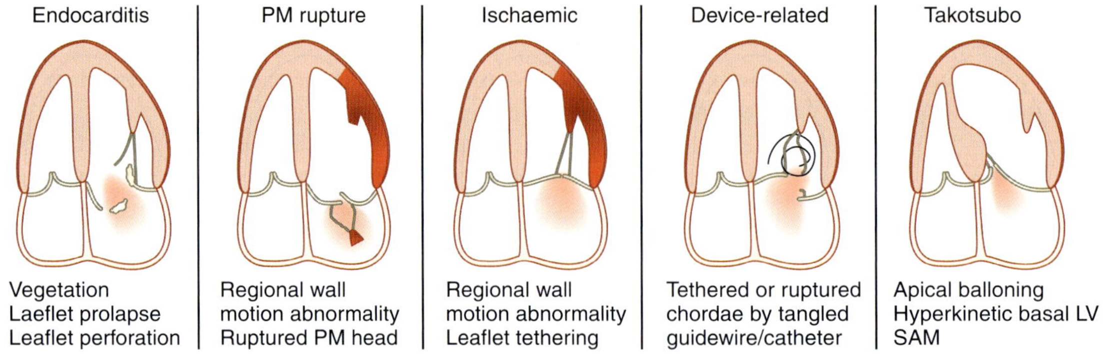

Fig. 2.5 Schematic of Causes of Acute Mitral Regurgitation. *LV*, Left ventricle; *PM*, papillary muscle; *SAM*, systolic anterior motion. (From Watanabe N. Acute mitral regurgitation. *Heart*. 2019;105[9]:671–677.)

TABLE 2.3 Stages of Chronic Primary Mitral Regurgitation

Stage	Definition	Valve Anatomy	Valve Hemodynamics[a]	Hemodynamic Consequences	Symptoms
A	At risk of MR	• Mild mitral valve prolapse with normal coaptation • Mild valve thickening and leaflet restriction	• No MR jet or small central jet area <20% LA on Doppler • Small vena contracta <0.3 cm	None	None
B	Progressive MR	• Moderate to severe mitral valve prolapse with normal coaptation • Rheumatic valve changes with leaflet restriction and loss of central coaptation • Prior IE	• Central jet MR 20%–40% LA or late systolic eccentric jet MR • Vena contracta <0.7 cm • Regurgitant volume <60 mL • Regurgitant fraction <50 % • ERO <0.40 cm^2 • Angiographic grade 1+ to 2+	• Mild LA enlargement • No LV enlargement • Normal pulmonary Pressure	None
C	Asymptomatic severe MR	• Severe mitral valve prolapse with loss of coaptation or flail leaflet • Rheumatic valve changes with leaflet restriction and loss of central coaptation • Prior IE • Thickening of leaflet with radiation heart disease	• Central jet MR >40% holosystolic eccentric jet MR • Vena contracta ≥0.7 cm • Regurgitant volume ≥60 mL • Regurgitant fraction ≥50% • ERO ≥0.40 cm^2 • Angiographic grade 3+ – 4+	• Moderate or severe LA enlargement • LA enlargement • Pulmonary hypertension may be present at rest or with exercise • C1: LVEF >60% and LVESD <40 mm • C2: LVEF ≤60% and/ or LVESD ≥40 mm	None
D	Symptomatic severe MR	• Severe mitral valve prolapse with loss of coaptation or flail leaflet • Rheumatic valve changes with leaflet restriction and loss of central coaptation • Prior IE • Thickening of leaflet with radiation heart disease	• Central jet MR >40% LA or holosystolic eccentric jet MR • Vena contracta ≥0.7 cm • Regurgitant volume ≥60 mL • Regurgitant fraction ≥50 % • ERO ≥0.40 cm^2 • Angiographic grade 3+ to 4+	• Moderate or severe LA enlargement • LV enlargement • Pulmonary hypertension present	• Decreased exercise tolerance • Exertional dyspnea

[a]Several valve hemodynamic criteria are provided for assessment of MR severity, but not all criteria for each category will be present in each patient. Categorization of MR severity as mild, moderate, or severe depends on data quality and integration of these parameters in conjunction with other clinical evidence.

ERO, Effective regurgitant orifice; *IE*, infective endocarditis; *LA*, left atrium/atrial; *LV*, left ventricular; *LVEF*, left ventricular ejection fraction; *LVESD*, left ventricular end-systolic dimension; *MR*, mitral regurgitation.

From Otto CM, Nishimura RA, Bonow RO, et al. 2020 ACC/AHA Guideline for the Management of Patients With Valvular Heart Disease: A Report of the American College of Cardiology/American Heart Association Joint Committee on Clinical Practice Guidelines. *J Am Coll Cardiol*. 2021;77(4):e25–e197.

TABLE 2.4 Stages of Secondary Mitral Regurgitation

Stage	Definition	Valve Anatomy	Valve Hemodynamics[a]	Associated Cardiac Findings	Symptoms
A	At risk of MR	• Normal valve leaflets, chords, and annulus in a patient with CAD or cardiomyopathy	• No MR jet or small central jet area <20% LA on Doppler • Small vena contracta <0.30 cm	• Normal or mildly dilated LV size with fixed (infraction) or inducible (ischemia) regional wall motion abnormalities • Primary myocardial disease with LV dilation and systolic dysfunction	• Symptoms attributable to coronary ischemia or HF may be present that respond to revascularization and appropriate medical therapy
B	Progressive MR	• Regional wall motion abnormalities with mild tethering of mitral leaflet • Annular dilation with mild tethering of mitral leaflet	• ERO <0.40 cm^2[b] • Regurgitant volume <60 mL • Regurgitant fraction <50%	• Regional wall motion abnormalities with reduced LV systolic function • LV dilation and systolic dysfunction attributable to primary myocardial disease	• Symptoms attributable to coronary ischemia or HF may be present that respond to revascularization and appropriate medical therapy
C	Asymptomatic severe MR	• Regional wall motion abnormalities and/or LV dilation with severe tethering of mitral leaflet • Annular dilation with severe loss of central coaptation of the mitral leaflets	• ERO ≥0.40 cm^2[b] • Regurgitant volume ≥60 mL[c] • Regurgitant fraction ≥50%	• Regional wall motion abnormalities with reduced LV systolic function • LV dilation and systolic dysfunction attributable to primary myocardial disease	• Symptoms attributable to coronary ischemia or HF may be present that respond to revascularization and appropriate medical therapy
D	Symptomatic severe MR	• Regional wall motion abnormalities and/or LV dilation with severe thethering of mitral leaflet • Annular dilation with severe loss of central coaptation of the mitral leaflets	• ERO ≥0.40 cm^2[b] • Regurgitant volume ≥60 mL[c] • Regurgitant fraction ≥50%	• Regional wall motion abnormalities with reduced LV systolic function • LV dilation and systolic dysfunction attributable to primary myocardial disease	• HF symptoms attributable to MR persist even after revascularization and optimization of medical therapy • Decreased exercise tolerance • Exertional dyspnea

2D, 2-Dimensional; *CAD*, coronary artery disease; *ERO*, effective regurgitant orifice; *HF*, heart failure; *LA*, left atrium; *LV*, left ventricular; *MR*, mitral regurgitation; *TTE*, transthoracic echocardiogram.

From Otto CM, Nishimura RA, Bonow RO, et al. 2020 ACC/AHA Guideline for the Management of Patients With Valvular Heart Disease: A Report of the American College of Cardiology/American Heart Association Joint Committee on Clinical Practice Guidelines. *J Am Coll Cardiol.* 2021;77(4):e25–e197.

[a]Several valve hemodynamic criteria are provided for assessment of MR severity, but not all criteria for each category will be present in each patient. Categorization of MR severity as mild, moderate, or severe depends on data quality and integration of these parameters in conjunction with other clinical evidence.

[b]The measurement of the proximal isovelocity surface area by 2D TTE in patients with secondary MR underestimates the true ERO because of the crescentic shape of the proximal convergence.

[c]May be lower in low-flow states.

Secondary Mitral Regurgitation as Proportionate or Disproportionate

Recent outcomes of major clinical trials Percutaneous Repair with the MitraClip Device for Severe Functional/Secondary Mitral Regurgitation (MITRA-FR) and the Cardiovascular Outcomes Assessment of the MitraClip Percutaneous Therapy (COAPT) have led to the question of when to intervene on the mitral valve in secondary or functional MR, which is by definition, not due to a problem with the mitral valve apparatus. Grayburn et al. proposed a way to distinguish this defining *proportionate* as MR proportionate to LV volume, which should respond to medical management of the LV. *Disproportionate* MR exceeding what was expected for a given LV volume would not be expected to be adequately treated by interventions aimed at reducing LV volume, and would benefit from intervention on the mitral valve.[30]

MITRAL STENOSIS

The vast majority of mitral stenosis worldwide is caused by sequalae of rheumatic heart disease. While rheumatic fever is now rare in the United States and industrialized countries, it continues to plague developing nations, and the resultant rheumatic valvular heart disease can present from teens in endemic areas to 50- to 70-year-old patients decades after having rheumatic fever. Rheumatic fever has a strong predilection for the female sex with 80% of those affected being women. Higher-income countries are seeing increasing proportions of mitral stenosis secondary to non-rheumatic annular calcifications extending onto the leaflets. Other rare causes of mitral stenosis include congenital stenosis of mitral valve leaflets, endocarditis with large vegetations, usually fungal, obstructing the orifice of the valve, tophaceous gout affecting the mitral valve leaflets, storage disorders, and drug induced.[7]

Rheumatic Mitral Stenosis

Rheumatic mitral stenosis is a slowly progressive disease characterized by a latent phase between the initial rheumatic illness and the development of valve stenosis. The length of the latent phase varies, being shorter in lower-income countries, likely due to recurrent carditis. Recurrent episodes of rheumatic fever can result in further valve damage shortening this latent period.[29] Acute and recurrent inflammation leads to fibrosis and calcification of valve leaflets, commissural fusion, and thickened/shortened chordae tendineae leading to mitral stenosis. The normal mitral valve area according to recent studies is approximately 10 cm^2 which is significantly larger than the widely accepted "normal" mitral annular area of 4 to 6 cm^2, allowing free flow of blood from the LA to the LV with a negligible pressure gradient.[3,14] In mitral stenosis, obstruction to this free flow of blood from the LA to the LV results in increased LA pressures and volumes. This is transmitted into the pulmonary circulation from the pulmonary veins to the capillary beds, where it results in increased hydrostatic pressure and pulmonary edema causing dyspnea. Hemoptysis may also occur in severe cases due to collateralization between pulmonary and bronchial veins, and high pressures leading to intraparenchymal rupture of bronchial vein.

Non-Rheumatic Mitral Stenosis

In first world countries, mitral stenosis is now more commonly caused by non-rheumatic mitral annular calcification (MAC). This is characterized by calcification of the mitral annulus extending inward onto the mitral leaflets, resulting in decreased annular area and increased rigidity of mitral leaflets. Unlike rheumatic mitral stenosis, there is no commissural fusion.[29]

Mitral Annular Calcification

MAC is a chronic, degenerative process common in the aging population, affecting greater than 40% of those ≥65 years of age compared to 8% to 15% in the general population.[31–33] MAC has an increased prevalence in females, those with chronic kidney disease, hypertension, left ventricular hypertrophy, MVP, atrial fibrillation; patients with calcific aortic stenosis; and patients with history of chest radiation. Increased stress on MV annulus and inflammation have been shown to lead to MAC. The pathogenesis of MAC occurs via osteoblastic phenotypes of valvular cells similar to that of atherosclerosis. MAC typically affects the posterior fibrous annulus; however, in those patients with history of chest radiation, MAC more commonly affects the anterior mitral annulus and the aortic-mitral intervalvular fibrosa.

In their retrospective cohort study, Pasca et al. found that the presence of calcific or degenerative mitral stenosis (DMS), even when mild, conferred a 53% 5-year mortality rate compared to 17% in age/gender matched general population. It was associated with elevated right atrial pressures and heart failure with normal LV function.[33] This makes sense as mitral stenosis is protective of the LV, and limits the volume the LV sees while increasing volume and pressure in the LA.

Earlier detection of calcium formation in valvular disease has been made possible by ^{18}F-sodium fluoride positron emission tomography (PET).[34] The signal is higher in areas of microcalcification, providing a marker of calcification activity. This differs from our traditional imaging modality of computed tomography (CT) which detects macroscopic, established calcium deposits. Massera et al. were able to show significant correlations between the uptake in this imaging modality, and new regions of macroscopic calcium deposition on CT 2 years later, suggesting the possibility of using this modality as a predictor of disease progression in MAC. They also found that higher baseline MAC correlated with increased disease activity and a faster rate of progression. This might suggest that calcium begets calcium and PET-CT may have a role in determining the still incomplete understanding of the pathophysiology of this condition.[32]

Other Causes of Mitral Stenosis

Radiation-induced valvular disease is one of the most common sequalae of mediastinal radiation. Mediastinal radiation is a commonly used treatment modality in many types of cancers including esophageal cancer, breast cancer, and lymphoma. The valves most affected are the aortic and mitral valves. While often developing many years after the completion of radiation treatment, this is a progressive condition with thickening and diffuse calcification of the valvular apparatus, often including the aortomitral curtain. The resultant physiology may be stenotic, regurgitant, or both. Severe MAC and porcelain aorta may also result and increase risk of paravalvular leak, embolic events from aortic manipulation, or even be considered inoperable.[35]

Iatrogenic mitral stenosis following mitral valve repair ranges in incidence from 9% to 54%.[36] Early postoperative mitral stenosis in degenerative mitral valve disease results from an undersized annuloplasty ring or excessive leaflet resection. This is somewhat in contrast to early postoperative mitral stenosis following repair for ischemic MR, which is thought to be more related to restricted leaflet motion from increased tethering combined with annuloplasty rings. Late postoperative mitral stenosis may result from leaflet fibrosis and pannus formation. This is thought to be related to foreign body reaction as histopathology has revealed giant cells containing intracytoplasmic ring material.[36] Postoperative mitral stenosis has also been related to the shape of the annuloplasty ring not matching the native saddle shape of the mitral valve annulus, as well as injury to the leaflets from the delivery apparatus starting a chain of inflammation and fibrosis. Iatrogenic mitral stenosis may also occur as a result of catheter-based procedures such as trans-catheter edge-to-edge repair (TEER) or even TAVR.[37,38]

Wilkins Score

Wilkins et al. showed in 1988 that the structure of the mitral valve and the subvalvular apparatus determined the outcome of balloon dilatation.[39] From this study, the Wilkins score was developed, which uses transthoracic echocardiography criteria to identify appropriate candidates for balloon valvuloplasty. This score is derived from the sum of the grades of four different categories: leaflet mobility, subvalvar (chordal) thickening, leaflet thickening, and leaflet calcification. Each category is given a grade of one to four, with four correlating with most pathologic finding. A Wilkins score of less than nine is amenable to balloon valvuloplasty.

Stages of Mitral Stenosis

The 2020 ACC/AHA Clinical Practice Guidelines define the stages of mitral stenosis as depicted in Table 2.5. The stages of mitral stenosis are determined by multiple factors such as patient symptoms, valve anatomy, valve hemodynamics, effects on the LA, and pulmonary pressures. Other concomitant conditions which may lead to similar symptoms should always be considered, such as diastolic dysfunction, compliance of the LA, and intrinsic pulmonary vascular disease.[29] Mitral stenosis is a progressive disease; however, worsening symptoms may result from changes in hemodynamics unrelated to increased stenosis of the mitral valve. Pregnancy, arrhythmias (particularly atrial fibrillation), fever, anemia, hyperthyroidism, and perioperative shifts should all be taken into consideration when a patient with mitral stenosis has worsening symptoms.

MIXED DISEASE

Mixed mitral valve disease refers to the combination of mitral stenosis and MR, and is usually seen in patients with rheumatic heart disease or severe MAC. Symptomatic mixed disease results from increased left atrial pressures as the LA takes on additional volume from MR in the setting of decreased outflow due to mitral stenosis. The resultant pathophysiology is described in the following section.

SEQUALAE OF MITRAL VALVE DISEASE

Pulmonary Hypertension

Both mitral stenosis and MR result in increased volume of blood and pressure in the LA. Elevated left atrial pressures result in two forms of pulmonary hypertension, with most patients developing passive pulmonary hypertension resulting from the transmission of elevated pressures from the LA to the venous capillary bed, resulting in increased hydrostatic pressure and pulmonary edema as previously described. The second type is reactive and affects approximately 40% of patients. Reactive pulmonary hypertension correlates with intimal fibrosis and medial hypertrophy of the pulmonary arterioles, decreasing the hydrostatic pressure gradient across the pulmonary capillary bed and decreasing pulmonary edema (Fig. 2.6).[14]

Heart Failure

Pulmonary hypertension correlates with increased right ventricular afterload requiring the right ventricle (RV) to generate

TABLE 2.5 Stages of Mitral Stenosis[a]

Stage	Definition	Valve Anatomy	Valve Hemodynamics	Hemodynamic Consequences	Symptoms
A	At risk of MS	Mild valve doming during diastole	Normal transmitral flow velocities	None	None
B	Progressive MS	• Rheumatic valve changes with commissural fusion and diastolic doming of the mitral valve leaflets • Planimetered mitral valve area >1.5 cm^2	• Increased transmitral flow velocities • Mitral valve area >1.5 cm^2 • Diastolic pressure half-time <150 ms	• Mild to moderate LA enlargement • Normal pulmonary pressure at rest	None
C	Asymptomatic severe MS	• Rheumatic valve changes with commissural fusion and diastolic doming of the mitral valve leaflets • Planimetered mitral valve area ≤1.5 cm^2	• Mitral valve area ≤1.5 cm^2 • Diastolic pressure half-time ≥150 ms	• Severe LA enlargement • Elevated PASP >50 mm Hg	None
D	Symptomatic severe MS	• Rheumatic valve changes with commissural fusion and diastolic doming of the mitral valve leaflets • Planimetered mitral valve area ≤1.5 cm^2	• Mitral valve area ≤1.5 cm^2 • Diastolic pressure half-time ≥150 ms	• Severe LA enlargement • Elevated PASP >50 mm Hg	• Decreased exercise tolerance • Exertional dyspnea

[a]This table depicts the stages of mitral stenosis based on anatomy, valve hemodynamics, hemodynamic consequences, and patient symptoms. The transmitral mean pressure gradient should be obtained to further determine the hemodynamic effect of the MS and is usually greater than 5 mm Hg in severe MS; however, because of the variability of the mean pressure gradient with the heart rate and forward flow, it has not been included in the criteria for severity.

LA, Left atrial; *MS*, mitral stenosis; *PASP*, pulmonary artery systolic pressure.

From Otto CM, Nishimura RA, Bonow RO, et al. 2020 ACC/AHA Guideline for the Management of Patients With Valvular Heart Disease: A Report of the American College of Cardiology/American Heart Association Joint Committee on Clinical Practice Guidelines. *J Am Coll Cardiol.* 2021;77(4):e25–e197.

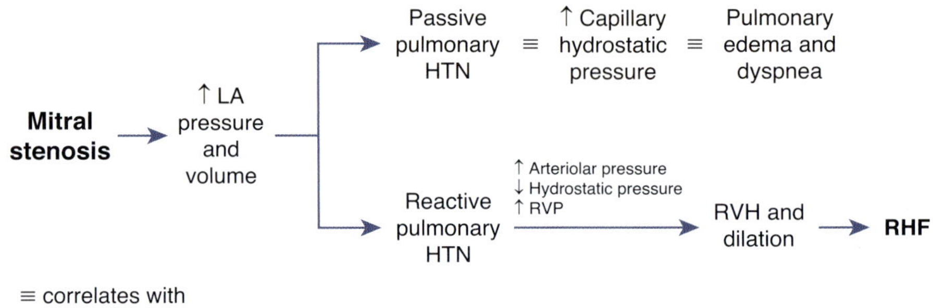

Fig. 2.6 Pathophysiology of Mitral Stenosis. Increased left atrial *(LA)* pressure and volume lead to either passive or reactive pulmonary hypertension. Passive originates in the venous system and results in pulmonary edema due to high hydrostatic pressure gradient at the pulmonary capillary bed. Reactive results in increased pulmonary arteriolar pressure, decreased pulmonary capillary bed hydrostatic pressure gradient thus decreased pulmonary edema. This results in increased right ventricular *(RV)* pressures, right ventricular hypertrophy *(RVH)* and dilation, and, ultimately, right heart failure *(RHF)*.

higher pressures. Chronic elevation in right ventricular pressures leads to right ventricular hypertrophy and dilation, and ultimately right heart failure.

Mitral valve area of less than 2 cm^2 is associated with hemodynamically significant reduction in left ventricular SV and CO due to decreased LV filling. Left ventricular systolic failure does not typically result from mitral stenosis, which could be said to be protective to the LV.

On the other hand, MR is progressive. Volume overload leads to LV wall stress which is initially ameliorated by the decreased afterload offered by low pressure LA. If the heart is able to maintain forward CO, it will transition from acute to compensated MR. The compensated stage, which may last from years to decades with an asymptomatic patient, is characterized by LV dilation maintaining normal wall stress and diastolic pressures.[6] Over time MR will lead to progressive LV dilation. This may be due to worsening MR, which may occur from increasing LV dimensions affecting the mitral valve apparatus, from the underlying mitral valve pathology, or a combination of factors. Ultimate LV failure results from increased wall stress, increased end-diastolic pressure, decreased myofiber content, and interstitial fibrosis.

Arrhythmia

Atrial arrhythmias, most commonly atrial fibrillation (AF), are an important sequalae of mitral valve disease. Chronically elevated left atrial pressure leads to left atrial dilation. This dilation can stretch the atrial conduction system resulting in atrial fibrillation. In mitral stenosis, the known effects of Rapid AFib, or AFib/RVR, are compounded. The amount of time for blood to pass through the already stenotic mitral valve is decreased, further limiting the amount of blood entering the LV, increasing LA pressure, and decreasing LV CO with possible associated hemodynamic instability. In MR, rapid heart rate increases the systolic regurgitation events per minute, increasing the burden of MR.

Pharmacologic treatment of atrial fibrillation includes anticoagulation, rate control, and/or rhythm control. In rheumatic mitral stenosis, the typical treatment for atrial fibrillation may be less effective due to rheumatic changes to the LA including progressive enlargement, and fibrosis of the atria itself in addition to internodal and interatrial tracts potentially including the sinoatrial node.[29]

Ventricular arrhythmias also occur as previously described in the section on malignant mitral valve prolapse.

Thromboembolic Events

Relative stagnation of blood flow in the LA is compounded by atrial fibrillation, predisposing the patient to atrial thrombus formation and risk of systemic thromboembolization, including, but not limited to, stroke. Rheumatic heart disease has a higher risk of embolization than other valvular disease. It has been speculated that rheumatic heart disease affects atrial muscle, increasing stasis and thrombus formation in the LA in addition to the left atrial appendage.[29]

Endocarditis

Mitral valve disease predisposes the patient to endocarditis of the mitral valve. Hemodynamic changes from structural abnormalities include turbulent flow and increased sheer stress. The increased stress on the valve tissues may result in endothelial damage, making the valve susceptible to bacterial invasion.[7]

SPECIAL POPULATIONS

Mitral Valve Disease in Pregnancy

Overall, maternal mortality has decreased over the last decade; however, cardiac maternal death has not.[40] Antenatal heart disease is primarily due to congenital heart disease in high-income, industrialized countries; whereas, rheumatic heart disease is the primary cause in low- and moderate-income countries.[41]

Physiologic and Hemodynamic Changes

Pregnancy results in extensive hemodynamic changes in healthy women such as increased blood volume, decreased blood viscosity/hemoglobin/hematocrit due to dilutional effects, decreased peripheral vascular resistance, decreased blood pressure, and increased heart rate.[41,42] Mitral stenosis is the most commonly encountered valvular disease in pregnancy and is highly susceptible to changes in volume and heart rate. Pregnant women have an increased pressure gradient across the stenotic mitral valve, which may lead to deterioration and need for intervention regardless of the severity of baseline mitral stenosis. This is due to the stenotic mitral valve hindering the heart's ability to increase CO in response to increased plasma volume and increased demands of uteroplacental blood flow. This results in increasing LA, pulmonary pressure, and heart failure with even mild mitral stenosis having a 15.8 % incidence, with 31.8% for moderate, and 48.1% for severe mitral stenosis according to study reviewing data from the international Registry of Pregnancy and Cardiac Disease.[40] Similarly, moderate to severe MR which is usually thought of as benign resulted in 23% of patients developing heart failure.

Spontaneous chordal rupture has been reported during the peripartum period.[43] One proposed mechanism is that hormonal changes may soften the mitral leaflets and annulus via changes in matrix metalloproteinase expression and deposition of matrix proteins. A bovine model of pregnancy valve changes also identified an increase in leaflet thickness with a 33% increase in leaflet area and a 25% increase in chordal attachments indicating structural remodeling of the valvular apparatus during pregnancy.

Thromboembolic Events in Prosthetic Valves

Pregnant women with mechanical heart valves are at increased risk of cardiovascular and neonatal events with only 58% having an event-free pregnancy with a live birth.[44] Favorable outcomes for both mother and baby are even more rare at 28%. While anticoagulation is associated with obstetric hemorrhage, miscarriage, and congenital malformations, thromboembolic events such as valve thrombosis may lead to maternal mortality. Postpartum cardiac interventions including ICD and/or pacemaker implantation, valve replacement, and need for left ventricular assist devices or heart transplantation are also increased. Guidelines for management of anticoagulation and risk/benefit to mechanical versus bioprosthetic valves in young female patients are lacking.

Most importantly we must realize that mothers with valvular heart disease need special evaluation and treatment during and after pregnancy, as they are at increased risk of many adverse events affecting both themselves and their baby.

Congenital Mitral Valve Disease

Congenital mitral valve disease primarily results in MR (72%), followed by mixed disease (15%), and mitral stenosis (13%).[45] Isolated congenital mitral valve disease affects less than 1% of infants born with a normal-sized LV. It is more commonly (60%) in conjunction with other cardiac anomalies such as atrioventricular canal defects, single ventricles, and Shone's syndrome.[46] A complete review of congenital mitral valve disease and the genetic syndromes that may result in mitral valve disease is beyond the scope of this chapter. We will focus on some of the more well-known conditions and the differences in how mitral valve disease is approached in congenital patients as opposed to adult patients.

Atrioventricular Canal Defects

Atrioventricular canal defects are the most common cause for mitral valve repair or replacement in pediatric patients.

TABLE 2.6 Rastell Classification of Complete Atrioventricular Canal Defects

Type A	Superior bridging leaflet is almost completely adherent to the left ventricle and is firmly attached on the ventricular septum by multiple chordal insertions
Type B	Superior bridging leaflet is attached over the ventricular septum by an anomalous papillary muscle of the right ventricle
Type C	Superior bridging leaflet is not attached to the ventricular septum (free-floating leaflet)

(Modified from Calabrò R, Limongelli G. Complete atrioventricular canal. *Orphanet J Rare Dis*. 2006;1:8.)

Atrioventricular (AV) canal defects, also referred to as endocardial cushion defects and atrioventricular septal defects (AVSDs) occur due to incomplete development of septal tissue and include a spectrum of disease from cleft mitral valve to complete AV canal.[7,47] Cleft mitral valve, as discussed in Type I Carpentier classification, usually occurs in the anterior leaflet and may occur in isolation, or as part of AV canal defect. Cleft mitral valve defects are frequently associated with abnormal chordal attachment to the membranous septum. Clefts can result in MR which is usually mild. Complete AV canal refers to a single atrioventricular valve bridging both the right and left sides of the heart, as well as atrial and ventricular septal defects.[47] The resultant superior bridging leaflet is the basis of the Rastelli classification of complete AV canal defects (Table 2.6).[48]

Shone's Complex

Complete Shone's complex was originally described in 1963 as the combination of parachute mitral valve, supravalvular ring of the LA, subaortic stenosis, and coarctation of the aorta.[49] Complete Shone's complex is extremely rare. More commonly seen would be incomplete Shone's complex, which is comprised of one left ventricular inflow lesion and one left ventricular outflow lesion, not necessarily one of those initially described by Dr. Shone above. Focusing on the mitral valve, parachute mitral valve occurs when the chordae are all attached to a single papillary muscle and usually results in mitral stenosis. Supravalvular ring of the LA was initially described as a circumferential ring of connective tissue arising from the base of the atrial surfaces of the mitral valve, protruding a variable amount into the inlet of the mitral valve with variable obstruction or mitral stenosis. It has been postulated that a proximal obstruction during fetal development predisposes to distal obstructions due to decreased flow. The proximal obstructions associated with Shone's syndrome have also been associated with hypoplastic LV potentially from the same mechanism. Regardless of ventricle size, a single ventricle repair may be required in these patients depending on the degree of obstruction occurring at multiple levels; therefore, both single- and bi-ventricular repairs have been reported.[50]

Isolated Congenital Mitral Valve Disease

Isolated congenital disease of the mitral valve is exceedingly rare. As previously noted, mitral cleft can be seen alone or in conjunction with AV canal defects and results in MR, usually mild. Parachute mitral valve is a frequent cause of congenital mitral stenosis, which results from the convergence of all chordae into a single papillary muscle. In this condition, the chordae are also shortened and thickened, restricting leaflet motion. It may also occur on its own or as part of obstructive left heart lesions or conotruncal anomalies such as the aforementioned Shone's syndrome.

Hammock mitral valve, or Arcade mitral valve, is a defect of the suspension of the mitral valve in which there may be no papillary muscle identified or numerous very small papillary muscles usually situated posteriorly. Leaflets are suspended by a network of chordae, possibly attaching directly to the ventricular wall.[47,51] This results in reduced interchordal space and restricted leaflet motion typically causing mixed-type disease. In its most severe form, the leaflets are attached directly to the papillary muscles with no space for blood to flow between the chordae.[45] Thus, blood entering this tunnel during LV ejection would be obligatorily regurgitant leading to progressive MR with or without concomitant stenosis.

The double orifice mitral valve (DOMV) accounts for approximately 1% of congenital heart disease. It is rarely isolated but rather found with AVSD (52%), obstructive left heart lesions (41%), or cyanotic heart defects.[45] DOMV is defined as a single, fibrous annulus with two orifices opening into the LV. Variations in the size of the orifices determine the amount of stenosis or regurgitation that results with MR being most common (43%), followed by mitral stenosis (13%), and mixed disease (6.5%).[7,45]

Surgery for Congenital Mitral Valve Disease

In pediatric patients, mitral valve repair is always preferred over replacement as long-term outcomes are superior. For this reason, marginal outcomes of repair are more accepted in congenital heart surgery than would be typically accepted in an adult repair. When operative result must err on one side or the other, MR is preferred over mitral stenosis as it is more receptive to medical management. Anticoagulation in pediatric patients can be difficult to manage, contributing to the preference for repair over replacement with mechanical valve.

SUMMARY

Mitral valve pathology can largely be broken down into regurgitant and stenotic disease with primary disease resulting from abnormalities of some portion of the mitral valve apparatus while secondary disease occurs due to abnormalities in other portions of the heart, namely the LA and LV. We have described the Carpentier classification of MR with some of the newer modifications to this classification, as well as the primary causes of mitral stenosis. One must also be aware of the pathophysiology of the mitral valve during pregnancy and the congenital malformations of the mitral valve.

CASE-BASED ASSESSMENT

A 59-year-old male presents with new onset heart failure and a new murmur. He had been seen 2 months ago at which time he had been diagnosed with a STEMI affecting the right coronary artery. Transthoracic ECHO at this time shows new significant mitral regurgitation.

What are the potential causes of his mitral regurgitation and the Carpentier classification of each?

See page 315 for the answers.

REFERENCES

1. Oliveira D, Srinivasan J, Espino D, et al. Geometric description for the anatomy of the mitral valve: a review. *J Anat.* 2020;237:209–224.
2. Karagodin I, Singh A, Lang RM. Pathoanatomy of mitral regurgitation. *Struct Heart.* 2020;4:254–263.
3. Topilsky Y. Mitral regurgitation: anatomy, physiology, and pathophysiology-lessons learned from surgery and cardiac imaging. *Front Cardiovasc Med.* 2020;7:84.
4. Saha A, Roy S. Papillary muscles of left ventricle-Morphological variations and it's clinical relevance. *Indian Heart J.* 2018;70: 894–900.
5. Carpentier A. Cardiac valve surgery—the "French correction. *J Thorac Cardiovasc Surg.* 1983;86:323–337.
6. El Sabbagh A, Reddy YNV, Nishimura RA. Mitral valve regurgitation in the contemporary era: insights into diagnosis, management, and future directions. *JACC Cardiovasc Imaging.* 2018;11:628–643.
7. Fishbein GA, Fishbein MC. Mitral valve pathology. *Curr Cardiol Rep.* 2019;21:61.
8. Aby ES, Rosol Z, Simegn MA. Mitral valve perforation in libman-sacks endocarditis: a heart-wrenching case of lupus. *J Gen Intern Med.* 2016;31:964–969.
9. de Groot-de Laat LE, McGhie J, Ren B, Frowijn R, et al. A modified echocardiographic classification of mitral valve regurgitation mechanism: the role of three-dimensional echocardiography. *J Cardiovasc Imaging.* 2019;27:187–199.
10. Levine RA, Hagége AA, Judge DP, et al. Mitral valve disease—morphology and mechanisms. *Nat Rev Cardiol.* 2015;12: 689–710.
11. Gertz ZM, Raina A, Saghy L, et al. Evidence of atrial functional mitral regurgitation due to atrial fibrillation: reversal with arrhythmia control. *J Am Coll Cardiol.* 2011;58:1474–1481.
12. Li Q, Liu Y, Zuo W, et al. Mechanisms, features, and significance of diastolic mitral regurgitation: a case series. *Eur Heart J Case Rep.* 2020;4:1–8.
13. Medical Advisory Secretariat. Extracorporeal lung support technologies—bridge to recovery and bridge to lung transplantation in adult patients: an evidence-based analysis. *Ontario Health Technol Assess Ser.* 2010;10:1–47.
14. Lilly LSHarvard Medical School. *Pathophysiology of heart disease: a collaborative project of medical students and faculty.* 5th ed. Baltimore, MD: Wolters Kluwer Health/Lippincott Williams & Wilkins; 2011:1 online resource.
15. Barlow JB, Pocock WA. The significance of late systolic murmurs and mid-late systolic clicks. *Md State Med J.* 1963;12:76–77.
16. Carpentier A, Chauvaud S, Fabiani JN, et al. Reconstructive surgery of mitral valve incompetence: ten-year appraisal. *J Thorac Cardiovasc Surg.* 1980;79:338–348.
17. Siordia JA. Current discoveries and interventions for Barlow's disease. *Curr Cardiol Rep.* 2016;18:73.

18. Garbi M, Garweg C. Arrhythmia in mitral valve prolapse: all roads lead to Rome. *J Am Coll Cardiol.* 2020;76:650–652.
19. Basso C, Perazzolo Marra M, Rizzo S, et al. Arrhythmic mitral valve prolapse and sudden cardiac death. *Circulation.* 2015;132:556–566.
20. Huttin O, Pierre S, Venner C, et al. Interactions between mitral valve and left ventricle analysed by 2D speckle tracking in patients with mitral valve prolapse: one more piece to the puzzle. *Eur Heart J Cardiovasc Imaging.* 2017;18:323–331.
21. Muthukumar L, Rahman F, Jan MF, et al. The Pickelhaube sign: novel echocardiographic risk marker for malignant mitral valve prolapse syndrome. *JACC Cardiovasc Imaging.* 2017;10: 1078–1080.
22. Zouridakis EG, Parthenakis FI, Kochiadakis GE, et al. QT dispersion in patients with mitral valve prolapse is related to the echocardiographic degree of the prolapse and mitral leaflet thickness. *Europace.* 2001;3:292–298.
23. Farb A, Tang AL, Atkinson JB, et al. Comparison of cardiac findings in patients with mitral valve prolapse who die suddenly to those who have congestive heart failure from mitral regurgitation and to those with fatal noncardiac conditions. *Am J Cardiol.* 1992;70:234–239.
24. Forteleoni A, Montereggi F, Sanna GD, et al. Traumatic mitral valve regurgitation: a case report and state-of-the-art review. *J Cardiovasc Med. (Hagerstown).* 2019;20:709–717.
25. Watanabe N. Acute mitral regurgitation. *Heart.* 2019;105:671–677.
26. Lancellotti P, Dulgheru R, Marchetta S, et al. Valve disease in heart failure: secondary but not irrelevant. *Heart Fail Clin.* 2019;15:219–227.
27. Shingu Y, Ooka T, Katoh H, et al. Feasibility and limitations of mitral valve repair, with or without left ventricular reconstruction in non-ischemic dilated cardiomyopathy. *J Cardiol.* 2018;71: 329–335.
28. Noack T, Borger MA. Commentary: prevention of systolic anterior motion after mitral repair in hypertrophic obstructive cardiomyopathy: one simple stitch fits all? *Semin Thorac Cardiovasc Surg.* 2020;32:269–270.
29. Otto CM, Nishimura RA, Bonow RO, et al. 2020 ACC/AHA Guideline for the Management of Patients With Valvular Heart Disease: Executive Summary: A Report of the American College of Cardiology/American Heart Association Joint Committee on Clinical Practice Guidelines. *J Am Coll Cardiol.* 2021;77:450–500.
30. Grayburn PA, Sannino A, Packer M. Proportionate and disproportionate functional mitral regurgitation: a new conceptual framework that reconciles the results of the MITRA-FR and COAPT trials. *JACC Cardiovasc Imaging.* 2019;12:353–362.
31. Bertrand PB, Mihos CG, Yucel E. Mitral annular calcification and calcific mitral stenosis: therapeutic challenges and considerations. *Curr Treat Options Cardiovasc Med.* 2019;21:19.
32. Massera D, Trivieri MG, Andrews JPM, et al. Disease activity in mitral annular calcification. *Circ Cardiovasc Imaging.* 2019;12:e008513.
33. Pasca I, Dang P, Tyagi G, et al. Survival in patients with degenerative mitral stenosis: results from a large retrospective cohort Study. *J Am Soc Echocardiogr.* 2016;29:461–469.
34. Tzolos E, Dweck MR. ^{18}F-Sodium Fluoride ^{18}F-NaF for imaging microcalcification activity in the cardiovascular system. *Arterioscler Thromb Vasc Biol.* 2020;40:1620–1626.
35. Ali K, Lee DJ, Adamson DL, et al. Radiation-induced dystrophic calcification and severe valvular stenosis: the central role of multimodality 3D cardiac imaging in disease assessment and planning of combined transcatheter aortic and mitral valve replacement. *BMJ Case Rep.* 2020;13.
36. Shabsigh M, Lawrence C, Rosero-Britton BR, et al. Mitral valve stenosis after open repair surgery for non-rheumatic mitral valve regurgitation: a review. *Front Cardiovasc Med.* 2016;3:8.
37. Al-Azizi K, Szerlip M. Mitral Stenosis After Mitraclip: How to Avoid and How to Treat. *Curr Cardiol Rep.* 2020;22:50.
38. Harries I, Chandrasekaran B, Barnes E, et al. Iatrogenic mitral stenosis following transcatheter aortic valve replacement (TAVR). *Indian Heart J.* 2015;67:60–61.
39. Wilkins GT, Weyman AE, Abascal VM, et al. Percutaneous balloon dilatation of the mitral valve: an analysis of echocardiographic variables related to outcome and the mechanism of dilatation. *Br Heart J.* 1988;60:299–308.
40. van Hagen IM, Thorne SA, Taha N, et al. Pregnancy outcomes in women with rheumatic mitral valve disease: results from the registry of pregnancy and cardiac disease. *Circulation.* 2018;137: 806–816.
41. French KA, Poppas A. Rheumatic heart disease in pregnancy: global challenges and clear opportunities. *Circulation.* 2018;137:817–819.
42. Perelshtein Brezinov O, Simchen MJ, Ben Zekry S, et al. Maternal and neonatal complications of pregnant women with mitral stenosis. *Isr Med Assoc J.* 2019;21:88–93.
43. Chiu FH, Yang CJ, Huang CK, et al. Spontaneous chordae tendineae rupture during peripartum. *Am J Emerg Med.* 2018;36 1127. e1–1127.e3.
44. Mahgoub A, Kotit S, Bakry K, et al. Thrombosis of mechanical mitral valve prosthesis during pregnancy: an ongoing "saga" in need of comprehensive solutions. *Glob Cardiol Sci Pract.* 2020;2020:e202032.
45. Seguela PE, Houyel L, Acar P. Congenital malformations of the mitral valve. *Arch Cardiovasc Dis.* 2011;104:465–479.
46. Mitruka SN, Lamberti JJ. Congenital heart surgery nomenclature and database project: mitral valve disease. *Ann Thorac Surg.* 2000;69:S132–S146.
47. Kaiser LR, Kron IL, Spray TL. *Mastery of Cardiothoracic Surgery.* 2nd ed. Philadelphia: Lippincott Williams & Wilkins; 2007.
48. Calabrò R, Limongelli G. Complete atrioventricular canal. *Orphanet J Rare Dis.* 2006;1:8.
49. Shone JD, Sellers RD, Anderson RC, et al. The developmental complex of "parachute mitral valve," supravalvular ring of left atrium, subaortic stenosis, and coarctation of aorta. *Am J Cardiol.* 1963;11:714–725.
50. Elmahrouk AF, Ismail MF, Arafat AA, et al. Outcomes of biventricular repair for shone's complex. *J Card Surg.* 2021;36:12–20.
51. Rajesh GN, Sajeer K, Nair A, et al. Hammock mitral valve: a rare cause of congenital mitral regurgitation—a case report. *Indian Heart J.* 2014;66:370–371.

3

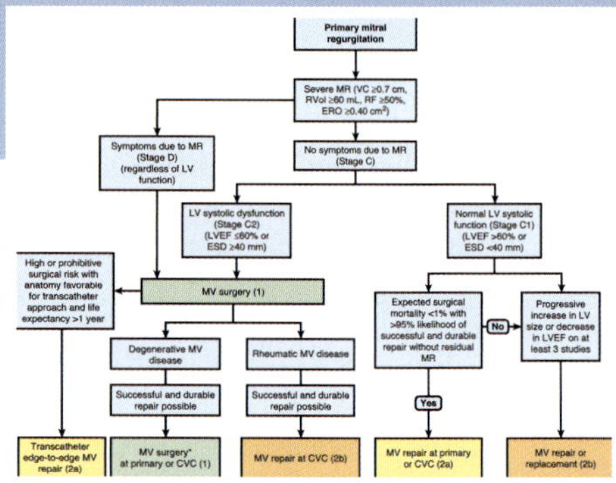

ACC/AHA Guidelines and Treatment Options for Mitral Valve Disease

Zach Rozenbaum, William A. Gray

CHAPTER OUTLINE

LEARNING OBJECTIVES

1. To review treatment options and mitral valve recommendations from the 2020 ACC/AHA Guideline for the Management of Patients With Valvular Heart Disease and discuss differences compared to the 2021 European Society of Cardiology/European Association for Cardio-Thoracic Surgery (ESC/EACTS) Guidelines for the Management of Valvular Heart Disease.

INTRODUCTION

Guidelines and recommendations for the treatment of valvular syndromes are periodically published by the American College of Cardiology (ACC) and the American Heart Association (AHA). In this chapter we will review the mitral valve (MV) recommendations from the 2020 ACC/AHA Guideline for the Management of Patients with Valvular Heart Disease[1] and discuss differences compared to the 2021 European Society of Cardiology/European Association for Cardio-Thoracic Surgery (ESC/EACTS) Guidelines for the Management of Valvular Heart Disease.[2]

ACC/AHA strength of recommendations are assigned Class I (strong), Class IIa (moderate), Class IIb (weak), Class III (no benefit), and Class IIIb (harm), whereas in the ESC the divisions are worded slightly differently: Class I (recommended), Class IIa (should be considered), Class IIb (may be considered), and Class III (is not recommended). The ACC/AHA Levels of Evidence are categorized as A (high quality), Level B-R (moderate quality), Level B-NR (nonrandomized moderate quality), Level C-LD (limited data), and Level C-EO (expert opinion), whereas in the ESC they are again slightly different, with Level A (multiple randomized control trials [RCTs]), Level B (single RCT or large nonrandomized studies), and Level C (expert opinion or small studies).

Criteria for determining severity of, and recommendations for, MV syndromes are discussed in a different chapter and include additional factors aside from valve function, such as comorbidities, surgical risk, and cardiac and extra-cardiac end-organ damage. Accordingly, guidelines will not only involve active surgical or interventional treatments, but also include conservative management, watchful waiting, periodic monitoring, and postprocedural care. Therefore, guidelines stress thorough initial and subsequent evaluations ought to be performed in order to continuously optimize and individualize treatment. Evaluation should encompass establishing the stage of the disease (Table 3.1), which takes into account symptomatology, physical examination, anatomy, severity, response of the ventricle and pulmonary circulation, and results of noninvasive and invasive testing as indicated. Finally, candidates for

TABLE 3.1 Stages of Valvular Heart Disease

Stage	Definition	Description
A	At risk	Patients with risk factors for development of VHD
B	Progressive	Patients with progressive VHD (mild to moderate severity and asymptomatic)
C	Asymptomatic severe	Asymptomatic patients who have the criteria for severe VHD
		CI: Asymptomatic patients with severe VHD in whom the LV or RV remains compensated
		CII: Asymptomatic patients with severe VHD with decompensation of the LV or RV
D	Symptomatic severe	Patients who have developed symptoms as a result of VHD

LV, Left ventricle; *RV*, right ventricle; *VHD*, valvular heart disease.
(From Otto CM, Nishimura RA, Bonow RO, et al. 2020 ACC/AHA Guideline for the management of patients with valvular heart disease: a report of the American College of Cardiology/American Heart Association Joint Committee on Clinical Practice Guidelines. *J Am Coll Cardiol*. 2021;77(4):e25–e197.)

interventions should be evaluated by a multidisciplinary heart valve team (MDT) (recommendation I, Level C-EO).

In a patient who is a candidate for intervention, risks should be calculated and discussed (recommendation I, Level C-EO) using an outcome score. In the US, the Society of Thoracic Surgeons (STS) score is most commonly used, although the European System for Cardiac Operative Risk Evaluation (EuroSCORE) II can also be considered (Table 3.2). A high surgical risk patient is, strictly speaking, defined as having an STS score above 8% for mortality. Other important determinations of surgical risk not necessarily accounted for in the surgical risk scores include two or more frailty indices of moderate-to-severe frailty (indices such as Katz Activities of Daily Living, and independence in ambulation), a major organ system compromise (cardiac or extra-cardiac) that is predicted not to improve postoperatively, or possible procedure-specific considerations, including the presence of tracheostomy, porcelain ascending aorta, chest malformation, arterial coronary graft adherent to posterior chest wall, prior sternotomy, severe chronic obstructive pulmonary disease (COPD), pulmonary hypertension, and hepatic dysfunction and radiation damage. Prohibitive surgical risk is defined as STS score above 50% for mortality or major morbidity, two or more frailty indices of moderate-to-severe frailty, three or more major organ system compromise that is predicted not to improve postoperatively, or severe procedure-specific impediments. Finally, multivalvular disease must be assessed, and indicators of futility, such as STS score for mortality over 15%, life expectancy of less than 1 year, and a poor candidate for rehabilitation, should also be considered.

TABLE 3.2 Risk Assessment for Surgical Valve Procedures

Criteria	Low-Risk SAVR (Must Meet ALL Criteria in This Column)	Low-Risk Surgical Mitral Valve Repair for Primary MR (Must Meet ALL Criteria in This Column)	High-Risk Surgical (Any One Criterion in This Column)	Prohibitive Surgical Risk (Any One Criterion in This Column)
STS-predicted risk of death[a]	<3% AND	<1% AND	>8% OR	Predicted risk of death or major morbidity (all-cause) >50% at 1 year OR
Frailty[b]	None AND	None AND	≥2 Indices (moderate to severe) OR	≥2 Indices (moderate to severe) OR
Cardiac or other major organ system compromise not to be improved postoperatively[c]	None AND	None AND	1–2 Organ systems OR	≥3 Organ systems OR
Procedure-specific impediment[d]	None	None	Possible procedure-specific impediment	Severe procedure-specific impediment

[a]Use of the STS predicted Risk of Mortality (http://riskcalc.sts.org/stswebriskcalc/#/) to predict risk in a given institution with reasonable reliability is appropriate only if institutional outcomes are within 1 standard deviation of the STS average observed/expected mortality ration for the procedure in question. The FUROSCORE II risk calculator may also be considered for use and is available at http://www.euroscore.org/calc.html.

[b]Seven frailty indices: Katz Activities of Daily Living (independence in feeding, bathing, dressing, transferring, toileting, and urinary continence) plus independence in ambulation (no walking aid or assistance required, or completion of a 5-m walk in <6 seconds). Other scoring systems can be applied to calculate no, mild, or moderate-to-severe frailty.

[c]Examples of major organ system compromise include cardiac dysfunction (severe LV systolic or diastolic dysfunction or RV dysfunction, fixed pulmonary hypertension); kidney dysfunction (chronic kidney disease, stage 3 or worse); pulmonary dysfunction (FEV_1, <50% or $DLCO_2$ <50% of predicted); central nervous system dysfunction (dementia, Alzheimer disease, Parkinson disease, cerebrovascular accident with persistent physical limitation); gastrointestinal dysfunction (Crohn disease, ulcerative colitis, nutritional impairment, or serum albumin <3.0); cancer (active malignancy); and liver dysfunction (any history of cirrhosis, variceal bleeding, or elevated INR in the absence of VKA therapy).

[d]Examples of procedure-specific impediments include presence of tracheostomy, heavily calcified (porcelain) ascending aorta, chest malformation, arterial coronary graft adherent to posterior chest wall, and radiation damage.*DLCO2*, Diffusion capacity for carbon dioxide; *FEV1*, forced expiratory volume in 1 second; *INR*, international normalized ratio; *LV*, left ventricular; *MR*, mitral regurgitation; *RV*, right ventricular; *SAVR*, surgical aortic valve replacement; *STS*, Society of Thoracic Surgeons; *VKA*, vitamin K antagonist.

(From Otto CM, Nishimura RA, Bonow RO, et al. 2020 ACC/AHA Guideline for the Management of Patients With Valvular Heart Disease: A Report of the American College of Cardiology/American Heart Association Joint Committee on Clinical Practice Guidelines. *J Am Coll Cardiol*. 2021;77(4):e25–e197.)

MITRAL REGURGITATION

Over the years, guidelines have had to accommodate the progression in therapeutic options as new technologies have emerged. Threshold for nonsurgical interventions is continuously lowered since there is less impact of traditional comorbidities on outcomes, and with greater technical expertise, better patient selection, and generational device improvements procedural complications have generally declined and clinical outcomes improved. Percutaneous therapies such as the U.S. Food and Drug Administration (FDA)-approved edge-to-edge repair, as well as current investigational valve implantation, annuloplasty, and technologies aiming at chordae repair strategies, have substantially impacted management of patients with mitral regurgitation (MR) in clinical practice. Aims of invasive treatment include alleviation of symptoms, interrupting the vicious cycle of left ventricular (LV) volume overload and its sequalae, and improving mortality outcomes.

MR can be divided into acute and chronic, and treatment options vary accordingly and may be influenced by the specific etiology of MR. A further mechanistic division, which is more relevant to the chronic MR, includes primary and secondary MR.

Acute Mitral Regurgitation

Whether acute MR results from leaflet perforation, chordal rupture, or rupture of the papillary muscle, acute LV volume overload, low forward flow, and pulmonary congestion ensue, along with the potential for acute hemodynamic decompensation. Initial management includes vasodilator therapy and intra-aortic balloon counter-pulsation (IABP) or other means of hemodynamic support. Both guidelines, ESC and ACA/AHA, suggest the possible use of diuretics; however, as there are no supporting data, firm recommendations were not issued. Undoubtedly, prompt MV surgery, preferably repair, is indicated when feasible, as it is lifesaving in many instances. Although surgery has been the traditional mode of management, there are emerging reports on successful urgent/emergent transcatheter interventions for severe acute MR.[3]

Chronic Mitral Regurgitation

Imaging

As noted above, chronic MR can be divided into primary or degenerative, and secondary or functional MR. Generally speaking, degenerative MR results from primary MV pathologies (may be more than one component), while functional MR results from associated chamber pathology. Transthoracic echocardiography (TTE) is indicated for initial screening and evaluation of primary MR (recommendation I, Level B-NR) and is quite accurate in determining the severity of regurgitation, whereas transesophageal echocardiography (TEE) is indicated both when TTE provides insufficient or discordant information, and to better define the anatomic pathology in detail (recommendation I, Level C-EO). Cardiac magnetic resonance (CMR) imaging is indicated when there is a discrepancy in regurgitant severity between the findings on clinical assessment and echocardiography since CMR volume—and derivative regurgitant—determinations are quite accurate (recommendation I, Level B-NR). Intraoperative or intraprocedural TEE is indicated to provide guidance and to evaluate the degree of regurgitation at the end of surgical MV repair (MVr), as even mild MR is a risk factor for late failure (Table 3.3). As with degenerative MR, TEE is indicated in advance of percutaneous repair of secondary chronic MR to determine suitability for the procedure (Table 3.4).

TABLE 3.3 Diagnostic Testing: Initial Diagnosis

Recommendations for Diagnostic Testing: Initial Diagnosis of Chronic Mitral Regurgitation

COR	LOE	Recommendations
I	B-NR	1. In patients with known or suspected primary MR, TTE is indicated for baseline evaluation of LV size and function, RV function, LA size, pulmonary artery pressure, and the mechanism and severity of primary MR (stages A–D).
I	C-EO	2. In patients with primary MR, when TTE provides insufficient or discordant information, TEE is indicated for evaluation of the severity of MR, mechanism of MR, and status of LV function (stages B–D).
I	B-NR	3. In patients with primary MR, CMR is indicated to assess LV and RV volumes and function and may help with assessing MR severity when there is a discrepancy between the findings on clinical assessment and echocardiography.
I	B-NR	4. In patients with severe primary MR undergoing mitral intervention, intraoperative TEE is indicated to establish the anatomic basis for primary MR (stages C and D) and to guide repair.

CMR, Cardiac magnetic resonance; *LA,* left atrium/left atrial; *LV,* left ventricle; *MR,* mitral regurgitation; *RV,* right ventricle; *TEE,* transesophageal echocardiography; *TTE,* transthoracic echocardiography.

(From Otto CM, Nishimura RA, Bonow RO, et al. 2020 ACC/AHA Guideline for the management of patients with valvular heart disease: a report of the American College of Cardiology/American Heart Association Joint Committee on Clinical Practice Guidelines. *J Am Coll Cardiol.* 2021;77(4):e25–e197.)

Periodic Monitoring

When monitoring patients with stage B (progressive) disease, echocardiography should be performed every 3 to 5 years with mild severity and every 1 to 2 years with moderate severity. Although most patients with severe asymptomatic disease (stage Class I) would increasingly be considered candidates for intervention (especially with ventricular findings), echocardiography should be performed every 6 to 12 months (recommendation Class I, Level B-NR). Additional parameters, such as serum biomarkers and global longitudinal strain (GLS) may be useful as well to guide timing of intervention (recommendation Class IIb, Level B-NR; Table 3.5). Moreover, in equivocal cases, hemodynamic exercise testing, invasive measurement, or cardiopulmonary exercise may be useful (recommendation Class IIb, Level of Evidence B-NR; Table 3.6).

Treatment of Primary Mitral Regurgitation

Class I indications for invasive treatment of severe primary MR include symptoms and LV dysfunction (defined as ejection

TABLE 3.4 Diagnosis of Chronic Secondary Mitral Regurgitation

Recommendations for Diagnosis of Secondary Mitral Regurgitation

COR	LOE	Recommendations
I	B-NR	1. In patients with chronic secondary MR (stages B–D), TTE is useful to establish the etiology and to assess the extent of regional and global LV remodeling and systolic dysfunction, severity of MR, and magnitude to pulmonary hypertension.
I	C-EO	2. In patients with chronic secondary MR (stages B–D), noninvasive imaging (stress nuclear/PET, CMR, or stress echocardiography), coronary CT angiography, or coronary arteriography is useful to establish etiology of MR to assess myocardial viability.
I	B-NR	3. In patients with chronic secondary MR with severe symptoms (stage D) that are unresponsive to GDMT who are being considered for transcatheter mitral valve interventions, TTE is indicated to determine suitability for the procedure.
I	C-EO	4. In patients with chronic secondary MR undergoing transcatheter mitral valve intervention, intraprocedural guidance with TEE is recommended.

CMR, Cardiac magnetic resonance; *CT,* computed tomography; *GDMT,* guideline-directed management and therapy; *LV,* left ventricle; *MR,* mitral regurgitation; *PET,* positron emission tomography; *TEE,* transesophageal echocardiography; *TTE,* transthoracic echocardiography.

(From Otto CM, Nishimura RA, Bonow RO, et al. 2020 ACC/AHA Guideline for the management of patients with valvular heart disease: a report of the American College of Cardiology/American Heart Association Joint Committee on Clinical Practice Guidelines. *J Am Coll Cardiol.* 2021;77(4):e25–e197.)

TABLE 3.5 Diagnostic Testing: Routing Follow-Up

Recommendations for Diagnostic Testing: Routine Follow-Up for Chronic Primary Mitral Regurgitation

COR	LOE	Recommendations
I	B-NR	1. For asymptomatic patients with severe primary MR (stages B and Cl), TTE is indicated every 6–12 months for surveillance of LV function (estimated by LVEF, LVEDD, and LVESD) and assessment of pulmonary artery pressure.
IIb	B-NR	2. In asymptomatic patients with severe primary MR (stages B and Cl), use of serum biomarkers and novel measurements of LV function, such as global longitudinal strain, may be considered as an adjunct to guide timing of intervention.

LV, Left ventricle; *LVEDD,* left ventricular end-diastolic diameter; *LVEF,* left ventricular ejection fraction; *LVESD,* left ventricular end-systolic diameter; *MR,* mitral regurgitation; *TTE,* transthoracic echocardiography.

(From Otto CM, Nishimura RA, Bonow RO, et al. 2020 ACC/AHA Guideline for the management of patients with valvular heart disease: a report of the American College of Cardiology/American Heart Association Joint Committee on Clinical Practice Guidelines. *J Am Coll Cardiol.* 2021;77(4):e25–e197.)

TABLE 3.6 Diagnostic Testing: Exercise Testing

Recommendation for Diagnostic Testing: Exercise Testing for Chronic Primary Mitral Regurgitation

COR	LOE	Recommendation
IIa	B-NR	In patients with primary MR (stages B and C) and symptoms that might be attributable to MR, hemodynamic exercise testing using Doppler echocardiography or cardiac catheterization or cardiopulmonary exercise testing is reasonable.

MR, Mitral regurgitation.

(From Otto CM, Nishimura RA, Bonow RO, et al. 2020 ACC/AHA Guideline for the management of patients with valvular heart disease: a report of the American College of Cardiology/American Heart Association Joint Committee on Clinical Practice Guidelines. *J Am Coll Cardiol.* 2021;77(4):e25–e197.)

fraction [EF] of 60% or less or left ventricular end-systolic diameter [LVESD] of 40 mm or more) to prevent further deterioration, preferably with repair and not replacement (Fig. 3.1). Intervention may also be considered in asymptomatic patients if a successful repair is likely (less than 5% failure expectancy) with very low mortality risk (recommendation Class IIa, Level of Evidence B-NR), when there is progressive increase in LV size or a decrease in EF (recommendation Class IIb, Level of Evidence C-LD). Despite accumulating data, transcatheter interventions are still recommended only for patients with high/prohibitive surgical risk (recommendation Class IIa, Level of Evidence B-NR; Table 3.7). Notwithstanding, while median operative mortality rates of MVr are 1%, operative mortality rates for MV replacement (MVR) are 5% and are even higher (9%) when combined with coronary artery bypass graft (CABG) or aortic valve replacement (AVR) (Table 3.8). Rheumatic MV disease is an outlier in terms of treatment of primary MR due to decreased suitability for repair, thereby often necessitating replacement.

Treatment of Secondary Mitral Regurgitation

In secondary MR, surgery has not been proven to decrease mortality and is largely reserved for symptomatic relief in selected cases, whereas transcatheter edge-to-edge intervention (TEER) has been shown to improve clinical outcomes and mortality based on The COAPT trial results. TEER is recommended for patients with LV EF of 20% to 49%, LVESD of 70 mm or less, and pulmonary artery systolic pressure (SPAP) of 70 mm Hg or less (recommendation Class IIa, Level of Evidence B-R), while surgery is recommended with LV EF of 20% to 49% unsuitable for TEER (recommendation Class IIb, Level of Evidence B-R) or for "atrial MR" (recommendation Class IIb, Level of Evidence B-NR; Fig. 3.2). Notably, in a recent trial, MVr had no apparent benefit over replacement in secondary MR at 2 years.[4] Finally, when CABG is undertaken, concomitant MVr should be performed when significant MR is present (recommendation Class IIa, Level of Evidence B-R).

Medical Management

Among patients in whom LV systolic dysfunction occurs and surgery is deferred in favor of conservative therapy, guideline-directed medical management (GDMT) for LV systolic dysfunction,

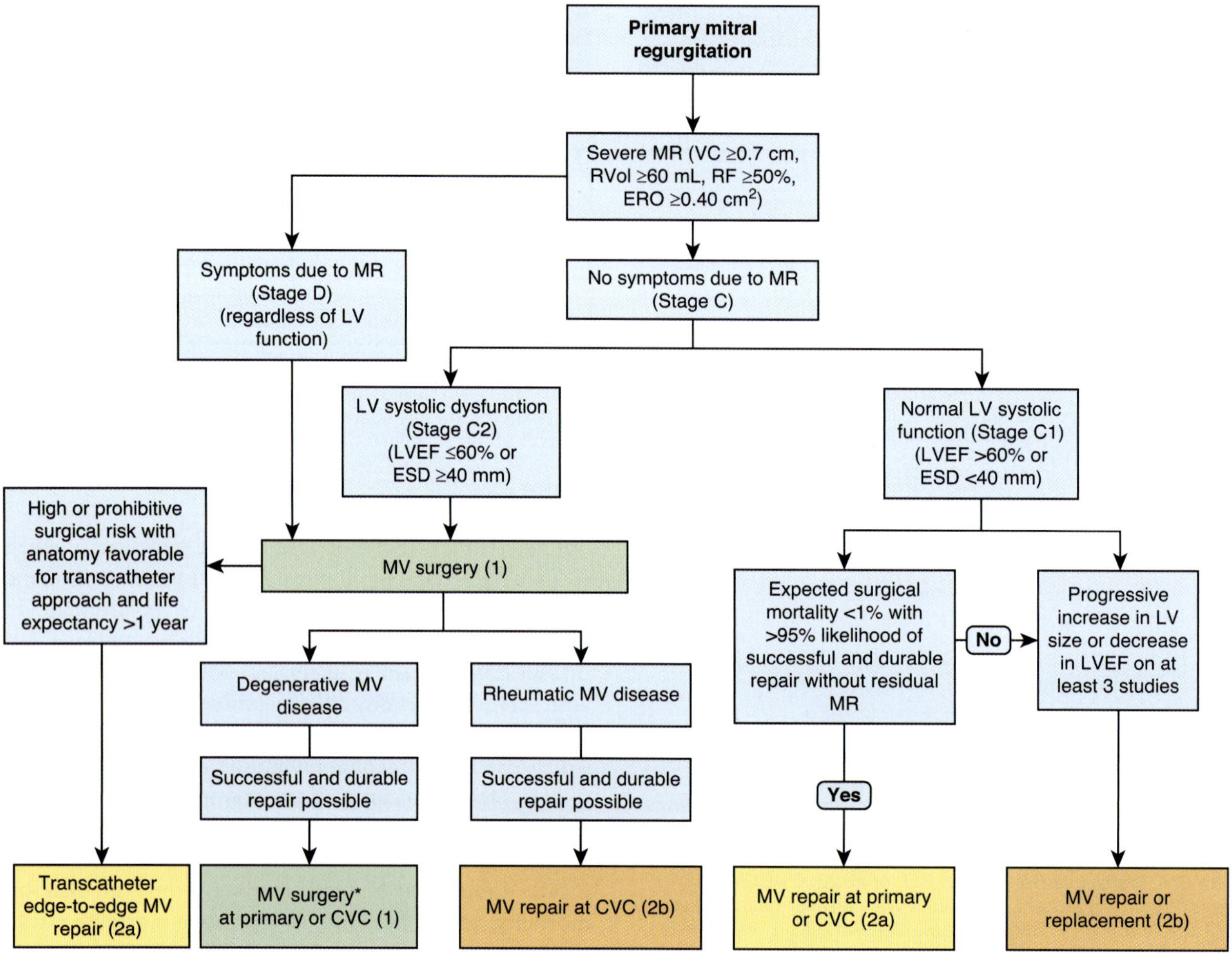

Fig. 3.1 Primary Mitral Regurgitation. *Mitral valve replacement if mitral valve repair is not possible. *CVC*, Comprehensive valve center; *ERO*, effective regurgitant orifice; *ESD*, end-systolic dimension; *LV*, left ventricle; *LVEF*, left ventricular ejection fraction; *MR*, mitral regurgitation; *MV*, mitral valve; *RF*, regurgitant fraction; *RVol*, regurgitant volume; *VC*, vena contracta. (From Otto CM, Nishimura RA, Bonow RO, et al. 2020 ACC/AHA Guideline for the management of patients with valvular heart disease: a report of the American College of Cardiology/American Heart Association Joint Committee on Clinical Practice Guidelines. *J Am Coll Cardiol.* 2021;77[4]:e25–e197.)

including beta-adrenergic blockade, angiotensin-converting enzyme inhibitors (ACEi)/angiotensin II receptor blockers (ARBs), and possibly aldosterone antagonists, is indicated (recommendation Class IIa, Level of Evidence B-NR; Table 3.9). With secondary MR where LV dysfunction is also prominent, there may be more evidence for use of angiotensin receptor neprilysin inhibitors (ARNIs) and biventricular pacing in addition to the above-mentioned medications (recommendation Class I, Level A; Table 3.10). Both guidelines, ESC and ACA/AHA, stress the importance of medical treatment of patients with symptomatic chronic secondary MR as an initial management strategy.

Post-Procedural Echocardiography

The minimal requirements for postprocedural echo are at 1 to 3 months postprocedure, and annually thereafter; for transcatheter MV repair (TMVr) and replacement (TMVR), after 1 year and then every 2 to 3 years for surgical MVr, at 5 and 10 years with a surgical bioprosthesis, but then annually, and only at an early post-operative time-point for a mechanical valve.

Differences Between ACC/AHA and ESC Guidelines

Similar to the ACC/AHA guidelines, ESC guidelines recommend invasive treatment for asymptomatic severe primary MR for patients with EF ≤of 60% or less or LVESD of 40 mm or greater. This is a revision from the previous 2017 guidelines which recommended LVESD of 45 mm as a cut-off, signifying earlier treatment indications. A major difference between guidelines is that ESC recommends surgery in primary asymptomatic severe MR with preserved LV function in case of new onset atrial fibrillation or SPAP greater than 50 mm Hg and high likelihood of durable repair, low surgical risk, and left atrial dilatation (recommendation strength IIa, Level of Evidence B; Fig. 3.3). Interestingly, in the same scenario, the 2017 ESC guidelines accepted flail leaflet as an alternative to left atrial dilatation; this was revised in the current version and is not regarded as an indication. Another difference with severe chronic secondary MR is the regard to LV assist device (LVAD) or heart transplant in patients with end stage LV or right ventricular (RV) failure. Results from the Mitra-Fr trial serve as an important basis for

TABLE 3.7 Intervention

Recommendations for Intervention for Chronic Primary Mitral Regurgitation

COR	LOE	Recommendations
I	B-NR	1. In symptomatic patients with severe primary MR (stage D), mitral valve intervention is recommended irrespective of LV systolic function.
I	B-NR	2. In asymptomatic patients with severe primary MR and LV systolic dysfunction (LVEF ≤60%, LVESD ≥40 mm) (stage CII), mitral valve surgery is recommended.
I	B-NR	3. In patients with severe primary MR for whom surgery is indicated, mitral valve repair is recommended in preference to mitral valve replacement when the anatomic cause of MR is degenerative disease, if a successful and durable repair is possible.
IIa	B-NR	4. In asymptomatic patients with severe primary MR and normal LV systolic function (LVEF ≥60% and LVESD ≤40 mm) (stage CI), mitral valve repair is reasonable when the likelihood of a successful and durable repair without residual MR is >95% with an expected mortality rate of <1%, when it can be performed at a primary or comprehensive valve center.
IIb	C-LD	5. In asymptomatic patients with severe primary MR and normal LV systolic function (LVEF >60% and LVESD <40 mm) (stage CI) but with a progressive increase in LV size or decrease in EF on ≥3 serial imaging studies, mitral valve surgery may be considered irrespective of the probability of a successful and durable repair.
IIa	B-NR	6. In severely symptomatic patients (NYHA Class III or IV) with primary severe MR and high or prohibitive surgical risk, transcatheter edge-to-edge repair (TEE) is reasonable if mitral valve anatomy is favorable for the repair procedure and patient life expectancy is at least 1 year.
IIb	B-NR	7. In symptomatic patients with severe primary MR attributable to rheumatic valve disease, mitral valve repair may be considered at a Comprehensive Valve Center by an experienced team when surgical treatment is indicated, if a durable and successful repair is likely.
III: Harm	B-NR	8. In patients with severe primary MR where leaflet pathology is limited to less than one half the posterior leaflet, mitral valve replacement should not be performed unless mitral valve repair has been attempted at a primary or comprehensive valve center and was unsuccessful.

EF, Ejection fraction; *LV,* Left ventricle; *LVEF,* left ventricular ejection fraction; *LVESD,* left ventricular end systolic diameter; *MR,* mitral regurgitation; *NYHA,* New York Heart Association.

(From Otto CM, Nishimura RA, Bonow RO, et al. 2020 ACC/AHA Guideline for the management of patients with valvular heart disease: a report of the American College of Cardiology/American Heart Association Joint Committee on Clinical Practice Guidelines. *J Am Coll Cardiol.* 2021;77(4):e25–e197.)

TABLE 3.8 Median Operative Mortality Rates for Specific Surgical Procedures (Society of Thoracic Surgeons Adult Cardiac Surgery Database, 2019)

Procedure	Mortality Rate (%)
AVR	2.2
AVR and CABG	4.0
AVR and mitral valve replacement	9.0
Mitral valve replacement	5.0
Mitral valve replacement and CABG	9.0
Mitral valve repair	1.0
Mitral valve repair and CABG	5.0

AVR, Aortic valve replacement; *CABG,* coronary artery bypass graft surgery; *STS,* Society of Thoracic Surgeons.

(From Otto CM, Nishimura RA, Bonow RO, et al. 2020 ACC/AHA Guideline for the management of patients with valvular heart disease: a report of the American College of Cardiology/American Heart Association Joint Committee on Clinical Practice Guidelines. *J Am Coll Cardiol.* 2021;77(4):e25–e197.)

proper exclusion of the futile patient, as these patients did not demonstrate benefit.[5] The absence of LVAD and heart transplant from explicit ACC/AHA recommendations could arise from the fact that management focus is shifted from valvulopathy towards heart failure in patients with advanced disease. Nevertheless, such options should be taken into consideration.

Future Perspectives

Currently in the United States, MitraClip is the only FDA-approved device for commercial use in percutaneous MVr, and it is the only transcatheter technique mentioned in both guidelines, a reality that is likely to change in upcoming revisions given the rapid evolution of novel devices, as annuloplasty (direct or indirect) approaches include the Carillon Mitral Contour System (Cardiac Dimensions, Washington, DC, USA), Cardioband Mitral System (Edwards Lifesciences, Irvine, California, USA), PASCAL System (Edwards Lifesciences, Irvine, CA, USA), and Millipede Mitral Annuloplasty System (Boston Scientific, Massachusetts, USA). Beating heart chordal repair approaches include the NeoChord system (NeoChord Inc., St. Louis Park, MN, USA) and the Harpoon system (Edwards Lifesciences, Irvine, CA, USA). Lastly, percutaneous MVR approaches include the Intrepid Valve (Medtronic, Minneapolis, MN, USA) and the Tendyne Valve (Abbott Vascular, Chicago, Il, USA), with several others in development. Most of the valve replacement strategies have started transapical but are transitioning to transseptal.

MITRAL STENOSIS

The patient profile with mitral stenosis (MS) differs from those with MR, as women are more likely to have valvular sequela of rheumatic fever, the incidence is low in high-income countries, and patients present at a younger age. Severe symptomatic disease is defined as mitral valve area (MVA) of 1.5 cm^2 or

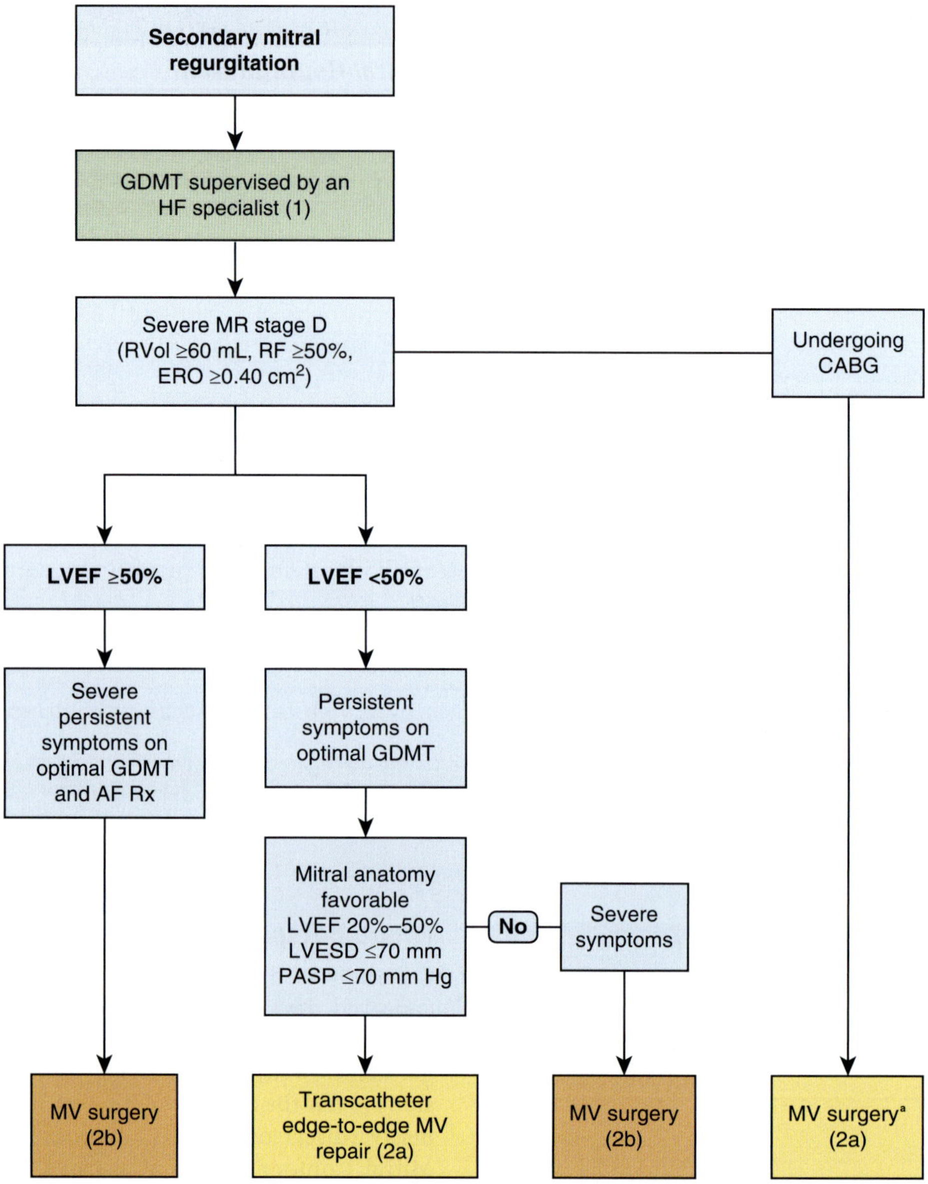

Fig. 3.2 Secondary Mitral Regurgitation. [a]Chordal-sparing MV replacement may be reasonable to choose over downsized annuloplasty repair. *AF*, Atrial fibrillation; *CABG*, coronary artery bypass graft; *ERO*, effective regurgitant orifice; *GDMT*, guideline-directed management and therapy; *HF*, heart failure; *LVEF*, left ventricular ejection fraction; *LVESD*, left ventricular end-systolic dimension; *MR*, mitral regurgitation; *MV*, mitral valve; *PASP*, pulmonary artery systolic pressure; *RF*, regurgitant fraction; *RVol*, regurgitant volume; *Rx*, medication. (From Otto CM, Nishimura RA, Bonow RO, et al. 2020 ACC/AHA Guideline for the management of patients with valvular heart disease: a report of the American College of Cardiology/American Heart Association Joint Committee on Clinical Practice Guidelines. *J Am Coll Cardiol.* 2021;77[4]:e25–e197.)

less and occurs with diastolic pressure half-time of 150 ms or more, which usually correlates to gradients of 6 to 10 mm Hg at a controlled heart rate. Another relatively common cause of MS is mitral annulus calcifications (MACs) in which leaflets may be calcified as well. Although MAC is a very common finding, only a small percent of patients have clinically meaningful MS. Patients with MAC are generally considerably older and incidence is higher in high-income countries.

Periodic Monitoring

TTE is the modality of choice for diagnosis and quantification of MS (recommendation Class I, Level of Evidence B-NR). When monitoring stage B (progressive) disease with MVA greater than 1.5 cm^2, echocardiography should be performed every 3 to 5 years. With severe asymptomatic disease (stage Class I), echocardiography should be performed every 1 to 2 years for MVA of 1 to 1.5 cm^2 and annually for MVA of less than 1 cm^2. When there is a discrepancy between echocardiography and symptoms, exercise echocardiography or invasive measurements should be pursued (recommendation Class I, Level of Evidence C-LD).

Treatment of Mitral Stenosis

The procedure of choice in rheumatic MS is percutaneous mitral balloon commissurotomy (PMBC) (recommendation

TABLE 3.9 Medical Therapy

Recommendations for Medical Therapy for Chronic Primary Mitral Regurgitation

COR	LOE	Recommendations
IIa	B-NR	1. In symptomatic or asymptomatic patients with severe primary MR and LV systolic dysfunction (stages CII and D) in whom surgery is not possible or must be delayed, GDMT for systolic dysfunction is reasonable.
III: No Benefit	B-NR	2. In asymptomatic patients with primary MR and normal LV systolic function (stages B and CI), vasodilator therapy is not indicated if the patient is normotensive.

GDMT, Guideline-directed management and therapy; *LV*, Left ventricle; *MR*, mitral regurgitation.

(From Otto CM, Nishimura RA, Bonow RO, et al. 2020 ACC/AHA Guideline for the management of patients with valvular heart disease: a report of the American College of Cardiology/American Heart Association Joint Committee on Clinical Practice Guidelines. *J Am Coll Cardiol.* 2021;77(4):e25–e197.)

TABLE 3.10 Medical Therapy

Recommendations for Medical Therapy for Secondary Mitral Regurgitation

COR	LOE	Recommendations
I	A	1. Patients with chronic severe secondary MR (stages C and D) and HF with reduced LVEF should receive standard GDMT for HF, including ACE inhibitors, ARBs, beta blockers, aldosterone antagonists, and/or sacubitril/valsartan, and biventricular pacing as indicated.
I	C-EO	2. In patients with chronic severe secondary MR and HF with reduced LVEF, a cardiologist expert in the management of patients with HF and LV systolic dysfunction should be the primary MDT member responsible for implementing and monitoring optimal GDMT.

ACE, Angiotensin-converting enzyme; *ARBs*, Angiotensin II Receptor Blockers; *GDMT*, guideline-directed management and therapy; *HF*, heart failure; *LV*, Left ventricle; *LVEF*, left ventricular ejection fraction; *MDT*, Multidisciplinary Heart Valve Team; *MR*, mitral regurgitation

(From Otto CM, Nishimura RA, Bonow RO, et al. 2020 ACC/AHA Guideline for the management of patients with valvular heart disease: a report of the American College of Cardiology/American Heart Association Joint Committee on Clinical Practice Guidelines. *J Am Coll Cardiol.* 2021;77(4):e25–e197.)

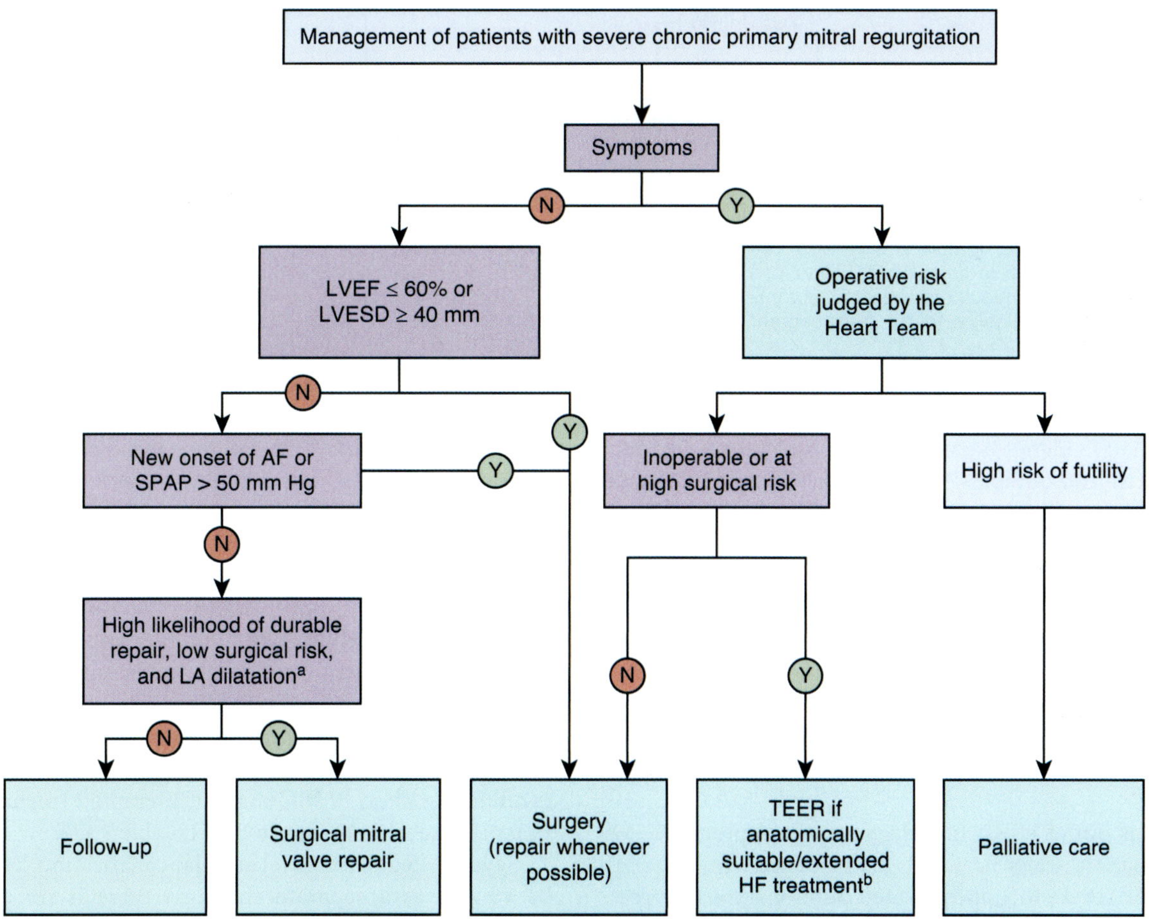

Fig. 3.3 Management of Patients With Severe Chronic Primary Mitral Regurgitation. [a]LA dilatation: volume index ≥60 mL/m^2 or diameter ≥55 mm at sinus rhythm. [b]Extended heart failure treatment included the following: CRT: ventricular assist devices; heart transplantation. *AF*, Atrial fibrillation; *HF*, heart failure; *LA*, left atrium/left atrial; *LVEF*, left ventricular ejection fraction; *LVESD*, left ventricular end-systolic diameter; *SPAP*, systolic pulmonary arterial pressure; *TEER*, transcatheter edge-to-edge repair. (From Vahanian A, Beyersdorf F, Praz F, et al. 2021 ESC/EACTS Guidelines for the management of valvular heart disease. *Eur Heart J* 2021.)

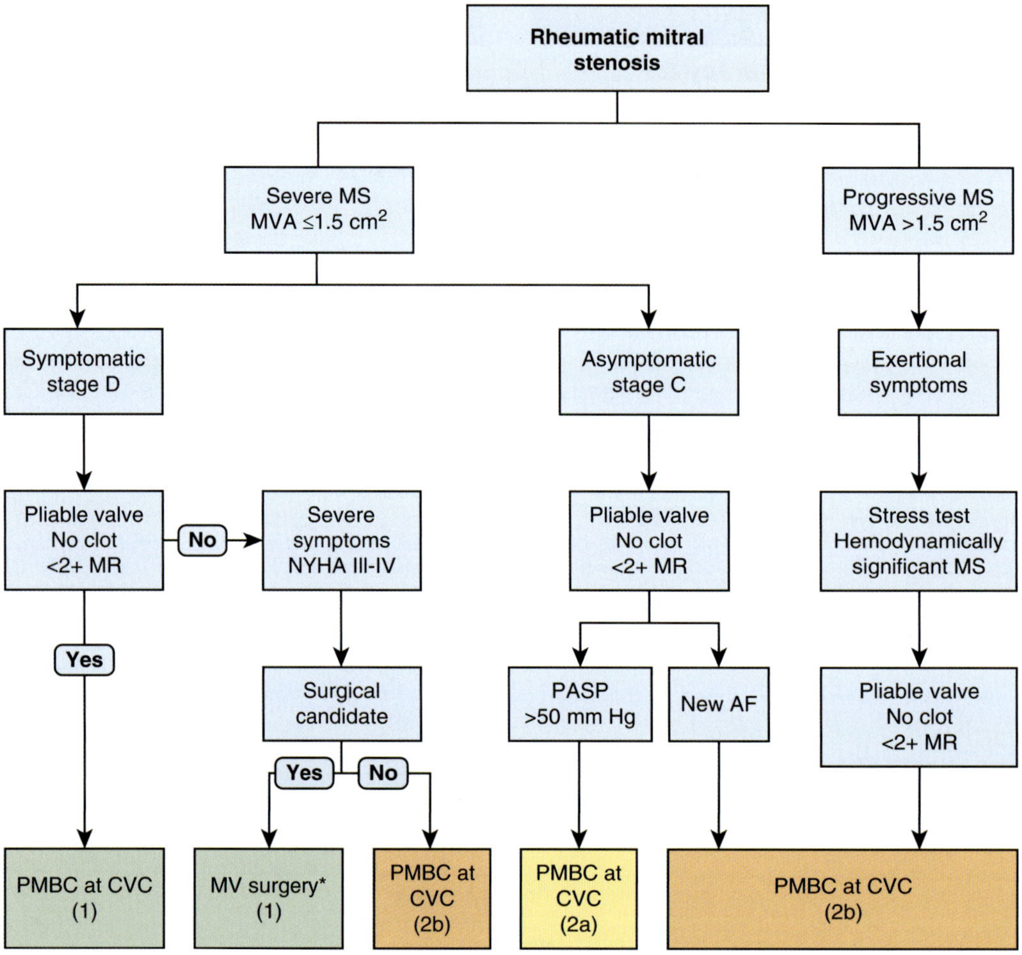

Fig. 3.4 Intervention for Mitral Stenosis. *Repair, commissurotomy, or valve replacement. *AF*, Atrial fibrillation; *CVC*, comprehensive valve center; *MR*, mitral regurgitation; *MS*, mitral stenosis; *MV*, mitral valve; *MVA*, mitral valve area; *NYHA*, New York Heart Association; *PASP*, pulmonary artery systolic pressure; *PMBC*, percutaneous mitral balloon commissurotomy. (From Otto CM, Nishimura RA, Bonow RO, et al. 2020 ACC/AHA Guideline for the management of patients with valvular heart disease: a report of the American College of Cardiology/American Heart Association Joint Committee on Clinical Practice Guidelines. *J Am Coll Cardiol.* 2021;77[4]:e25–e197.)

Class I, Level of Evidence A), which in the well-selected patient is both effective and durable. Prior to intervention, TEE should be performed to evaluate MR severity (which may be underestimated due to shadowing of calcifications) as well as rule out LA thrombus (recommendation Class I, Level of Evidence C-LD), because both pose contraindications to PMBC. Next, a procedural prediction score, such as the Wilkins score, should be performed. Anatomical factors include leaflet mobility, thickening, and calcifications, and sub-valvular fusion. Patient characteristics and other cardiac structures' function must also be taken into consideration as they are predictive of outcome success.

Indications for PMBC include severe symptomatic MS (recommendation Class I, Level of Evidence A; Fig. 3.4), asymptomatic severe MS, and elevated pulmonary artery pressure (recommendation Class IIa, Level of Evidence B-NR) or new onset atrial fibrillation (recommendation Class IIb, Level of Evidence C-LD), and moderate symptomatic MS if wedge pressure or MV gradients are high (>25 mm Hg and >15 mm Hg, respectively) during exercise (recommendation Class IIb, Level of Evidence C-LD), because these patients were shown to improve clinically after PMBC. Moreover, earlier treatment allows prevention of long term sequalae, such as irreversible pulmonary artery hypertension (termed the "second stenosis"), left atrial enlargement, and/or fibrosis.

Patients who are not candidates for PMBC or have undergone an unsuccessful PMBC should undergo surgical commissurotomy (open or closed), or alternative replacement (recommendation Class I, Level of Evidence B-NR). Finally, in patients with severe symptomatic MS who are not optimal candidates for PMBC in terms of anatomy but are not surgical candidates either, PMBC may be attempted (recommendation Class IIb, Level of Evidence B-NR; Table 3.11).

Severe MS due to mitral annular calcification (MAC) should be viewed as a separate entity, as there is no commissural fusion and calcifications are generally limited to the annulus and leaflet bases, so the recognized mechanism (commissural "cracking") in PMBC is not present. As these anatomic characteristics are usually less favorable, procedural risks may be higher and effectiveness and durability considerably less than

TABLE 3.11 Intervention

Recommendations for Intervention for Rheumatic Mitral Stenosis

COR	LOE	Recommendations
I	A	1. In symptomatic patients (NYHA Class II, III, or IV) with severe rheumatic MS (mitral valve area 1.5 cm^2, stage D) and favorable valve morphology with less than moderate (2+) MR[a] in the absence of LA thrombus, PMBC is recommended if it can be performed at a comprehensive valve center.
I	B-NR	2. In severely symptomatic patients (NYHA Class III or IV) with severe rheumatic MS (mitral valve are \$1.5 cm^2, stage D) who (1) are not candidates for PMBC, (2) have failed a previous PMBC, (3) require other cardiac procedures, or (4) do not have access to PMBC, mitral valve surgery (repair, commissurotomy, or valve replacement) is indicated.
IIa	B-NR	3. In asymptomatic patients with severe rheumatic MS (mitral valve are $\leq$1.5 cm^2, stage C) and favorable valve morphology with less than 2+ MR in the absence of LA thrombus who have elevated pulmonary pressures (pulmonary artery systolic pressure >50 mm Hg), PMBC is reasonable if it can be performed at a comprehensive valve center.
IIb	C-LD	4. In asymptomatic patients with severe rheumatic MS (mitral valve area $\leq$1.5 cm^2, stage C) and favorable valve morphology with less than 2+/ MR[a] in the absence of LA thrombus who have new onset of AF, PMBC may be considered if it can be performed at a comprehensive valve center.
IIb	C-LD	5. In symptomatic patients (NYHA Class II, III, or IV) with rheumatic MS and a mitral valve area >1.5 cm^2, if there is evidence of hemodynamically significant rheumatic MS on the basis of a pulmonary artery wedge pressure >25 mm Hg or a mean mitral valve gradient >15 mm Hg during exercise, PMBC may be considered if it can be performed at a comprehensive valve center.
IIb	B-NR	6. In severely symptomatic patients (NYHA Class II or IV) with severe rheumatic MS (mitral valve area $\leq$1.5 cm^2, stage D) who have a suboptimal valve anatomy and who are not candidates for surgery or are at high risk for surgery, PMBC may be considered if it can be performed at a comprehensive valve center.

[a]2+ on a 0 to 4+ scale according to Sellar's criteria or less than moderate by Doppler echocardiography.

AF, Atrial fibrillation; *LA,* left atrium/left atrial; *MR,* mitral regurgitation; *MS,* mitral stenosis; *NYHA,* New York Heart Association; *PMBC,* percutaneous mitral balloon commissurotomy

(From Otto CM, Nishimura RA, Bonow RO, et al. 2020 ACC/AHA Guideline for the management of patients with valvular heart disease: a report of the American College of Cardiology/American Heart Association Joint Committee on Clinical Practice Guidelines. *J Am Coll Cardiol.* 2021;77(4):e25–e197.)

PMBC in rheumatic patients. Therefore, cases should be extensively studied and discussed before the decision on intervention (recommendation Class IIb, Level of Evidence C-LD). The treatment of choice is surgical, most often MVR. Percutaneous transcatheter valve-in-MAC[6] is an emerging promising alternative; however, this procedure is not commonly performed as outcomes are uncertain yet.

Post-Procedural Echocardiography

The minimal requirements for postprocedural echo are at baseline (1 to 3 months post-procedure), thereafter annually for TMVr and TMVR, after 1 and then every 2 to 3 years for surgical MVr, at 5 and 10 years with surgical bio-prostheses, but then annually, and only at baseline for a mechanical valve.

Medical Management

Rate control may be beneficial for symptoms of patients with severe MS (recommendation Class IIa, Level of Evidence A), particularly in the setting of atrial fibrillation (recommendation Class IIa, Level of Evidence C-LD) unless an underlying chronotropic incompetence exists. Obviously, anticoagulation is warranted with atrial fibrillation (with Vitamin K antagonist), as well as with LA thrombus, or a prior embolic event (recommendation Class I, Level of Evidence C-LD).

Differences Between ACC/AHA and ESC Guidelines

A major difference between the ACC/AHA and ESC guidelines is in indications for intervention. Aside from the previously mentioned indications, ESC guidelines also recommend PMBC in the asymptomatic patient with an embolic event, dense spontaneous contrast in the left atrium, a need for non-cardiac surgery, and desire for pregnancy (recommendation Class IIa, Level of Evidence C). Another difference is contraindications for PMBC. Most are mentioned in both guidelines; however, they are well defined in the ESC, and consist of MVA greater than 1.5 cm^2, more than mild MR, severe or bi-commissural calcification, absence of commissural fusion, severe concomitant aortic valve disease or severe combined tricuspid stenosis and regurgitation requiring surgery, and concomitant coronary artery disease requiring bypass surgery.

Future Perspectives

Despite decline in incidence, non-rheumatic MS is still encountered in high-income countries due to aging populations. Additional transcatheter valves are to be tested and may be able to expand treatment options in both rheumatic and non-rheumatic MS.

CASE-BASED ASSESSMENT

1. According to the ACC/AHA guidelines, what are the Class I indications for treatment of severe primary mitral regurgitation?
   A. Symptoms
   B. Left ventricular ejection fraction ≤60%
   C. Left ventricular end-systolic diameter ≥40 mm
   D. Asymptomatic but low procedural risk
   E. A, B, C
   F. All of the Above
2. In severe secondary mitral regurgitation, when is surgery preferred over transcatheter intervention?
   A. Always
   B. For LV EF of 20% to 49%
   C. For LV EF of 20% to 49% with left ventricular end-systolic dimension >70 mm
   D. For "atrial MR"
   E. For concomitant CABG
   F. C, D, E
   G. D, E
   H. All of the above
3. After mitral valve repair annual echocardiography follow-up is sufficient.
   A. True
   B. False
4. What is the procedure of choice for severe symptomatic rheumatic mitral stenosis?
   A. Surgical mitral valve repair
   B. Surgical mitral valve replacement
   C. Percutaneous mitral balloon commissurotomy
   D. Conservative management
5. When is surgical treatment recommended as Class I indication for severe symptomatic rheumatic mitral stenosis?
   A. Surgery is the procedure of choice
   B. In case of new onset atrial fibrillation
   C. In case of progressive mitral stenosis and a stress test showing hemodynamically significant mitral stenosis
   D. In case percutaneous mitral balloon commissurotomy is contraindicated

See page 315 for the answers.

REFERENCES

1. Otto CM, Nishimura RA, Bonow RO, et al. 2020 ACC/AHA Guideline for the Management of Patients With Valvular Heart Disease: A Report of the American College of Cardiology/American Heart Association Joint Committee on Clinical Practice Guidelines. *Circulation*. 2021;143:e72–e227.
2. Vahanian A, Beyersdorf F, Praz F, et al. 2021 ESC/EACTS Guidelines for the management of valvular heart disease. *Eur Heart J*. 2022, Feb 14;43(7):561–632.
3. Estevez-Loureiro R, Shuvy M, Taramasso M, et al. Use of Mitra-Clip for mitral valve repair in patients with acute mitral regurgitation following acute myocardial infarction: Effect of cardiogenic shock on outcomes (IREMMI Registry). *Catheter Cardiovasc Interv*. 2021;97:1259–1267.
4. Goldstein D, Moskowitz AJ, Gelijns AC, et al. Two-year outcomes of surgical treatment of severe ischemic mitral regurgitation. *N Engl J Med*. 2016;374:344–353.
5. Obadia JF, Messika-Zeitoun D, Leurent G, et al. Percutaneous Repair or Medical Treatment for Secondary Mitral Regurgitation. *N Engl J Med*. 2018;379:2297–2306.
6. Guerrero M, Eleid M, Foley T, et al. Transseptal transcatheter mitral valve replacement in severe mitral annular calcification (transseptal valve-in-MAC). *Ann Cardiothorac Surg*. 2018;7:830–833.

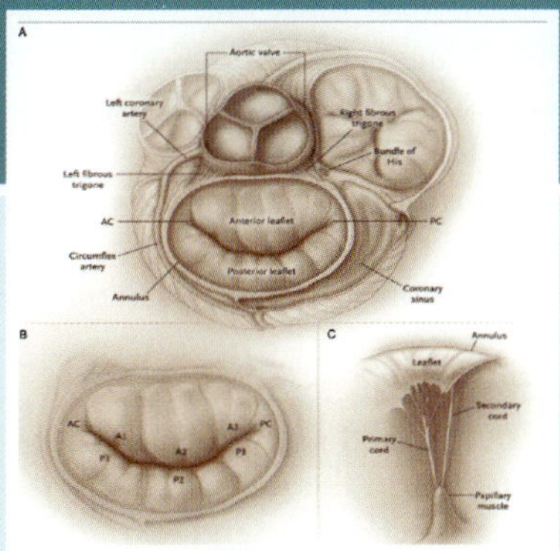

4

Physical Examination

Sehrish Memon, William A. Gray

CHAPTER OUTLINE

LEARNING OBJECTIVES

- Define anatomic components of the mitral valve apparatus
- Describe the etiology of two main types of mitral valve pathology, i.e., mitral stenosis and mitral regurgitation; their mechanistic effects on mitral valve leaflets and physical examination findings.

THE MITRAL VALVE

Anatomy

Mitral valve apparatus components include: two main leaflets, anterior and posterior, each with three distinct scallops (A1, A2, A3, and P1, P2, P3), mitral annulus, chordae tendinae (primary, attached to valve free edge, and secondary, attached to ventricular leaflet surface), and papillary muscles connecting mitral valve leaflets to left ventricle (Fig. 4.1). There are two papillary muscles, and each provides chordae tendinae to both mitral valve leaflets. Anterolateral papillary muscle usually has one body but receives dual coronary artery blood supply from left anterior descending and diagonal or obtuse marginal branch of left circumflex artery. The posteromedial papillary muscle has two bodies, receives blood supply from either left circumflex or right coronary artery (dependent upon which is dominant) and is more prone to injury from myocardial infarction due to single coronary artery blood supply.

Physical Examination

Mitral Stenosis

Mechanism. Thickened, distorted, and stiffened mitral valve leaflets leading to insufficient opening during diastole.

Etiology: Rheumatic fever from a remote group A beta-hemolytic streptococcus infection, age-related calcification, infective endocarditis, granulomatous infiltration. The different etiologies lead to separate mechanisms for the valvular stenosis. For example, a rheumatic valve will have commissural fusion resulting in leaflet restriction, whereas a senile calcific valve will largely preserve commissural opening but will present with annular calcification (reducing annular size without creating a significant gradient), which can then also involve body of the leaflet restricting leaflet motion.

Murmur (Fig. 4.2)

Location: Apex

Radiation: Little to none

Intensity: Grade 1 to 4

Heart sound associated findings: S1 accentuated in early MS due to increased Left Atrium (LA) pressure promoting leaflet excursion, but may become softened in severe MS as valve closure is reduced by the advanced stenotic process and valvular restriction. S1 may occasionally be palpable at the apex.

Opening snap (OS) follows S2 and low pitched early-to-mid decrescendo diastolic murmur, referred to as a rumble. The closer the OS is to S2, the worse the stenosis.

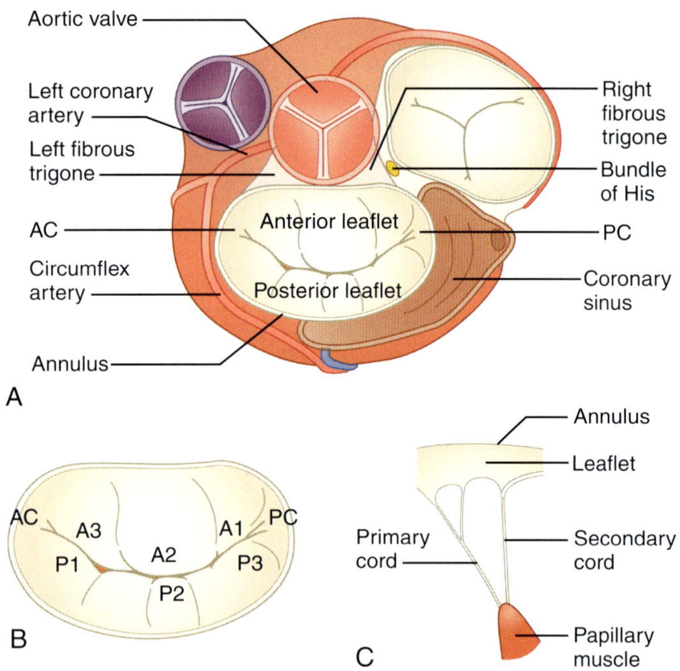

Fig. 4.1 (A) Mitral valve and surrounding cardiac structures in "surgeons view" orientation. (B) Anterior and posterior mitral valve leaflets with A1, A2, A3, and P1, P2, P3 scallops each. Anterior commissure *(AC)* located at lateral aspect (A1/P1 scallop) and posterior commissure *(PC)* located at medial aspect (A3/P3 scallop). (C) Primary chordae attached to free edge of mitral valve leaflet and secondary chordae attached to ventricular surface of leaflets. (Redrawn from Verma S, Mesana TG. Mitral-valve repair for mitral-valve prolapse. *N Engl J Med.* 2009;361:2261–2269.)

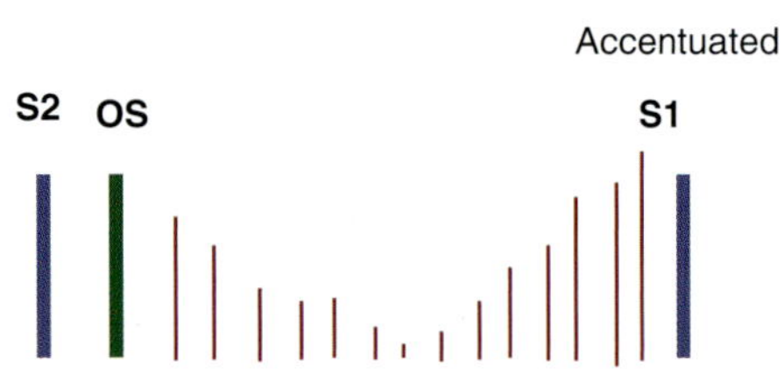

Fig. 4.2 Mitral Stenosis. *OS,* Opening snap.

If sinus rhythm is present, a late diastolic crescendo murmur is present related to atrial contraction. This will be absent if the patient is in atrial fibrillation.

If pulmonary hypertension present, P2 accentuated and right ventricular impulse may be palpable.

Special considerations: Auscultatory sounds may be difficult with mild mitral stenosis or low cardiac output. Auscultation may be enhanced by placing patient in left lateral decubitus position and using bell part of stethoscope. Exercise may accentuate murmur.

Mitral Regurgitation

Mechanism. Failure of complete mitral valve leaflet closure during ventricular systole resulting in regurgitation of blood from left ventricle into left atrium. Left atrial pressure and volume overload leads to pulmonary congestion, and ventricular volume overload can progress to left ventricular dilation and dysfunction.

Etiology: Two broad categories encompass most mitral regurgitation (MR) causes: degenerative (primary) and functional (secondary). These etiologic distinctions may be discernable by nuanced physical exam findings (see below).

Degenerative MR is related to valve prolapse or chordal rupture with resultant flail leaflet due to either tissue laxity (e.g., Barlow's) or age-related tissue degeneration (i.e., fibroelastic degeneration [FED]).

In functional MR, the mitral valve is itself normal, but its architecture is distorted due to left atrium or left ventricular dilation (or both), which lead to dysfunction in the mitral valve supporting structures (papillary muscles, chordea tendonea) which can tether the valve leaflets and prevent closure. Functional MR can also result from Left Ventricle (LV) and/or LA enlargement, leading to associated enlargement in mitral valve annular size and leaflet malcoaptation.

Rheumatic valve disease, infective endocarditis, and dynamic/transient MR related to ischemia are less common causes.

General Physical Exam Considerations

Since, especially in younger patients with degenerative MR, there may be an associated connective tissue disease at play, it will be important to assess for these clinically and/or genetically because many can have important implications beyond the mitral valve. Examples include Ehlers-Danlos syndrome, Marfan syndrome, Loeys-Dietz syndrome, osteogenesis imperfecta, and pseudoxanthoma elasticum. In addition, thyrotoxic Grave's disease and pectus excavatum can also be an etiological cause of MR and should be evident on physical exam.

Murmur: Functional MR (Fig. 4.3)

Location: Apex

Radiation: Most commonly to left axilla and less commonly to left sternal border

Quality: Harsh and holosystolic

Intensity: Soft to loud, loud associated with apical thrill

Heart sound associated findings: Decreased S1 due to lack of complete mitral valve (MV) closure. Presence of apical S3 reflective of left ventricular volume overload. Increased and sustained apical impulse amplitude in functional MR or in late-stage degenerative MR.

Murmur: Degenerative MR (Fig. 4.4)

Location: Apex

Radiation: Generally does not radiate

Quality: In mitral valve prolapse (MVP), a medium-pitched, mid-systolic click is often accompanied by a late systolic murmur from sudden tensing of mitral valve apparatus as leaflets prolapse into left atrium.

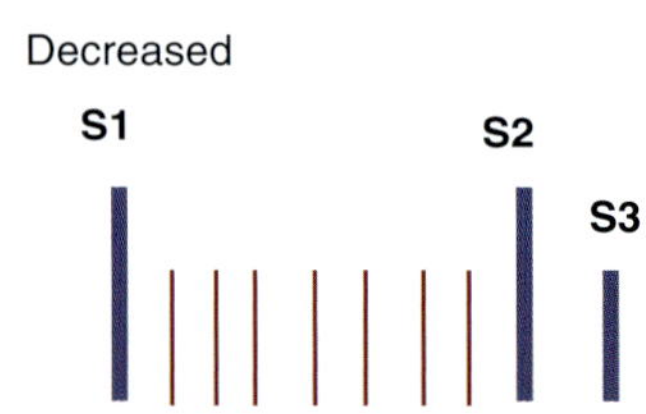

Fig. 4.3 Mitral Regurgitation.

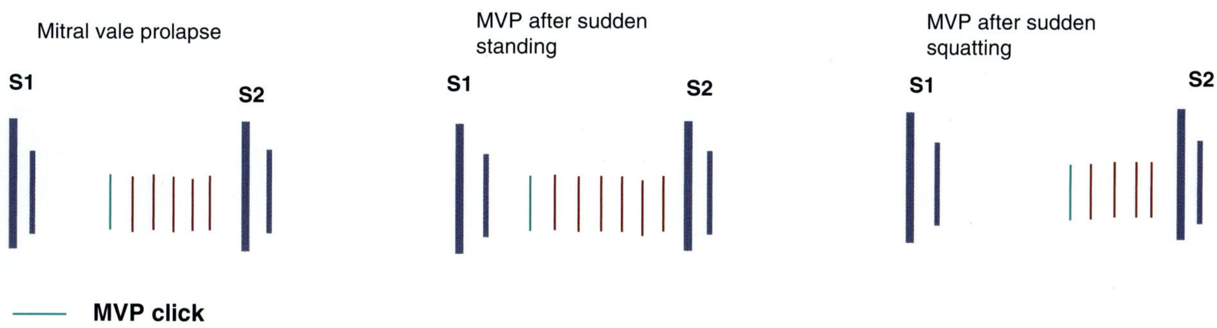

Fig. 4.4 Mitral Valve Prolapse *(MVP).*

Heart sounds with physiologic maneuvers: Standing decreases end-diastolic volume and click-murmur occurs earlier in systole, shortly after S1. Squatting increases end-diastolic volume causing click-murmur complex to move toward second heart sound.

Physical Examination: A Case Based Assessment

1. What is false regarding the anatomy of mitral valve apparatus?
   A. Mitral valve consists of two main leaflets, each with three distinct scallops.
   B. A1/P1 scallops are located at lateral aspect of anterior commissure.
   C. Primary chordae tendinae are attached to ventricular surface of leaflets.
   D. Posteromedial papillary muscle is more prone to injury from myocardial infarction due to single coronary artery blood supply.
2. What is true regarding the physical exam findings of the murmur of mitral valve stenosis?
   A. S1 is soft during early pathologic process of mitral valve stenosis while it is accentuated in late more severe disease.
   B. S1 is accentuated in early mitral stenosis disease and soften late in disease process.
   C. Mitral stenosis murmur is a high-pitched mid-to-late decrescendo diastolic murmur.
   D. The farther the opening snap from S2, the worse the stenosis.
3. What is false regarding the murmur findings of mitral valve prolapse?
   A. Medium pitched, located at the apex and generally does not radiate.
   B. Mid-systolic click is often accompanied by late systolic murmur.
   C. Squatting increases end-diastolic volume and click-murmur moves towards S2.
   D. Standing increases end-diastolic volume and click-murmur occurs later in systole.

See page 315 for the answers.

BIBLIOGRAPHY

1. Verma S, Mesana TG. Mitral-valve repair for mitral-valve prolapse. *N Engl J Med.* 2009;361:2261–2269.
2. Bickley LS. The cardiovascular system. *Bate's Guide to Physical Examination and History Taking* Lippincott Williams & Wilkins Publication; 2012:279–335.
3. Holmes K, Gibbison B, Vohra HA. Mitral valve and mitral valve disease. *BJA Educ.* 2017;17(1):1–9.
4. Maganti K, Rigolin VH, Sarano ME, et al. Valvular heart disease: diagnosis and management. *Mayo Clin Proc.* 2010;85(5):483–500.
5. Mann DL, Zipes DP, Libby P, et al. *Braunwald's Heart Disease: A Textbook of Cardiovascular Medicine.* 10th ed. Philadelphia, PA: Elsevier/Saunders; 2015.
6. Delling FN, Vasan RS. Epidemiology and pathophysiology of mitral valve prolapse new insights into disease progression, genetics, and molecular basis. *Circulation.* 2014;129(21):2158–2170.

5

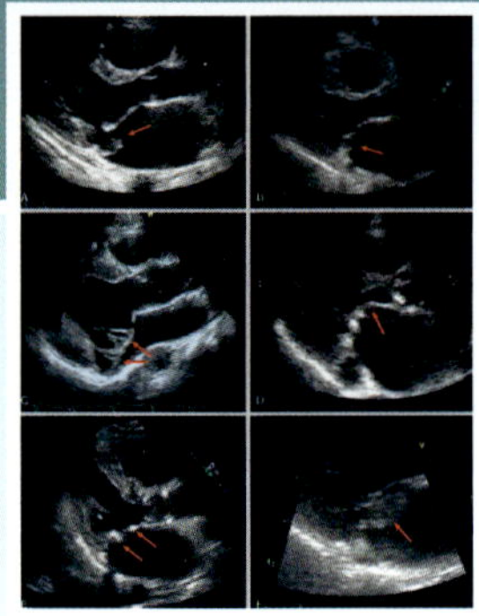

Transthoracic Echocardiogram

Sandra V. Abramson, Gwyneth McNeill

CHAPTER OUTLINE

LEARNING OUTCOMES

- Comprehensively assess the mitral valve apparatus and the left ventricle to distinguish degenerative versus functional mitral regurgitation as they are different disease processes with different prognoses and different treatments.
- Evaluate the severity of mitral regurgitation using an integrated approach as no single parameter is accurate. It is essential to evaluate color-flow Doppler (flow convergence, vena contracta, color jet area), pulsed-wave Doppler (mitral inflow, pulmonary venous flow), and continuous-wave Doppler (mitral regurgitation envelope).
- Determine the compensatory mechanisms of the heart to a volume overloaded state. Assess left ventricular size and function, left atrial size, right ventricular size and function, and right ventricular systolic pressure. It is unlikely to have severe, chronic mitral regurgitation with normal-sized chambers.
- Resolve all hemodynamic issues (volume status, blood pressure, tachycardia, atrial fibrillation) before a final determination of mitral regurgitation severity is made.
- Consider additional testing such as transesophageal echocardiography, cardiac magnetic resonance imaging, and exercise echocardiography if there is discordance between 2D and Doppler findings, discordance between clinical assessment and MR severity, or suboptimal image quality.

Kollaborate link: https://www.kollaborate.tv/link?id=61ae2a9c70360

INTRODUCTION

Transthoracic echocardiography (TTE) is the best screening modality to assess the structure and function of the mitral valve and its hemodynamic effects on the left ventricle (LV), left atrium (LA), and the right heart. Accurate assessment of the severity and mechanism of the mitral valve pathology determines patient prognosis and the timing and type of intervention. It is important to identify whether the mitral regurgitation (MR) is due to an abnormal mitral valve (primary, degenerative), pathology of the ventricle, atria, or annulus (secondary, functional), or a combination of both (mixed etiology).[1–3] Primary MR must be distinguished from secondary MR as surgical and transcatheter options may differ depending on the etiology. It is essential to use Doppler to assess multiple parameters for MR severity including regurgitant color-flow jet, vena contracta width (VCW), proximal isovelocity surface area (PISA), MR jet profile, mitral inflow, pulmonary vein flow, and flow quantitation.[1–3] Additional testing may be required if the severity or mechanism of MR cannot be established despite a good quality, complete TTE. Transesophageal echocardiogram (TEE) should be performed if the mechanism of MR is unclear, but it should not be relied upon to assess MR severity due to the favorable hemodynamic changes that occur with the administration of sedation. If the severity is unclear, consider cardiac magnetic resonance imaging or stress testing.[4]

STANDARD MITRAL VALVE EVALUATION

Meticulous interrogation of the mitral valve apparatus is essential to assess the mechanism and etiology of the pathology and to individualize the timing and treatment of the mitral valve disease. It is important to visualize leaflets, annulus, chordae, and papillary muscles to assess their contribution to the pathology. Abnormal leaflet pathology includes thickening, calcification, prolapse, flail, vegetation, and masses. Significant calcification of the mitral leaflets makes surgical and transcatheter valve repair difficult. Abnormal subvalvular morphology includes calcification, ruptured chordae, chordal fusion, vegetations, and masses. Mitral annulus must be evaluated for dilatation and calcification. If the mitral apparatus is normal, primary MR is unlikely.

The mitral valve should be evaluated in at least five views: parasternal long axis (PSLA), parasternal short-axis mitral valve level (PSSA), apical 4-chamber (A4C), apical 2-chamber (A2C), and apical long axis (ALA) for morphology (Fig. 5.1) and regurgitation severity. Two-dimensional (2D) imaging is used to assess valvular structure while Doppler (color-flow, pulsed-wave, and continuous-wave) is used to assess the severity of MR (Fig. 5.2). Three-dimensional (3D) applications have increased the accuracy of localization of valve pathology predominantly using TEE since the current lower spatial and temporal resolution has limited its evaluation during TTE.[5,6] There are several methods that should be used to assess the severity of the MR, and the final interpretation should integrate all the methods, as no single method should be completely relied upon. It is important to be aware of the strengths and limitations of each method (Table 5.1). MR is very dynamic and responsive to loading conditions such as volume status, blood pressure, heart rate, medications, and pacemakers which all should be optimized before making the final decision about the severity of the mitral valve disease.[1–3,7]

Carpentier classification of the etiology of MR based on leaflet motion should be used to describe the precise anatomical pathology and mechanism.[8] Carpentier type I represents MR with normal leaflet motion and includes perforation or cleft (primary MR) and MR due to dilated annulus (secondary MR). Carpentier type II includes excessive leaflet motion such as prolapse or flail (primary MR). Type IIIa describes rheumatic disease with leaflet restriction in both systole and diastole (primary MR). Type IIIb is seen in dilated cardiomyopathy with restricted motion only in systole (secondary MR) (Fig. 5.3).

MITRAL REGURGITATION

Mechanism of Mitral Regurgitation

Primary Mitral Regurgitation (Degenerative)

MR is considered primary when there is abnormal structure of the mitral valve apparatus (Table 5.2). In primary, degenerative MR, the specific pathology and location must be identified. It is important to methodically image the leaflets, chordae, and papillary muscle for thickening, prolapse, flail, tethering, and calcifications (Fig. 5.4). Specific scallops can be identified on TTE, but only if on-axis views are obtained. The anterior and posterior leaflets are divided into three anatomic segments from medial to lateral (A3, A2, A1 and P3, P2, P1). The two leaflets meet at the medial and lateral commissures. Parasternal long-axis view shows the middle scallops of both leaflets (A2 and P2) (see Fig. 5.1). The parasternal short-axis view demonstrates medial scallops on the left (A3, P3) and lateral scallops on the right (A1, P1). The A4C usually demonstrates P1 and A2/A3, but angulation will change which scallops are visualized. Anterior angulation demonstrates A1/P1 while inferior angulation will show A3/P3. The A2C view shows posteromedial and anterolateral commissures and demonstrates P3, A2, P1 from left to right. More accurate localization of pathology requires a TEE. As treatment options increase, there will be specific treatment tailored to specific pathology. For example, if there is a torn chord, the treatment may be an insertion of synthetic chords, either surgically or transcatheter approach.

When primary MR is accompanied by a normal-sized LV and LA, it is unlikely to be severe, unless an acute leaflet flail is present.[1–3] Primary MR is unlikely if the mitral valve is normal.

Mitral valve prolapse (Carpentier type II). Myxomatous degeneration is a spectrum of pathology that is the most common cause of primary MR in developed countries.[9] It can range from fibroelastic deficiency with thin leaflets with one prolapsed/flailed segment to Barlow's disease with billowy leaflets and multiple prolapsing segments. Mitral valve prolapse (MVP) is present when the body of the leaflet is displaced 2 mm beyond the mitral annular diameter into the LA as seen in the parasternal long-axis view (see Fig. 5.4B). MVP should not be assessed in the apical views due to the saddle shape of the annulus which will result in a false appearance of the leaflets being displaced beyond the annular plane.

Barlow's disease. Barlow's disease results from an excess of myxomatous tissue leading to thick, bulky, redundant leaflets with elongated chordae resulting in bileaflet, multi segmental prolapse (see Fig. 5.4C).[10] The MR associated with Barlow's disease is frequently late-systolic MR seen as a "flash" (not holosystolic) on color flow and a non holosystolic jet on continuous-wave Doppler interrogation of the MR jet (Fig. 5.18C). Transcatheter therapy of MR due to Barlow's disease may differ from MVP as edge-to-edge repair may not be beneficial in these patients with multi segmental prolapse.

Flail leaflet (Carpentier type II). Flail leaflets are part of the MVP spectrum[2] and occur when the edge of the leaflet, not just the body, moves into the LA during systole. Rupture of the primary chords is usually present. Flail leaflet is usually associated with an eccentric jet of severe MR. The direction of the jet

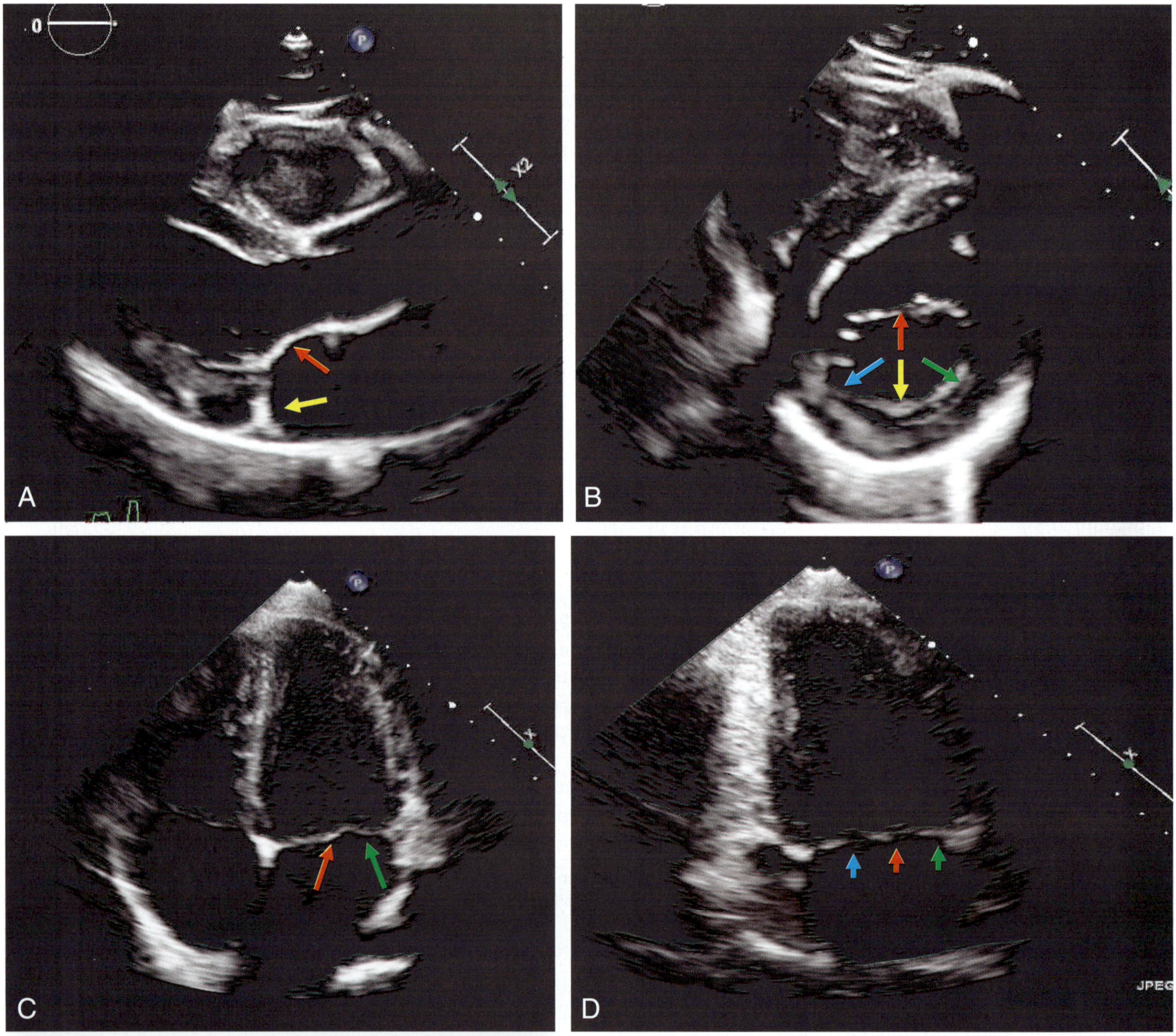

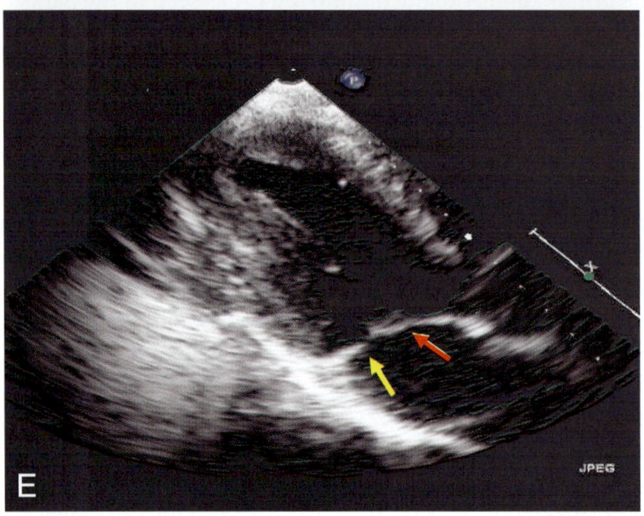

Fig. 5.1 **Normal Mitral Leaflets: Four Views.** There are four standard views to assess the mitral valve during a transthoracic echocardiogram. Both the anterior and posterior leaflets are visualized in each view. (A) Parasternal long-axis view. The anterior leaflet is always closest to the aortic valve. A2 *(red arrow)* and P2 *(yellow arrow)* are seen in this view. (B) Parasternal short-axis mitral valve level view. The anterior leaflet is on the top of the screen. Posterior leaflet is divided into three separate scallops. From lateral to medial scallops, P1 *(green arrow)*, P2 *(yellow arrow)*, and P3 *(blue arrow)*. A1, A2 *(red arrow)*, and A3 are the portion of the anterior leaflet corresponding to the specific posterior leaflet scallop. (C) Apical 4-chamber view. Anterior leaflet is closest to the right ventricle. Usually, P1 and A2/A3 are seen in this view but angulation may change the specific scallop visualized. Anterior angulation will visualize A1/P1 while inferior angulation will visualize A3/P3. (D) Apical 2-chamber view shows both anterolateral and posteromedial commissures and demonstrates P3 *(blue arrow)*, A2 *(red arrow)*, and P1 *(green arrow)*. (E) Apical long-axis view. Normal leaflets should be thin, noncalcified, and mobile. Transesophageal echocardiogram may be required to determine specific scallop involvement.

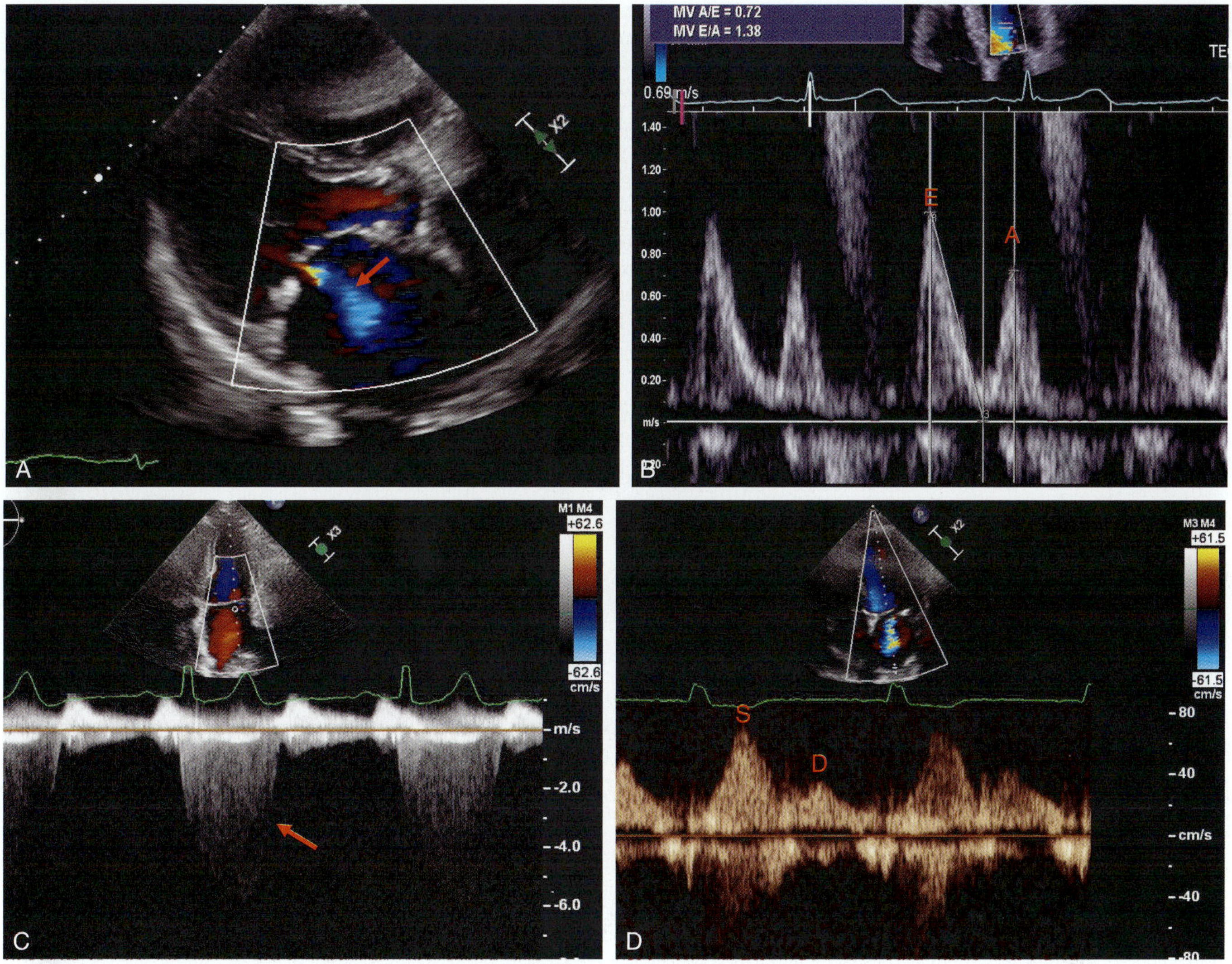

Fig. 5.2 Normal Doppler Flow in Mild Mitral Regurgitation. Doppler is used to assess the severity of mitral regurgitation. Mild mitral regurgitation is a normal finding in 50% of patients. (A) Color-flow imaging demonstrates a small blue flame *(red arrow)* emanating from the mitral leaflet tips in systole occupying less than 20% of the left atrium. (B) Normal pulsed-wave Doppler of mitral inflow demonstrates E wave slightly greater than A wave. (C) Continuous-wave Doppler demonstrates a faint or incomplete mitral regurgitation envelope *(red arrow)* demonstrating a small number of red blood cells involved in the regurgitation. (D) Normal pulmonary vein flow demonstrating systolic predominance (S>D) suggestive of normal left atrial pressures.

aids in determining the leaflet pathology. Although the regurgitant jet area (RJA) may not occupy 50% of the LA, the marked eccentricity of the jet is specific for severe regurgitation (see Figs. 5.4A, 5.5, 5.7, 5.10, Videos 5.1–5.6 and 5.13–5.18).

Perforation, cleft (Carpentier type I). There may be normal leaflet motion in patients with a congenital cleft or perforation due to healed endocarditis, but there is regurgitation through the defect in the leaflets. Identification of clefts usually requires a TEE. Currently, this is not amenable to percutaneous mitral valve repair.

Rheumatic (Carpentier type IIIa). Rheumatic mitral leaflets demonstrate diffuse leaflet thickening and commissural fusion associated with some degree of mitral stenosis (MS). Both systolic and diastolic leaflet restriction is present due to fused commissures and retracted chordae. Classic hockey-stick morphology of anterior leaflet with restricted posterior leaflet is usually present (see Fig. 5.4D).[2] Due to the presence of MS with thickened, calcified leaflets, percutaneous repair is currently not recommended in MR due to rheumatic disease.

Arrhythmic mitral valve prolapse. Although MVP is common and usually benign, with outcome predominantly determined by the severity of the MR, there is a rare form that is associated with sudden cardiac death. Our understanding of this malignant subset of MVP is incomplete, but it is associated with frequent ventricular arrhythmias, mitral annular disjunction (MAD), leaflet redundancy, and T-wave inversions and is independent of MR severity.[11] MAD is an abnormal

TABLE 5.1 Strengths and Limitations of Common Echocardiographic Parameters of Mitral Regurgitation Severity[a]

Parameter	Strengths	Limitations
Valve morphology	Flail leaflets or ruptured papillary muscles are specific for severe MR	Other findings are nonspecific
Regurgitant color flow	Easy to use; evaluates spatial orientation of MR jet, differentiates mild versus severe	Subject to technical and hemodynamic variation; can be underestimated with wall-impinging jets: image quality-dependent
Vena contracta width	Quick and easy to use; independent of hemodynamic and instrumentation factors; applies to eccentric Jets; can differentiate mild versus severe MR	Not applicable to multiple jets; intermediate values require confirmation; small measurement errors can lead to big changes; 2D measure of a 3D structure; limited lateral resolution
Proximal isovelocity surface area (PISA)	Can be applied to eccentric jets (when angle-corrected); not affected by etiology of MR; quantitative; provides both lesion severity (EROA) and volume data (RVol)	Not valid with multiple jets; provides peak flow and maximal EROA; interobserver-variability; errors in radius measurement are squared; multiple potential sources of measurement error
Flow quantitation-PW	Quantitative; valid in multiple jets and eccentric jets; provides both lesion severity (EROA, RF) and volume data (RVol)	Time consuming; measurement of flow at MV annulus less reliable with calcified MV and/or annulus; not valid with concomitant significant AR unless pulmonic site is used; requires measurement at multiple sites, which introduces errors
Jet profile-CW	Simple, readily available, easy assessment of MR timing	Qualitative; complementary data; complete signal difficult to obtain in eccentric jet; gain-dependent
Peak mitral E velocity	Simple, readily available, A-wave dominance excludes severe MR	Influenced by LA pressure/compliance, LV relaxation, MV area, and AF; complementary data only, does not quantify MR severity
Pulmonary vein flow	Simple; systolic now reversal is specific for severe MR	Influenced by LA pressure, AF; not accurate if MR jet directed into the sampled vein; absence does not rule out severe MR
LA and LV size	Enlargement sensitive for chronic severe MR, important for outcomes; normal size virtually excludes severe chronic MR	Enlargement seen in other conditions (nonspecific); may be normal in acute, severe MR

[a]A comprehensive approach where multiple parameters are evaluated must be used to assess MR severity. The strengths and limitations of each parameter are listed here. No single method to assess MR severity is accurate alone. All methods should be assessed and analyzed before arriving at a final interpretation. It is also necessary to assess LV, LA, and RV to understand the hemodynamic impact of the MR on the heart chambers.

AF, atrial fibrillation; *AR*, aortic regurgitation; *CW*, continuous wave; *EROA*, effective regurgitant orifice area; *LA*, left atrium; *LV*, left ventricle; *MR*, mitral regurgitation; *MV*, mitral valve; *RF*, regurgitant fraction; *RV*, right ventricular; *RVol*, regurgitant volume.

(From Bonow RO, et al. 2020 Focused update of the 2017 ACC expert consensus decision pathway on the management of mitral regurgitation. *J Am Coll Cardiol*. 2020;75:2236–2270.)

atrial displacement of the mitral valve leaflet hinge point in which the annulus becomes detached from the ventricular myocardium (Fig. 5.6).[12] Cardiac magnetic resonance to assess for presence and extent of myocardial fibrosis is necessary for risk stratification.

Acute mitral regurgitation. Careful assessment of the LV, LA, right ventricle, and right ventricular (RV) systolic pressure is essential in determining the severity of the MR and its chronicity. Acute MR is less common than chronic MR and patients usually present in hemodynamic distress. Acute MR is usually due to ruptured chordae tendinae, ruptured papillary muscle, or leaflet destruction due to endocarditis. If the LV and LA are normal sizes, significant chronic MR is unlikely, but acute MR may be present (Fig. 5.7).[2,13] Doppler assessments of color RJA, effective regurgitant orifice area (EROA), regurgitant volume (RVol), regurgitant fraction (RF), and mitral inflow will be inaccurate due to low driving pressure from high left atrial pressure and hypotension. Imaging of a flail leaflet with a normal-sized LV, hyperdynamic systolic function associated with decreased stroke volume (SV), and systolic reversal in pulmonary veins should confirm the diagnosis of acute, severe MR even if a large MR jet is not seen by color-flow imaging.[13] Careful measurements of the LA and LV volumes performed according to the American Society of Echocardiography (ASE) Guidelines by 2D method of disks (modified Simpson's method) or 3D is crucial for differentiating acute versus chronic MR (Fig. 5.8).[6,14] All measurements should be indexed to body surface area. Chronic MR is almost always associated with dilated left-sided chambers (see Videos 5.1–5.6).

Secondary Mitral Regurgitation (Functional)

Secondary (functional) MR is a distinct disease process due to ventricular pathology in which the valve leaflets and chordae are structurally normal, although minimal abnormalities such as nonspecific leaflet thickening and mild calcification may be present.[15-18] Secondary MR is much more complicated because the left ventricular dilatation and systolic dysfunction are frequently the cause rather than the result of the MR. In some patients, it may be an indicator of a diseased ventricle, whereas in others, it may contribute to further progression of LV

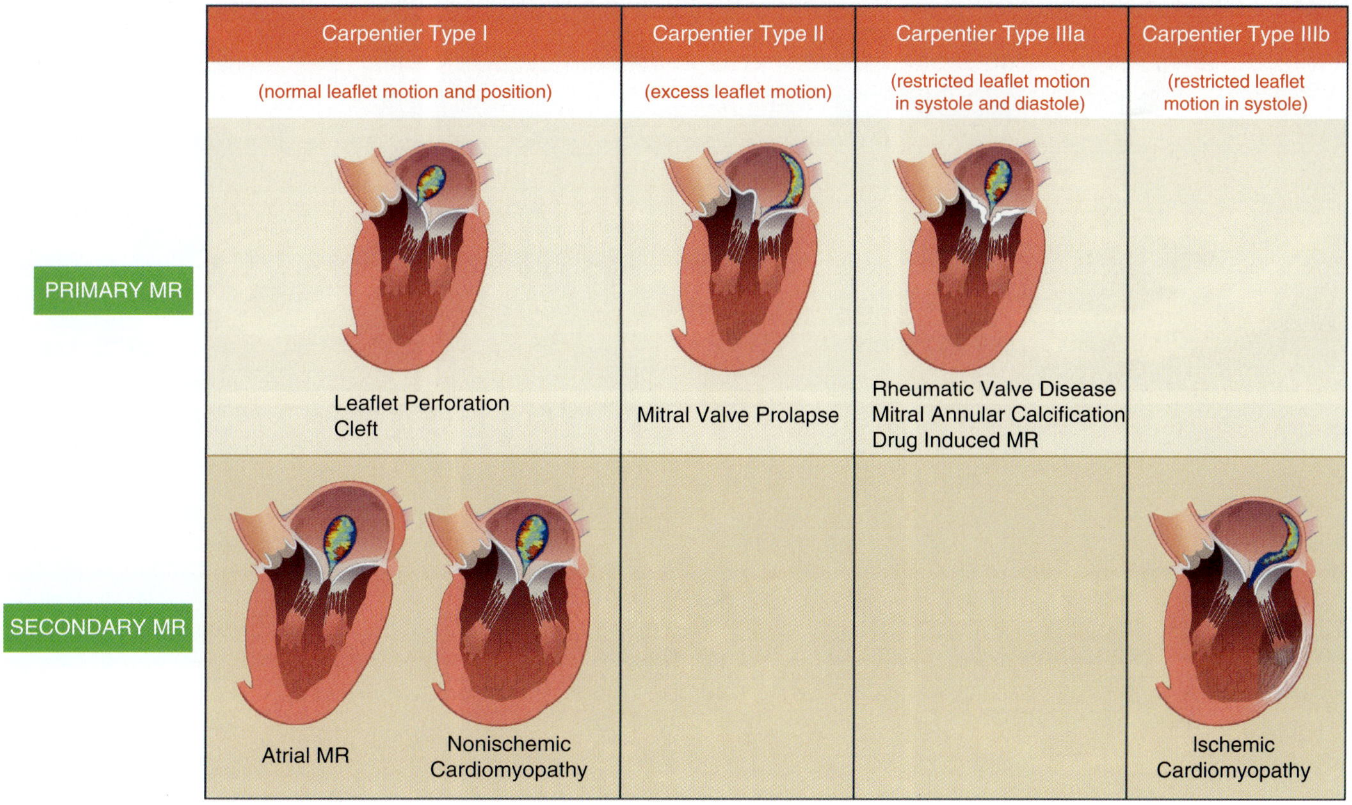

Fig. 5.3 Carpentier Classification of the Etiology of Mitral Regurgitation. Primary and secondary mitral valve regurgitation (MR) groupings with their respective Carpentier's functional classification. Carpentier type I represents normal leaflet motion and position. Carpentier type II represents excess leaflet motion. Carpentier type IIIa represents restricted leaflet motion in systole and diastole. Carpentier type IIIb represents restricted leaflet motion in systole. (From El Sabbagh A, Reddy YNV, Nishimura RA. Mitral valve regurgitation in the contemporary era. *JACC Cardiovasc Imaging.* 2018;11[4]: 628–643.)

dysfunction.[1] Functional MR is associated with a worse prognosis than degenerative MR.

Functional MR is usually a consequence of LV remodeling with ventricular dilatation, annular dilatation, papillary muscle displacement, leaflet tethering, and malcoaptation of leaflets due to chordal stretching (see Table 5.2).[15–18] In the presence of a dilated cardiomyopathy, it may be difficult to determine whether the MR is the cause of the dilated cardiomyopathy or a result of the dilated cardiomyopathy and simply a marker of poor prognosis. As the LV dilates, the papillary muscles become displaced and restrict leaflet mobility, resulting in more MR. "MR begets MR" as the saying goes. Proportionate MR refers to the "appropriate" amount of MR you would expect after considering the LV end-diastolic volume, ejection fraction, and RF. Disproportionate MR, when the MR severity is more severe than would be predicted by the size of the LV alone, may differentiate those patients who will benefit from an intervention from those whose ventricles will not recover.[19] Functional MR may occur with normal leaflet motion (Carpentier type I) due to a dilated annulus, but it may also be seen with restricted leaflets (Carpentier type IIIb) due to adverse LV remodeling from ischemic or nonischemic cardiomyopathy. Symmetric bileaflet tethering due to LV remodeling occurring in nonischemic cardiomyopathies usually results in a central jet. Asymmetric posterior leaflet tethering due to inferior wall remodeling in an ischemic cardiomyopathy frequently results in a posteriorly directed jet (Fig. 5.9). A significant posterior jet may also be seen with an isolated inferior/inferolateral infarction due to a restricted posterior leaflet despite relative preservation of LV size and function. If the posterior leaflet is restricted with the anterior leaflet overriding it, this is still considered secondary MR. Several methods have been proposed to assess the amount of leaflet restriction including tenting area, a measurement of the area between the leaflet tips and the annulus, and coaptation depth, the maximal distance from the leaflet tip to the annular plane.[15,16] Secondary MR is significantly affected by preload, afterload, and heart rate/rhythm. Atrial fibrillation may worsen secondary MR due to increased atrial stretch and annular dilatation. Functional MR is extremely sensitive to loading conditions and the MR severity should be re-evaluated after guideline-directed medical therapy has been instituted and cardiac resynchronization therapy has been considered. Anesthetic agents tend to optimize LV filling and decrease MR which necessitates that secondary MR severity be assessed by TTE rather than TEE (see Videos 5.7–5.12 and 5.19–5.23).

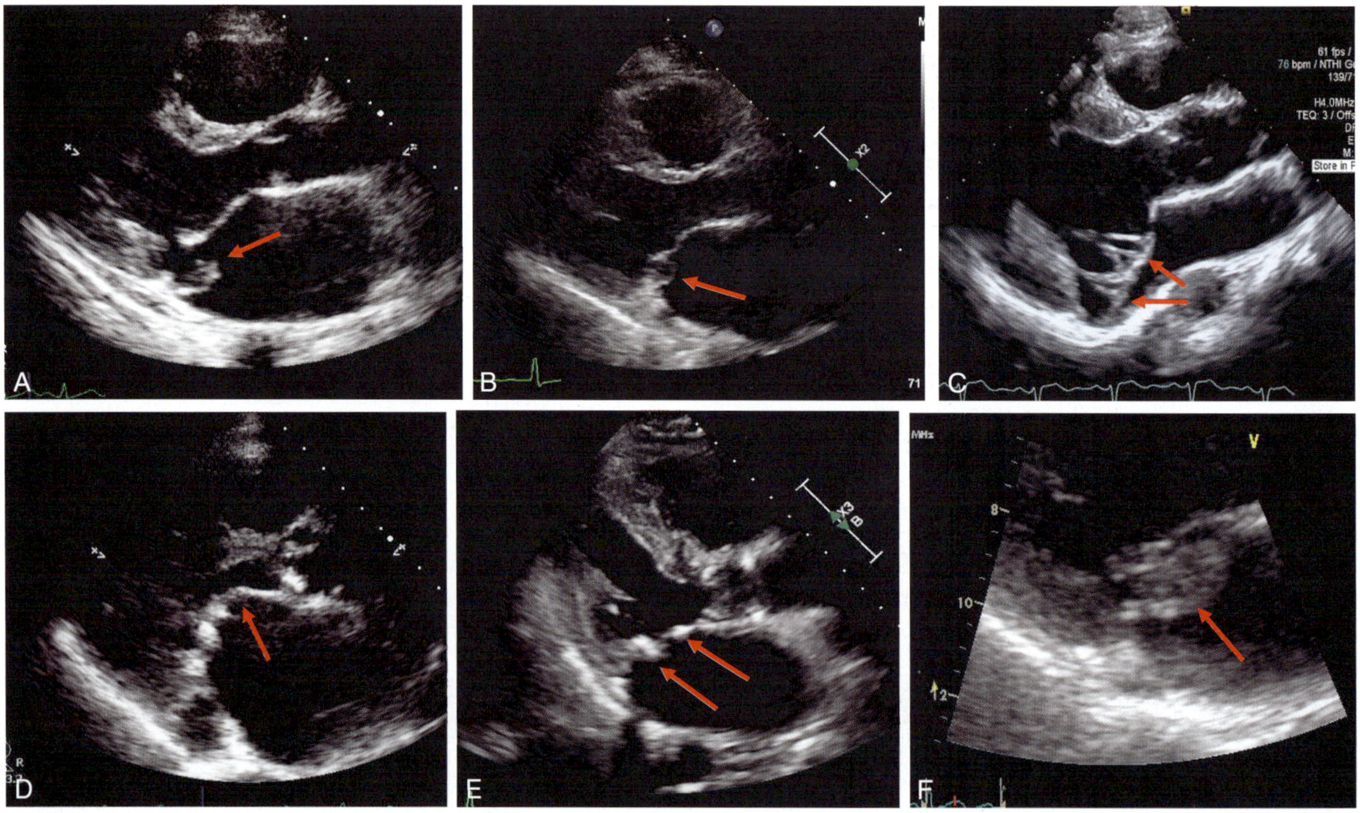

Fig. 5.4 **Various Mechanisms of Mitral Regurgitation.** Leaflets must be assessed for: (A) flail when the tip of the leaflet is directed into the left atrium, (B) prolapse when the body of the leaflet is displaced 2 mm beyond the mitral annular diameter into the left atrium as seen in the parasternal long-axis view. (C) Barlow's disease with billowy leaflets and multi segmental prolapse. (D) Rheumatic leaflets are thickened, restricted with a hockey-stick appearance of the anterior leaflet. (E) Leaflet calcifications on both the anterior and posterior leaflets, and (F) large vegetation attached to anterior leaflet.

Mixed Etiology

Mixed MR due to both primary and secondary causes is also possible. A sudden onset of shortness of breath in a patient with a dilated, ischemic cardiomyopathy may signal a ruptured chordae with a flail leaflet (Fig. 5.10). Also, long-standing untreated severe MR due to prolapse may result in dilated cardiomyopathy (see Videos 5.13–5.18).

Assessment of Mitral Regurgitation Severity

An integrative approach is necessary to accurately assess the severity of chronic MR. It is important to identify several variables consistent with severe MR rather than simply one or two. Ten criteria for severe MR should be evaluated in every patient-color RJA, VCW, PISA, mitral inflow, MR jet profile, pulmonary venous waveform, RV (fraction), leaflet morphology, and LV size and function (Fig. 5.11).[1–3,7,20–23] If the TTE has suboptimal image quality, consider TEE to more accurately identify mechanism and severity. If multiple parameters are discordant, consider cardiac magnetic resonance imaging to measure RV, RF, LV size, and LV function.

Color-Flow Doppler

Color-flow Doppler (CFD) is the primary method for assessing regurgitation severity. Three aspects of the regurgitant jet are identified-flow convergence on the LV aspect of the valve PISA, VCW at the narrowest part of the jet, and the regurgitant color jet area in the LA. It is important to analyze all three aspects of the MR jet (Fig. 5.12).

Regurgitant color jet area. CFD assessment of the ratio of the mitral regurgitant color jet area compared with the left atrial size is the easiest but least accurate way to grade the severity of MR. It was initially proposed that the ratio of the RJA to the left atrial area in the apical views greater than 50% is consistent with severe MR, but this method is fraught with many issues. Visual assessment of the color-flow area should never be the only method used to assess the MR severity as it is unreliable when used alone to grade the severity of the MR.[20–23] The use of the MR jet area alone overestimates MR severity when compared with cardiac magnetic resonance imaging.[4] Central jets (due to loss of viscous friction forces) will always appear larger in the LA, which overestimates severity; thus, you should rely more on quantitative data when you have a central jet.[20–23] When a jet is eccentric and wall-hugging (Coanda effect), it is more likely to be severe and due to leaflet pathology, which can be identified by the direction of the jet.[2,21,22] Despite equivalent hemodynamic severity, eccentric wall-hugging jets appear much smaller than central jets and therefore may be overlooked. The direction of the color-flow jet may aid in identifying the mechanism of MR.

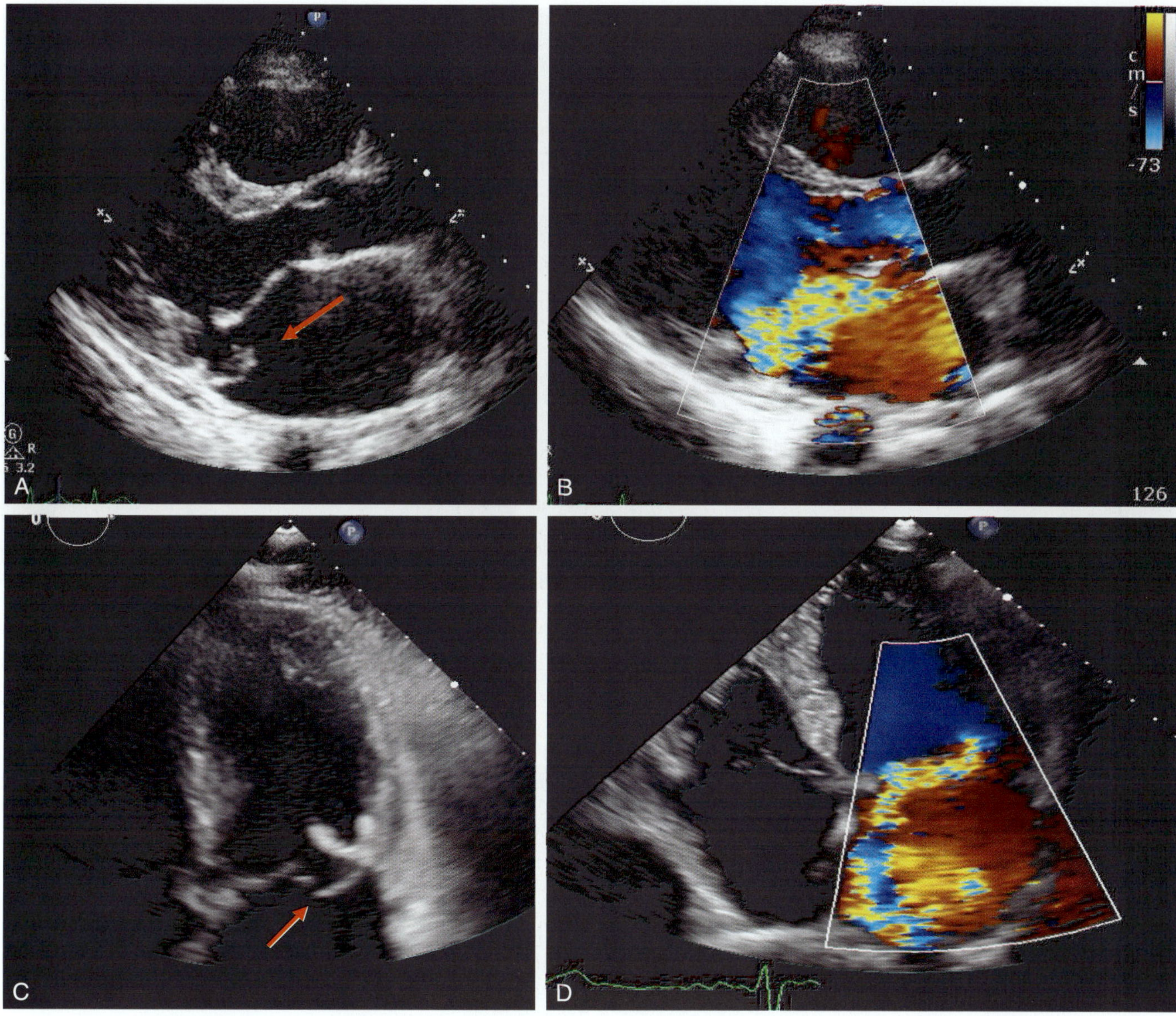

Fig. 5.5 **Posterior (P2) Flail.** Example of 2D and color-flow imaging of a flail of the posterior leaflet. (A) Parasternal long axis with red arrow pointing to flail P2 segment. P2 segment does not coapt at the annulus; instead leaflet tip falls into the left atrium. (B) Using color-flow Doppler in the same patient as A, the direction of the jet is away from the flailed posterior leaflet segment. (C) Posterior leaflet flail *(red arrow)* adjacent to a large posterior calcium shelf that would make edge-to-edge transcatheter repair difficult. (D) Color-flow Doppler demonstrating an eccentric jet with flow directed away from the flail posterior leaflet.

An anteriorly directed jet is usually due to a posterior leaflet flail/prolapse or a restricted anterior leaflet, while a posteriorly directed jet is most commonly due to flail/prolapse of anterior leaflet or restricted posterior leaflet (see Figs. 5.5, 5.7, 5.9–5.10). These Coanda jets may be missed or underappreciated. An eccentric, wall-hugging jet should be differentiated from a jet that is just a little off center. Horizontal splaying of the mitral regurgitant jet, likely due to a side-lobe artifact, may also be a clue to the presence of severe MR.[24–26]

The size of the MR jet is significantly affected by hemodynamics and machine settings (Box 5.1). A high velocity jet due to hypertension or aortic stenosis will appear significantly larger than a lower velocity jet. Therefore, MR jets assessed only by CFD will appear larger in hypertensive patients and smaller in critically ill patients with a low driving force. A hypertensive patient with mild MR may have a larger jet area than a critically ill hypotensive patient with acute, severe MR. If a study shows severe MR while the patient is hypertensive, volume overloaded, or abnormal rhythm/rate, the study should be repeated when the patient is normotensive, euvolemic, or sinus rhythm. Always report the blood pressure, heart rate, and heart rhythm during the exam. Pre-operative TTE in an experienced lab is preferable to intraoperative TEE to assess the severity of MR as anesthetic agents improve hemodynamics, thus decreasing the

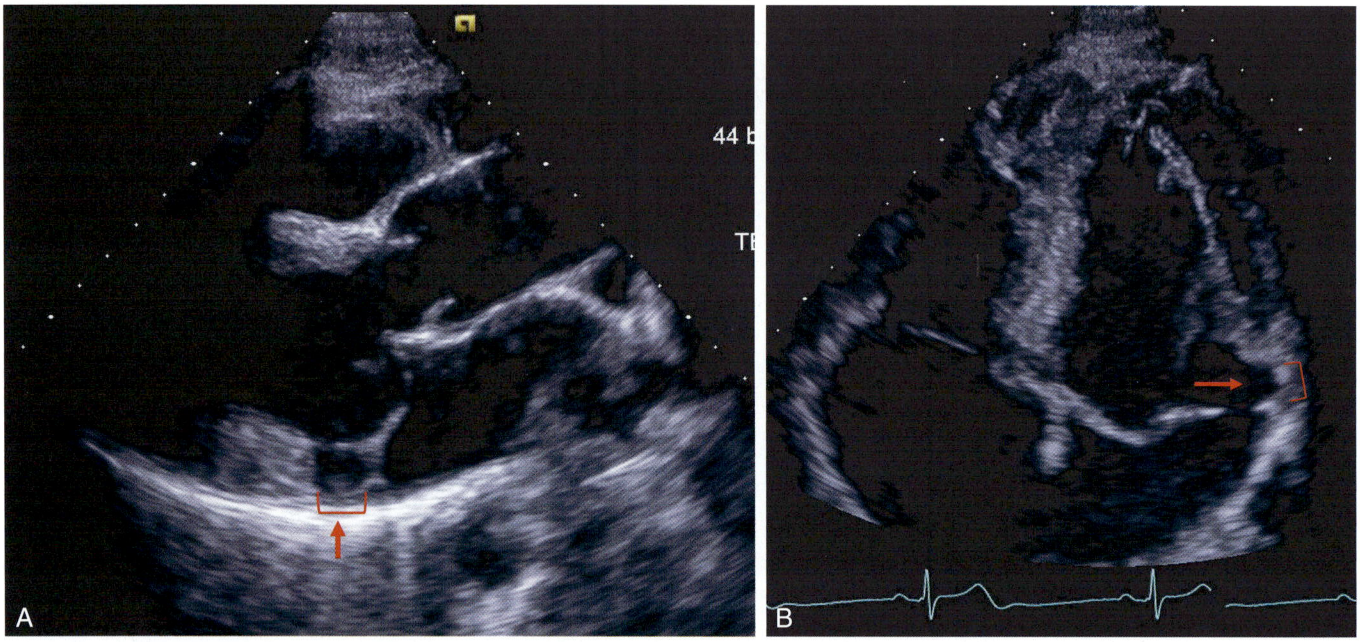

Fig. 5.6 Mitral Annular Disjunction. Mitral annular disjunction (MAD) occurs when the posterolateral mitral annulus becomes detached from the posterolateral ventricular myocardium during systole. MAD is associated with arrhythmic mitral valve prolapse. The red arrow points to the MAD which is the space between the posterior annulus and the myocardium. (A) Parasternal long-axis view. (B) Apical 4-chamber view.

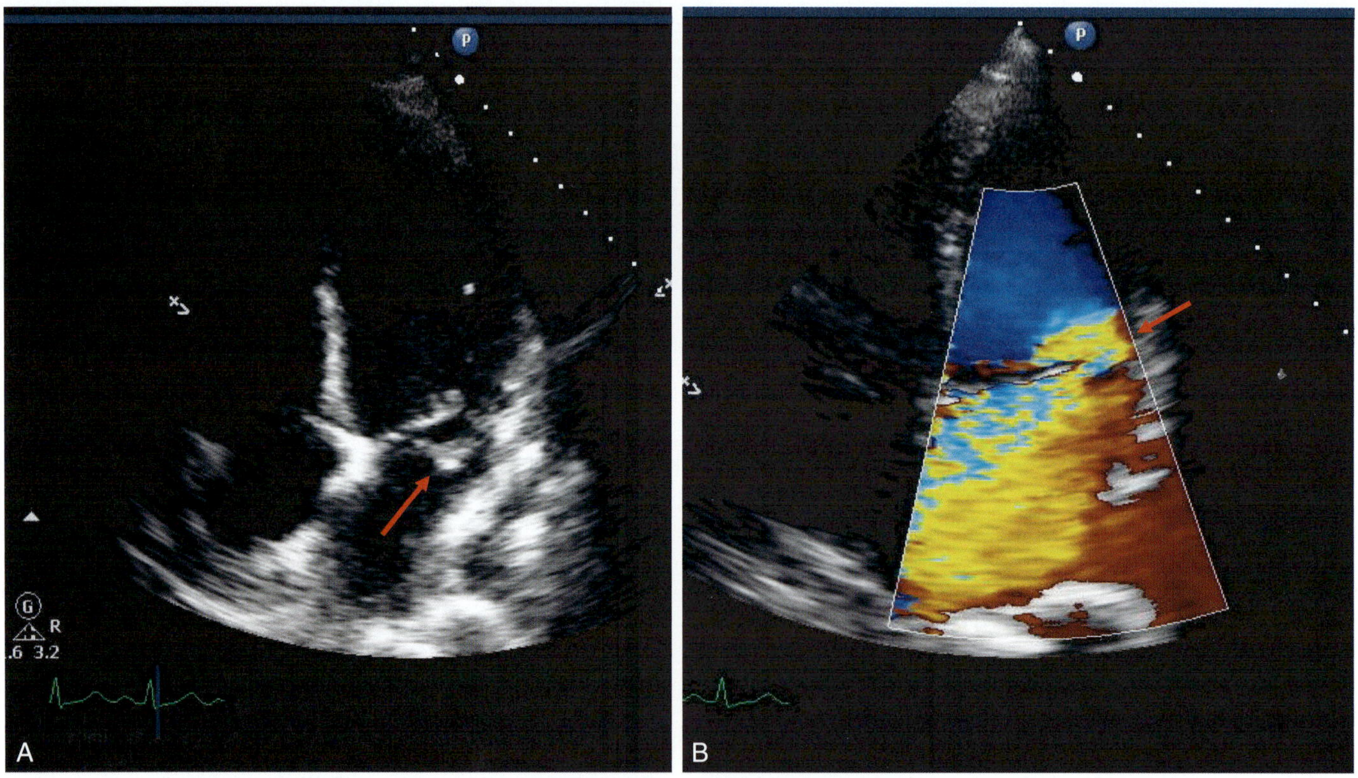

Fig. 5.7 Acute Mitral Regurgitation-Severe Mitral Regurgitation With Normal Left Ventricle/Left Atrium Size. (A) Apical 4-chamber demonstrating flail P2 segment resulting in acute, severe mitral regurgitation (MR). The normal-sized, hyperdynamic left ventricle and normal-sized left atrium support this acute pathology. The red arrow points to the flail P2 segment. (B) Color-flow Doppler imaging demonstrating severe MR directed away from the flail segment. Large proximal isovelocity surface area effective regurgitant orifice area is visualized.

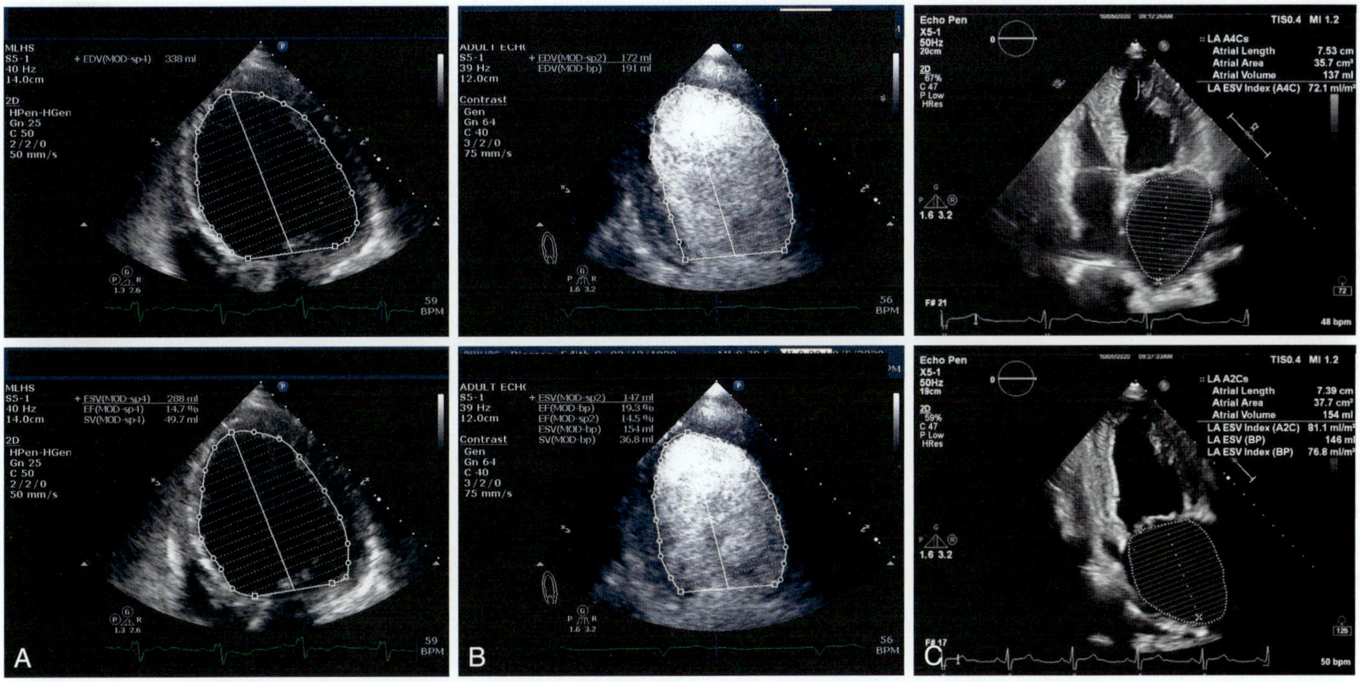

Fig. 5.8 **Left Ventricular/Left Atrium chamber size.** Simpson's method of disks assessment for left ventricle (LV) size and function and left atrium (LA) size must be assessed for every patient. The sonographer traces the endocardial border at end-diastole and end-systole to estimate a left ventricular end-diastolic volume (LVEDV) and left ventricular end-systolic volume (LVESV) from which the ejection fraction is calculated. (A) Apical 4-chamber showing LVEDV 338 mL and LVESV 288 mL, yielding an EF of 15%. (B) Apical 2-chamber with opacification from a different patient showing LVEDV 172 mL and LVESV 147 mL, yielding an EF of 14.5%. (C) Severely dilated left atrium with a biplane indexed volume of 76.8 m/m^2.

MR severity. It is also important to make sure all the machine settings are optimized while performing a cardiac ultrasound. If the Nyquist limit is set inappropriately low, the jet will appear erroneously larger than if the Nyquist limit is set correctly (50 to 70 cm/s).

Proximal isovelocity surface area-flow convergence. Flow acceleration of the red blood cells as they approach the regurgitant orifice of the mitral valve is represented by a series of concentric hemispheric shells seen on color-flow imaging. As the RV increases, the size of the hemisphere increases.[2] Visual absence of flow convergence at a normal Nyquist limit is consistent with mild MR. PISA is only accurate when you can visualize the entire hemisphere, which requires angulation of the probe to obtain the largest PISA visually. Thus, in functional MR where the regurgitant orifice is often crescentic along the entire coaptation surface rather than a discrete circular orifice, PISA may not be accurate. To optimize the PISA, we magnify the valve and shift the aliasing velocity to between 20 and 40 cm/s which increases the size of the radius of the hemisphere, decreasing our measurement error. Small errors in measuring the radius lead to major errors in calculating an EROA due to squaring of the radius. PISA should be measured in mid-systole when the RV is at its peak. The radius of the hemisphere is measured, and using the aliasing velocity, the peak flow rate is calculated. EROA is calculated by dividing the peak flow rate by the peak velocity of the regurgitant jet using the equation:

$$\text{EROA} = (2\pi r^2 \cdot \text{Va})/\text{V}_{\text{regurgitant jet}}$$

where Va is the aliasing velocity (mL/s) and $\text{V}_{\text{regurgitant jet}}$ is the peak velocity of the MR jet (cm/s). The MR RV can be calculated by multiplying the EROA by the velocity time integral (VTI) of the MR jet (Fig. 5.13).

An EROA $\geq$.40 cm^2 is considered severe, while mild MR is an EROA $\leq$.20 cm^2. PISA is a good quantitative assessment, but it is technically difficult, hard to reproduce, and cannot be applied to all pathologies. The sonographer is heavily relied upon for this measurement. PISA is more accurate for central jets and circular orifices than eccentric jets and noncircular orifices. It has limited accuracy in non holosystolic jets because if the regurgitation only occurs during half of systole, then the true EROA is only half of the calculated EROA. PISA assessment may be inaccurate with functional etiology where the orifice is crescentic due to the valve leaking along the entire coaptation surface rather than a discrete orifice.[16] This underestimation of PISA in functional MR may explain why smaller EROAs are associated with a worse prognosis. An accurately performed PISA-derived effective regurgitant orifice correlates best with cardiac magnetic resonance predictors of the severity of MR.[4,27]

Vena contracta width. Vena contracta width is the narrowest portion of the regurgitant jet as it emerges from the orifice. It is measured on a magnified view of the parasternal long axis

TABLE 5.2 Primary Versus Secondary Mitral Regurgitation[a]

		SECONDARY MR[b]	
Primary MR[b]		**Regional LV Dysfunction**	**Global LV Dysfunction**
Etiology	Myxomatous or calcific leaflet degeneration	Inferior myocardial infarction	Nonischemic cardiomyopathy, large anterior or multiple myocardial infarctions
LV remodeling	Global, if severe chronic MR	Primarily inferior wall	Global dilation with increased sphericity
LA remodeling	Moderate to severe if chronic MR	Variable	Usually severe
Annulus	Dilated, preserved dynamic function	Mild to no dilation, less dynamic	Dilated, flattened, nondynamic
Leaflet morphology:	Yes/moderate, severe	No/mild	No/mild
• Thickening	Usually present	No	No
• Prolapse or flail	Variable	No/mild	No/mild
• Calcification			
Tethering pattern	None	Asymmetric	Symmetric
Systolic tenting	None	Increased	Markedly increased
Papillary muscle distance	Normal	Increased posterior papillary-intervalvular fibrosa distance	Increased interpapillary muscle distance
MR jet direction	Eccentric or central	Posterior	Usually central
CWD	May be late systolic (if MVP) or uniform if flail or with calcific degeneration	Density usually uniform throughout systole	Biphasic pattern, with increased density in early- and late-systolic flow and mid-systolic dropout
PISA	Often hemispheric	Often not hemispheric	Often not hemispheric; may be biphasic

[a]In addition to evaluating the morphology of the mitral leaflets for thickening, prolapse, flail, and calcifications, the left ventricle must be assessed for size, ejection fraction, and regional wall motion abnormalities to aid in differentiating primary versus secondary MR.

[b]Primary and secondary MR may coexist. (From Zoghbi WA, et al. Recommendations for noninvasive evaluation of native valvular regurgitation: a report from the American Society of Echocardiography developed in collaboration with the society for cardiovascular magnetic resonance. *J Am Soc Echocardiogr.* 2017;30:303–371.)

CWD, Continuous-wave Doppler; *LA*, left atrium; *LV*, left ventricle; *MR*, mitral regurgitation; *MVP*, mitral valve prolapse; *PISA*, proximal isovelocity surface area.

perpendicular to leaflet closure.[10] A2C view should never be used for this measurement as this view is parallel to the coaptation line which will overestimate all CFD measurements, especially the vena contracta measurement.[23] VCW is reliable for both central and eccentric jets with a width less than .3 cm, indicating mild MR and a width ≥.7 cm specific for severe MR (Fig. 5.14).[20]

Pulsed-Wave Doppler

Mitral inflow. Using pulsed-wave Doppler with the sample volume placed at the leaflet tips in an A4C view, a spectral display of the mitral inflow is obtained. In a normal patient, flow during LV relaxation (E wave) is greater than the flow with atrial contraction (A wave). As the SV across the mitral valve increases, the E wave will increase. An elevated E wave of 1.2 to 1.5 m/s in sinus rhythm is sensitive, but not specific for severe MR.[28] A wave dominance almost always excludes severe MR. Increased E wave can be seen in other processes such as MS, diastolic dysfunction, high cardiac output, and prosthetic valves. In secondary MR, it may be difficult to determine if the increased E wave is due to elevated LV filling pressures or severe MR (Fig. 5.15).[13]

Pulmonary vein flow. Pulmonary vein flow demonstrates the hemodynamic consequences of MR as it represents the differential pressures between the LA and the pulmonary veins. Normal pulmonary vein flow shows atrial reversal (if normal sinus rhythm is present) followed by an S wave during systole and a D wave during diastole. Systolic flow should be greater than diastolic flow in mild MR, while the left atrial pressure remains low. As the left atrial pressure increases, the pulmonary vein systolic flow decreases and the diastolic flow increases. Systolic blunting (S<D) is seen with moderate MR but also may be seen in atrial fibrillation due to decreased atrial compliance. In disease processes with poor LA compliance as in atrial fibrillation, there is frequently no forward flow during systole with no S wave visualized. As the left atrial pressure increases with severe MR, systolic reversal is present. It is important to sample both left, and right-sided pulmonary veins and to avoid sampling a specific pulmonary vein if the regurgitant jet is flowing into that pulmonary vein. If the LA is massively dilated, systolic reversal may not be present in the pulmonary veins. The presence of systolic flow reversal in two pulmonary veins is specific for severe MR (Fig. 5.16).

Regurgitant volume and regurgitant fraction. RV and RF can be measured by using SV, PISA, and volumetric methods.[a] The pulsed-wave Doppler method compares the SV across the mitral

[a]References 2, 8, 13, 16, 20, 23.

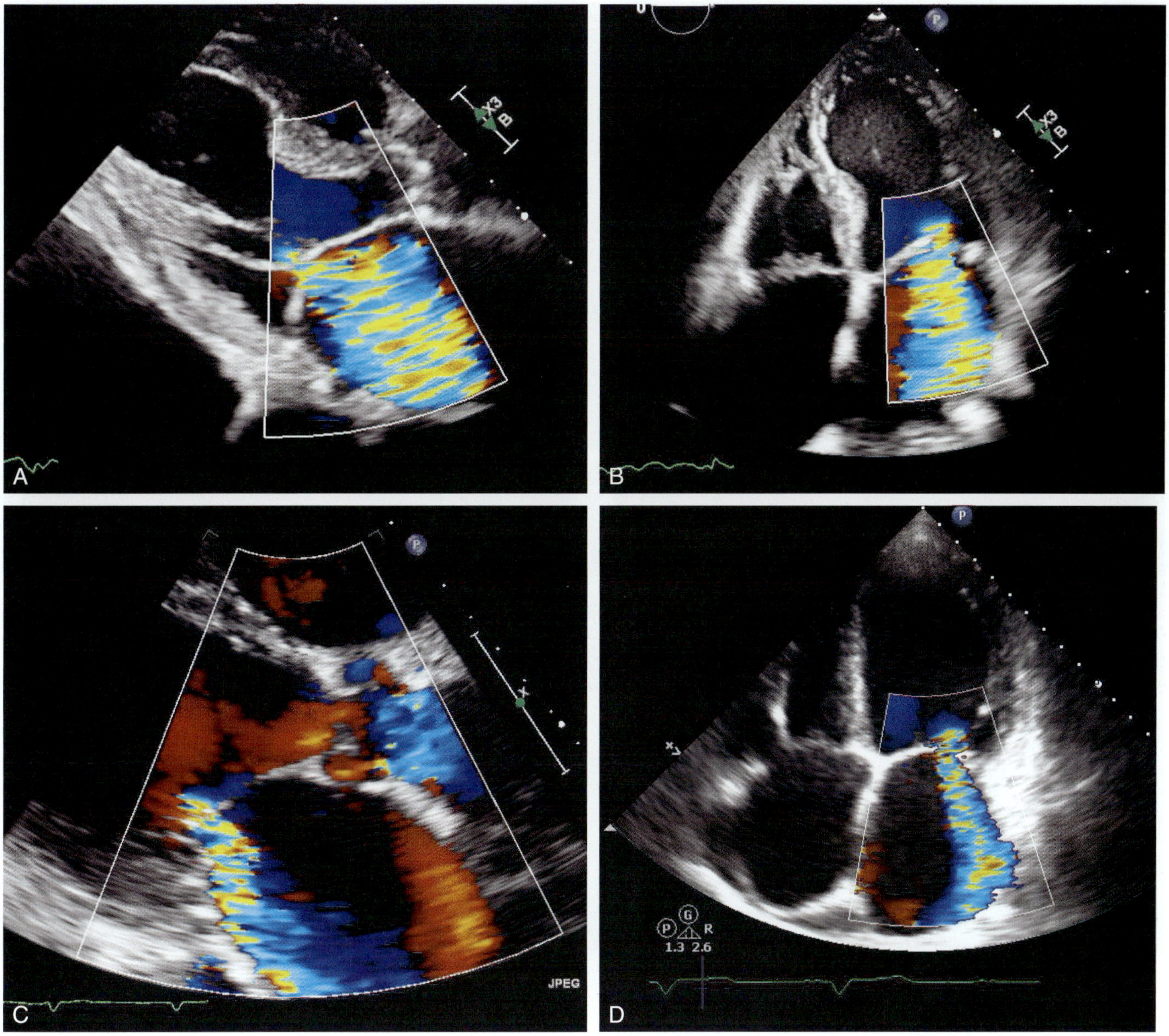

Fig. 5.9 Severe Functional Mitral Regurgitation With Central Jet Versus Eccentric Jet. (A) Color-flow imaging in a parasternal long axis (PSLA) view demonstrates a large central mitral regurgitation (MR) jet which usually occurs with symmetric bileaflet tethering seen in a nonischemic cardiomyopathy. Despite similar regurgitant volumes, a central jet will appear larger than an eccentric jet due to lack of wall constraints. It is necessary to integrate other measurements in your final assessment of MR severity. (B) Apical 4-chamber view demonstrating severe MR with large, central jet. (C) Large eccentric, posteriorly directed jet due to asymmetric leaflet tethering in an ischemic cardiomyopathy seen in a PSLA view. Although the jet does not occupy greater than 50% of the left atrium, the wall-hugging aspect is consistent with severe MR. (D) Severe MR due to an eccentric, posteriorly directed jet in an apical 4-chamber view. This eccentric jet demonstrates the Coanda effect.

valve with the SV across another "normal" valve, usually the aortic valve (Fig. 5.17). The valve with which it is being compared must have less than mild regurgitation for this method to be accurate. SV across any valve is the product of the cross-sectional area (CSA) and the VTI measured by pulsed Doppler at the annulus.[b]

$$SV = CSA \times VTI = \pi r^2 \times VTI$$

SV across the aortic valve is calculated from the left ventricular outflow tract (LVOT) diameter obtained in the PSLA and the LVOT pulsed-wave Doppler obtained in the apical 5-chamber or 3-chamber view. SV across the mitral valve is obtained in the 4-chamber view where the sample volume is placed in

[b]References 2, 8, 13, 16, 20, 23.

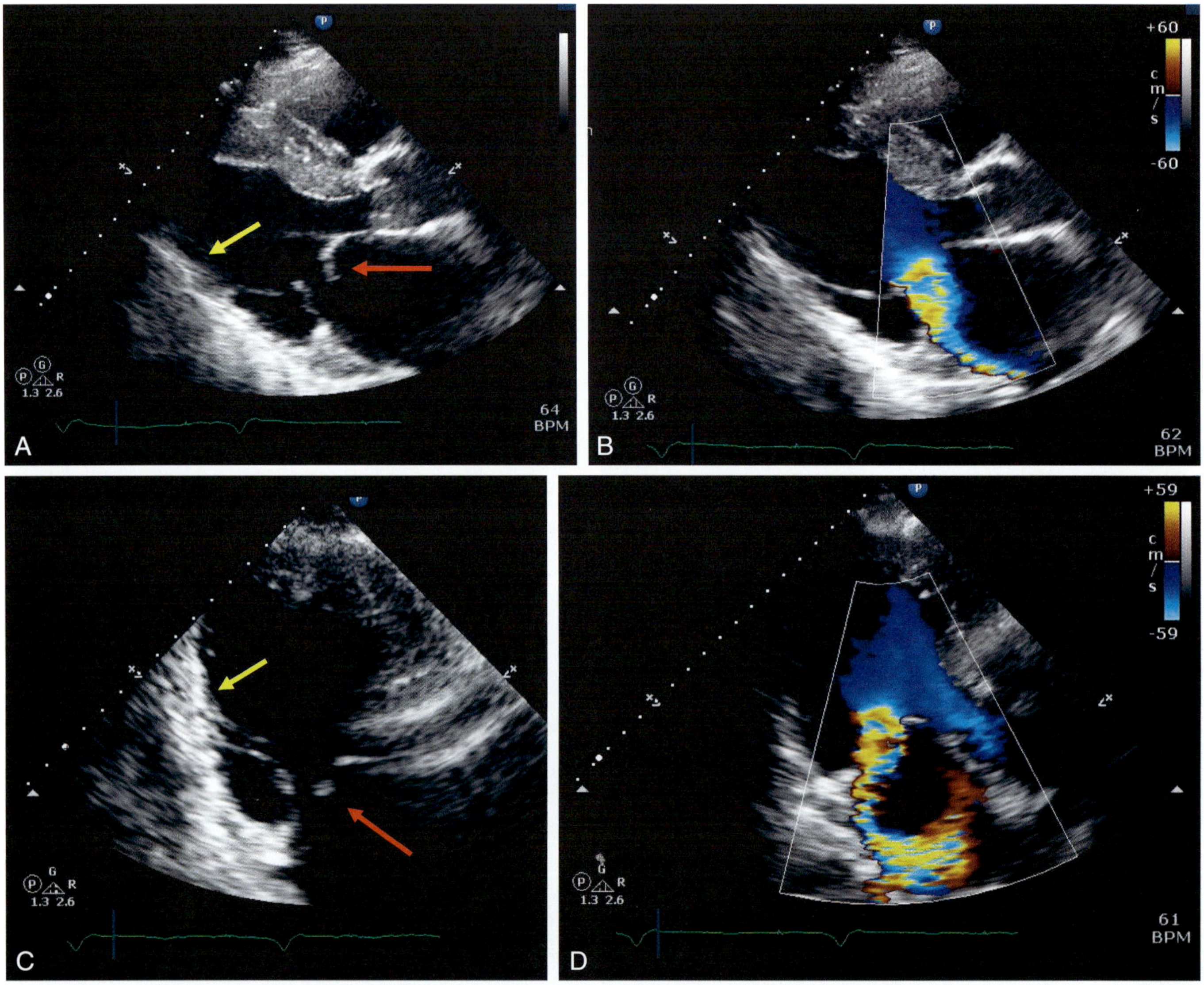

Fig. 5.10 Mixed Etiology. (A) This patient had known ischemic cardiomyopathy, as evidenced by the thin and scarred inferolateral wall *(yellow arrow)*, and presented with an acute flail of the anterior leaflet *(red arrow)*. Parasternal long-axis view. (B) Posteriorly directed jet is due to a flail/prolapse of the anterior leaflet, as seen in this patient. Direction of regurgitant jet aids in determining pathology. (C) Apical 2-chamber view demonstrating inferior scar *(yellow arrow)* and flail leaflet *(red arrow)*. (D) Apical long-axis showing eccentric, posteriorly directed jet.

the mitral annulus (not at the leaflet tips which is used for measuring diastolic function) at the same level where the mitral annular diameter is measured. SV is calculated using the continuity equation:

$$SV = A1'' \, V1 = A2'' \, V2$$

where A1 is the LVOT area, V1 is the VTI from the LVOT PW, A2 is the mitral annular area, V2 is VTI from the mitral valve PW at the annulus.

$$MRRegVol = SV_{MV} - SV_{LVOT}$$

RV is obtained by subtracting the LVOT SV from the mitral SV.

$$MRRegFraction = RV_{MV} / SV_{MV}$$

RF is obtained by dividing the MV SV by the RV.

An alternative volumetric method calculates total SV using 2D or 3D measurements subtracting left ventricular end-systolic volume (LVESV) from left ventricular end-diastolic volume (LVEDV) and then subtracting the aortic valve SV to estimate the RV.[c] RV can also be calculated using PISA EROA by multiplying the MR VTI by the EROA.

RV ≥60 cc's and RF ≥50% are considered severe. Mild MR is a RV less than 30 mL and RF less than 30%.

All of these methods are difficult to reproduce due to multiple measurements in different locations and at

[c]References 2, 8, 13, 16, 20, 23.

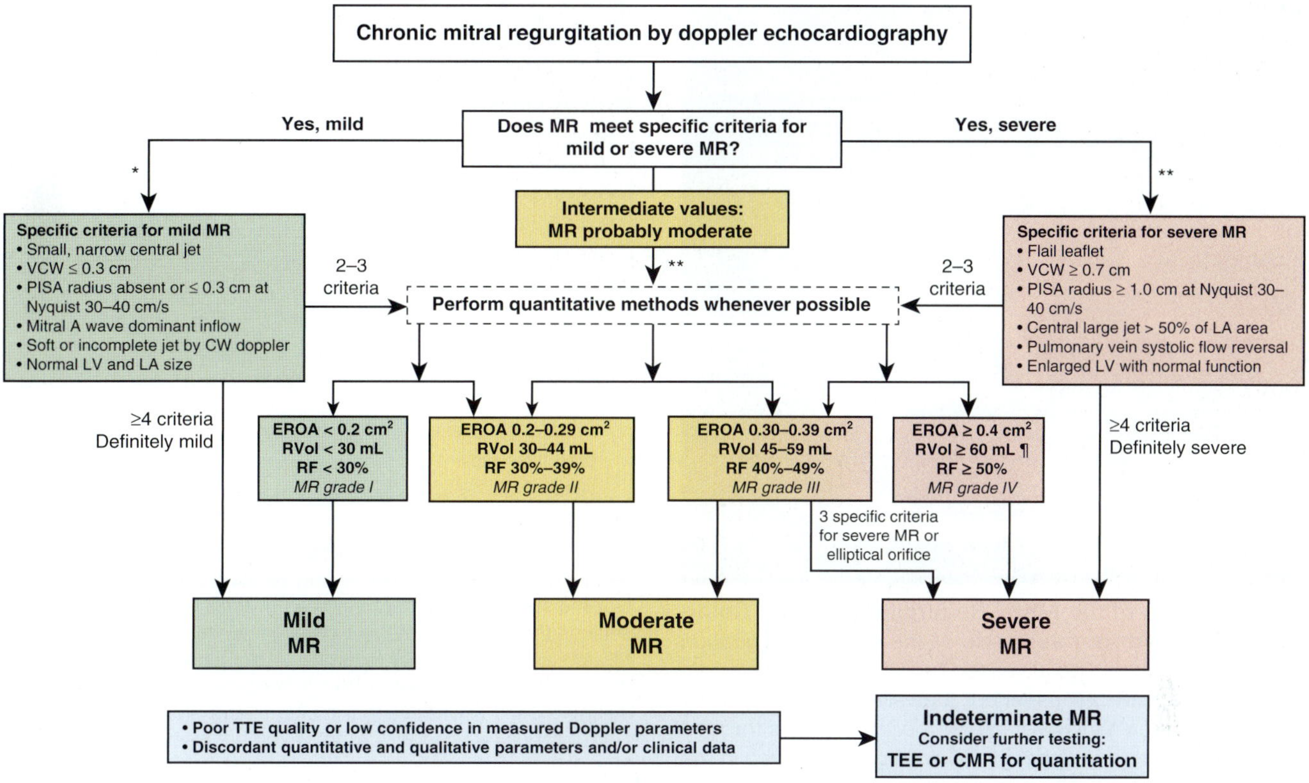

*	Beware of underestimation of MR severity in eccentric, wall impinging jets; quantitation is advised
**	All values for EROA by PISA assume holosystolic MR; single frame EROA by PISA and VCW overestimate non-holosystolic MR
¶	Regurgitant volume for severe MR may be lower in low flow conditions.

Fig. 5.11 Algorithm for the Integration of Multiple Parameters of Mitral Regurgitation Severity. Decision tree for assessing the severity of chronic MR by TTE. Additional considerations: (1) When uncertainty exists regarding MR severity based on clinical and echocardiographic assessment (i.e., mild to moderate or moderate to severe), consider further testing. (2) Further testing may include right and left heart catheterization, stress echo, TEE, or CMR in select circumstances. (3) Color Doppler can often overestimate MR. This is most common with high blood pressure, high LV systolic pressure in AS or HOCM, peak velocities ≥6.0 m/s, or single-frame measurements (PISA, VCW, VCA) in non holosystolic MR. (4) Color Doppler can also underestimate MR severity. This is most common with high LA pressures, low LV ejection fraction, or large LA/LV volumes. (5) Adjunctive criteria that support mild MR include a soft or incomplete MR jet on CW Doppler, normal PA systolic pressure, or MR duration less than 30% of systole. (6) Adjunctive criteria that support severe MR include a dense triangular CW Doppler profile, a well-aligned CW MR jet velocity less than 4.5 m/s indicating high LAP, dilated LA or LV with no other cause, PA systolic pressure greater than 50 mm Hg with no other cause, and systolic PV flow reversal and significant mitral inflow E-wave dominance with high velocity (>1.2 to 1.5 m/s) in the absence of mitral stenosis. *AS*, aortic stenosis; *CMR*, cardiovascular magnetic resonance; *CW*, color wave; *EROA*, effective regurgitant orifice area; *HOCM*, hypertrophic obstructive cardiomyopathy; *LA*, left atrium; *LAP*, left atrial pressure; *LV*, left ventricle; *MR*, mitral regurgitation; *PA*, pulmonary artery; *PISA*, proximal isovelocity surface area; *PV*, pulmonary valve; *RF*, regurgitant fraction; *RVol*, regurgitant volume; *TEE*, transesophageal echocardiogram; *TTE*, transthoracic echocardiogram; *VCA*, vena contracta area; *VCW*, vena contracta width. (From Zoghbi WA, Adams D, Bonow RO, et al. Recommendations for noninvasive evaluation of native valvular regurgitation: a report from the American Society of Echocardiography developed in collaboration with the society for cardiovascular magnetic resonance. *J Am Soc Echocardiogr.* 2017;30:303–371.)

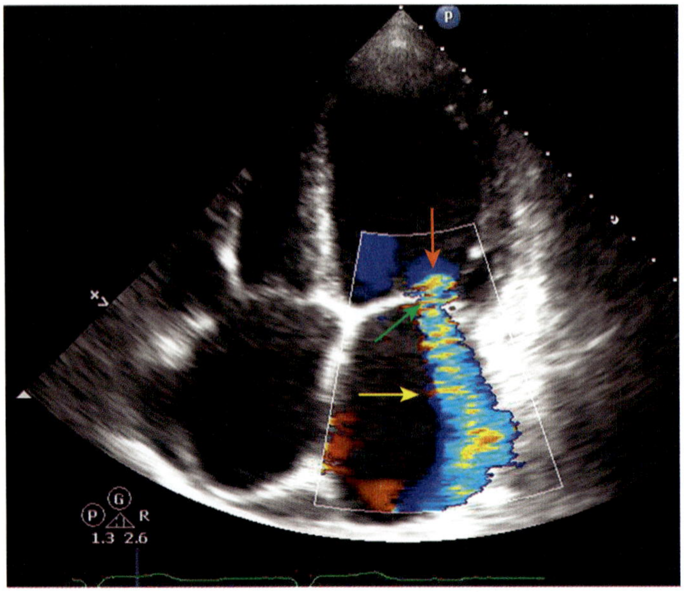

Fig. 5.12 **Three Parts of the Mitral Regurgitation Using Color-flow Doppler.** There are three parts of the mitral regurgitation (MR) color jet that should be assessed for MR severity-flow convergence on the ventricular aspect of the valve *(red arrow),* vena contracta width of the narrowest part of the jet as it goes through the valve *(green arrow),* and the color-flow regurgitant area in the left atrium *(yellow arrow).* Coanda effect is demonstrated by this eccentric, wall-hugging posterolaterally directed jet.

BOX 5.1 Hemodynamic and Technical Factors That Affect Mitral Regurgitation Color Jet Area[a]

Regurgitant volume
LV systolic pressure
Central vs wall-hugging jet
Heart rhythm and rate
LA size and compliance
Regurgitant orifice size and shape
Influence of co-existing flow streams
Technical Factors
- Gain setting
- Scale
- Frame rate, sector size
- Color flow maps
- Vendor

[a]Mitral regurgitation (MR) color-flow jet area should never be the sole method used to assess MR severity as there are many patient issues (volume status, blood pressure, heart rhythm, heart rate) and machine settings that will affect the size of the jet in the left atrium. For example, MR jets assessed only by regurgitant color jet area will appear larger in hypertensive patients and smaller in hypotensive patients. *LA*, Left atrium; *LV*, left ventricle. (Modified from Lang RM, et al. *ASE's Comprehensive Echocardiography*. 2nd ed. Elsevier; 2015:486, Box 116.2.)

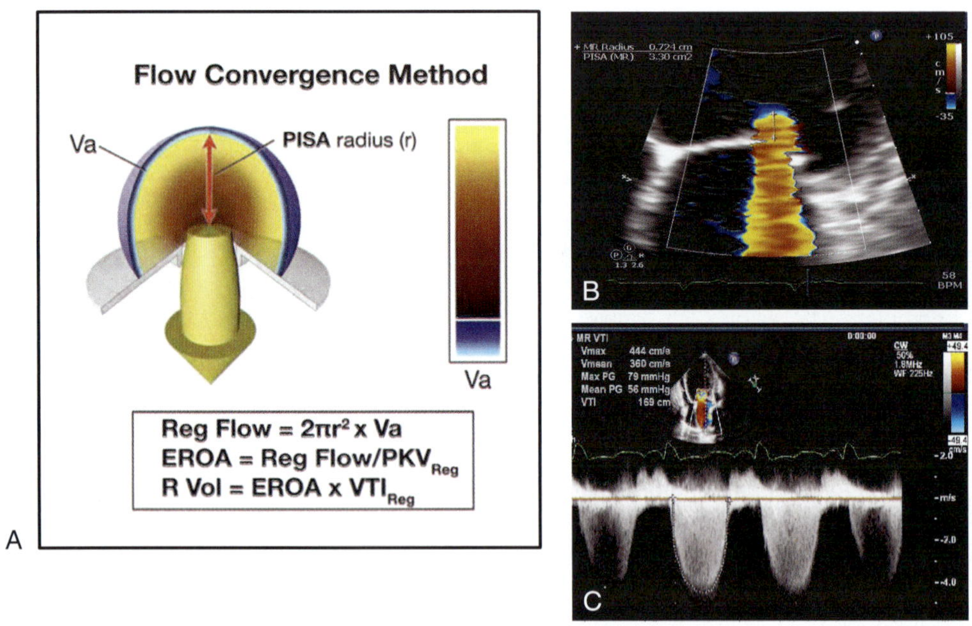

Fig. 5.13 **Flow Convergence Method.** (A) Schematic representation of the flow convergence method *(PISA).* (B) The example on the right shows the measurement of the PISA radius after adjusting the aliasing velocity which temporally corresponds to the maximal jet velocity by color-flow Doppler. The radius of the hemisphere is .72 cm, the aliasing velocity is 35 cm/s. (C) The peak MR velocity is 444 cm/s. Using the equation in A, the EROA = $2\pi r r^2 \times V_a$ = $[2\pi \times (.72)^2 \times 35]/444$ = .24 cm^2. Regurgitant volume = .24 × 169 = 40 mL. These values are consistent with moderate mitral regurgitation. *EROA*, Effective regurgitant orifice area. (From Zoghbi WA, Adams D, Bonow RO, et al. Recommendations for noninvasive evaluation of native valvular regurgitation. *JASE*. 2017;30:313, Fig. 5.)

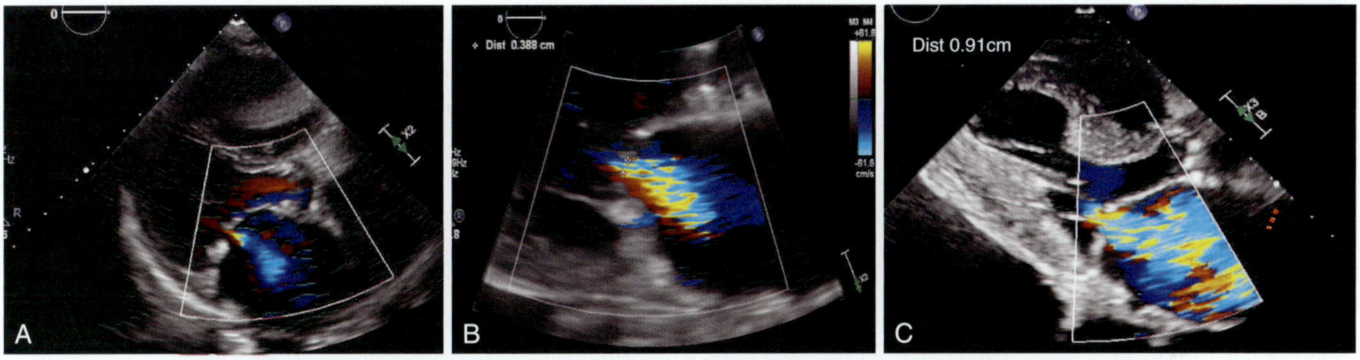

Fig. 5.14 **Vena Contracta Width.** Vena contracta is the narrowest portion of the regurgitant flow that occurs at the regurgitant orifice. Vena contracta width (VCW) less than .3 cm is mild and greater than .7 cm is severe. (A) Mild mitral regurgitation (MR) with a VCW too small to measure. (B) Moderate MR with a VCW .38 cm. (C) Severe MR with a VCW .91 cm.

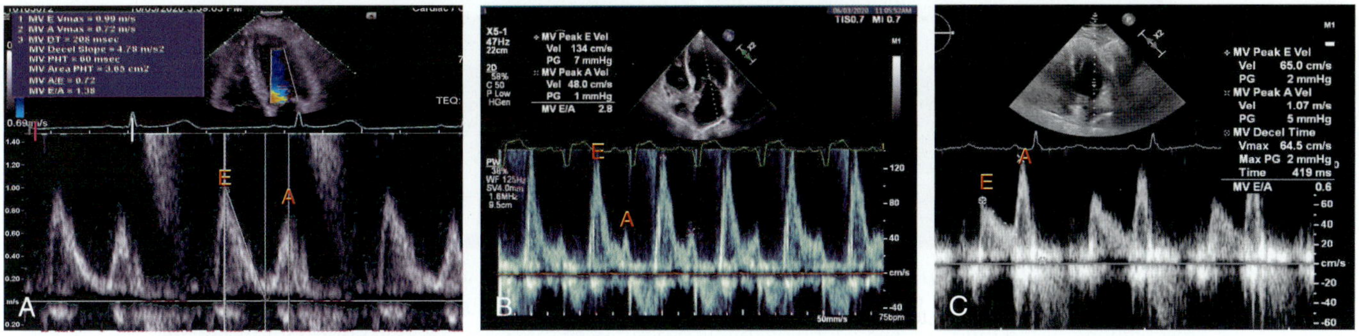

Fig. 5.15 **Various Patterns of Mitral Inflow.** (A) Normal mitral inflow demonstrates an E wave between .8 to 1.2 cm/s. (B) As the mitral regurgitation (MR) severity increases, the E wave increases. This pattern is frequently seen with severe MR. E wave greater than 1.2 cm/s is abnormal and may be due to significant MR but other pathology can also result in elevated E waves such as mitral stenosis, diastolic dysfunction and high output states. (C) It is unlikely to have significant MR when the E wave is less than the A wave.

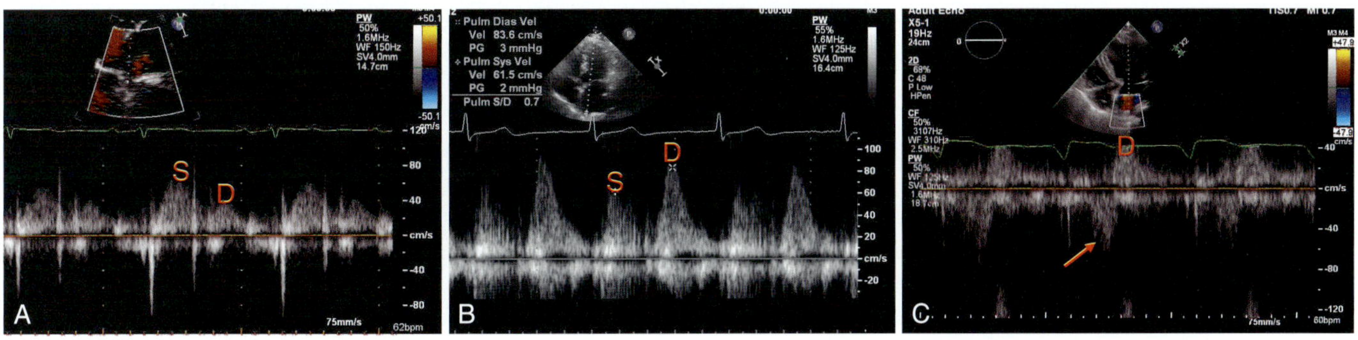

Fig. 5.16 **Pulmonary Venous Flow.** (A) In a normal heart with normal left atrial pressures, pulmonary vein systolic flow *(S)* is greater than diastolic *(D)* flow. (B) With increasing left atrial pressures, the systolic wave decreases resulting in systolic blunting with moderate mitral regurgitation (MR). (C) Systolic reversal is specific for severe MR *(red arrow)*. The specific pulmonary vein where the MR jet is flowing into should not be sampled.

different times during the cardiac cycle. But they all assess the MR during the entirety of systole. The advantage of these techniques is that they are valid with multiple jets and eccentric jets.

Continuous-Wave Doppler

Jet timing, morphology, and intensity. Continuous-wave Doppler of MR must be obtained in the apical views to ensure alignment with the flow to obtain the most accurate depiction

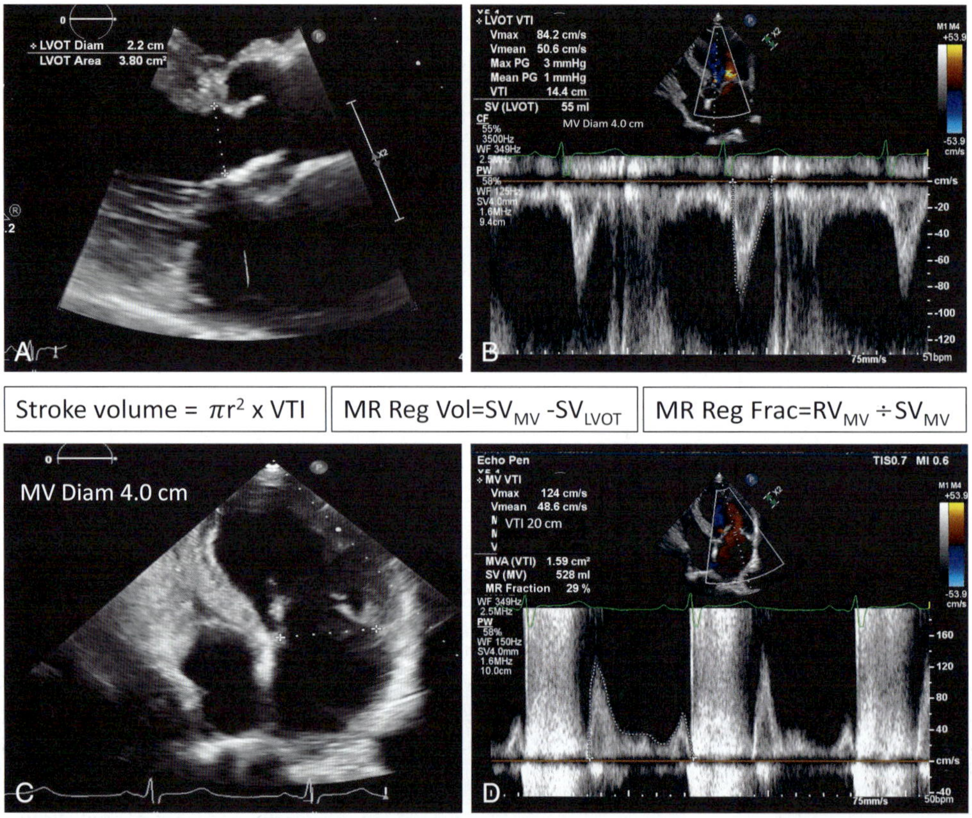

Fig. 5.17 Regurgitant Volume and Regurgitation Fraction. Stroke volume = $\pi r^2 \times$ VTI. MR Reg Vol = $SV_{MV} - SV_{LVOT}$. MR Reg Frac = $RV_{MV} \div SV_{MV}$. Regurgitant volume and regurgitant fraction calculations of the LVOT and MV annulus in this patient with massive MR. It is important to obtain measurements at the same time in the cardiac cycle (mid-systole for LVOT) and the same location (PW sample volume at the mitral annulus for MV). (A) LVOT diameter is measured at the base of the aortic leaflets in mid-systole in the PSLA view. (B) Sample volume of LVOT pulsed-wave Doppler should be obtained at .8 to 1.0 cm above the aortic valve, prior to the acceleration of flow through the aortic valve. SV LVOT is 55 mL (d = 2.2 cm, VTI =14.4 cm). (C) Mitral annular diameter should be measured in diastole during the maximal opening of the mitral valve. (D) Sample volume of the mitral valve must be placed at the annulus, rather than the usual placement at the leaflet tips. SV MV is 251 mL (d = 4.0 cm, VTI = 20 cm). Regurgitant volume ($SV_{MV} - SV_{LVOT}$) of 196 mL and regurgitant fraction (RV_{MV}/SV_{MV}) of 78% is consistent with severe mitral regurgitation. *LVOT,* Left ventricular outflow tract; *MR,* mitral regurgitation; *MV,* mitral valve; *PSLA,* parasternal long axis; *PW,* pulsed wave; *RV,* right ventricular; *SV,* stroke volume; *VTI,* velocity time integral.

of the jet. The jet must be accurately interrogated as erroneous interpretations will be made if the spectral tracing is not obtained parallel to the flow. It is important to assess the timing of the jet and to demonstrate that it is holosystolic. Severe MR will always be holosystolic. It is unlikely to have severe MR with a late-systolic jet.[10] Barlow's disease frequently has late-systolic MR that, since the regurgitation is only occurring during a small portion of systole, makes it difficult to have a large total RV. The morphology of the MR jet on spectral display is normally parabolic (Fig. 5.18). An early peaking or triangular-shape envelope suggests severe MR with rapid equilibration of the transmitral gradient (V-wave cut-off sign). The density of the CW jet, which represents the number of red blood cells reflecting the signal, can be compared with the density of the mitral inflow (representing the antegrade flow across the valve) after the gains have been adjusted. If the density of the MR jet (below the baseline) is equal to the density of the mitral inflow (above the baseline), it suggests severe MR. If it is incomplete or faint, the regurgitation is likely trace or mild. Eccentric jets may make it difficult to obtain a complete CW waveform as it is difficult to get parallel to the jet. MR jet peak velocity reveals no useful information about MR severity, but it does reveal clues about the hemodynamic state. Usually, the peak MR velocity is between 4.5 and 5.5 m/s corresponding to an LV to LA gradient of 80 to 120 mm Hg using the Bernoulli equation. A low MR velocity (≤4 m/s) suggests low blood pressure and/or high left atrial pressures, while a high MR velocity (>6 m/s) suggests elevated LV systolic pressure due to systemic hypertension or aortic stenosis.

Associated Hemodynamic Consequences

Left Ventricle

Left ventricular volume and function should always be included in the assessment of MR, as it is useful for determining the need and timing of intervention (see Fig. 5.8). LV volumes should ideally be

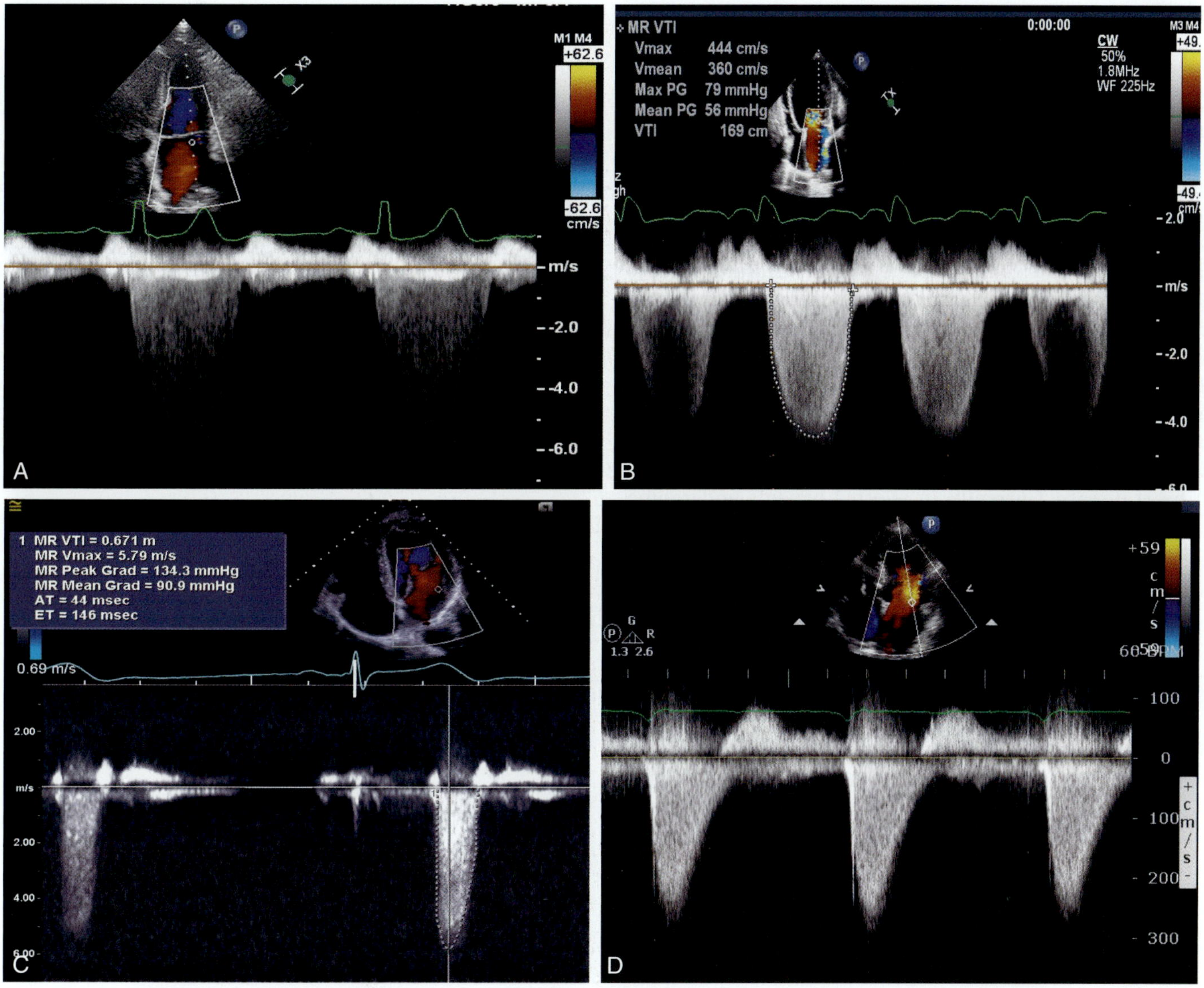

Fig. 5.18 **Continuous-Wave Doppler of Mitral Regurgitation Jet.** Examination of the mitral regurgitation (MR) envelope as assessed by continuous-wave (CW) Doppler. (A) A faint jet as compared with the antegrade flow above the baseline consistent with mild MR. (B) A dense CW jet, with an intensity similar to antegrade flow, consistent with severe MR. (C) A late-systolic jet frequently seen in Barlow's disease which is almost never severe mitral regurgitation. Only the dense part of the MR CW profile should be traced for use in quantification. (D) A triangular jet rather than a parabolic MR envelope with a low peak velocity (<3 m/s), which is consistent with acute, severe MR in a hemodynamically unstable patient.

assessed using 3D, but 2D Simpson's method of disks may also be used if 3D is unavailable.[1-3,7,14] Volumes should always be indexed to body size. Increased LV volumes are an expected consequence of chronic, severe MR. In functional MR, the relationship between LV size and MR severity is much more intertwined, making it difficult to assess if the LV dilatation is the cause or the result of the MR. Assessment of LV systolic dysfunction is important as it demonstrates how the LV adapts to the increased volumes. Patients with severe MR who develop an ejection fraction (EF) ≤60% have already developed LV dysfunction.[29,30] Patients with extremely poor systolic function may not benefit from an intervention, although this specific EF has not yet been determined for transcatheter therapies. Global longitudinal strain may be useful in identifying myocardial dysfunction earlier than a decrease in ejection fraction.[31,32] Dilatation of the LV is a supportive sign of significant valvular regurgitation and not a specific sign.[2]

Left Atrium

Left atrial volumes should always be included in the assessment of MR. LA volumes are superior to left atrial dimensions in evaluating dilatation and predicting outcomes.[33] Left atrial volumes should always be increased with chronic, severe MR, but left atrial dilatation does not imply severe MR as it occurs in many other disease processes such as atrial fibrillation, hypertension, diastolic dysfunction, and cardiomyopathies. A normal left atrial volume may exclude chronic, severe MR (see Fig. 5.8).

Right Heart

Echocardiography evaluation of the right heart, including RV size and function, tricuspid annular size, severity of tricuspid regurgitation (TR), and pulmonary artery systolic pressure should be assessed. Right ventricle should be assessed for size and function. RV function may be assessed using 2D area change, Tricuspid annular planar systolic excursion (TAPSE), and tissue Doppler imaging of the tricuspid annulus (S′).[2,7,13,34] RV size is measured using linear dimensions, as its unusual shape is not conducive to the same volume measurements as with the LV. TAPSE measures the lateral descent of the tricuspid annulus and is a surrogate for RV function. TAPSE greater than 1.6 cm is consistent with normal RV systolic function (Fig. 5.19). Functional TR is frequently observed in the advanced stage of left-sided valvular heart disease.[35,36] Functional TR is usually due to tricuspid annulus dilatation caused by RV dilatation and dysfunction due to pulmonary hypertension from left heart disease. Currently, in selected patients undergoing surgical treatment for severe MR, it is recommended to repair the tricuspid valve at the same setting.[34,37–39] We do not know how that will be applied to transcatheter interventions in the future. Remodeling of the right heart in response to elevated pulmonary artery systolic pressure is the likely cause of functional TR.[34,36,38] As the right heart dilates, further RV remodeling leads to more dilatation resulting in papillary muscle displacement and leaflet tethering which worsens RV dilatation and TR. Severely dilated right ventricle with severely decreased systolic function is unlikely to improve with a mitral valve intervention. TR severity is determined by similar methods of MR including the size of the color RJA, VCW, and EROA using PISA (Fig. 5.20).

Pulmonary hypertension is necessary to assess mitral valve disease for both prognostic predictions and treatment options. Noninvasive assessment of RV systolic pressure applying the modified Bernoulli equation to the peak velocity of TR is essential in every patient.

$$\Delta P = 4V^2$$

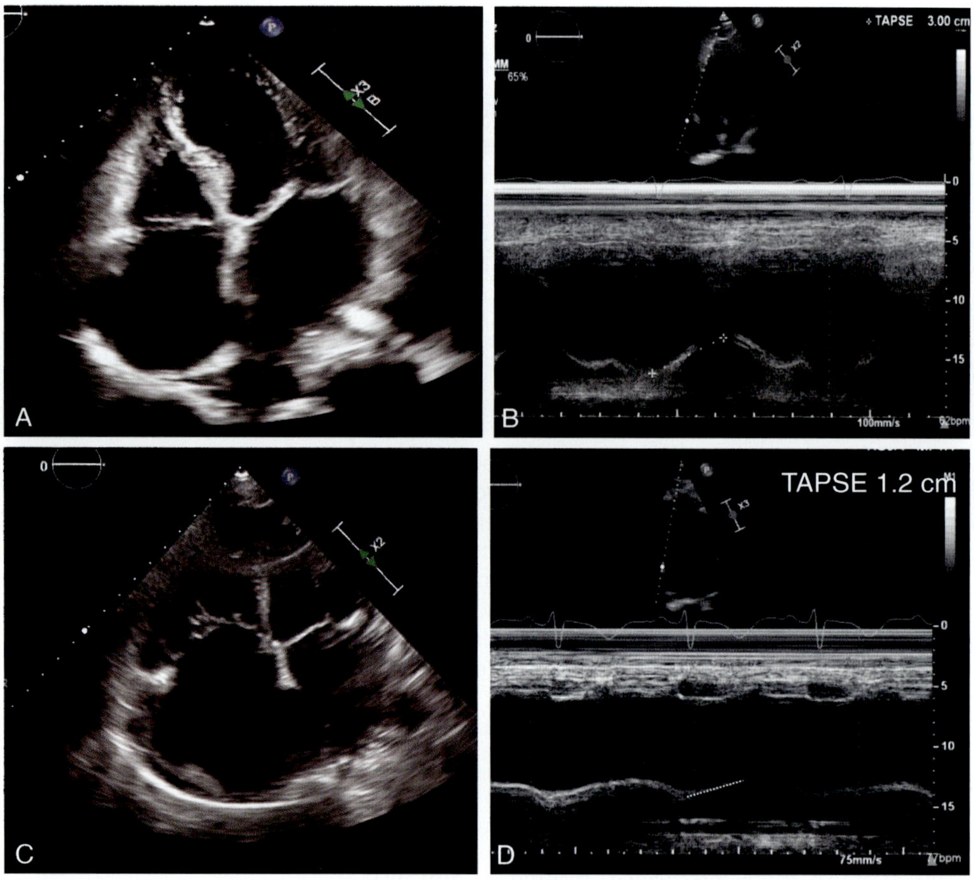

Fig. 5.19 **Right Ventricular Size and Tricuspid Annular Planar Systolic Excursion.** (A) Normal right ventricular (RV) size. RV volume should always appear smaller than the left ventricular (LV) volume in an apical 4-chamber view. The apex of the heart is comprised solely of the LV apex. (B) Quantitative assessment of the right ventricle involves tricuspid annular planar systolic excursion (TAPSE) which can be used as a surrogate for RV function, measuring the lateral descent of the tricuspid annulus. TAPSE >1.6 cm is consistent with normal RV systolic function. (C) Severely dilated right ventricle is demonstrated by a larger volume than the LV volume. Also, the apex of the heart is comprised of the RV. (D) Abnormal TAPSE demonstrating decreased RV systolic function.

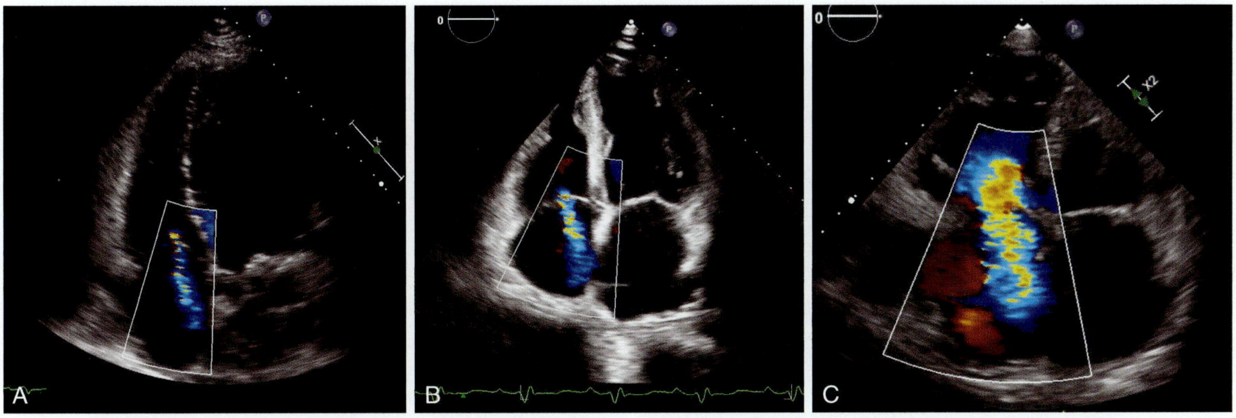

Fig. 5.20 Tricuspid Regurgitation Severity. Tricuspid regurgitation (TR) severity is assessed using color regurgitant jet area with mild occupying less than 25% right atrium (RA), and severe occupying greater than 50% RA. Tricuspid regurgitation is very sensitive to volume status. Pulmonary hypertension cannot be assessed using color-flow imaging. (A) Mild TR. (B) Moderate TR. (C) Severe TR.

Here, ΔP is the peak gradient across the tricuspid valve calculated by multiplying the square of the peak TR velocity obtained using CW Doppler by 4 (Fig. 5.21). The mean right atrial pressure, assessed non invasively using the inferior vena cava size and respiratory variation, is added to the peak gradient to obtain the estimated RV systolic pressure. If the inferior vena cava (IVC) is normal size (<2.1 cm) and collapses more than 50% with inspiration, the right atrial pressure is assumed to be 3 mm Hg. When the IVC is dilated (>2.1 cm) and collapses less than 50% with inspiration, the right atrial pressure is assumed to be elevated at 15 mm Hg. If the IVC is normal size but does not vary with respiration, or is dilated and collapses with inspiration, the estimated right atrium (RA) pressure is 8 mm Hg (Fig. 5.22).[34] The presence of pulmonary hypertension in the absence of other causes is evidence of compensatory mechanisms.

Integrative Approach

No single echocardiographic parameter has the measurement precision or reproducibility to serve as the sole arbiter of MR severity.[2,3,7] Many physicians assess MR severity based solely on the regurgitant color-flow area, which is incorrect. CFD should be your starting point that integrates multiple factors before arriving at a final determination.[1–3] An algorithm developed by consensus opinion from the ASE 2017 Guidelines for valvular regurgitation proposes having four of six specific criteria as evidence for severe MR (Box 5.2).[2,27] If fewer than four criteria are present, MR should be quantified using EROA, RV, or RF.[2,27] When discrepant measurements exist, re-examine all technical and hemodynamic reasons looking for inaccuracies to explain the contradiction. If discrepancies cannot be resolved, consider magnetic resonance imaging. When MR is holosystolic, properly measured values of EROA ≧.4 cm^2, RV ≧ 60 mL, RF ≧50% are highly specific for severe MR. Properly measured values of EROA less than .2 cm^2, RV ≦30 mL, RF ≦30% are highly specific for mild MR.[2,13] Final assessment of the severity of MR should also consider the hemodynamic state of the patient.

MITRAL STENOSIS

TTE is the primary modality to assess the severity and mechanism of MS and evaluate other structures relevant to prognosis and timing of intervention including LV size and function, LA size and function, RV size and function, and RV systolic pressure.[40] Although complete assessment of the mitral valve is possible by TTE, further imaging may be required such as a TEE for suboptimal image quality or left atrial appendage thrombus and a stress echocardiogram when symptoms appear worse than the resting echo suggests.

Leaflet Morphology

MS is usually due to rheumatic disease in developing countries or calcific disease in developed nations. Less common etiologies include systemic lupus erythematosus, carcinoid, radiation and rare congenital lesions such as parachute mitral valve, cor triatriatum, and supravalvular ring.

Rheumatic Mitral Stenosis

Rheumatic heart disease is the most common cause of MS worldwide. Rheumatic involvement of the mitral valve results in thickened leaflets, decreased mobility, commissural fusion, chordal shortening, and calcifications in the valvular and subvalvular apparatus. PSLA is the ideal view to visualize thickened leaflets (>5 mm), restricted posterior leaflet motion, and anterior leaflet doming (hockey-stick appearance) (Fig. 5.23). The disease process starts at leaflet tips and progresses toward the papillary muscle. Significant commissural fusion is the hallmark of rheumatic MS, best visualized on a parasternal short-axis view. Varying degrees of MR associated with rheumatic MS must be carefully assessed prior to determining appropriate therapy. Associated MR should be accurately quantitated when moderate or severe. When the severities of both stenosis and regurgitation are balanced, indications for interventions rely more on the consequences of combined stenosis

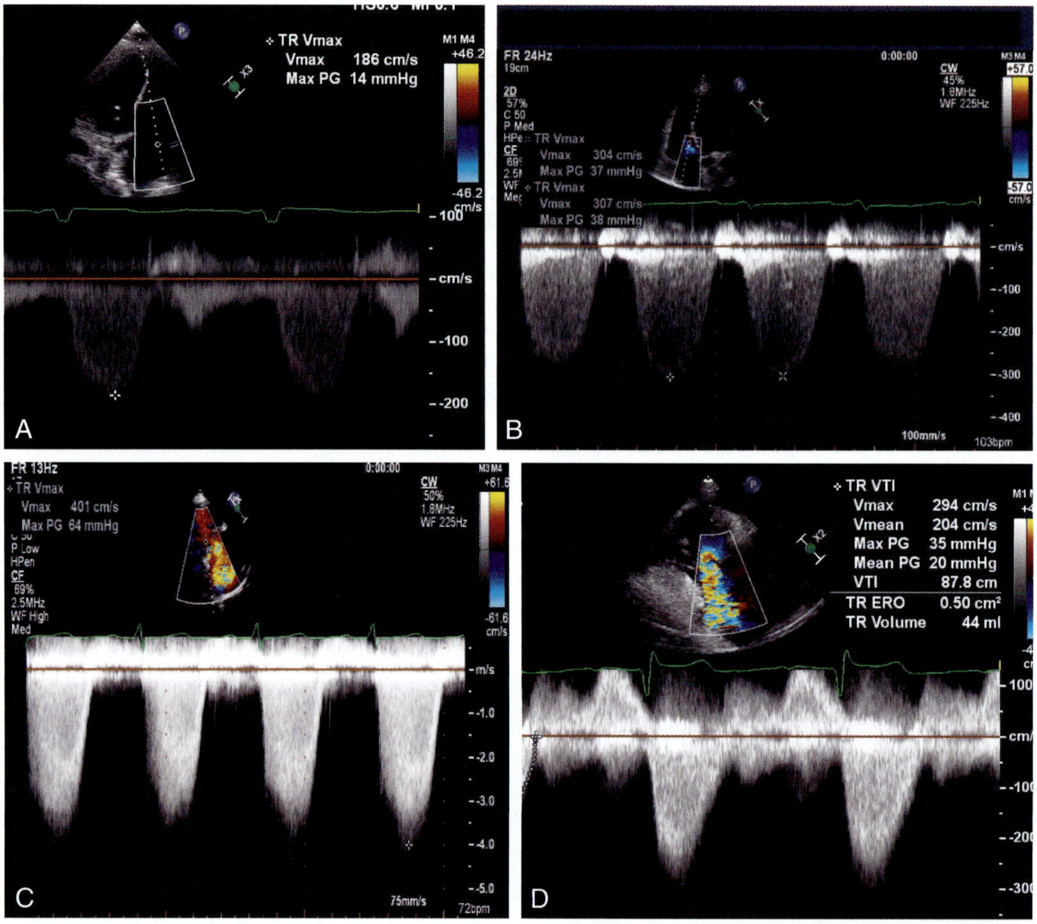

Fig. 5.21 Assessment of Pulmonary Hypertension Using Tricuspid Regurgitation Envelope. Assessment of the tricuspid regurgitation (TR) profile including the peak velocity helps in assessing how the right ventricle and pulmonary circuit are handling the left-sided valvular disease. Right ventricular systolic pressure is assessed by measuring the velocity across the tricuspid valve and converting it to a gradient using the modified Bernoulli equation. $PG = 4V^2$ where PG is the peak gradient across the tricuspid valve and V is the peak velocity of the TR jet. (A) The peak gradient of the tricuspid valve is $4 \times (1.88)^2 = 14$ mm Hg. This gradient is then added to the estimate of the right atrium pressure using the IVC diameter. The faint envelope of the TR jet is consistent with mild TR. (B) The peak velocity of the TR jet is 3 m/s, which correlates to a trans tricuspid gradient of 36 mm Hg. (C) The marked intensity of the TR envelope is consistent with severe TR. The elevated peak velocity of 4 m/s reveals severe pulmonary hypertension. (D) The triangular shape of this TR jet is consistent with severe tricuspid regurgitation with a single chamber physiology. The RVSP will be significantly underestimated using the peak TR jet and thus cannot be estimated in this situation.

and regurgitation, as assessed by exercise tolerance and mean gradient, than any single individual index of severity of stenosis or regurgitation.[41] Balloon mitral valvuloplasty, which splits the fused commissures, is only beneficial in rheumatic MS, not calcific MS.[42]

TTE criteria for identifying appropriate candidates with rheumatic MS for successful valvuloplasty are based on the Wilkins score which assesses leaflet thickening, leaflet mobility, leaflet calcification, and subvalvular thickening graded on a scale from 0 (normal) to 4 (severe). Wilkins score ranges from 0 to 16 with an appropriate candidate having a score ≤8 with mild MR and no intracardiac thrombus visualized on TEE (Table 5.3).[40–44]

Calcific Mitral Stenosis

Contrary to rheumatic MS, calcific MS occurs when the calcium from the annulus encroaches onto the base of the leaflet and then progresses toward the tips, sparing the free edges of the leaflets (see Fig. 5.23). Usually, the mitral leaflets are only minimally involved but heavy calcification can significantly restrict leaflet mobility resulting in severe calcific MS. Calcific MS has become increasingly prevalent with increasing life expectancy.[45] There is usually associated calcium in the LVOT, aortic valve, and chordae. There is no chordal thickening or commissural fusion. Calcific MS is frequently mild and rarely severe.[36] Patients with calcific MS are typically elderly and debilitated with multiple comorbidities. Mitral valve area (MVA)

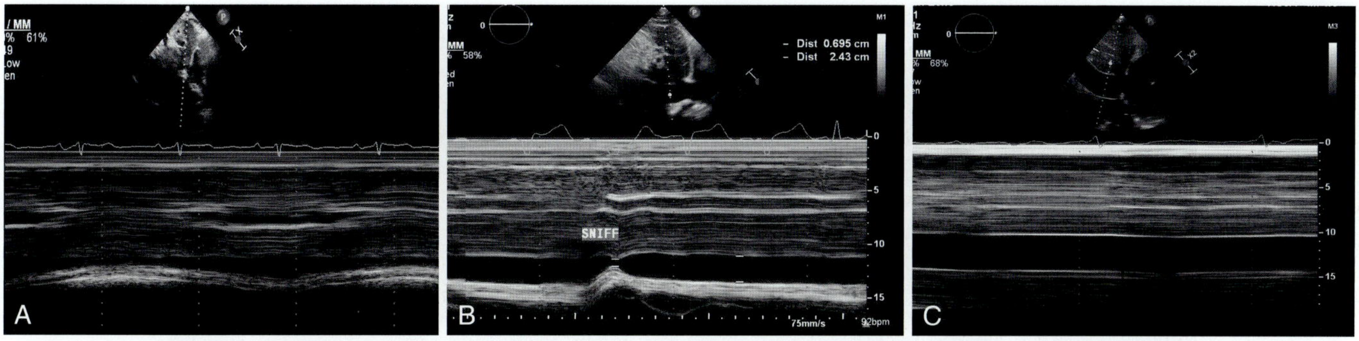

Fig. 5.22 Using IVC to Estimate Right Atrial Pressure. Noninvasive estimate of the right atrial pressure uses IVC diameter and respiratory variation. (A) Right atrial pressure is estimated at 3 mm Hg if IVC is less than 2.1 cm and varies greater than 50% with inspiration. (B) Right atrial pressure is estimated at 8 mm Hg when IVC is normal size without respiratory variation or is dilated with greater than 50% respiratory variation. (C) Right atrial pressure is estimated at 15 mm Hg if IVC is greater than 2.1 cm and varies less than 50% with normal inspiration. The use of the IVC to non invasively estimate right atrial pressure is invalid with mechanical ventilation.

BOX 5.2 Specific Criteria for Severe Mitral Regurgitation[a]

Specific criteria consistent with severe MR[b]

1. Flail leaflet
2. VCW ≥0.7 cm
3. PISA radius ≥1.0 cm at Nyquist limit of 30–40 cm/s
4. Central large jet >50% of LA area
5. Pulmonary vein systolic flow reversal
6. Enlarged left ventricle with normal function

Quantitative measures consistent with severe MR

EROA ≥0.4 cm^2

RVol ≥60 mL

RF ≥50%

[a]Initially, six specific criteria should be assessed. If four out of six specific criteria are present, then severe MR is present. If fewer than four specific criteria are present, then the three additional quantitative measures should be performed to confirm severity.

[b]Definitely severe if at least four specific criteria are present.

EROA, Effective regurgitant orifice area; *LA*, left atrium; *MR*, mitral regurgitation; *PISA*, proximal isovelocity surface area; *RF*, regurgitant fraction; *RVol*, regurgitant volume; *VCW*, vena contracta width.

(From Hung J, Zeng X, Little SH. Quantifying mitral regurgitation: how much should we lean on PISA? *J Am Soc Echocardiogr.* 2018;31(9):1000–1001.)

assessment is challenging in patients with calcific MS. Direct 2D planimetry is difficult due to the heavy calcification. The pressure half-time (PHT) method is inaccurate due to the associated diastolic dysfunction among the elderly. The continuity method is the preferred method in these patients, although an integrated approach should be attempted.[40,41,45] It is necessary to identify the etiology of the MS as certain treatments such as balloon valvuloplasty are contraindicated in calcific MS.

Quantification of Mitral Stenosis

In addition to leaflet morphology, complete echocardiographic assessment of MS should include the mean transmitral gradient, MVA using planimetry and pressure half-time, and secondary changes of relevant chambers including left atrial size, and right heart size, function, and pulmonary artery pressures (Table 5.4).[40]

Transmitral Pressure Gradients

Mean gradient. There is an inverse correlation between the MVA and the diastolic pressure gradient between the LA and the LV. As the MVA decreases, the transmitral diastolic gradient increases. Mitral valve gradient is assessed in the apical views aligning the continuous-wave Doppler to obtain the highest jet velocity. The envelope is traced to calculate a mean mitral valve gradient (Fig. 5.24).[40] Assessment of gradients assumes a normal SV and a normal heart rate. Changes in cardiac output such as anemia, fever, pregnancy, and tachycardia may temporarily increase the gradient without a change in the mitral valve orifice.[42] If the patient is in atrial fibrillation with varying R-R intervals, at least five cardiac cycles should be measured and averaged. Mitral valve gradients were not included in the most recent valvular guidelines due to variability with heart rate and SV, but severe MS is usually associated with a mean gradient greater than 10 mm Hg (Table 5.5).[46] If the patient's symptoms are out of proportion to the findings on the resting echo, consider exercise stress testing.

Mitral Valve Area

Planimetry. When the mitral valve is visualized using 2D echocardiography in a parasternal short axis at the leaflet tips, a tracing of the mitral valve orifice in mid-diastole can be obtained. This is a direct measurement of the anatomic area that is accurate and independent of other confounding variables such as valvular regurgitation or LV diastolic function. Since it may be difficult to determine where the leaflet tips are, 3D planimetry is considered the echocardiographic gold standard for the MVA.[47] This assessment may be difficult when leaflets are heavily calcified. There is a typical fish mouth appearance with rheumatic etiology due to commissural fusion. A normal MVA is 4 to 6 cm^2. Severe MS is a valve area of ≤1.5 cm^2.

Pressure Half-Time

PHT is the time required for the transmitral gradient to reach half of its initial value. As the MVA decreases, pressure half-time increases because it requires more time to flow through a stenotic

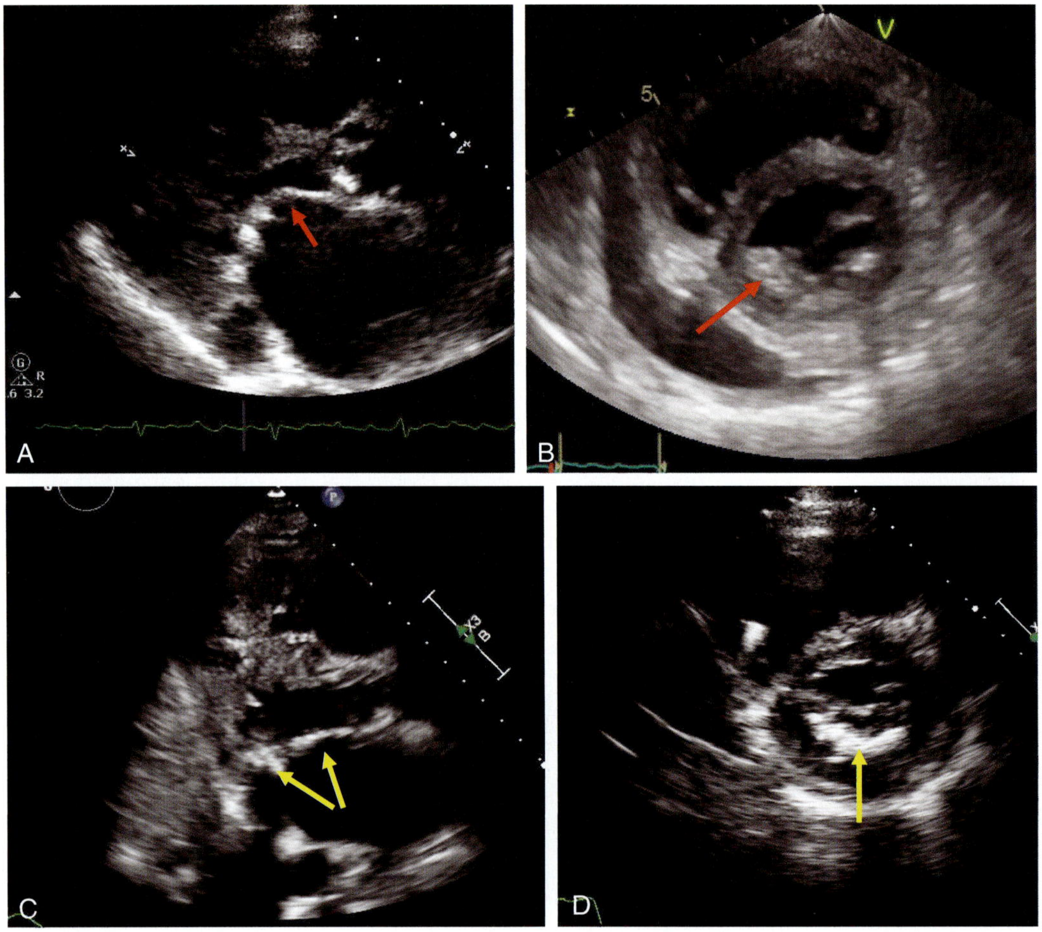

Fig. 5.23 Rheumatic Versus Calcific Mitral Stenosis. (A) Hockey-stick *(red arrow)* appearance of anterior mitral leaflets is consistent with rheumatic mitral stenosis. The hallmark of rheumatic mitral stenosis is commissural fusion, but significant calcification may also be present. (B) Parasternal short-axis mitral valve level showing commissural fusion of medial commissure *(red arrow).* (C) Calcific mitral stenosis starts at the annulus and extends into the base of the leaflets. Parasternal long axis shows heavy calcification of the anterior and posterior mitral leaflets *(yellow arrows).* (D) Significant mitral annular calcium extending into the posterior mitral leaflet.

TABLE 5.3 Assessment of Mitral Valve Anatomy According to the Wilkins Score[a,b]

Grade	Mobility	Thickening	Calcification	Subvalvular Thickening
1	Highly mobile valve with only leaflet tips restricted	Leaflets near normal in thickness (4–5 mm)	A single area of increased echo brightness	Minimal thickening just below the mitral leaflets
2	Leaflet mid and base portions have normal mobility	Mid-leaflets normal, considerable thickening of margins (5–8 mm)	Scattered areas of brightness confined to leaflet margins	Thickening of chordal structures extending to one-third of the chordal length
3	Valve continues to move forward in diastole, mainly from the base	Thickening extending through the entire leaflet (5–8 mm)	Brightness extending into the mid-portions of the leaflets	Thickening extended to distal third of the chords
4	No or minimal forward movement of the leaflets in diastole	Considerable thickening of all leaflet tissue (>8–10 mm)	Extensive brightness throughout much of the leaflet tissue	Extensive thickening and shortening of all chordal structures extending down to the papillary muscles

[a]The total score is the sum of the four items and ranges between 4 and 16.

[b]The Wilkins score is used to predict the feasibility of balloon valvuloplasty in rheumatic mitral stenosis assessing for leaflet mobility, thickening, calcification, and subvalvular calcification. The Wilkins score is the sum of the score (1 to 4) assigned to each variable. A score of less than 8 predicts a good valvuloplasty result. Contraindications to balloon valvuloplasty include greater than mild MR, calcific mitral stenosis and left atrial or left atrial appendage thrombus seen on transesophageal echocardiogram. (From Baumgartner H, Hung J, Bermejo J, et al. Echocardiographic assessment of valve stenosis: EAE/ASE recommendations for clinical practice. *J Am Soc Echocardiogr.* 2009;22(1):1–23, Table 5.)

TABLE 5.4 Evaluation of Mitral Stenosis[a,b]

Measurement	Units	Formula/Method	Concept	Advantages	Disadvantages
Valve Area					
• Planimetry by 2D echo	cm^2	Tracing mitral orifice using 2D echo	Direct measurement of anatomic MVA	Accuracy independence from other factors	• Experience required • Not always feasible (poor acoustic window, severe valve calcification)
• Pressure half-time	cm^2	$220 / T_{1/2}$	Rate of decrease of transmitral flow is inversely proportional to MVA	Easy to obtain	Dependence on other factors (AR, LA compliance, LV diastolic function . . .)
• Continuity equation	cm^2	$MVA = (CSA_{LVOT})(VTI_{Aortic})/VTI_{Mitral}$	Volume flows through mitral and aortic orifices are equal	Independence from flow conditions	• Multiple measurements (source of errors) • Not valid if significant AR or MR
• PISA	cm^2	$MVA = \pi(r^2)(V_{Aliasing}) / \text{peak } V_{Mitral} \alpha / 180^\circ$	MVA assessed by dividing mitral volume flow by the maximum velocity of diastolic mitral flow	Independence from flow conditions	Technically difficult
Mean gradient	mm Hg	$\Delta P = \sum 4v^2 / N$	Pressure gradient calculated from velocity using the Bernoulli equation	Easy to obtain	Dependent on heart rate and flow conditions
Systolic pulmonary artery pressure	mm Hg	$sPAP = 4v^2_{Tricuspid} + \text{RA pressure}$	Addition of RA pressure and maximum gradient between RV and RA	Obtained in most patients with MS	• Arbitrary estimation of RA pressure • No estimation of pulmonary vascular resistance
Mean gradient and systolic pulmonary artery pressure at exercise	mm Hg	$\Delta P = \sum 4v^2 / N$ $sPAP = 4v^2_{Tricuspid} + \text{RA pressure}$	Assessment of gradient and sPAP for increasing workload	Incremental value in assessment of tolerance	• Experience required • Lack of validation for decision-making
Valve resistance	Dyne sec^{-1} cm^{-5}	__MVres = $P_{Mitral} / (CSA_{LVOT})(VTI_{Aortic}) / DFT)$	Resistance to flow caused by MS	Initially suggested to be less flow-dependent, but not confirmed	• No prognostic value • No clear threshold for severity • No additional value vs valve area

[a]Assessment of mitral stenosis should include inspection of leaflet anatomy, planimetry in the short axis (2D or 3D), mean transmitral gradient, pressure half-time, and pulmonary artery systolic pressure.

[b]Level of recommendations: (1) appropriate in all patients *(yellow)*; (2) reasonable when additional information is needed in selected patients *(green)*; and (3) not recommended *(blue)*.

AR, Aortic regurgitation; *CSA*, cross-sectional area; *DFT*, diastolic filling time; *LA*, left atrium; *LV*, left ventricle; *LVOT*, left ventricular outflow tract; *MR*, mitral regurgitation; *MS*, mitral stenosis; *MVA*, mitral valve area; *MVres*, mitral valve resistance; Δ*P*, gradient; *sPAP*, systolic pulmonary artery pressure; *r*, the radius of the convergence hemisphere; *RA*, right atrium; *RV*, right ventricle; *T1/2*, pressure half-time; *v*, velocity; *VTI*, velocity time integral; *N*, number of instantaneous measurements.

(From Baumgartner H, Hung J, Bermejo J, et al. Echocardiographic assessment of valve stenosis: EAE/ASE recommendations for clinical practice. *J Am Soc Echocardiogr*. 2009;22(1):17).

orifice. In the absence of MS, the PHT is decreased as the LV and LA equilibrate rapidly. PHT is easily obtained by acquiring a CW Doppler through the mitral valve and measuring the downslope of the E wave. Short cardiac cycles should be avoided as there may not be enough time for pressure to decrease. If there are two slopes visualized, the initial slope should be ignored and the subsequent slope measured.[40,41] In atrial fibrillation, PHT from five beats should be averaged due to varying R-R intervals. PHT method overestimates MVA when the initial gradient is extremely high such as patients with large ASDs, severe aortic

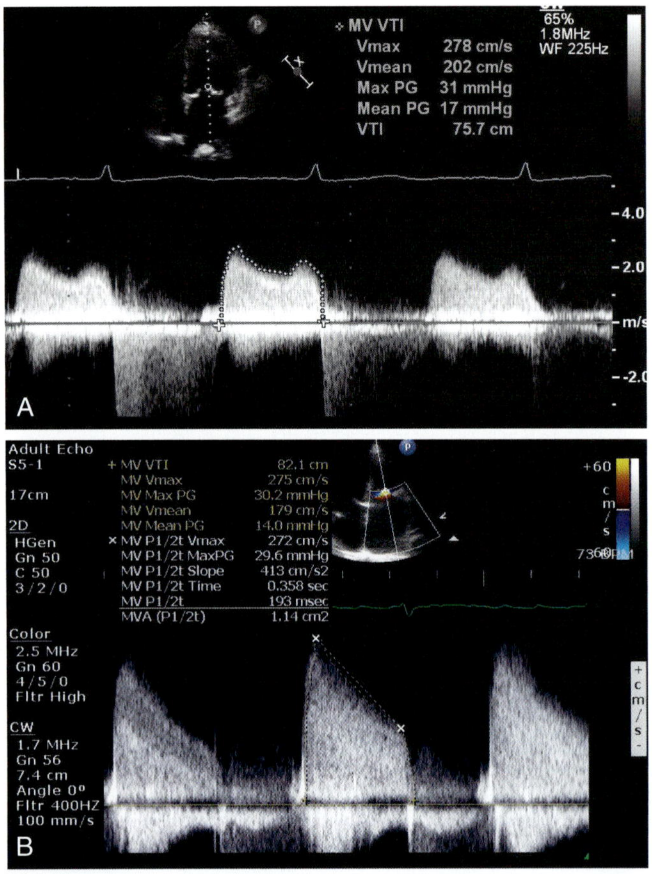

Fig. 5.24 Mitral Stenosis-Pressure Half-Time and Mean Gradient. (A) Mitral inflow envelope is obtained using continuous-wave Doppler from any apical view, which is then traced to obtain a mean transmitral gradient. Severe mitral stenosis is present with a mean gradient of 17 mm Hg at a heart rate of 60 beats/min. Mitral gradients are dependent on diastolic filling time, so heart rate should always be included when discussing mean transmitral gradients. (B) As the valve area decreases, the time required for the left ventricle and left atrium gradients to equilibrate will increase, as measured by pressure half-time (PHT). PHT of 201 m/s yields a mitral valve area of 1.09 cm^2 using the equation MVA = 220/PHT. *MVA,* Mitral valve area.

regurgitation, and diastolic dysfunction. PHT should not be used to assess the MVA immediately post balloon valvuloplasty as the non compliant LV needs time to recover.[48] The empiric equation is MVA (cm^2) = 220/PHT (ms) (see Fig. 5.24).

Continuity equation. In the absence of significant regurgitant lesions, SV across one valve should equal the SV across any other valve. Diastolic SV across the mitral valve should be the same as the systolic stoke volume across the aortic valve. This technique is independent of flow but is cumbersome as multiple measurements are involved. It is not valid if there is significant regurgitation of either the mitral or aortic valve.[40,41] Avoid using the continuity equation in atrial fibrillation due to the multiple measurements and varying R-R intervals. Using the continuity equation (explained in RVs) and knowing three of the variables, the MVA can be calculated (see Table 5.4) as.

$$SV_{MV} = SV_{LVOT}, \text{ thus } MVA \times MV\ VTI = LVOT\ area \times LVOT\ VTI$$

Solving for MVA yields the following equation:

$$MVA = (LVOT\ area \times LVOT\ VTI)/MV\ VTI$$

Proximal isovelocity surface area. Using the same principle as for MR, as the blood flow increases as it approaches a stenotic orifice, it will result in a series of hemispheric rings. Since these rings are not complete hemispheres due to the restriction of the leaflets, the angle of the leaflets must be considered in this calculation.[40,41,49] These measurements are technically difficult to accurately perform. The flow convergence equation for MS includes the angle between the mitral leaflets on the atrial side: $MVA = 2\pi r^2\ V_a/V_1 \times (\theta/180)$ where θ is the angle between the two leaflets in diastole, V_a is the aliasing velocity, and V_1 is the peak MS velocity obtained by CW (see Table 5.4).

Associated Hemodynamic Consequences

See Right Heart in the above section on Assessment of Mitral Regurgitation Severity.

Transthoracic echo is essential to assess the right heart complications of MS including RV failure and pulmonary hypertension. RV size and function must be assessed using 2D/3D imaging of dedicated RV views including volume calculations, TAPSE, and tissue Doppler imaging of lateral tricuspid annulus (RV S′). RV systolic pressure should be assessed using the tricuspid regurgitant jet (see Figs. 5.19–5.22). RV dysfunction and severe pulmonary hypertension are associated with a worse prognosis in patients with MS. TTE also allows assessment of the aortic and tricuspid valve for concurrent rheumatic involvement. Although rheumatic involvement of the aortic valve usually results in aortic stenosis, tricuspid involvement may result in stenosis or regurgitation. TR is more commonly due to RV enlargement resulting in functional TR.

SUMMARY

The etiology of MS should be determined in all patients as therapeutic interventions may differ according to various pathology. Minimally, a mean transmitral diastolic gradient and MVA using direct planimetry and PHT should be performed. If there is discrepant information, consider MVA assessment by the continuity equation or PISA methods. The presence and severity of MR and secondary changes involving LV, LA, and right heart must also be considered.

TABLE 5.5 Stages of Mitral Stenosis[a]

Stage	Definition	Valve Anatomy	Valve Hemodynamics[b]	Hemodynamics Consequences	Symptoms
A	At risk of MS	• Mild valve doming during diastole	• Normal transmitral flow velocity	• None	• None
B	Progressive MS	• Rheumatic valve changes with commissural fusion and diastolic doming of the mitral valve leaflets • Planimetered MVA >1.5 cm^2	• Increased transmitral flow velocities • MVA >1.5 cm^2 • Diastolic pressure half-time <150 ms	• Mild-moderate LS enlargement • Normal pulmonary pressure at rest	• None
C	Asymptomatic severe MS	• Rheumatic valve changes with commissural fusion and diastolic doming of the mitral valve leaflets • Planimetered MVA ≤1.5 cm^2 • (MVA ≤1.0 cm^2 with very severe MS)	• MVA ≤1.5 cm^2 • (MVA ≤1.1 cm^2 with very severe ms) • Diastolic pressure half-time ≥150 ms • (Diastolic pressure half-time ≥220 ms with very severe MS)	• Severe LA enlargement • Elevated PASP >30 mm Hg	• None
D	Symptomatic severe MS	• Rheumatic valve changes with commissural fusion and diastolic doming of the mitral valve leaflets	• MVA ≤1.5 cm^2 • (MVA ≤1.0 cm^2 with very severe MS) • Diastolic pressure half-time ≥150 ms • (Diastolic pressure half-time ≥220 ms with very severe MS)	• Severe LA enlargement • Elevated PASP >30 mm Hg	• Decreased exercise tolerance • Exertional dyspnea

[a]Stages of rheumatic mitral valve disease ranging from at risk of MS (Stage A) to severe symptomatic MS (Stage D). Each stage is defined by valve anatomy, hemodynamics, LA size, RV systolic pressure, and symptoms. Mean transmitral pressure gradient is not included due to its variability with heart rates, but severe mitral stenosis will usually correspond to a gradient greater than 10 mm Hg.

[b]The transmitral mean pressure gradient should be obtained to further determine the hemodynamic effect of the MS and is usually greater than 5 to 10 mm Hg in severe MS; however, due to the variability of the mean pressure gradient with heart rate and forward flow, it has not been included in the criteria for severity.

LA, left atrial; *MS*, mitral stenosis; *MVA*, mitral valve area; and *PASP*, pulmonary artery systolic pressure; *RV*, right ventricule.(From Nishimura RA, Otto CM, Bonow RO, et al. 2014 ACC/AHA Guidelines for the management of patients with valvular heart disease. *J Am Coll Cardiol.* 2014;63:2438–2488.)

CASE-BASED ASSESSMENT

An 82-year-old female with recent anterior ST-elevation myocardial infarction treated with percutaneous coronary intervention of mid percutaneous coronary intervention of mid left anterior descending coronary artery (mid-LAD) presents to the office with worsening dyspnea on exertion. She denies chest discomfort at the visit today. Her blood pressure is 105/65 mm Hg, pulse is 82 beats/min, and oxygen saturation is 94% on room air. An echocardiogram was performed (see Figs. 5.25–5.27 and Videos 5.19–5.24):

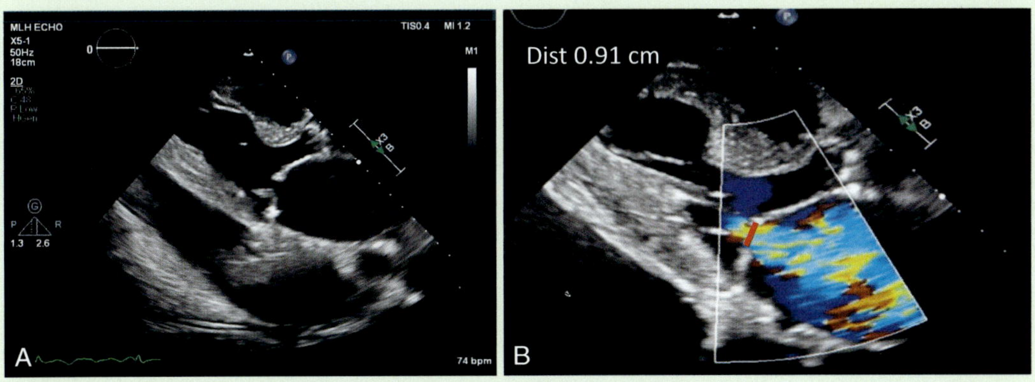

Fig. 5.25 Parasternal Long-Axis View. Still frame of a 2D parasternal long-axis view. (A) Failure of anterior and posterior mitral leaflets to coapt. Left pleural effusion is also visualized. (B) Color-flow regurgitant jet occupies greater than 50% of the left atrium. Vena contracta width is .9 cm.

Continued

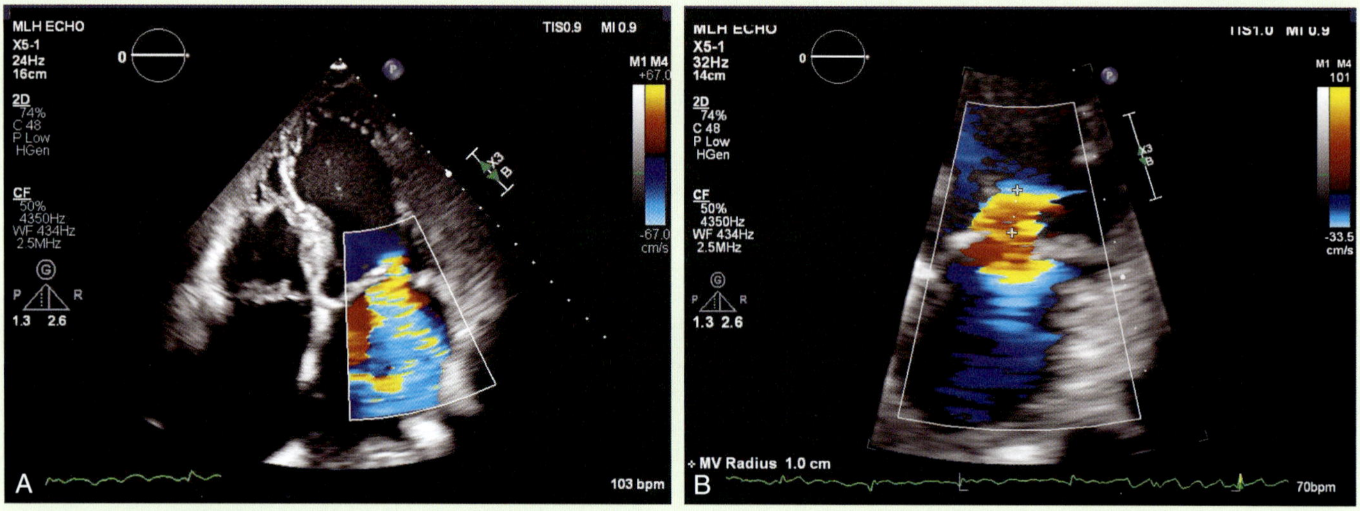

Fig. 5.26 **Apical 4-Chamber.** (A) Still frame of an apical 4-chamber view. Color-flow regurgitant jet occupies greater than 50% of the left atrium. (B) Zoomed-in view after changing Nyquist limit demonstrating proximal isovelocity surface area radius of 1 cm at an aliasing velocity of 33.5 cm/s.

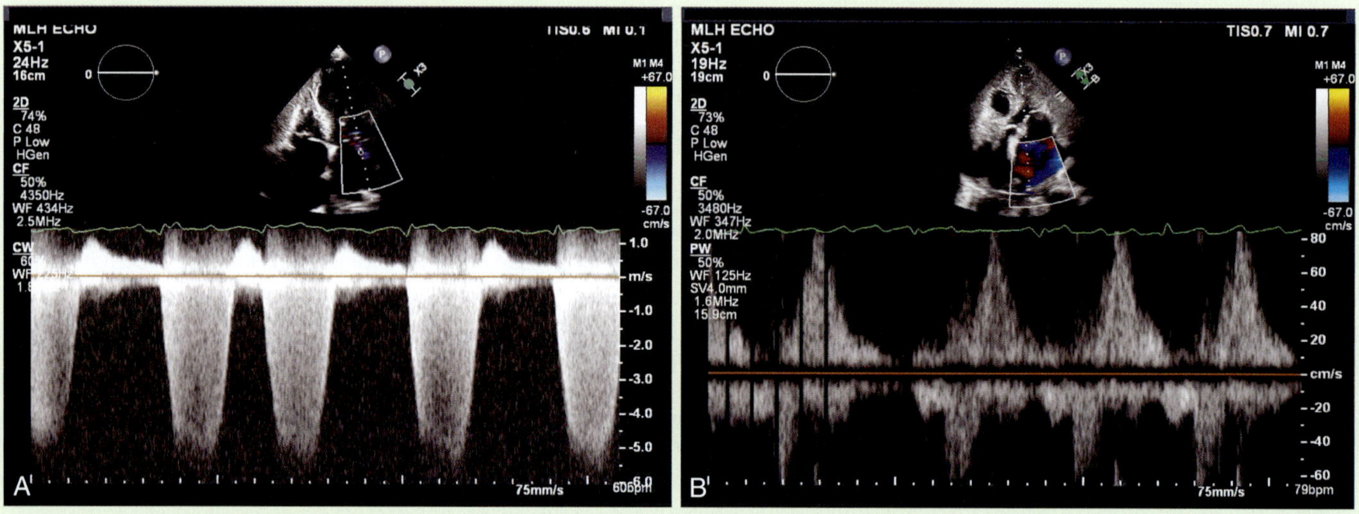

Fig. 5.27 (A) Continuous-wave Doppler of the mitral regurgitation (MR) jet demonstrates an MR envelope similar in intensity with the antegrade mitral inflow above the baseline. (B) Pulsed-wave Doppler of the pulmonary vein showing systolic reversal.

Questions

1. What is the mechanism of the mitral regurgitation?
   a. Primary MR due to flail leaflet
   b. Primary MR due to prolapsed posterior leaflet
   c. Secondary (functional) MR due to ischemic cardiomyopathy
   d. Unable to determine, consider other imaging for work-up
2. What is the severity of the mitral regurgitation?
   a. Mild
   b. Moderate
   c. Severe
   d. Unable to assess
3. What left ventricle remodeling findings are specific for chronic, severe mitral regurgitation?
   a. Dilated left ventricular cavity
   b. Concentric left ventricular hypertrophy
   c. Normal left ventricular cavity size, but a dilated left atrial size should be present
   d. Normal left ventricular cavity size, but a dilated right ventricle should be present
4. What would you expect the E wave of the mitral inflow to be in this case (measured in m/s)?
   a. Less than 0.8 m/s
   b. Between 0.8 and 1.0 m/s
   c. Greater than 1.2 m/s
   d. Unable to predict
5. What is the next step in treating this patient's mitral regurgitation?
   a. Medication such as diuretics and then re-evaluate MR severity
   b. TEE to assess etiology of MR more accurately
   c. Cardiac MRI to determine severity of MR more accurately
   d. Schedule for surgery

See page 315 for the answers.

REFERENCES

1. Bonow RO, O'Gara PT, Adams DH, et al. 2020 focused update of the 2017 ACC expert consensus decision pathway on the management of mitral regurgitation. *J Am Coll Cardiol.* 2020;75:2236–2270.
2. Zoghbi WA, Adams D, Bonow RO, et al. Recommendations for noninvasive evaluation of native valvular regurgitation: a report from the American Society of Echocardiography developed in collaboration with the society for cardiovascular magnetic resonance. *J Am Soc Echocardiogr.* 2017;30:303–371.
3. Baumgartner H, Falk V, Bax JJ, et al. 2017 ESC/EATS Guidelines for the Management of Valvular Heart Disease. *Eur Heart J.* 2017;38:2739–2791.
4. Uretsky S, Argulian E, Supariwala A, et al. A comparative assessment of echocardiographic parameters for determining primary mitral regurgitation severity using magnetic resonance imaging as a reference standard. *JASE.* 2018;31:992–999.
5. Grayburn PA, She L, Roberts BL, et al. Comparison of transesophageal and transthoracic echocardiographic measurements of mechanism and severity of mitral regurgitation in ischemic cardiomyopathy (from the STICH trial). *Am J Cardiol.* 2015;116(6):913–918.
6. Messika-Zeitoun D, Bellamy M, Avierinos JF, et al. Left atrial remodeling in mitral regurgitation-methodologic approach, physiological determinants, and outcome implications: a prospective quantitative Doppler-echocardiographic and electron beam-computed tomographic study. *Eur Heart J.* 2007;28:1773 –181.
7. Nishimura RA, Otto CM, Bonow RO, et al. 2017 AHA/ACC focused update of the 2014 AHA/ACC guideline for the management of patients with valvular heart disease: a report of the American College of Cardiology/American Heart Association Task Force on Clinical Practice Guidelines. *J Am Coll Cardiol.* 2017;70:252–289.
8. Sabbagh AE, Reddy YN, Nishimura R. Mitral valve regurgitation in the contemporary era. *JACC Cardiovasc Imaging.* 2018;11(4):628–643.
9. Griffin BP. Myxomatous mitral valve disease. In: Otto CM, Bonow RO, eds. *Valvular Heart Disease.* Philadelphia: Saunders; 2009:243–259.
10. Topilsky Y, Michelena H, Bichara V, et al. Mitral valve prolapse with mid-late systolic mitral regurgitation: pitfalls of evaluation and clinical outcome compared with holosystolic regurgitation. *Circulation.* 2012;125:1643–1651.
11. Esssayagh BE, Saggag A, Antoine C, et al. Presentation an outcome of arrhythmic mitral valve prolapse. *J Am Coll Cardiol.* 2020;76(6):637–649.
12. Lee AP-W, Jin C-N, Fan Y, et al. Functional implication of mitral annular disjunction in mitral valve prolapse: a quantitative dynamic 3D echocardiographic study. *JACC Cardiovasc Imaging.* 2017;10:1424–1433.
13. Lancellotti P, Moura L, Pierard LA, et al. European Association of Echocardiography recommendations for the assessment of valvular regurgitation. Part 2: mitral and tricuspid regurgitation (native valve disease). *Eur J Echocardiogr.* 2010;11:307.
14. Lang RM, Badano LP, Mor-Avi V, et al. Recommendations for cardiac chamber quantification by echocaradiography in adults: an updated for the American Society of Echocardiography and the European Association of Echocardiography and the European Association of Cardiovascular Imaging. *J Am Soc Echo.* 2015;28:1–39.
15. Levine RA, Schwammenthal E. Ischemic mitral regurgitation on the threshold of a solution: from paradoxes to unifying concepts. *Circulation.* 2005;112:745–758.
16. Grayburn PA, Carabello B, Hung J, et al. Defining "severe" secondary mitral regurgitation: emphasizing an integrated approach. *J Am Coll Cardiol.* 2014;64:2792–2801.
17. Gelsomino S, van Garsel, Luca F, et al. Left ventricular strain in chronic ischemic mitral regurgitation; mechanisms and echocardiographic classification. *J Am Soc Echocardiogr.* 2013;26:370–380.
18. Levine RA, Messas E, Nathan NS, et al. New understanding of ischemic mitral regurgitation: the marionette and its masters. *Eur J Echocardiogr.* 2004;15:313–317.
19. Grayburn PA, Sannino A, Packer M. Proportionate and disproportionate functional mitral regurgitation: a new conceptual framework that reconciles the results of the MITRA-FR and COAPT trials. *JACC Cardiovasc Imaging.* 2019;12:353–362.
20. Zoghbi WA, Enriquez-Sarano M, Foster E, et al. Recommendations for evaluation of the severity of native valvular regurgitation with two-dimensional and Doppler echocardiography. *J Am Soc Echocardiogr.* 2003;16:777–802.
21. Enriquez-Sarano M, Tajik AJ, Bailey KR, et al. Color flow imaging compared with quantitative Doppler assessment of severity of mitral regurgitation: influence of eccentricity of jet and mechanism of regurgitation. *J Am Coll Cardiol.* 1993;21:1211–1219.
22. Grayburn PA, Weissman NJ, Zamorano JL. Quantitation of mitral regurgitation. *Circulation.* 2012;126:2005–2017.
23. Tharendiranathan P, Phelan D, Collier P, et al. Quantitative assessment of mitral regurgitation: how best to do it. *JACC Cardiovasc Imaging.* 2012;5:1161–1175.
24. -Bertrand PB, Nagata Y, Namasivayam M, et al. The artifact that tells the truth: color doppler splay unmasking significant mitral regurgitation. *J Am Soc Echocardiogr.* 2020;33(10):1220–1222.
25. Chen CG, Thomas JD, Anconina J, et al. Impact of impinging wall jet on color Doppler quantification of mitral regurgitation. *Circulation.* 1991;84:712–720.
26. Wiener PC, Friend EJ, Bhargav R, et al. Color Doppler splay: a clue to the presence of significant mitral regurgitation. *J Am Soc Echocardiogr.* 2020;33(10):1212–1219 e1.
27. Hung J, Zeng X, Little S. Quantifying mitral regurgitation: how much should we lean on PISA?. *J Am Soc Echocardiogr.* 2018;31:1000–1001.
28. Quader N, Katta P, Najib MQ, et al. Effect of mitral inflow pattern on diagnosis of severe mitral regurgitation in patients with chronic organic mitral regurgitation. *J Cardiovasc Ultrasound.* 2013;21(4):165–170.
29. Tribouilloy C, Rusinaru D, Szymanski C, et al. Predicting let ventricular dysfunction after valve repair for mitral regurgitation due to leaflet prolapse: additive value of left ventricular end-systolic dimension to ejection fraction. *Eur J Echocardiogr.* 2011;12: 702–710.
30. Quintana E, Suri RM, Thalji NM, et al. Left ventricular dysfunction after mitral valve repair-the fallacy of "normal" preoperative myocardial function. *J Thorac Cardiovasc Surg.* 2014;148: 2752–2760.
31. Lancellotti P, Cosyns B, Zacharakis D, et al. Importance of left ventricular longitudinal function and functional reserve in patients with degenerative mitral regurgitation: assessment by two-dimensional speckle tracking. *J Am Soc Echocardiogr.* 2008;21:1331–1336.
32. Witkowski TG, Thomas JD, Debonnaire PJ, et al. Global longitudinal strain predicts left ventricular dysfunction after mitral valve repair. *Eur Heart J Cardiovasc Imaging.* 2013;14:69–76.
33. Messika-Zeitoun D, Bellamy M, Avierinos JF, et al. Left atrial remodeling in mitral regurgitation-methodologic approach, physiological determinants, and outcome implications: a prospective

quantitative Doppler-echocardiographic and electron beam-computed tomographic study. *Eur Heart J.* 2007;28:1773–1781.
34. Rudski LG, Wyman WL, Afialo J, et al. Guidelines for the echocardiographic assessment of the right heart in adults: a report from the American Society of Echocardiography. *J Am Soc Echocardiogr.* 2010;23:685–713.
35. Bruce CJ, Connolly HM. Right-sided valve disease deserves a little more respect. *Circulation.* 2009;119:2726–2734.
36. Nath J, Foster E, Heidenreich PA. Impact of tricuspid regurgitation on long-term survival. *J Am Coll Cardiol.* 2004;43:405–409.
37. Dreyfus GD, Corbi PJ, Chan KM, et al. Secondary tricuspid regurgitation or dilatation: which should be the criteria for surgical repair?. *Ann Thorac Surg.* 2005;79:127–132.
38. Van de Veire NR, Braun J, Delgado V, et al. Tricuspid annuloplasty prevents right ventricular dilatation and progression of tricuspid regurgitation in patients with tricuspid annular dilatation undergoing mitral valve repair. *J Thorac Cardiovasc Surg.* 2011;141:1431–1439.
38. Chikwe J, Itagaki S, Anyanwu A, et al. Impact of concomitant tricuspid anuloplasty on tricuspid regurgitation, right ventricular function and pulmonary artery hypertension after repair of mitral valve prolapse. *J Am Coll Cardiol.* 2015;65:1931–1938.
40. Baumgartner H, Hung J, Bermejo J, et al. Echocardiographic assessment of valve stenosis: EAE/ASE recommendations for clinical practice. *J Am Soc Echocardiogr.* 2009;22(1):1–23.
41. Vahanian A, Baumgartner H, Bax J, et al. Guidelines on the management of valvular heart disease: the task force on the management of valvular heart disease of the European Society of Cardiology. *Eur Heart J.* 2007;28:230–268.
42. Carabello BA. Modern management of mitral stenosis. *Circulation.* 2005;112(3):432–437.
43. Wilkins GT, Weyman AE, Abascal VM, et al. Percutaneous balloon dilatation of the mitral valve: an analysis of echocardiographic variables related to outcome and the mechanism of dilatation. *Br Heart J.* 1988;60:299–308.
44. Nunes MC, Tan TC, Elmariah S, et al. The echo score revisited: Impact of incorporating commissural morphology and leaflet displacement to the prediction of outcomes for patients undergoing percutaneous mitral valvuloplasty. *Circulation.* 2014;129:886–895.
45. Kato N, Padang R, Scott CG, et al. The natural history of severe calcific mitral stenosis. *J Am Coll Cardiol.* 2020;75(24):3048–3057.
46. Nishimura RA, Otto CM, Bonow RO, et al. 2014 ACC/AHA Guidelines for the management of patients with valvular heart disease. *J Am Coll Cardiol.* 2014;63:2438–2488.
47. Schlosshan D, Aggarwal G, Mathur G, et al. Real-time 3D transesophageal echocardiography for the evaluation of rheumatic mitral stenosis. *JACC Cardiovasc Imaging.* 2011;4(6):580–588.
48. Thomas JD, Wilkins GT, Choong CY, et al. Inaccuracy of mitral pressure half-time immediately after percutaneous mitral valvotomy. Dependence of transmitral gradient and left atrial and ventricular compliance. *Circulation.* 1988;78(4):980–993.
49. Rodriguez L, Thomas JD, Monterroso V, et al. Validation of the proximal flow convergence method. Calculation of orifice area in patients with mitral stenosis. *Circulation.* 1993;88(3):1157–1165.

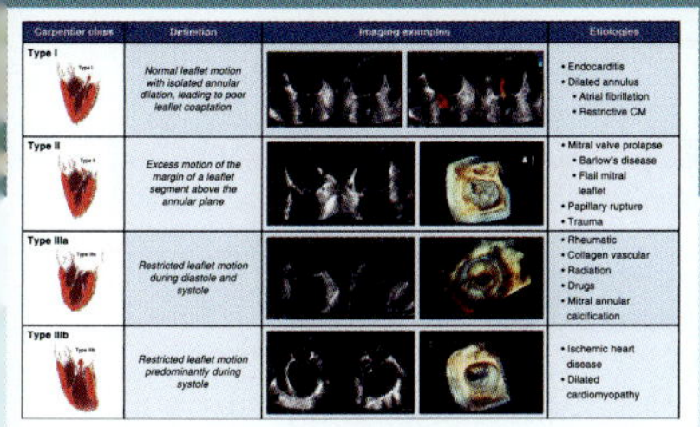

6

Diagnostic Tools: Transesophageal Echocardiography for Mitral Valve

Rebecca T. Hahn

CHAPTER OUTLINE

LEARNING OBJECTIVES

- Transesophageal echocardiography is the imaging modality of choice to evaluate the mitral valve complex prior to transcatheter interventions
- A comprehensive assessment of the mitral valve for interventions includes defining the morphology, etiology, and severity of disease
- Quantifying mitral regurgitation severity at baseline, intraprocedurally, and at follow-up requires a multi-parametric and multi-modality (two- [2D] and three-dimensional [3D]) echocardiographic assessment.

INTRODUCTION

With the addition of transcatheter edge-to-edge repair (TEER) for mitral regurgitation (MR) to the current American College of Cardiology/American Heart Association Guideline for the Management of Patients With Valvular Heart Disease[1] transcatheter mitral interventions have become an essential treatment option for patients with both primary and secondary MR. Transesophageal echocardiography (TEE) is the imaging modality of choice for determining anatomic suitability for[1,2] and procedural guidance.[3,4] The role of three-dimensional (3D) TEE for defining complex mitral anatomical details[5–9] and MR severity has become indisputable.[10] A number of other transcatheter devices are also in development or clinical trials. The basic TEE imaging protocol[2] prior to intervention will be discussed as well as the anatomic considerations for mitral valve (MV) transcatheter therapies.

GENERAL TRANSESOPHAGEAL ECHOCARDIOGRAPHY IMAGING PROTOCOL FOR THE MITRAL VALVE

Mid-Esophageal Views (Table 6.1)

Due to the oblique orientation of the mitral apparatus relative to the anatomical axes of the body, the anterior and posterior mitral valve (MV) leaflets are oriented in a more anterosuperior and posteroinferior position.[11,12] The esophagus is positioned directly posterior to the lateral roof of the left atrium (LA). Thus to position the probe over the dome of the LA with the annulus perpendicular to the insonation beam, one will typically use right flexion and retroflection. With the annulus perpendicular to the ultrasound beam and centered in the sector, continuous mechanical rotation or simultaneous biplane imaging results in on-axis imaging of the MV from all views. The mid-esophageal

TABLE 6.1 Standard Mid-Esophageal Imaging Planes of the Mitral Valvel

TEE view	Three-D model	2D TEE example	Acquisition	Structures imaged
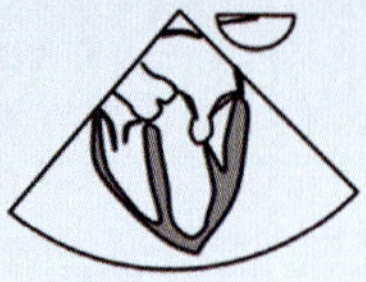 **ME five chamber**	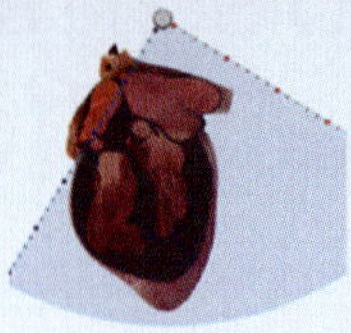	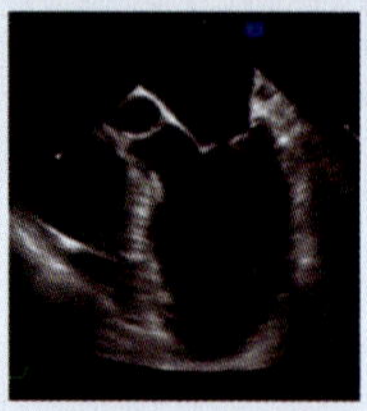	**Transducer angle:** ~ 0 to 20° **Level:** Mid-esophageal **Maneuver** (from prior image): NA	Aortic value LVOT Left atrium Right atrium Left ventricle Right ventricle IVS Mitral valve (A1/2, P1/2) Tricuspid valve
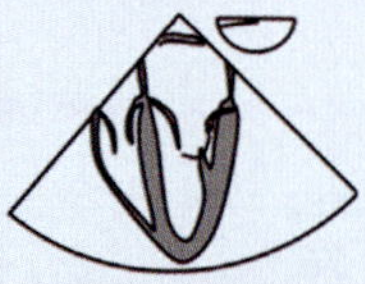 **ME four chamber**	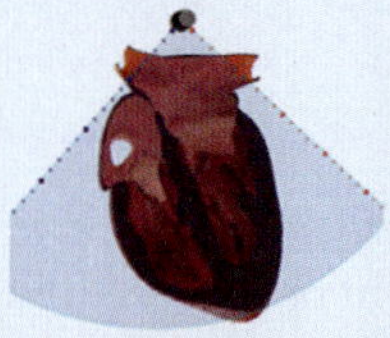	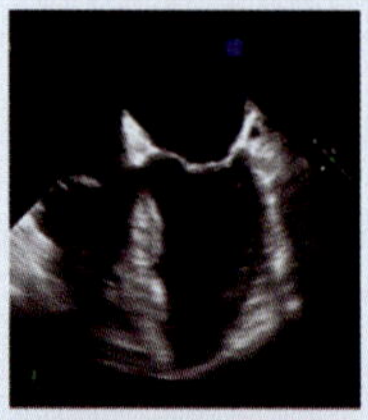	**Transducer angle:** ~ 0 to 10° **Level:** Mid-esophageal **Maneuver** (from prior image): Advance ± retroflex	Left atrium Right atrium IAS Left ventricle Right ventricle IVS Mitral valve (A2/3, P1/2) Tricuspid valve
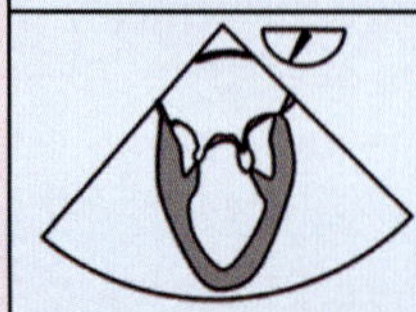 **ME intercommissural**	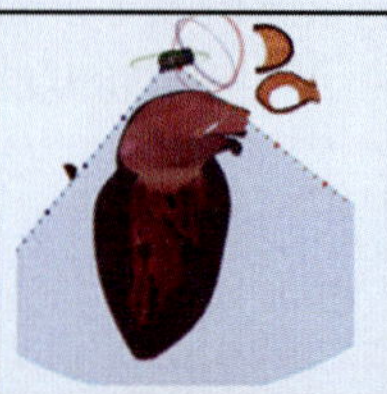	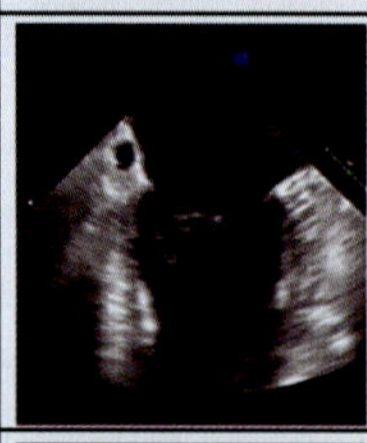	**Transducer angle:** ~ 60 to 75° **Level:** Mid-esophageal **Maneuver** (from prior image): NA	Left atrium Coronary sinus Left ventricle Mitral valve (P3, A2, P1) Papillary muscles Chordae tendinae
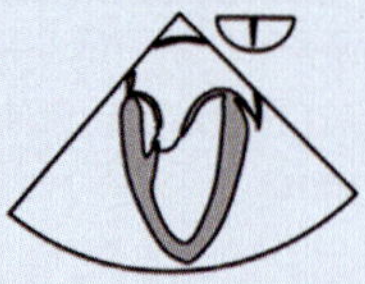 **ME two chamber**	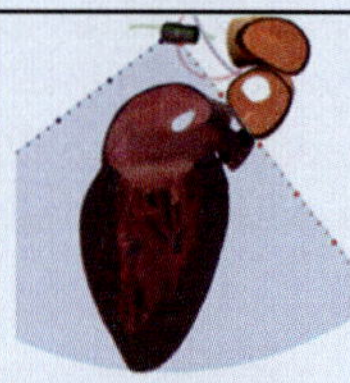	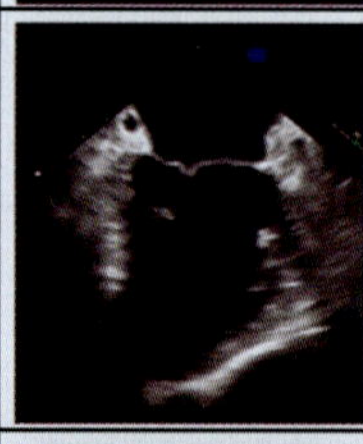	**Transducer angle:** ~ 80 to 100° **Level:** Mid-esophageal **Maneuver** (from prior image): NA	Left atrium Coronary sinus Left atrial appendage Left ventricle Mitral valve (P3, A2/A1)
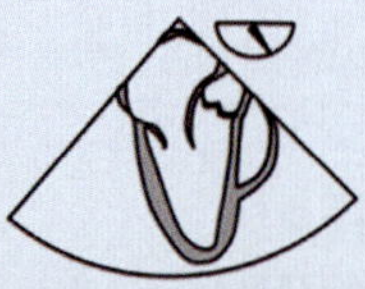 **ME three chamber**	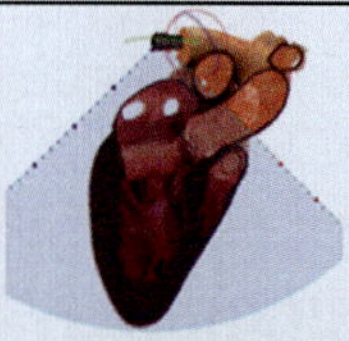	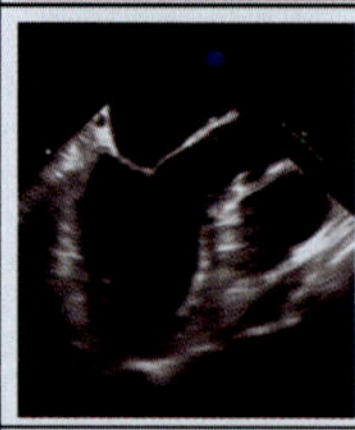	**Transducer angle:** ~ 110 to 130° **Level:** Mid-esophageal **Maneuver** (from prior image): NA	Left atrium Left ventricle LVOT RVOT Mitral valve (A2, P2) Aortic value Proximal ascending aorta
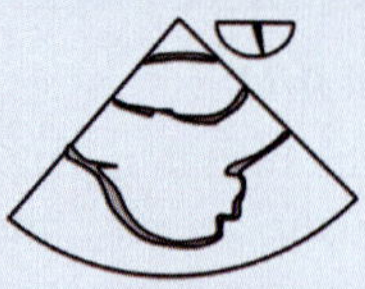 **ME bicaval**	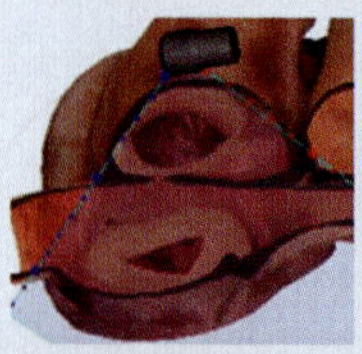	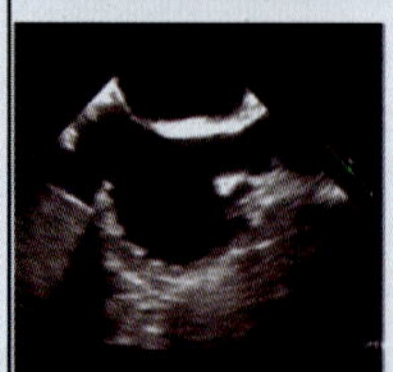	**Transducer angle:** ~ 90 to 120° **Level:** Mid-esophageal **Maneuver** (from prior image): Withdraw	Left atrium Right atrium/appendage IAS Superior vena cava Inferior vena cava
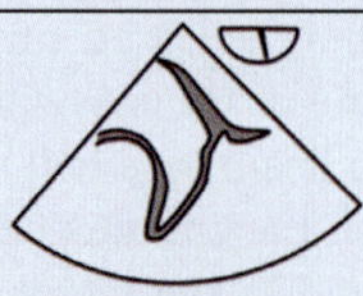 **ME left atrial appendage and let pulmonary veins**	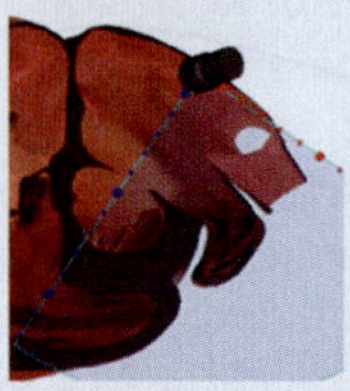	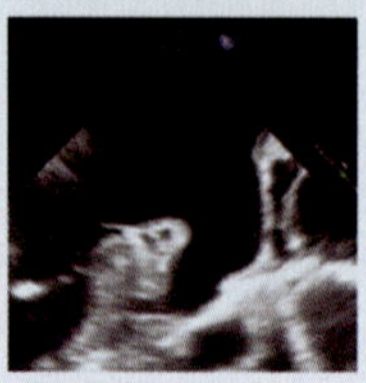	**Transducer angle:** ~ 0 to 120° **Level:** Mid-esophageal **Maneuver** (from prior image): Advance	Left atrial appendage Left upper pulmonary vein

Abbreviations: IAS = interatrial septum, IVS = interventricular septum, LVOT = left ventricular outflow tract, ME = mid esophageal, RVOT = right ventricular outflow tract

(Modified from Hahn RT, Abraham T, Adams MS, et al. Guidelines for performing a comprehensive transesophageal echocardiographic examination: recommendations from the American Society of Echocardiography and the Society of Cardiovascular Anesthesiologists. *J Am Soc Echocardiogr.* 2013;26(9):921–264.)

(ME) 4-chamber view is usually acquired with a mechanical rotation of 0 to 20 degrees. Withdrawing the probe (and/or anteflexion) will bring the lateral commissure into view while advancing the probe (and/or retroflection) images more medial structures. The ME mitral commissural view (50 to 70 degrees) should aim for a symmetric display of papillary muscle heads and chords. Clockwise and counterclockwise rotation of the TEE probe moves the imaging plane anteriorly and posteriorly, respectively. The left atrial appendage (LAA) offers a clear landmark for the anterolateral commissure and the A_1/P_1 scallops, whereas the atrial septum is adjacent to the posteromedial commissure and the A_3/P_3 scallops. Biplane imaging from the ME commissural view images the ME long-axis view in the orthogonal view. A biplane sweep from the A_1/P_1 (lateral) scallops on the right side of the screen to the A_3/P_3 (medial) scallops on the left side of the screen images the entire line of coaptation. The single plane ME long-axis view (120 to 140 degrees) typically images the A_2/P_2 scallops; however, the clockwise rotation will image the medial commissure, and counterclockwise rotation will image the lateral commissure. Because the relationship of the MV and aortic valve AV is variable, aligning the AV in the ME long-axis view may not always image the same scallops, and confirmation using 3D imaging is always recommended.

Understanding the orientation of the 2D biplane and 3D rendered image is integral to identifying MV pathology. From the ME commissural view (50 to 70 degrees), the acquired 3D volume is rotated to view the MV view from the atrial perspective with the aorta at the 6 o'clock position. To generate the surgical en-face view, the image is then rotated 180 degrees to position the aortic valve at 12 o'clock and the posterior MV leaflet in the far field. Because of this 180-degree rotation, the A_1/P_1 (lateral) scallops are on the left side of the screen, and the A_3/P_3 (medial) scallops are on the right side of the screen: opposite to the 2D imaging described above.

The following parameters should be acquired from the ME views: color Doppler of the MR with and without baseline shift, continuous-wave (CW) Doppler for transmitral diastolic and systolic spectral flow profiles, pulse-wave (PW) Doppler at the mitral leaflet tips and annular plane, PW Doppler of the pulmonary vein inflow, and 3D volumes with and without color Doppler. From these acquisitions, the following can be measured: mitral inflow E velocity, vena contracta and MR jet size, peak/mean transmitral gradients, pressure halftime, MR VTI, planimetry of the valve area or vena contracta area,[13] quantitation of regurgitant volume. Doppler interrogation of the pulmonary venous inflow should be performed on both left and right veins.

Transgastric Views (Table 6.2)

Although ME 3D imaging of the MV has replaced transgastric (TG) imaging for identification of leaflet pathology and location of the regurgitant orifice, this level of imaging can still be used to confirm MV pathology (with and without color Doppler), visualize the sub-valvular apparatus (chordae and papillary muscle), perform CW Doppler measurements, particularly with eccentric (typically commissural) jets, and quantify forward stroke volume (across the left ventricular [LV] or right ventricular [RV] outflow tract).

TABLE 6.2 Standard Transgastric Imaging Planes of the Mitral Valve

TEE view	Three-D model	2D TEE example	Acquisition	Structures imaged
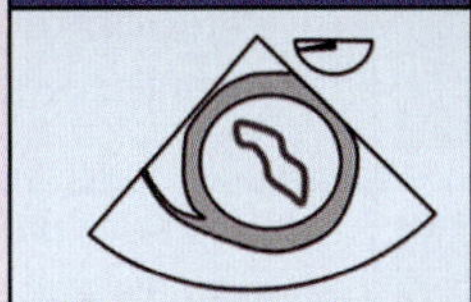 **TG basal short-axis**	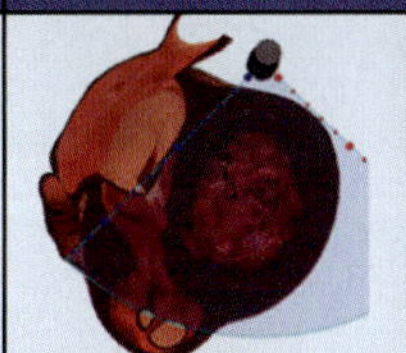	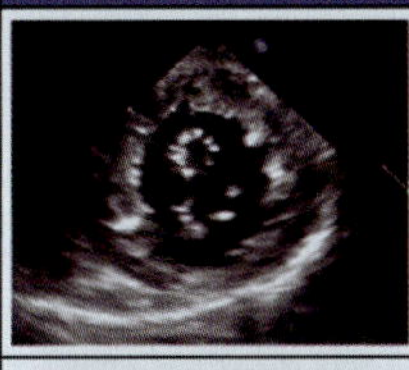	**Transducer angle:** ~ 0 to 20° **Level:** Transgastric **Maneuver** (from prior image): Advance ± anteflex	Left ventricle (base) Right ventricle (base) Mitral valve (short-axis) Tricuspid valve (short-axis)
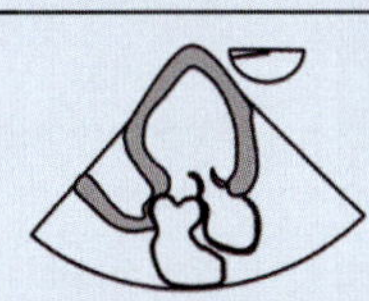 **DT five chamber**	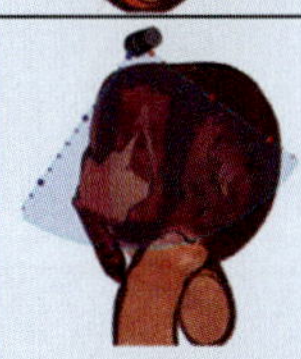	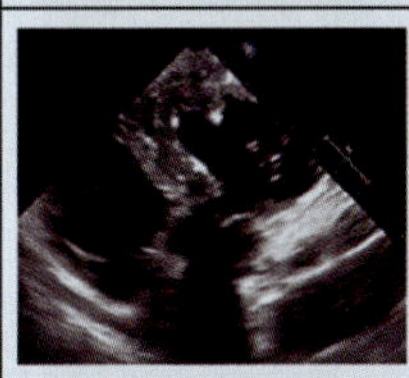	**Transducer angle:** ~ 0 to 20° **Level:** Transgastric **Maneuver** (from prior image): Left- flex, advance, anteflex	Left ventricle Left ventricular outflow tract Right ventricle Aortic valve Aortic root Mitral valve
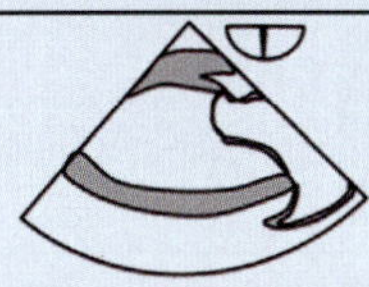 **TG two chamber**	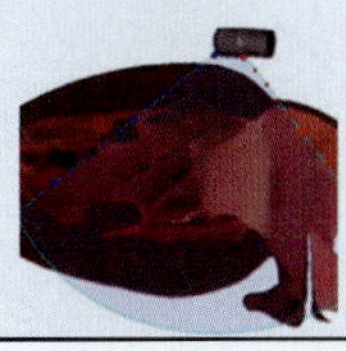	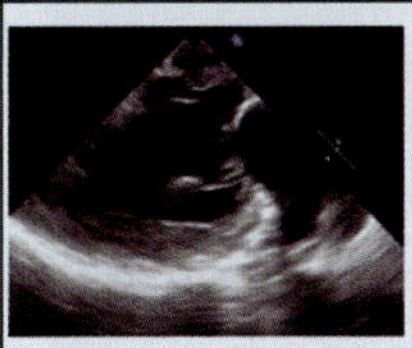	**Transducer angle:** ~ 90 to 110° **Level:** Transgastric **Maneuver** (from prior image): Neutral flexion, withdraw	Left ventricle Left atrium/appendage Mitral valve

Abbreviations: DT = deep transgastric, TG = transgastric

(Modified from Hahn RT, Abraham T, Adams MS, et al. Guidelines for performing a comprehensive transesophageal echocardiographic examination: recommendations from the American Society of Echocardiography and the Society of Cardiovascular Anesthesiologists. *J Am Soc Echocardiogr.* 2013;26(9):921–964.)

SPECIFIC TRANSESOPHAGEAL ECHOCARDIOGRAPHY IMAGING PROTOCOL FOR THE MITRAL VALVE INTERVENTIONS

Assessment of Mitral Valve Leaflets

The morphologic classification for MR based on leaflet mobility is the Carpentier classification (Fig. 6.1).[14] Type I MR involves normal mobility of leaflets with poor coaptation due to annular dilation or perforation or cleft/indentations of a leaflet. Type II MR involves excessive excess motion of the margin of a leaflet segment above the annular plane. Type III disease is associated with restricted mobility of leaflets, resulting in the coaptation of leaflets in the ventricular level. This attenuated mobility can be diastolic and systolic (Type IIIa) or just systolic (Type IIIb).

In addition to the classification of leaflet mobility, MR is also classified as primary or secondary disease. Although primary MR may be caused by Carpentier Type I (perforation or cleft) and Type IIIA (leaflet/chordal thickening) diseases, mitral valve prolapse (Type II) is the most common cause of chronic primary MR and is defined by an overriding of the annulus by a leaflet edge with a displacement of the coaptation point into the atrium. Leaflet 'flail' implies coaptation failure with eversion of the free edge of a leaflet into the LA, usually consequent to chordal rupture. The two main etiologies of secondary MR are annular dilatation or atriogenic MR (Carpentier Type I) and leaflet tethering from a ventricular disease (Carpentier IIIA). A number of mechanisms may contribute to malcoaptation of the MV leaflets in secondary MR: (1) global and/or regional LV dilatation/dysfunction, which decreases the closing forces of the leaflets, (2) displacement of the papillary muscles with tethering of the leaflets into the ventricular cavity which outweighs the closing forces, (3) dilatation and dysfunction of the annulus, and (4) inadequate leaflet adaptation to ventricular or atrial enlargement.[15–18] The anatomic features associated with these mechanisms thus predict the assessment of MR severity (Table 6.3) as well as recurrence following surgical repair: mitral leaflet tethering and restricted closure, asymmetric displacement and abnormal contraction of the LV wall underlying the papillary muscles, decreased shortening of the distance between the papillary muscles and increased LV sphericity.[16,19]

Multiple parameters may be used to determine anatomic feasibility for TEER devices. These include the location of the primary MR jet or leaflet abnormality, coaptation depth, coaptation length, coaptation (or flail) gap, and malcoaptation width. In addition, the presence of clefts or deep folds, multiple prolapsing segments or MR jets, very large coaptation gaps or widths, calcification or marked restriction of leaflet mobility, and small mitral orifice areas may all reduce the chances of an optimal TEER result. Leaflet lengths will also determine the feasibility of TEER device stability, and depending on the device, >7 to 10 mm of leaflet length may be required.

Assessment of Mitral Annulus

The mitral annulus is not a single, well-defined ring of connective tissue but is instead a multifaceted structure made up of the

Carpentier class	Definition	Imaging examples	Etiologies

Type I 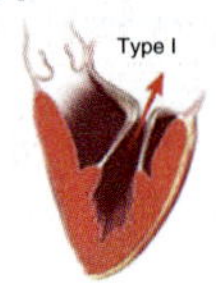	*Normal leaflet motion with isolated annular dilation, leading to poor leaflet coaptation*	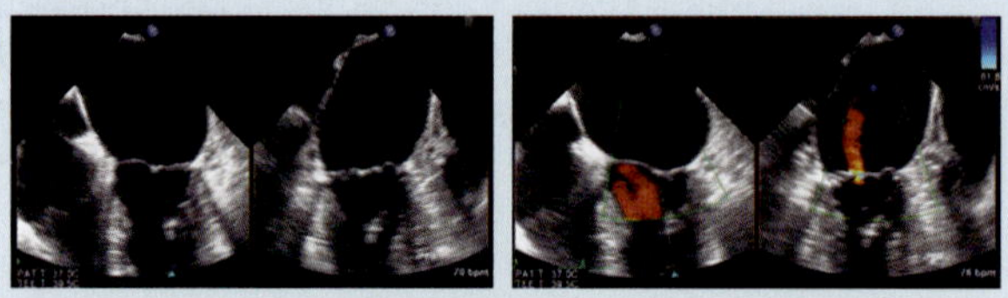	• Endocarditis
			• Dilated annulus
			  • Atrial fibrillation
			  • Restrictive CM

Type II 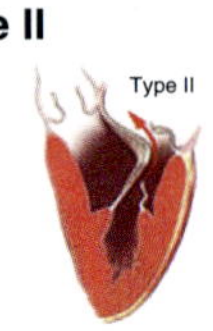	*Excess motion of the margin of a leaflet segment above the annular plane*	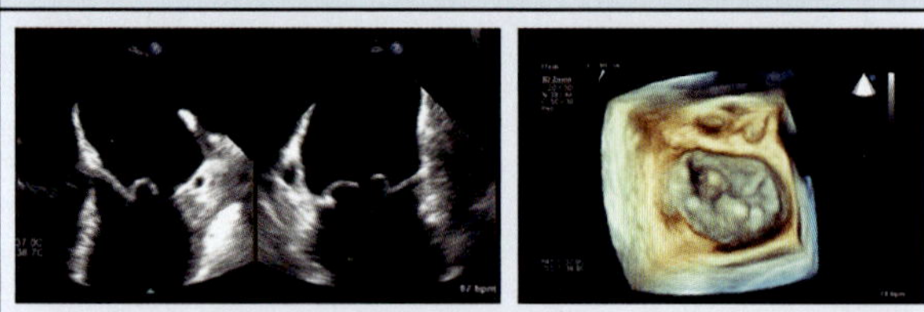	• Mitral valve prolapse
			  • Barlow's disease
			  • Flail mitral leaflet
			• Papillary rupture
			• Trauma

Type IIIa 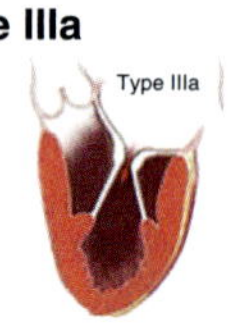	*Restricted leaflet motion during diastole and systole*	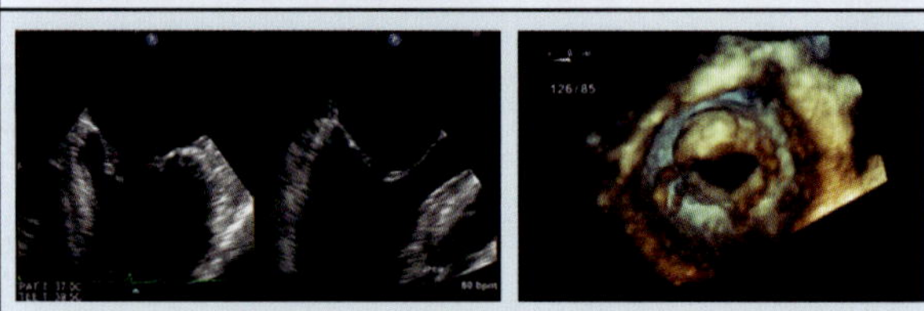	• Rheumatic • Collagen vascular • Radiation • Drugs • Mitral annular calcification
Type IIIb 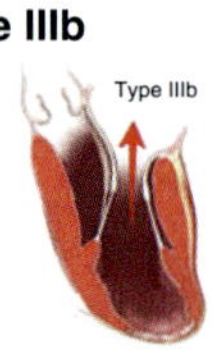	*Restricted leaflet motion predominantly during systole*	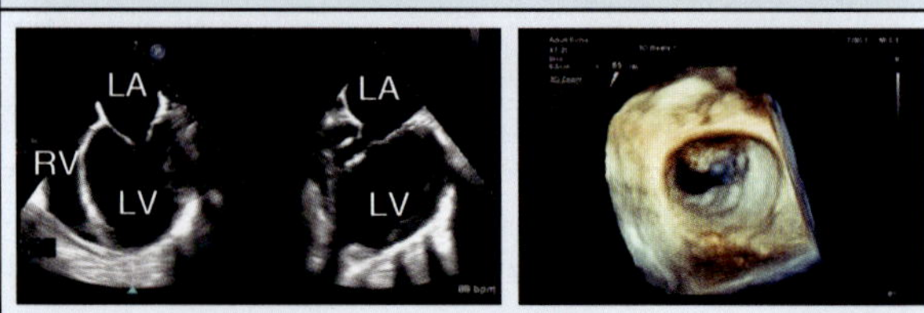	• Ischemic heart disease • Dilated cardiomyopathy

Fig. 6.1 Examples of the Carpentier Classification of Leaflet Mobility (after Carpentier A. Cardiac valve surgery–the "French correction". J Thorac Cardiovasc Surg 1983;86:323-37).

TABLE 6.3 Mitral Valve Apparatus, Cardiac Remodeling and Jet Characteristics in Primary and Secondary Mitral Regurgitation

	Primary MR[a]	Secondary MR[a]	
Etiology	Myxomatous or calcific leaflet degeneration	Inferior myocardial Infarction	Nonischemic cardiomyopathy, large anterior or multiple MI's
LV remodeling	Global, if severe chronic MR	Primarily inferior wall	Global dilation with increased sphericity
LA remodeling	Moderate to severe if chronic MR	Variable	Usually severe
Annulus	Dilated, preserved dynamic function	Mild to no dilation, less dynamic	Dilated, flattened, nondynamic
Leaflet morphology:			
• Thickening	Yes/moderate, severe	No/mild	No/mild
• Prolapse or flail	Usually present	No	No
• Calcification	Variable	No/mild	No/mild
Tethering pattern	None	Asymmetric	Symmetric
Systolic tenting	None	Increased	Markedly increased
Papillary muscle distance	Normal	Increased posterior papillary-intervalvular fibrosa distance	Increased interpapillary muscle distance
MR jet direction	Eccentric or central	Posterior	Usually central
CW Doppler jet	May be late systolic (if MVP) or uniform if flail or with calcific degeneration	Density usually uniform throughout systole	Biphasic pattern, with increased density in early and late systolic flow and mid-systolic dropout
PISA	Often hemispheric	Often not hemispheric	Often not hemispheric; may be biphasic

[a]Primary and secondary MR may coexist.

(From Zoghbi WA, Adams D, Bonow RO, et al. Recommendations for non-invasive evaluation of native valvular regurgitation: a report from the American Society of Echocardiography developed in collaboration with the Society for Cardiovascular Magnetic Resonance. *J Am Soc Echocardiogr.* 2017;30:303–371.)

convergence of several components: the atrial and ventricular muscular walls, the hinge line of the mitral leaflets, the epicardial adipose tissue, a discontinuous semi-circle of fibrous tissue on its posterior aspect and a band of connective tissue at its anterior aspect.[20] Because it forms the convergence of the atrial and ventricular myocardium, the posterior annulus may dilate in the setting of either LV or LA dilatation and is also prone to age-related degenerative calcification. The severity of calcification of the annulus, leaflets, and attached chordae may influence transcatheter device choice.

Although annular repair devices currently are limited to the treatment of secondary MR, transcatheter mitral valve replacement (TMVR) has been performed in both primary and secondary disease.[21] Thus a full characterization of the annulus is important, including annular motion, the severity of calcification, annular dimensions (commissural and anteroposterior), and annular size (perimeter, diameters, and areas) using both 2D and 3D imaging. Significant calcification at the site of device anchoring (whether annulus or leaflet) may be an exclusion criterion for device placement. Mitral annular disjunction is a variant of degenerative MR in which a wide separation between the atrial–MV junction and the basal LV myocardium is noted[22], and devices that rely on anchoring at the mitral annulus must redefine the most appropriate anchor zone (i.e., leaflet hinge or basal myocardium). Annular devices that implant anchors within the annulus or a device within the coronary sinus require an analysis of the adjacent anatomy, including the right coronary artery.

Additional Imaging Requirements for Transcatheter Annular Repair or Mitral Valve Replacement

Whether a transseptal or transapical approach is used, the intracardiac access site must be fully assessed. Preprocedural planning for devices using a transseptal approach should include a comprehensive evaluation of the interatrial septum for ideal transseptal puncture site, presence of an interatrial shunt, or other structural abnormalities (i.e., prominent Eustachian valve or Chiari network).

The site of anchoring may also generate specific imaging requirements. With most current devices, there is a risk of left ventricular outflow tract (LVOT) obstruction depending on the vertical dimensions of the device and the interaction with the native anatomy (i.e., the intact mitral valve apparatus, interventricular septum, and LV outflow tract). To analyze the risk of LV outflow tract obstruction with a TMVR, the anatomy of the LV outflow tract near the virtual distal extent of the device should be evaluated in both diastole and systole. Although computed tomography is the imaging modality of choice to assess the risk of obstruction,[23] the angle between the mitral annulus and LV outflow tract or aortic valve annulus (mitral-aortic angle) can also be measured by TEE. An angle of <120 degrees is considered a risk for LV outflow tract obstruction following TMVR.[24]

Both right and left atrial appendages should be thoroughly imaged to exclude intracavitary thrombus. The use of simultaneous biplane imaging may be helpful, although associated with lower temporal and spatial resolution. Spontaneous contrast may be difficult to distinguish from a newly formed thrombus, and a commercial ultrasound enhancing agent may be helpful. Since percutaneous balloon mitral commissurotomy (PBMC) is performed via a transseptal approach, it is also important to assess the interatrial septum for features that would affect the ease of transseptal puncture, such as a highly mobile fossa or severe lipomatous hypertrophy.

ASSESSMENT OF MITRAL REGURGITATION SEVERITY

Similar to all valvular regurgitation assessments by echocardiography, an integrative approach is needed in the overall evaluation of residual MR after mitral valve interventions. Recent guidelines have outlined TEE imaging for MR severity at baseline (Table 6.4), during (Table 6.5) and after (Table 6.6) transcatheter devices are placed.[25] Standard methods have significant limitations (Table 6.7) due to Doppler flow acceleration and acoustic artifacts from devices. In the post-transcatheter edge-to-edge repair setting, multiple mitral regurgitation jets may be difficult to assess on TEE color Doppler imaging due to

TABLE 6.4 Grading the Severity of Chronic Mitral Regurgitation by Echocardiography

MR Severity[a]	Mild	Moderate		Severe
Structural				
MV morphology	**None or mild leaflet abnormality** (e.g., mild thickening, calcifications or prolapse, mild tenting)	Moderate leaflet abnormality or moderate tenting		**Severe valve lesions** (Primary: flail leaflet, ruptured papillary muscle, severe retraction, large perforation; Secondary: severe tenting, poor leaflet coaptation)
LV and LA size[b]	Usually normal	Normal or mildly dilated		Dilated[c]
Qualitative Doppler				
Color flow jet area[d]	**Small, central, narrow, often brief**	Variable		**Large central jet** (>50% of LA) or eccentric wall-impinging jet of variable size
Flow convergence[e]	**Not visible, transient or small**	Intermediate in size and duration		**Large throughout systole**
CW Doppler jet	**Faint/partial**/parabolic	Dense but partial or parabolic		Holosystolic/dense/ **triangular**
Semi-quantitative				
Vena contracta width (mm)	<0.3	Intermediate		**≥0.7 (>0.8 for biplane)[f]**
Pulmonary vein flow[g]	**Systolic dominance** (May be blunted in LV dysfunction or AF)	Normal or systolic blunting		Minimal to no systolic flow/ **Systolic flow reversal**
Mitral inflow[h]	**A-wave dominant**	Variable		E-wave dominant (>1.2 m/s}
Quantitative[i,j]				
EROA, 2D PISA (cm^2)	<0.20	0.20–0.29	0.30–0.39	≥0.40 (may be lower in secondary MR with elliptical ROA)
Regurgitant volume (mL)	<30	30–44	45–59	≥60 (maybe lower in low flow conditions)
Regurgitant fraction (%)	< 30	30–39	40–49	≥50

[a]All parameters have limitations, and an integrated approach must be used that weighs the strength of each echocardiographic measurement. All signs and measures should be interpreted in an individualized manner that accounts for body size, sex, and all other patient characteristics.
[b]This pertains mostly to patients with primary MR.
[c]LV and LA can be within the "normal" range for patients with acute severe MR or with chronic severe MR who have a small body size, particularly women, or with small LV size preceding the occurrence of MR.
[d]With Nyquist limit 50–60 cm/s.
[e]Small flow convergence is usually <0.3 cm, and large is ≥1 cm at a Nyquist limit of 30–40 cm/s.
[f]For average between apical 2- and 4-chamber views.
[g]Influenced by many other factors (LV diastolic function, atrial fibrillation, LA pressure).
[h]Most valid in patients >50 years old and are influenced by other causes of elevated LA pressure.
[i]Discrepancies between EROA, regurgitant fraction, and regurgitant volume may arise in the setting of low or high flow states
[j]Quantitative parameters can help sub-classify the moderate regurgitation group.
Bolded qualitative and semi-quantitative signs are considered specific for their MR grade.
CW, Continuous wave; *EROA*, effective regurgitant orifice area; *LA*, left atrium; *LV*, left ventricle; *MR*, mitral regurgitation; *MV*, mitral valve; *TVI*, time velocity integral.
(From Zoghbi WA, Adams D, Bonow RO, et al. Recommendations for non-invasive evaluation of native valvular regurgitation: a report from the American Society of Echocardiography developed in collaboration with the Society for Cardiovascular Magnetic Resonance. *J Am Soc Echocardiogr* 2017;30:303–371.)

TABLE 6.5 Transesophageal Echocardiography Parameters Useful in Determining Residual Mitral Regurgitation Severity During the Procedure

Parameter	Caveats
General Echo Findings	
Spontaneous Echo Contrast in LA	• Appearance of spontaneous contrast after MV intervention suggests significant reduction in MR severity
LVEF	• Decline in LVEF after MV intervention suggests significant MR reduction, absent other causes (ischemia, pacemaker-related, etc)
Color Doppler	
Color Doppler Jet (size, number of jets, location, eccentricity)	• Easy to obtain with a comprehensive, systematic approach • Difficult to assess multiple and eccentric jets • Jet area affected by eccentricity, technical and hemodynamic factors (especially driving velocity)
Flow convergence	• Large flow convergence denotes significant residual MR whereas a small or no flow convergence suggests mild MR • Difficult to use in presence of multiple jets or very eccentric jets, or may be masked by the device
Vena Contracta Width (VCW)	• VCA ≥ 0.7 cm specific for severe MR • Difficult to use in the presence of multiple small jets or very eccentric jets for which orifice shape is not well delineated
Spectral Doppler	
Pulmonary Vein Flow Pattern	• Flow reversal >1 vein specific for severe MR • Change in pattern (increase in forward systolic flow) can help confirm MR reduction
CW Doppler Profile of MR jet (contour, density, peak velocity and VTI)	• Dense, triangular pattern suggests severe MR • May be hard to line up CW Doppler properly in flail leaflet or very eccentric jet after intervention (consider using transgastric windows)
Mitral Inflow Pattern	• In sinus rhythm, a mitral A wave dominant flow excludes severe MR • Decrease in mitral E velocity and VTI suggests reduction in MR severity
Pulsed Doppler of LVOT (deep transgastric view)	• IIncrease in LVOT velocity and VTI after procedure suggests MR reduction
Quantitation	
General Consideration	• More difficult to perform • Procedure-specific limitations in quantitation (i.e. post edge-to-edge repair)
EROA by PISA	• Not recommended after edge-to-edge repair or to assess prosthetic paravalvular regurgitation because assumption of hemispheric proximal flow convergence is violated by the device/sewing ring and noncircular shape of the regurgitant orifice. • PISA often underestimates MR severity in the presence of multiple jets or markedly eccentric jets.
Vena Contracta Area (VCA) by 3D Color Doppler Planimetry	• Lower temporal and spatial resolution may require multi-beat acquisitions • May be used for multiple regurgitant jets and irregular orifice shapes • May be less accurate if regurgitant orifice is non-planar • Regurgitant volume can be calculated
Quantitative Doppler	• Given inherent reduction in mitral valve area, PW Doppler to quantify diastolic stroke volume is not accurate

CW, Vena contracta width; *CWD*, continuous-wave Doppler; *EROA*, effective regurgitant orifice area; *LA*, left atrium; *LV* = left ventricle/ventricular; *LVEF*, left ventricular ejection fraction; *LVOT*, left ventricular outflow tract; *PISA*, proximal isovelocity surface area; *PW* = pulsed wave; *SEC*, spontaneous echo contrast; *TEE*, transesophageal echocardiography; *VCA*, vena contracta area; *VTI*, velocity-time integral.
Modified from Zoghbi WA, Asch FM, Bruce C, Gillam LD, Grayburn PA, Hahn RT, et al. Guidelines for the Evaluation of Valvular Regurgitation After Percutaneous Valve Repair or Replacement: A Report from the American Society of Echocardiography Developed in Collaboration with the Society for Cardiovascular Angiography and Interventions, Japanese Society of Echocardiography, and Society for Cardiovascular Magnetic Resonance. *J Am Soc Echocardiogr*. 2019;32(4):431–475.

artifacts from the device(s). Additionally, if jets are entrained by the devices, excessive jet spray could cause an overestimation of mitral regurgitant severity. Following MitraClip (Abbott Vascular, Santa Clara, CA), an assessment of residual regurgitation can be made by 3D color Doppler.[26] Pulmonary vein systolic flow should be imaged at baseline and follow-up. Pulmonary artery systolic pressure should be estimated as previously described.[27]

Assessing the diastolic gradients and resulting mitral orifice area after device implantation should also be performed. Current ACC/AHA guidelines state that severe disease is defined by a mitral valve area of ≤1.5 cm^2 without mention of mean gradients.[1] Echocardiographic guidelines emphasize that for native disease, the valve area is the most accurate assessment of stenosis, with supportive evidence from mean gradients.[28] The surgical and transcatheter literature has been conflicting with respect to residual mean transmitral gradient and outcomes. In a single-site study of TEER for MR (70% with secondary MR), an increased residual invasive gradient >5 mm Hg

TABLE 6.6 Parameters for Grading Mitral Regurgitation Severity by Transesophageal Echocardiography or Transthoracic Echocardiography During or After Transcatheter Mitral Valve Therapy

Parameter	Mild	Moderate	Severe
General Principles	Multiple criteria for mild MR improve specificity Change from baseline is crucial	There are no specific criteria for moderate MR Usually considered moderate when criteria are intermediate between mild and severe with no specific signs for severe MR Reverse LV remodeling despite a large color flow jet is likely moderate, not severe MR	Multiple criteria for severe MR is highly specific Failure of multiple parameters to improve from baseline Failure of LV end-diastolic volume to improve suggests persistent severe MR
Structural			
Morphology	Device appropriately positioned/ expected or normal valve motion	No specific criteria	Abnormal device position/flail valve (single leaflet device attachment, dehiscence, incomplete TMVR expansion, etc.)
LA and LV volumes	Reduction in size from baseline or normalization	Minimal change	Enlarged with no change/worsening from baseline, particularly in primary MR
Qualitative			
Color Doppler Jet (size, number, eccentricity)	1 or 2 small jets with no visible flow convergence	More than mild but does not meet severe criteria	Large central jet/multiple jets Eccentric jet(s) of any size wrapping around LA
Flow Convergence Size[a]	None or small	Intermediate	Large
Mitral Inflow Pattern	In sinus rhythm, A-wave dominant	No specific criteria	No specific criteria
Pulmonary Vein Flow Pattern[b]	Normal	Blunted systolic flow	Systolic flow reversal
CW Doppler of MR jet (density, contour)	Faint, parabolic contour	No specific criteria	Dense, triangular contour
Semi-Quantitative			
Vena Contracta Width (VCW) (cm)	Single jet with VCW ≤0.3	Single jet with VCW 0.4–0.6	Any jet with VCW ≥0.7 or ≥2 moderate jets
Quantitative			
Vena Contracta Area (VCA) by 3D Planimetry (cm^2)[c]	Single jet with VCA <0.2	Single jet with VCA 0.2–0.39	Any jet or combined VCA ≥ 0.4 or ≥2 moderate jets
EROA by PISA (cm^2)	EROA <0.2 (Note: not recommended after TEER)	EROA 0.2–0.39 (Note: not recommended after TEER)	EROA ≥0.4 (Note: not recommended after TEER)
Regurgitant Volume[d]	<30 mL	30–59	≥60 mL (may be lower in low flow states)
Regurgitant Fraction (%)	<30%	30%–49%	≥50%

[a]All parameters have limitations, and an integrated approach must be used that weighs the strength of each echocardiographic measurement. All signs and measures should be interpreted in an individualized manner that accounts for body size, hemodynamics, and other patient characteristics.
[b]Influenced by many other factors (LV diastolic function, atrial fibrillation, LA pressure).
[c]By color Doppler.
[d]Total stroke volume (inclusive of the RVol) is calculated from LV volumes. Use of 3D echocardiography and preferably contrast echocardiography is recommended to avoid underestimation of LV volumes, RVol, and RF. RVol cut-offs may be lower in low flow states.
CW, Continuous wave; *EROA*, effective regurgitant orifice area; *LA*, left atrium; *LV*, left ventricle; *MR*, mitral regurgitation; *PISA*, proximal isovelocity surface area; *TMVR*, transcatheter mitral valve replacement; *VCA*, Vena contracta area; *VCW*, vena contracta width.
(Modified from Zoghbi WA, Asch FM, Bruce C, et al. Guidelines for the evaluation of valvular regurgitation after percutaneous valve repair or replacement: a report from the American Society of Echocardiography developed in collaboration with the society for cardiovascular angiography and interventions, Japanese Society of Echocardiography, and society for cardiovascular magnetic resonance. *J Am Soc Echocardiogr.* 2019;32(4):431–745.)

TABLE 6.7 Limitations of Parameters to Assess Mitral Regurgitation Severity After Transcatheter Mitral Valve Interventions

Parameter	Limitations
Color Doppler Mitral Regurgitation (MR) Jet	Multiple jets can lead to falsely overestimating MR Device artifacts complicate interpretation of color flow Doppler jet area TMVR central valvular regurgitation due to cusp malfunction less difficult to assess but often difficult or not possible to identify, localize and quantify PVR by TTE. TEE needed. Eccentric jets difficult to evaluate and maybe harder to detect if out of imaging plane
EROA or RVol by PISA	Not validated for multiple jets, double orifice mitral valves, or eccentric jets for transcatheter mitral devices
Vena Contracta Width	Not validated for multiple jets Not validated for double orifice mitral valve
Vena Contracta Area (3D)	May be useful after MitraClip, but limited studies available
Volumetric EROA or RVol	Time-consuming Technically difficult Multiple measurements may compound errors Requires excellent endocardial definition May underestimate LV volume due to foreshortening of LV Stroke volume calculated from MV annular plane—MV annular dimension and pulse-wave sampling are altered by MitraClip Stroke volume calculated from LVOT—if LVOT is not circular, defining true stroke volume maybe inaccurate Stroke volume calculated across the RVOT may be used if aortic regurgitation or VSD present
Pulmonary Vein Flow	Diastolic inflow dominance may continue if left atrial hypertension is present due to persistent MR or LV dysfunction with an elevated Pulmonary vein flow reflects left atrial pressure, so it is affected by more factors than MR severity It may also be altered by hypovolemia—significant lowering of left atrial pressure will lessen or eliminate the V-wave or Change the Doppler flow pattern from S dominant to D dominant
Mitral Inflow Pattern	E-wave dominance not only reflects changes in MR severity but loading conditions If LA pressure increases—E dominance is likely to also increase Not interpretable in presence of atrial fibrillation
CW Doppler	Pattern and intensity reflect LV driving pressure as well as MR severity
PASP	Generally, drops if elevated prior to the MitraClip placement It will not drop if there is intrinsic pulmonary hypertension, so specificity is limited

(From Zoghbi WA, Asch FM, Bruce C, et al. Guidelines for the evaluation of valvular regurgitation after percutaneous valve repair or replacement: a report from the American Society of Echocardiography developed in collaboration with the society for cardiovascular angiography and interventions, Japanese Society of Echocardiography, and society for cardiovascular magnetic resonance. *J Am Soc Echocardiogr.* 2019;32(4):431–475.)

(echocardiographic gradient >4.4 mm Hg) was a significant predictor of outcome (all-cause mortality, left ventricular assist device, mitral valve replacement, or redo procedure) on multi-variable analysis after adjustment for N-terminal pro–B-type natriuretic peptide, age, and remaining mitral regurgitation (hazard ratio: 2.3; 95% confidence interval: 1.4 to 3.8; $P = 0.002$).[29] A recent post hoc analysis of the COAPT trial, however, showed that following TEER for secondary MR, higher MVGs on discharge did not adversely affect the 2-year composite endpoint of all-cause mortality or HF hospitalization or symptomatic and functional improvement.[30] Higher mean gradient (>3 mm Hg) following surgical repair for primary MR is associated with reduced functional capacity and quality of life[31] and risk of reintervention.[32] However, following surgical restrictive annuloplasty for secondary disease, mean gradients are not associated with outcomes.[33] It is thus possible that mean transmitral gradients following interventions may differ depending on the initial disease process and that lower gradients (<5 mm Hg) are optimal following device therapy for primary MR but less predictive in secondary MR. The assessment of the diastolic MV area by 2D or 3D planimetry may be the most accurate assessment of post-device mitral stenosis since pressure halftime is not validated in this patient population. Given the poor outcomes associated with surgical MV areas <0.9 cm^2/m^2, this result should be avoided following device therapy when possible with optimal valve area >2.0 cm^2 or >1.2 cm^2/m^2.[34]

CONCLUSION

Transesophageal echocardiography is the imaging modality of choice to evaluate the mitral valve complex prior to transcatheter interventions. A comprehensive assessment of the mitral valve for interventions includes defining the morphology, etiology, and severity of disease. Quantifying mitral regurgitation severity at baseline, intraprocedurally, and at follow-up requires a multi-parametric and multi-modality (2D and 3D) echocardiographic assessment. When appropriate, patients with an initial echocardiographic assessment of moderate or greater MR, should be referred to a Level I valve center for further quantitation and management.[1]

CASE-BASED ASSESSMENT

1. The current American College of Cardiology/American Heart Association Guideline for the Management of Patients With Valvular Heart Disease has added transcatheter edge-to-edge repair (TEER) for mitral regurgitation (MR) as a possible therapeutic option for both primary and secondary disease. Which of the following statements is true?
   A. Anatomic appropriateness of TEER is a criterion for consideration of this therapy.
   B. Echocardiography is a class I diagnostic test for the assessment of valvular morphology and function.
   C. Transesophageal echocardiography (TEE) is the imaging modality of choice for determining anatomic suitability for and procedural guidance of the TEER device.
   D. All of the above.
2. Which of the following parameters is not typically used to determine anatomic feasibility for TEER devices?
   A. Location of the primary MR jet and associated leaflet abnormality.
   B. Systolic reversal of pulmonary venous inflow.
   C. Coaptation depth and length.
   D. Flail gap and malcoaptation width.

See page 315 for the answers.

REFERENCES

1. Otto CM, Nishimura RA, Bonow RO, et al. 2020 ACC/AHA guideline for the management of patients with valvular heart disease: executive summary: a report of the American College of Cardiology/American Heart Association joint committee on clinical practice guidelines. *J Am Coll Cardiol.* 2021;77(4):450–500.
2. Hahn RT, Saric M, Faletra FF, et al. Recommended Standards for the performance of transesophageal echocardiographic screening for structural heart intervention: from the American Society of Echocardiography. *J Am Soc Echocardiogr.* 2022;35(1);1-76. doi:10.1016/j.echo.2021.07.006. Epub ahead of print. PMID: 34280494.
3. Silvestry FE, Rodriguez LL, Herrmann HC, et al. Echocardiographic guidance and assessment of percutaneous repair for mitral regurgitation with the Evalve MitraClip: lessons learned from EVEREST I. *J Am Soc Echocardiogr.* 2007;20(10):1131–1140.
4. Feldman T, Foster E, Glower DD, et al. Percutaneous repair or surgery for mitral regurgitation. *N Engl J Med.* 2011;364(15):1395–1406.
5. Levine RA, Handschumacher MD, Sanfilippo AJ, et al. Three-dimensional echocardiographic reconstruction of the mitral valve, with implications for the diagnosis of mitral valve prolapse. *Circulation.* 1989;80(3):589–598.
6. Topilsky Y, Vaturi O, Watanabe N, et al. Real-time 3-dimensional dynamics of functional mitral regurgitation: a prospective quantitative and mechanistic study. *J Am Heart Assoc.* 2013;2(3):e000039.
7. Grewal J, Suri R, Mankad S, et al. Mitral annular dynamics in myxomatous valve disease: new insights with real-time 3-dimensional echocardiography. *Circulation.* 2010;121(12):1423–1431.
8. Watanabe N, Ogasawara Y, Yamaura Y, et al. Mitral annulus flattens in ischemic mitral regurgitation: geometric differences between inferior and anterior myocardial infarction: a real-time 3-dimensional echocardiographic study. *Circulation.* 2005;112(suppl 9):I458I462.
9. Zeng X, Nunes MC, Dent J, et al. Asymmetric versus symmetric tethering patterns in ischemic mitral regurgitation: geometric differences from three-dimensional transesophageal echocardiography. *J Am Soc Echocardiogr.* 2014;27(4):367–375.
10. Tsang W, Lang RM. Three-dimensional echocardiography is essential for intraoperative assessment of mitral regurgitation. *Circulation.* 2013;128(6):643–652; discussion 52.
11. Theriault-Lauzier P, Andalib A, Martucci G, et al. Fluoroscopic anatomy of left-sided heart structures for transcatheter interventions: insight from multislice computed tomography. *JACC Cardiovasc Interv.* 2014;7(9):947–957.
12. Anderson RH, Kanani M. Mitral valve repair: critical analysis of the anatomy discussed. *Multimed Man Cardiothorac Surg.* 2007(102) mmcts.2006.002147.
13. Cobey FC, Ferreira R, Ursprung WW, et al. A novel approach to assess the three-dimensional anatomy of a mitral valve regurgitant jet orifice. *J Cardiothorac Vasc Anesth.* 2017;31(1):169–173.
14. Carpentier A. Cardiac valve surgery—the "French correction. *J Thorac Cardiovasc Surg.* 1983;86(3):323–337.
15. Dulgheru R, Magne J, Lancellotti P, et al. Dynamic ischaemic mitral regurgitation and the role of stress echocardiography. *J Cardiovasc Echogr.* 2013;23(1):10–17.
16. Levine RA, Hagége AA, Judge DP, et al. Mitral valve disease—morphology and mechanisms. *Nat Rev Cardiol.* 2015;12(12):689–710.
17. Bertrand PB, Schwammenthal E, Levine RA, et al. Exercise dynamics in secondary mitral regurgitation: pathophysiology and therapeutic implications. *Circulation.* 2017;135(3):297–314.
18. Kimura T, Roger VL, Watanabe N, et al. The unique mechanism of functional mitral regurgitation in acute myocardial infarction: a prospective dynamic 4D quantitative echocardiographic study. *Eur Heart J.* 2019;20(4):396–406.
19. Lancellotti P, Moura L, Pierard LA, et al. European Association of Echocardiography recommendations for the assessment of valvular regurgitation. Part 2: mitral and tricuspid regurgitation (native valve disease). *Eur J Echocardiogr.* 2010;11(4):307–332.
20. Faletra FF, Leo LA, Paiocchi VL, et al. Anatomy of mitral annulus insights from non-invasive imaging techniques. *Eur Heart J Cardiovasc Imaging.* 2019;20(8):843–857.
21. Bapat V, Rajagopal V, Meduri C, et al. Early experience with new transcatheter mitral valve replacement. *J Am Coll Cardiol.* 2018;71(1):12–21.
22. Lee AP-W, Jin C-N, Fan Y, et al. Functional implication of mitral annular disjunction in mitral valve prolapse. A quantitative dynamic 3d echocardiographic study. *JACC Cardiovasc Imaging.* 2017;10(12):1424–1433.
23. Blanke P, Naoum C, Dvir D, et al. Predicting LVOT obstruction in transcatheter mitral valve implantation: concept of the Neo-LVOT. *JACC Cardiovasc Imaging.* 2017;10(4):482–485.
24. Bapat V, Pirone F, Kapetanakis S, et al. Factors influencing left ventricular outflow tract obstruction following a mitral

valve-in-valve or valve-in-ring procedure, part 1. *Catheter Cardiovasc Interv*. 2015;86(4):747–760.
25. Zoghbi WA, Asch FM, Bruce C, et al. Guidelines for the Evaluation of valvular regurgitation after percutaneous valve repair or replacement: a report from the American Society of Echocardiography developed in collaboration with the Society for Cardiovascular Angiography and Interventions, Japanese Society of Echocardiography, and Society for Cardiovascular Magnetic Resonance. *J Am Soc Echocardiogr*. 2019;32(4):431–475.
26. Altiok E, Hamada S, Brehmer K, et al. Analysis of procedural effects of percutaneous edge-to-edge mitral valve repair by 2D and 3D echocardiography. *Circ Cardiovasc Imaging*. 2012;5(6):748–755.
27. Quinones MA, Otto CM, Stoddard M, et al. Recommendations for quantification of Doppler echocardiography: a report from the Doppler Quantification Task Force of the Nomenclature and Standards Committee of the American Society of Echocardiography. *J Am Soc Echocardiogr*. 2002;15(2):167–184.
28. Baumgartner H, Hung J, Bermejo J, et al. Echocardiographic assessment of valve stenosis: EAE/ASE recommendations for clinical practice. *J Am Soc Echocardiogr*. 2009;22(1):1–23 quiz 101–2.
29. Neuss M, Schau T, Isotani A, et al. Elevated mitral valve pressure gradient after mitraclip implantation deteriorates long-term outcome in patients with severe mitral regurgitation and severe heart failure. *JACC: Cardiovasc Interv*. 2017;10(9):931–999.
30. Halaby R, Herrmann HC, Gertz ZM, et al. Effect of mitral valve gradient after mitraclip on outcomes in secondary mitral regurgitation: results from the COAPT trial. *JACC Cardiovasc Interv*. 2021;14(8):879–889.
31. Chan KL, Chen SY, Chan V, et al. Functional significance of elevated mitral gradients after repair for degenerative mitral regurgitation. *Circ Cardiovasc Imaging*. 2013;6(6):1041–1047.
32. Tomšič A, Hiemstra YL, Arabkhani B, et al. Risk factors and clinical significance of elevated mitral valve gradient following valve repair for degenerative disease. *Eur J Cardiothorac Surg*. 2020;57(2):293–299.
33. Bertrand PB, Gutermann H, Smeets CJ, et al. Functional impact of transmitral gradients at rest and during exercise after restrictive annuloplasty for ischemic mitral regurgitation. *J Thorac Cardiovasc Surg*. 2014;148(1):183–187.
34. Magne J, Mathieu P, Dumesnil JG, et al. Impact of prosthesis-patient mismatch on survival after mitral valve replacement. *Circulation*. 2007;115(11):1417–1425.

7

Special Imaging Considerations for Transcatheter Mitral Therapy

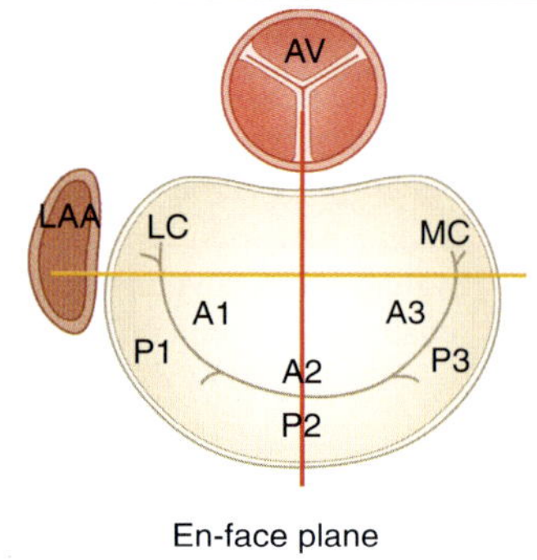

Leo Marcoff, Konstantinos P. Koulogiannis

CHAPTER OUTLINE

LEARNING OBJECTIVES

1. Understand the general principles and specific imaging techniques involved in screening for mitral transcatheter edge-to-edge repair (TEER).
2. Understand the imaging sequence and specific goals of intraprocedural imaging at each stage in TEER.
3. Recognize procedural complications and imaging challenges during TEER.

INTRODUCTION

Imaging plays an essential role in structural transcatheter interventions revealing intracardiac landscape and events throughout the diagnostic work-up, procedural planning, intraprocedural guidance, and follow-up. Unlike transcatheter aortic valve replacement (TAVR), mitral interventions cannot be performed under sole fluoroscopic guidance because fluoroscopy cannot adequately visualize soft tissues such as the endocardial surface and mitral leaflets. Cardiac computed tomography angiography (CTA) enables precise anatomic measurements and assessment of calcification to plan TMVR, but is stationary, does not provide real-time imaging including hemodynamic data, and has suboptimal temporal resolution compared to echo. Echocardiography has been the primary tool in the structural imager's armamentarium. Portable and safe, it provides illuminating anatomic and hemodynamic information about the heart and circulation in general - all in real-time. Current transcatheter mitral interventions rely heavily on echocardiography for procedural guidance.

Complexities of intracardiac navigation and maneuvering safely around the delicate structures of the heart require specific skillset and imaging expertise. Structural imaging has emerged as a new subspecialty within the neighboring fields of cardiology and anesthesiology.[1,2] Specific training requirements for structural imagers emphasize expertise in interpreting cardiac hemodynamics, functioning in a fast-paced environment of the operating room, and applying advanced echocardiographic skills, including 3D reconstructive techniques.[2]

Three-dimensional (3D) echocardiography is now omnipresent in structural imaging. In addition to providing spectacular volume-rendered images of intracardiac landscapes, 3D reconstruction generates any pre-defined 2D imaging plane, thus ensuring complete visualization of intracardiac structures and allowing for more accurate and precise measurements.

In this chapter, we describe and illustrate special echocardiographic methods and techniques on the example of transcatheter edge-to-edge repair (TEER)—currently the only Food and Drug Administration (FDA)-approved device-based transcatheter mitral intervention. In addition, we review special imaging considerations for some of the approved TMVR (CE mark only) and transcatheter annuloplasty platforms. The chapter's structure maps onto the clinical course of events in transcatheter valve therapy: screening, pre-procedural planning, the procedure itself, and the follow-up.

SCREENING

The goal of screening is to determine MR mechanism, MR severity, and the feasibility of transcatheter repair. In TEER, screening is accomplished using both transthoracic echocardiogram (TTE) and transesophageal echo (TEE). The two modalities complement each other by their opposite vantage points: anterior for TTE and posterior for TEE. Thus, while TEE provides superior visualization of the basal (posterior) cardiac structures, including the mitral valve and left atrium (LA), TTE is best to evaluate ventricular size and function and to assess right-sided structures in most cases. Data from both modalities are integrated in the final anatomic and physiologic assessment.

The Mitral Axis

The surgical view of the mitral valve has been used as the frame of reference for transcatheter mitral interventions (Fig. 7.1). The mitral valve in the surgical view is seen en-face from a hovering perspective in LA. The aortic valve positioned at the top (12 o'clock position) defines the antero-posterior axis, and the two commissures where the bases of the anterior and posterior leaflets meet define the medial-lateral axis. The echocardiographic views that map onto the mitral axes are (1) ***the commissural view*** (medial-lateral axis), (2) ***the long-axis view*** (antero-posterior axis), and (3) ***the en-face view***—the 3D (surgical) or the 2D short-axis view (see Fig. 7.1). Achieving the precise "on-axis" orientation of echocardiographic views is fundamental to locating pathology and procedural guidance.

The Commissural View

In the commissural view, also known as bicommissural or commissure-to-commissure (CC) view, the mitral scallops are completely separated: the P1 and P3 are seen on opposite sides, with the A2 "flying in the air" in the center (Fig. 7.2). Given that the commissures are aligned in this view, the heads of both papillary muscles, postero-medial and antero-lateral, are normally seen. The CC view lays out the entire line of coaptation, from

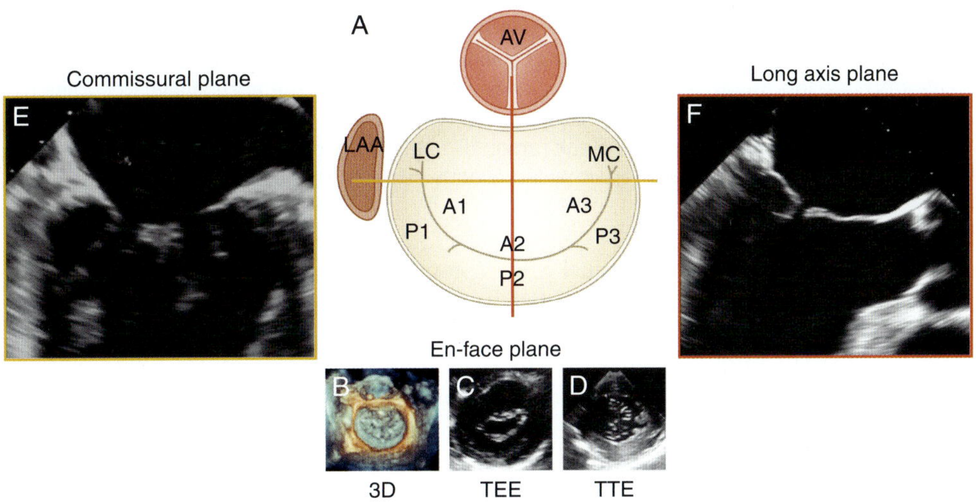

Fig. 7.1 The Mitral Valve Axis and Cardinal Planes. The surgical view of the mitral valve from the left atrium (LA) serves as the general frame of reference for mitral interventions and beyond (A and B). The 3D volume-rendered view is rotated so that the AV occupies the 12 o'clock position (B). In this orientation, the commissures lay on both sides at 3 and 9 o'clock positions, and the left atrial appendage occupies the 9 to 10 o'clock region (A and B). In addition to the 3D surgical view, the reference en-face (short-axis) plane can also be obtained from the parasternal window on transthoracic echocardiogram (TTE) (C) and the shallow transgastric window on transesophageal echo (TEE) (D). The commissural plane (A, E, *yellow line*) displays both commissures and the entire coaptation line, useful to localize all MR jets. The long-axis plane (A, F, *red line*) is orthogonal to commissural and connects the most anterior and most posterior points in each cut across the commissural plane. *AV,* Aortic valve; *LAA,* left atrial appendage; *LC,* lateral commissure; *MC,* medical commissure.

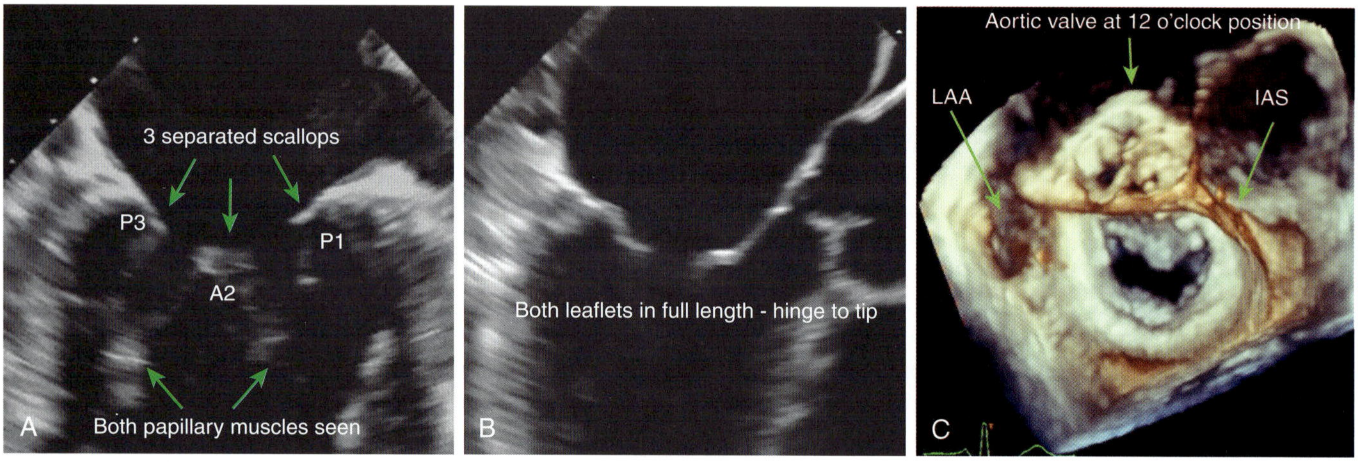

Commissural View (Medial-Lateral Plane)	**Long Axis View** (Anterior-Posterior Plane)	**Surgical View** (En-Face Plane)
1. Resolves MR into individual regurgitant jets 2. Demonstrates location of each jet on the coaptation line 3. Useful baseline view for mitral 3D acquisitions displaying full width of the coaptation line	1. Best view to evaluate the grasping zone for local leaflet length, leaflet thickening, focal calcification, flail gap, etc) 2. Serves as the source view for important Doppler interrogations (spectral Doppler of the antegrade mitral flow, MR, VCW, and PISA)	1. Best view to asses indentations and clefts 2. Provides a global perspective of the mitral space 3. Confirms location of pathology, including commissural disease

Fig. 7.2 The key mitral views correspond to the orthogonal planes of the mitral reference framework in Fig. 7.1: commissural, long-axis, and en-face. The commissural view (AO is defined by the complete separation of the scallops: *P1, A2,* and *P3,* from lateral to medial side. Reflecting the fact that papillary muscles reside directly below each commissure, portions of both papillary muscles should appear in the on-axis view. The orthogonal long-axis view (B), obtained directly or using biplane, demonstrates both leaflets in their full length, from hinge to tip. If the long-axis cut is midline, the left ventricular outflow tract will be fully open in most cases. (C) The en-face surgical view gives a hovering perspective of the mitral valve from the left atrium and by convention is oriented so that the aortic valve occupies the 12 o'clock position, the left atrial appendage *(LAA)* is at 9 to 10 o'clock, and the interatrial septum usually spans the 1 to 3 o'clock region. Practical applications of these key views are listed below each panel. *PISA,* Proximal isovelocity surface area.

lateral to medial commissure. In this view, the individual MR jets can be located and compared to each other—an essential task in selecting targets for intervention. Since the coaptation line is curved, slight rotation of the TEE probe is often needed to arrive at jet origins: clockwise to reach anteriorly, counterclockwise to focus on the posterior portions of the coaptation line.[3]

The Long-axis View

The long-axis (LAX) view is a single orthogonal cut across the medial-lateral axis at a particular location on the coaptation line (see Fig. 7.2). The midline (on-axis) LAX view will show A2 and P2 scallops as well as the fully opened left ventricular outflow tract (LVOT). To reach medially, the TEE probe is rotated clockwise, while counterclockwise rotation will shift the viewing plane laterally.[3] The LAX view demonstrates specific segments of both leaflets and the profile of the MR jet at that location (see Fig. 7.2).

The En-Face View

The surgical view reveals the entire circumference of the mitral annulus, a full view of the coaptation line, including both commissures, and the atrial surfaces of both leaflets (see Fig. 7.2). The volume-rendered image is rotated to bring the aortic valve (AV) to the 12 o'clock position.[4] Once aligned, the volume may need to be tilted slightly to fully expose both leaflets and commissures. In addition to the surgeon's view, a 2D short-axis view at the level of mitral leaflet tips provides axial reference, particularly when 3D imaging is not available or suboptimal.

Additional Views

Mid-esophageal 5-, 4-, and 2-chamber views and the corresponding transthoracic views complement the key mitral views and are part of the comprehensive echo exam.[3,5] Occasionally, non-standard views are required to elucidate pathology not adequately captured in conventional views. Ultimately, the best view is the one that provides an unequivocal answer to the specific clinical question.

The Role of the Three-dimensional Reconstructive Techniques

The current 3D technology provides lower spatial and temporal resolution compared to 2D and does not replace a dedicated 2D

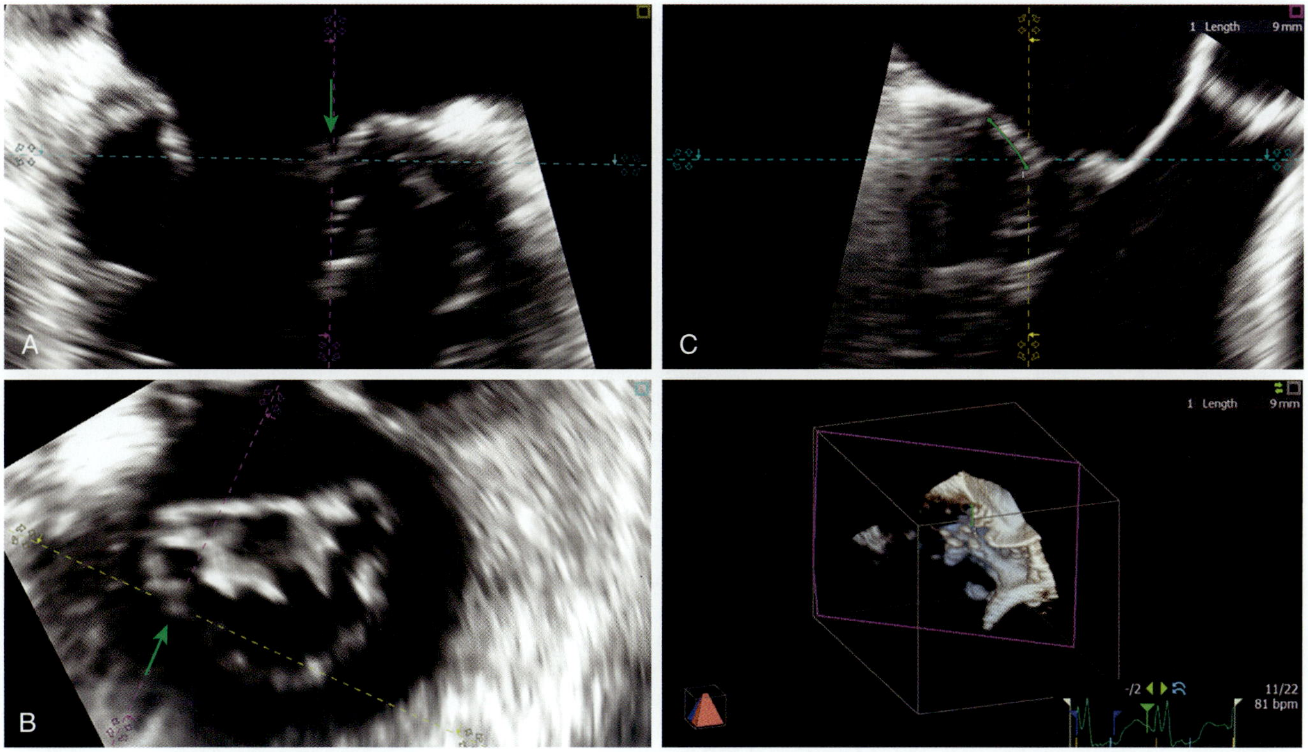

Fig. 7.3 3D Multiplanar Reconstruction. 3D allows the reconstruction of any 2D plane captured within the pre-defined region of interest. 3D software allows simultaneous view and manipulation of the three orthogonal planes (A– C). In this example, the intended grasping zone at the A1P1 coaptation *(green arrows)*. The position of the long-axis plane of interest *(purple line)* is first defined in the commissural view (A) and then adjusted to be perpendicular to the local segment of the coaptation line in the en-face view (B). Thus, generated long-axis view (C) allows measurement of the posterior leaflet length in the exact location of the intended grasp. Note that both spatial and temporal resolution of 3D are currently inferior to 2D and settings should be optimized at the time of acquisition for reliable measurements.

echo assessment.[4] In conjunction with 2D and Doppler echocardiography, 3D echo is a highly valuable tool for clarifying MR mechanism, severity, and feasibility for transcatheter therapy. 3D reconstructive techniques allow multiplanar reconstruction of any specific 2D plane from the acquired 3D volume (Fig. 7.3).[6] If the key views were not captured adequately by conventional 2D imaging, they can be reconstructed from the 3D volume. For offline reconstruction, the 3D data must be in the "raw" or native format, which includes the entire pyramidal 3D volume of data, as opposed to the flat unmanipulable volume-rendered reference view. The 3D volume should include the entire mitral annulus, leaflets, and the subvalvular apparatus. For 3D color Doppler acquisitions, the entire origin of the target regurgitant jet should be included in the volume for adequate analysis. In the end, quality 3D color Doppler imaging depends on a narrowly tailored compromise between the spatial and temporal resolution (optimized settings, multibeat acquisition), state-of-the-art ultrasound equipment, and the echocardiographer's experience.

Mitral Regurgitation Mechanism

The ***Carpentier classification*** is based on abnormalities of leaflet motion and covers a wide range of mital regurgitation (MR) etiologies—both common and rare (Fig 7.4).[7] Mitral regurgitation can also be classified broadly as ***primary*** or ***secondary***, based on whether the MR is due to primary abnormalities of the valve itself or the MR is secondary to extrinsic distortion of the mitral apparatus due to abnormal left ventricle and/or the LA.[8] The most common subtype of primary MR seen in current US clinical practice is ***degenerative MR (DMR)*** due to prolapsed or flail leaflets (Carpentier type II). The most common secondary MR is ***functional (FMR)*** due to (left ventricle (LV) dilatation and systolic dysfunction (Carpentier type IIIb) (see Fig. 7.4).

Another relatively common type of secondary MR—but distinct from FMR—is the ***atrial functional MR (AFMR)*** or pure annular dilatation (Carpentier type I) (see Fig. 7.4).[9] AFMR is distinct from FMR because the left ventricular ejection fraction (LVEF) is normal, and the pathologic substrate is dilatated LA and the mitral annulus. Annular dilatation is said to be present when the maximum antero-posterior annular diameter measured in the parasternal long-axis view is greater than 35 mm or the ratio of antero-posterior annular diameter to the length of the anterior leaflet is greater than 1.3.[10] As the annulus dilates, it flattens from its normal saddle-shape configuration which results in systolic straightening of the mitral leaflets without

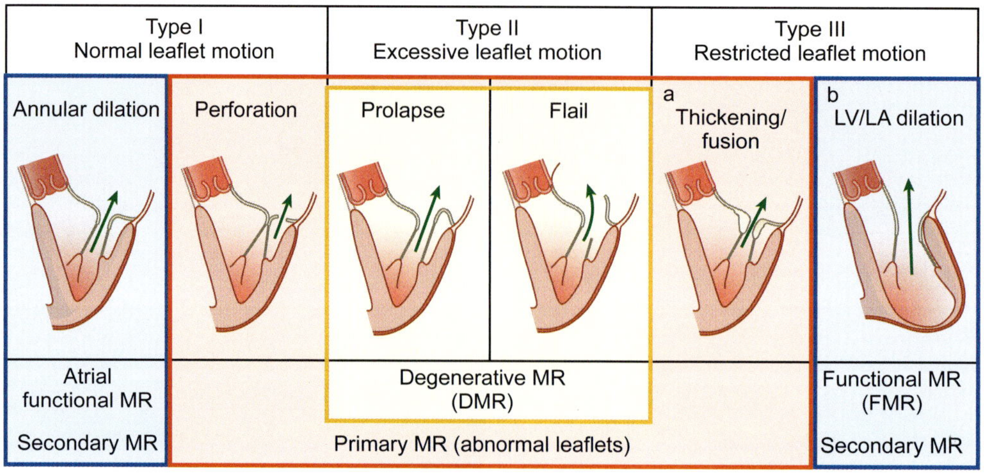

Fig. 7.4 Integrated Classification of MR Mechanism. The Carpentier classification of MR mechanism is based on leaflet motion and includes both common (e.g., prolapse) as well as uncommon etiologies (e.g., perforation). Other practical clinical classifications of MR mechanisms can be nested inside the Carpentier classification. Mitral regurgitation can be broadly classified as ***primary*** *(red box)*, in which case the pathology resides within the valve itself, or ***secondary*** *(blue boxes)* due to structural changes in the LV or LA stretching various portions of the MV apparatus. Primary MR due to prolapse or flail is referred to as ***degenerative MR*** (gold box, Carpentier type II)). Secondary MR due to LV systolic dysfunction is referred to as ***functional MR*** (right-most column, Carpentier type IIIb). Another notable subtype is ***atrial functional MR*** (left-most column, Carpentier type IIIa), in which the primary cause of MR is progressive annular dilatation as part of left atrium (LA) enlargement, often in the setting of chronic atrial fibrillation. Atrial functional MR (Carpentier type I) is characterized by normal leaflet motion and by preserved LV systolic function—in contrast to functional MR (Carpentier type IIIb) caused by LV systolic dysfunction and leaflet tethering. (Modified from Zoghbi WA, Adams D, Bonow RO, et al. Recommendations for noninvasive evaluation of native valvular regurgitation: a report from the American society of echocardiography developed in collaboration with the society for cardiovascular magnetic resonance. *J Am Soc Echocardiogr.* 2017;30[4]:303–371.)

prolapse (<2 mm billowing above the annulus).[11] The regurgitant jet has a "functional" appearance with a wide central jet due to diffuse malcoaptation. AFMR is commonly seen in the setting of LV diastolic dysfunction or atrial fibrillation.[9] Other, less common etiologies such as MR due to rheumatic disease, mitral annular calcification, drug-induced valvulopathies, Libman-Sacks endocarditis, and infective endocarditis are less common and rarely suitable for TEER.

MR Severity

Integrative Approach

Reliable grading of mitral regurgitation severity is complex because the reference "gold standard" is yet to be discovered. Although several specific criteria for MR severity have been established, none can be used as a sole determinant of MR grade because of multiple technical and hemodynamic caveats.[8] Qualitative assessment of the jet size on color Doppler, a widely used method in clinical practice, has proven to be unreliable outside of clear-cut cases where MR is very mild or very severe.[8,12] As a result, multiple datapoints obtained by different methods should be collected and included in the final analysis (Table 7.1 and Fig. 7.5). The methods include quantitative, semiquantitative, and qualitative Doppler assessments (color, spectral, quantitative, 3D color), as well as indirect clues to MR severity such as LV and LA chamber size, pulmonary vein flow profile, pulmonary artery systolic pressures, and right-sided function.[8] The final integrative assessment of MR severity also takes into account data quality and applicability in a particular case. The ultimate goal is to determine whether MR answer the practical clinical question: whether MR is clinically severe MR or nonsevere MR, because only the severe MR, coupled with symptoms and/or its detrimental effects on LV or upstream, is an indication for invasive treatment.[12,13] This distinction is clear in the presence of multiple specific criteria but less so when none or only a few are present (see Fig 7.5).

Specific Criteria

Specific criteria for mild MR include small, narrow centrally directed jet, vena contracta width (VCW) ≤3 mm, proximal isovelocity surface area (PISA) radius less than 3 mm at a Nyquist limit of 30 to 40 cm/s, A-wave-dominant mitral inflow, and normal LV and LA size (see Fig 7.5). These features are not consistent with chronic severe mitral regurgitation.[8] Conversely, VCW ≥7 mm, PISA radius ≥10 mm at Nyquist 30 to 40 cm/s, very large central jet filling greater than 50% of the LA area in a standard view, and dilated LV with normal systolic function

TABLE 7.1 Grading the Severity of Chronic MR by Echocardiography

	MR SEVERITY[a]			
	Mild	**Moderate**		**Severe**
Structural				
MV morphology	None or mild leaflet abnormality (e.g., mild thickening, calcifications or prolapse, mild tenting)	Moderate leaflet abnormality or moderate tenting		Severe valve lesions (primary: flail leaflet, ruptured papillary muscle, severe retraction, large perforation; secondary: severe tenting, poor leaflet coaptation)
LV and LA size[b]	Usually normal	Normal or mild dilated		Dilated[c]
Qualitative Doppler				
Color flow jet area[d]	Small, central, narrow, often brief	Variable		Large central jet (>50% of LA) or eccentric wall-impinging jet of variable size
Flow convergence[e]	Not visible, transient, or small	Intermediate in size and duration		Large throughout systole
CWD jet	Faint/partial/parabolic	Dense but partial or parabolic		Holosystolic/dense/triangular
Semiquantitative				
VCW (cm)	<0.3	Intermediate		≥0.7 (>0.8 for biplane)[f]
Pulmonary vein flow[g]	Systolic dominance (may be blunted in LV dysfunction or AF)	Normal or systolic blunting[g]		Minimal to no systolic flow/systolic flow reversal
Mitral inflow[h]	A-wave dominant	Variable		E-wave dominant (>1.2 m/s)
Quantitativett.[i,j]				
EROA, 2D PISA (cm²)	<0.20	0.20–0.29	0.30–0.39	≥0.40
				(may be lower in secondary MR with elliptical ROA)
RVol (mL)	<30	30–44	40–49	≥60
(may be lower in low-flow conditions)				
RF (%)	<30	30–39	45–59	≥50

[a]All parameters have limitations, and an integrated approach must be used that weighs the strength of each echocardiographic measurement. All signs and measures should be interpreted in an individualized manner that accounts for body size, sex, and all other patient characteristics
[b]This pertains mostly to patients with primary MR.
[c]LV and LA can be within the "normal" range for patients with acute severe MR or with chronic severe MR who have small body size, particularly women, or with small LV size preceding the occurrence of MR.
[d]With Nyquist limit 50 to 70 cm/s.
[e]Small flow convergence is usually less than 0.3 cm, and large is ≥1cm at a Nyquist limit of 30 to 40 cm/s.
[f]For average between apical 2- and 4-chamber views.
[g]Influenced by many other factors (LV diastolic function, atrial fibrillation, LA pressure).
[h]Most valid in patients greater than 50 years old and is influenced by other causes of elevated LA pressure.
[i]Discrepancies among EROA, RF, and RVol may arise in the setting of low or high flow states.
[j]Quantitative parameters can help subclassify the moderate regurgitation group.
From Zoghbi WA, Adams D, Bonow RO, et al. Recommendations for noninvasive evaluation of native valvular regurgitation: a report from the American Society of Echocardiography developed in collaboration with the society for cardiovascular magnetic resonance. *J Am Soc Echocardiogr.* 2017;30(4):303–371.
Bolded qualitative and semi-quantitative signs are considered specific for their MR grade. *LA,* left atrium; *ROA*, regurgitant orifice area.

in the absence of significant aortic regurgitation. Flail leaflet is another specific criterion for severe MR, although small flails may sometimes be associated with less than 3+ MR.[14]

Quantitative Criteria

The three quantitative parameters used clinically to describe valvular regurgitation are the ***effective regurgitant orifice area (EROA)***, ***the regurgitant volume***, and ***the regurgitant fraction*** (see Table 7.1 and Fig 7.5).[8] The regurgitant volume can be calculated from EROA and vice versa using MR velocity-time integral (VTI) obtained by continuous-wave Doppler. The EROA can be obtained by various Doppler techniques: PISA, direct planimetry of the 3D vena contracta area (3D VCA), and quantitative Doppler. The first two methods use color Doppler to capture the EROA at a single moment with the assumption that the EROA remains relatively constant throughout systole. However, if there is a significant systolic variation in the size of the regurgitant orifice or if MR is not holosystolic, then using

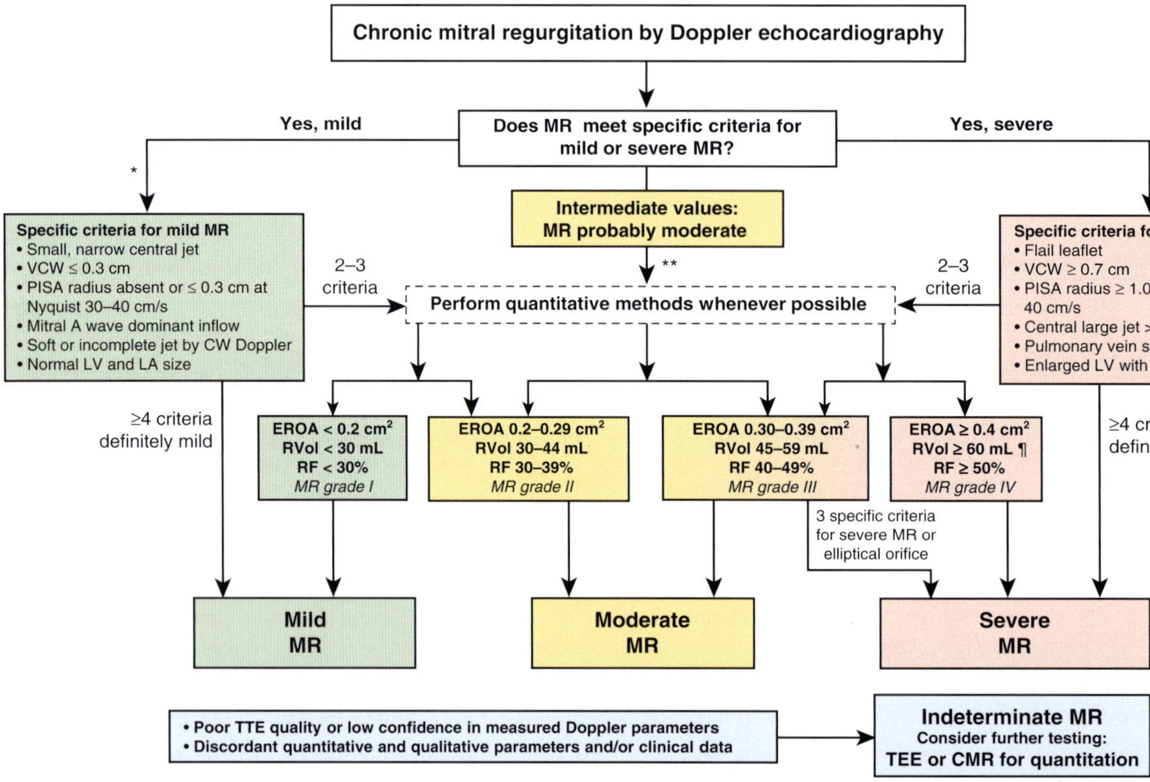

*	Beware of underestimation of MR severity in eccentric, wall impinging jets; quantitation is advised
**	All values for EROA by PISA assume holosystolic MR; single frame EROA by PISA and VCW overestimate non-holosystolic MR
¶	Regurgitant volume for severe MR may be lower in low flow conditions.

Fig. 7.5 Integrative Approach to Grading Mitral Regurgitation. This flowchart sorts out mild and severe MR by multiple specific criteria and centers on the more difficult task of splitting the intermediate range into clinically relevant categories of mild, moderate, and severe MR. Since no single parameter is pathognomonic for either category, multiple qualitative and quantitative parameters are combined prior to a final diagnosis. *ROA*, Regurgitant orifice area. Bolded qualitative and semiquantitative signs are considered specific for their MR grade. *All parameters have limitations, and an integrated approach must be used that weighs the strength of each echocardiographic measurement. All signs and measures should be interpreted in an individualized manner that accounts for body size, sex, and all other patient characteristics. †This pertains mostly to patients with primary MR. ‡LV and LA can be within the "normal" range for patients with acute severe MR or with chronic severe MR who have small body size, particularly women or with small LV size preceding the occurrence of MR. §With Nyquist limit 50 to 70 cm/s.
kSmall flow convergence is usually less than 0.3 cm, and large is $ 1 cm at a Nyquist limit of 30 to 40 cm/s. {For average between apical 2- and 4-chamber views. #Influenced by many other factors (LV diastolic function, atrial fibrillation, LA pressure). **Most valid in patients greater than 50 years old and is influenced by other causes of elevated LA pressure. ††Discrepancies among EROA, regurgitant fraction (RF), and regurgitant volume (RVol) may arise in the setting of low or high flow states. ‡‡Quantitative parameters can help subclassify the moderate regurgitation group. *EROA*, Effective regurgitant orifice area; *LA*, left atrium; *TEE*, transesophageal echo; *TTE*, transthoracic echocardiogram; *PISA*, proximal isovelocity surface area.
(Reproduced from Zoghbi WA, Adams D, Bonow RO, et al. Recommendations for noninvasive evaluation of native valvular regurgitation: a report from the American society of echocardiography developed in collaboration with the society for cardiovascular magnetic resonance. *J Am Soc Echocardiogr.* 2017;30[4]:303–371.)

unadjusted instantaneous EROA to calculate the regurgitant volume will result in error. In contrast, quantitative Doppler estimates the regurgitant volume as the difference between the forward LV stroke volume and the total volume entering the LV in diastole. The regurgitant volume can then be divided by the MR VTI to obtain the mean EROA. In addition, the regurgitant volume can be divided by the total LV stroke volume to estimate the regurgitant fraction. Although well suited to handle systolic variation in EROA, as well as multiple and eccentric jets, quantitative Doppler is limited by multiple geometric assumptions and requires expertise for reliable results.[8]

Semiquantitative Criteria

Several semiquantitative criteria are also included in the integrative assessment of MR (see Table 7.1). Of these, the VCW is another instantaneous color Doppler method of approximating the EROA in a single dimension (orthogonal measurements can be averaged if EROA is elliptical).[8] Intermediate values for VCW are not particularly useful, but the extremes—VCW ≤3 mm or ≥7 mm—are used as specific criteria for mild and severe MR, respectively. Functional MR presents a special challenge for classic color Doppler techniques (VCW, PISA) because the jet origin is typically wide and elliptical violating the circular orifice assumption inherent to these methods. Since the major diameter of FMR's elliptical orifice is in the commissural view (approximated by the standard 2-chamber view on TTE), the average of VCW in 2- and 4-chamber views may be used on TTE with biplane VCW less than 0.8 mm used as specific criteria for severe MR.[8] Methods that do not require geometric assumptions about the shape of regurgitant orifice, including quantitative Doppler and 3D VCA planimetry, are better suited to estimate EROA in FMR than 2D methods.[15–17]

Other supplemental criteria include mitral inflow patterns on pulsed wave Doppler. Late diastolic predominance (A-dominant inflow) is frequently seen with nonsevere MR, while the dominance of flow in early diastole (E-wave) is seen in chronic severe MR.[8] In systole, the left atrial pressure increases sharply with significant MR impeding or reversing the normally antegrade flow in the pulmonary veins. Accordingly, the pulmonary vein flow pattern is used as a semiquantitative criterion to assess the impact of MR on systolic left atrial pressure.[18] Pulmonary venous flow reversal is more specific when present in more than one vein.[8]

Pitfalls of Color Doppler

Color Doppler is an essential tool to detect MR and assess its geographic distribution. The size of the color Doppler jet depends on multiple technical factors, not the least of which are color gain and scale. Similarly, applying low flow optimization settings, normally used to detect nonturbulent (venous) flow, to the high-velocity MR jets results in unwanted detection of the entrained nonregurgitant blood and larger total MR jet. Jet size can also be influenced by hemodynamic factors, which increase the driving force behind MR and the momentum of the jet. The higher the jet momentum (determined in large part by jet velocity), the larger the corresponding jet area on color Doppler.[8] This can be seen with large EROAs, central (unconstrained) jets, and abnormally high jet velocity, often as a result of systemic hypertension (Fig. 7.6). Accordingly, hypotension is a frequent cause of underestimation of true MR severity in the setting of low flow state or general anesthesia.[19]

Total MR severity may also be overestimated if the amount of regurgitation varies during systole due to a dynamic regurgitant orifice. The two most common forms of MR—functional and degenerative—often demonstrate a significant variation of MR flow through systole.[20,21] A prolapse may not result in significant MR until the late systole when malcoaptation occurs. Functional MR is often biphasic: a sharp peak in very early systole followed by a late systolic peak.[22] Nonholosystolic MR can be recognized on color Doppler, facilitated by frame-by-frame analysis and color m-mode, and by an incomplete continuous-wave Doppler envelope (see Fig. 7.6). Volumetric methods (e.g., quantitative Doppler) account for systolic variation and are better suited to assess MR severity in these situations but are subject to their own limitations.[8]

Highly eccentric jets present a challenge to color Doppler due to frequently nonparallel alignment and rapid loss of momentum upon contact with the LA wall, resulting in a deceptively small color jet area. A notable color Doppler pattern is the "flat and wide" mosaic appearance of the regurgitant jet filling the periannular space. These jets can be seen in association with flail segments (see Fig. 7.6). The small jet area can lead to a significant underestimation of MR. A "flat and wide" jet, particularly in the presence of pulmonary vein systolic flow reversal, triangular MR CW Doppler envelope, or acute systolic heart failure, warrants further investigation to clarify MR severity, usually with TEE. This is distinct from the color Doppler "splay," a broadening of the basal portion of the jet on color Doppler representing a sidelobe artifact from high flow regions of the MR jet, which also suggests significant MR.[23]

In a minority of cases, the uncertainty about MR severity may require a cardiac MRI and/or stress echo to resolve it. Cardiac MRI can provide a reproducible quantitative assessment of MR, including the regurgitant fraction, and is currently recommended when echo is nondiagnostic or discrepant with clinical findings.[8] In addition, MRI provides reliable measurements of LV and right ventricle (RV) volumes as well as ejection fraction. Stress echo can potentially demonstrate exercise-induced MR not evident from resting studies and assess pulmonary artery systolic pressures during exercise.

Feasibility Assessment

Echocardiography alone allows comprehensive feasibility assessment for TEER repair. Screening studies should demonstrate adequate baseline mitral valve area (MVA) that would allow MR reduction to ≤2+ without pathologic stenosis, adequate leaflet tissue for secure grasp, and a clear transseptal path for delivery catheters to the mitral valve (Table 7.2).

Baseline Mitral Valve Area

Multiple studies have reported worse clinical outcomes in patients with TEER-induced hemodynamically significant mitral stenosis.[24,25] Therefore, it is important to accurately estimate the baseline MVA. Although gradients are reflective of the MVA, they also depend on cardiac output and therefore should always be interpreted in the context of the heart rate and LV stroke volume. The pressure half-time method has limited applicability outside of the rheumatic population.[26] The continuity equation is not valid in the setting of significant MR.[8] Planimetry of the MVA is independent of hemodynamics but requires some expertise to capture the optimal echocardiographic plane for direct planimetry (Fig. 7.7). This is most reliably done with 3D multiplanar reconstruction using the double oblique technique (Fig. 7.8).[27–30] The desired short-axis plane with the largest mitral valve opening is reconstructed by aligning two orthogonal long-axis planes with the leaflet tips. Both spatial and temporal resolution are important for reliable planimetry of the MVA. Adequate spatial resolution helps reliably identify leaflet tips' margins, and adequate temporal resolution ensures that the largest MV opening is captured. The region of

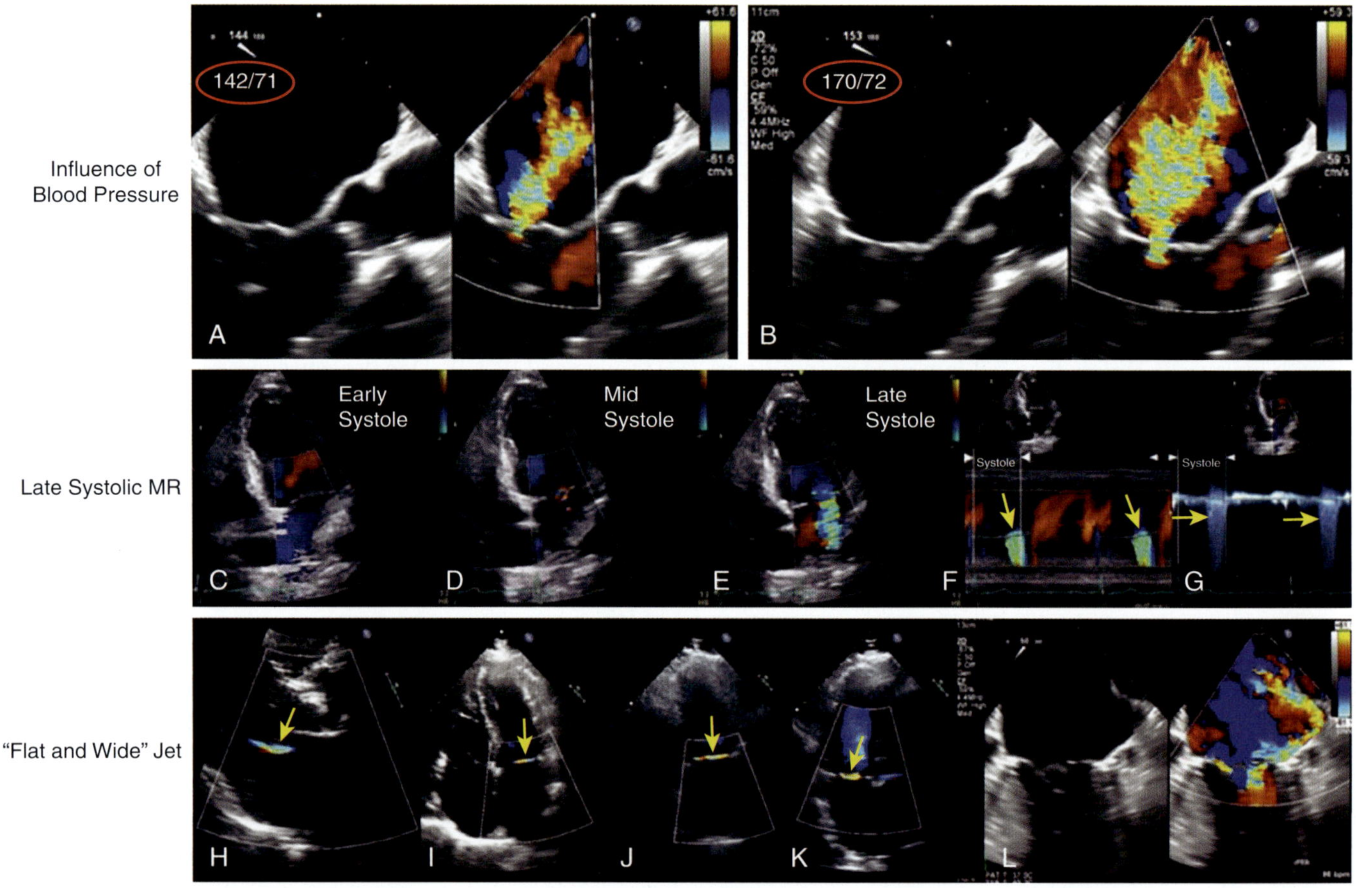

Fig. 7.6 Pitfalls of Color Doppler. (A and B) Systemic hypertension increases afterload, which increases the velocity and momentum of the MR jet, which in turn increases the size of the jet on color Doppler. In this example increase in systolic blood pressure by 28 mm Hg results in a significantly larger color jet area. (C–G) Another common pitfall is failure to account for the systolic variation of MR. In this patient with mitral valve prolapse, there is hardly any color jet area in the early and mid-systole (C and D) until a large jet appears in the late systole (E), corresponding to the timing of maximal prolapse. The nonholosystolic presence of MR can be more easily appreciated on color M-mode (F, *arrows*) and CW Doppler (G, *arrows*). Extrapolation of the color jet area or color Doppler-derived parameters (e.g., vena contracta, proximal isovelocity surface area, and 3D vena contracta area) to the entire systole will overestimate the true MR severity. (H–L) Highly eccentric jets may escape detection in standard transthoracic echocardiogram views and present only as a small "flat and wide" jet area at the mitral annulus (H–K, *arrows*). Subsequent transesophageal echo in the same patient reveals severe MR as a highly eccentric jet hugging the left atrium wall (L). (Reproduced from Marcoff L, Gillam LD. Role of the imager in transcatheter mitral valve repair. *Curr Cardiol Rep.* 2020;22[10]:120.)

TABLE 7.2 Anatomic Feasibility of the Edge-to-Edge Transcatheter Mitral Valve Repair

Optimal	Rarely Feasible
Focal disease: Single MR jet at A2P2	Barlow's disease with multiple significant jets
MVA >4.0 cm^2[a]	MVA <3.5 cm^2
Posterior leaflet length >10 mm	Posterior leaflet length <7 mm
No leaflet calcification in the grasping area	Severe calcification in the grasping area
Flail gap <10 mm; Flail width <15 mm	Wide regurgitant orifice when limited to one device
	Cleft in the grasping area
	Large coaptation gap[b]
	Rheumatic MV disease, leaflet perforation, endocarditis

[a]Measured by planimetry, preferably 3D multiplanar reconstruction.
[b]New generation transcatheter edge-to-edge devices capable of grasping each leaflet independently may allow treating larger coaptation gaps.

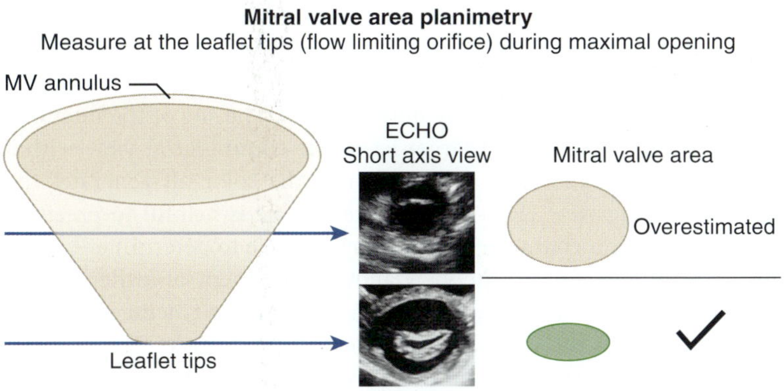

Fig. 7.7 Planimetry of the Mitral Valve Area. Since creating pathologic stenosis is a dreaded complication of TEER, an accurate estimate of the MVA is required prior to the procedure. The mitral valve can be represented schematically as a funnel that narrows down at the leaflet tips level. Thus, a "blind" short-axis plane at any other level will result in overestimation of the MVA by varying degrees, depending on the distance from the leaflet tips.

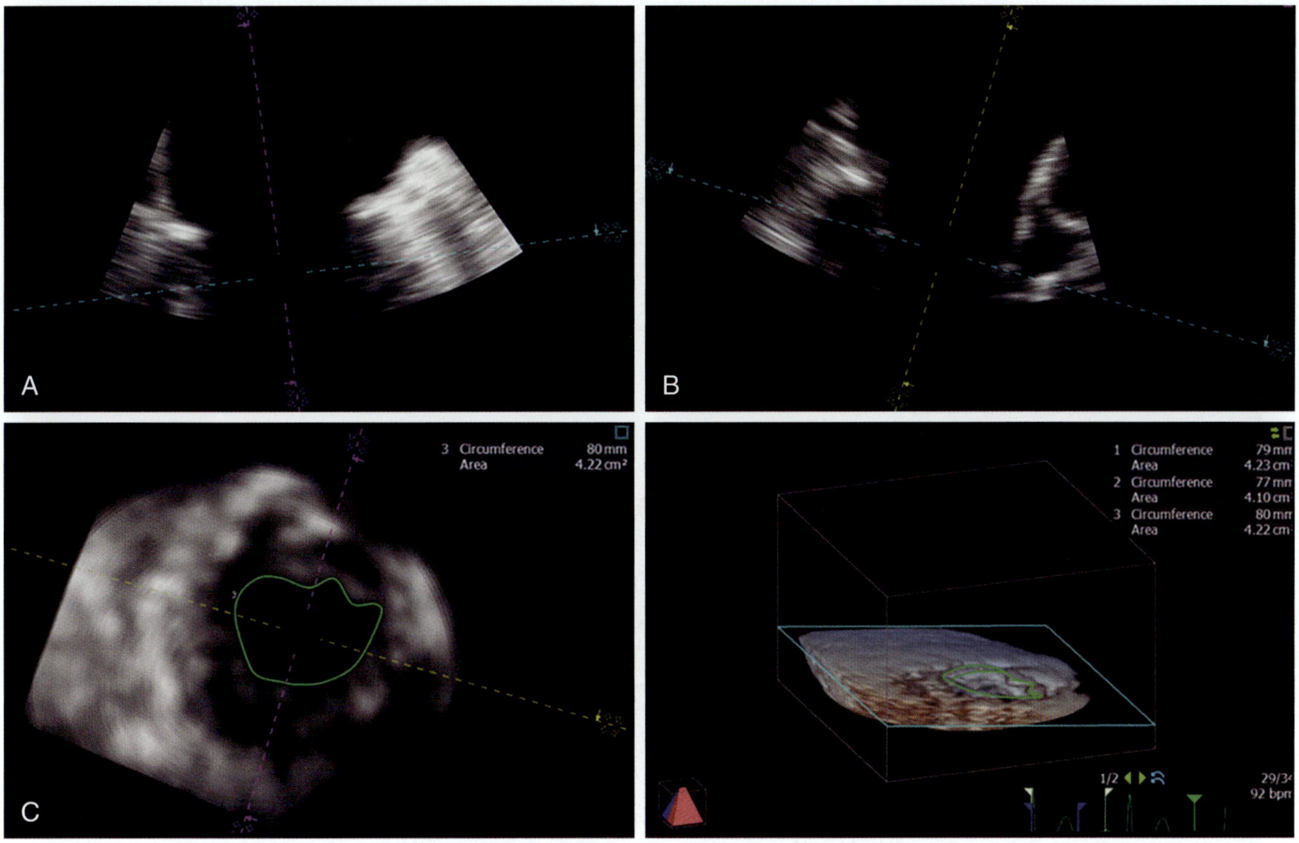

Fig. 7.8 Planimetry of the Mitral Valve Area Using 3D Multiplanar Reconstruction. Three-dimensional data allow reconstruction of the narrowest portion of the mitral inflow at the leaflet tips—the optimal plane for 2D planimetry of mitral valve area (MVA). After selecting the frame with maximal mitral valve opening, the short-axis plane *(blue)* is positioned at the leaflet tips in two orthogonal views (A and B). This process generates the optimal 2D short-axis plane for MVA planimetry (C).

interest can be extended vertically to include leaflet tips without significantly reducing the frame rate, in contrast to changing the width of the region.

Biplane imaging is a feature available with 3D transducers and is useful for MVA planimetry if multiplanar reconstruction cannot be performed. The biplane cursor is positioned across the mitral leaflet tips in the early diastole within the parasternal long-axis view on TTE. This will generate the defined short-axis plane for MVA planimetry. Although inferior to 3D multiplanar reconstruction (MPR) for lack of control of the coronal plane, the biplane method still ensures at least partial alignment with leaflet tips. In contrast, using the single plane of 2D TTE requires careful scanning of the LV base in the parasternal short axis to align with the mitral leaflet tips and depends on the sonographer's expertise to identify the optimal plane for planimetry. The 2D planimetry has been shown to overestimate the MVA compared to 3D echo and invasive Gorlin MVA.[30,31] Reliable estimate of the baseline MVA is essential for procedural planning, particularly in cases likely to require more than one device (e.g., large flail segments, multiple target jets).

Selecting the Target Jet

While visual identification of the target jet on color Doppler is usually straightforward, precisely locating the jet origin can be challenging if imaging off-axis. Jet direction is often a clue to the general location of pathology, but the target is the jet origin on the coaptation line corresponding to the vena contracta in the commissural view. This view can be adjusted by a slight rotation of the probe clockwise or counterclockwise to bring out the different segments of the curved coaptation line and optimize individual jets.[3] Multiple jets are frequent and may present separate TEER targets, depending on how widely they are separated on the coaptation line. In FMR, color Doppler often reveals the confluence of adjacent jets into a single elliptical origin which can be considered a single TEER target.

Grasping Area Survey

Generating grasping view. The grasping view is the specific long-axis plane showing both leaflets at the site of the intended grasp. Bisecting the target jet in the commissural view with a biplane cursor and then switching the color off generates the grasping view (Fig. 7.9). This technique is helpful to precisely locate and characterize the grasping zone to determine the feasibility of TEER. The view allows assessment of leaflet length, the degree of prolapse or tethering, leaflet calcification, and chords in the actual area of the intended grasp. 3D MPR allows reconstruction of on-axis views and planimetry of the 3D VCA, particularly useful if the acquired 2D views are off-axis (see Fig. 7.9).

Posterior leaflet length. The posterior leaflet is the shortest of the two leaflets, and its length can be a limiting factor in TEER. Current TEER devices rely on capturing enough leaflet tissue to engage the full array of the frictional elements in order to sustain the cyclic load. Inadequate leaflet insertion may result

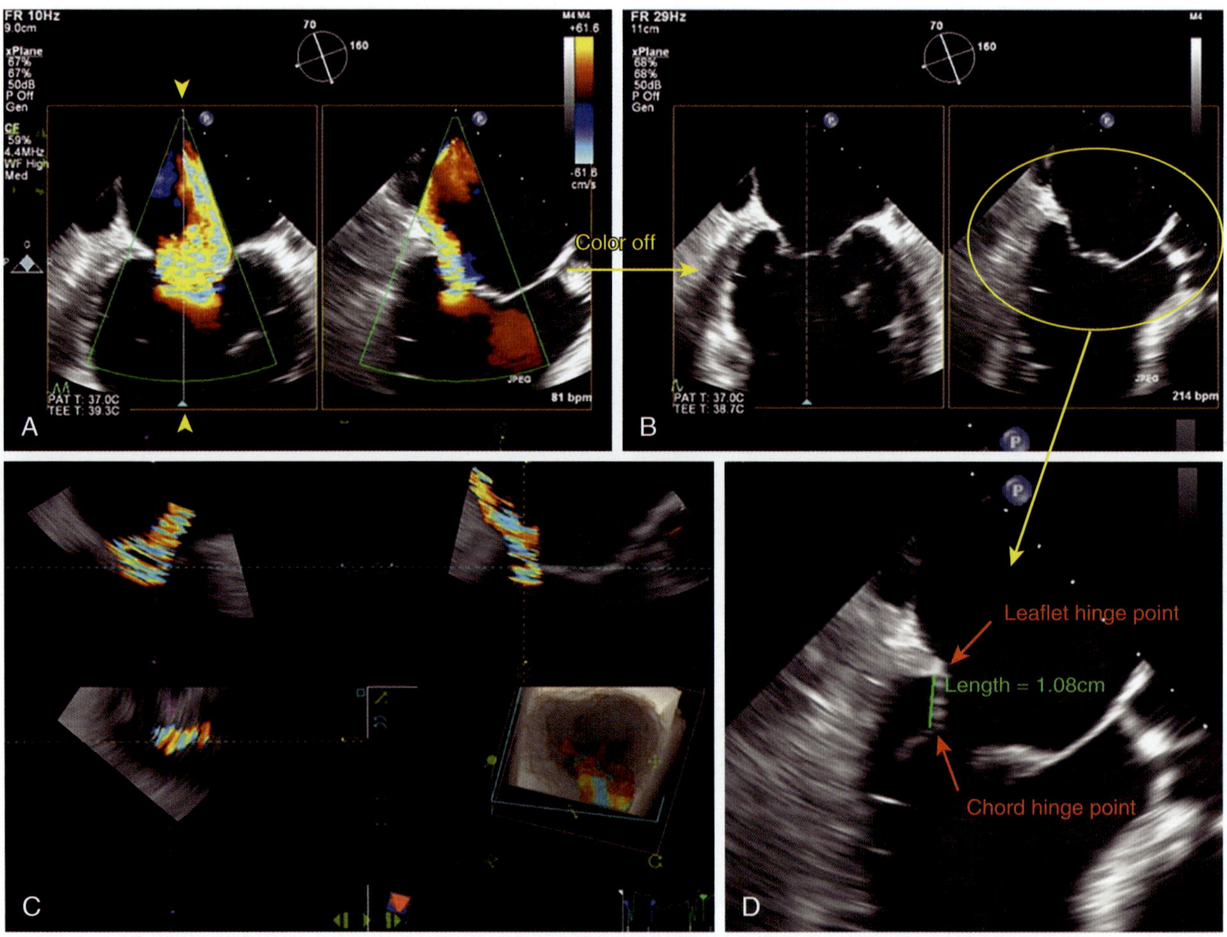

Fig. 7.9 Generating Grasping View. The grasping view can be generated by placing the biplane cursor *(arrowheads)* across the middle of the target jet on color Doppler (A). The orthogonal long-axis grasping view will appear in the secondary plane (A, *right panel*). While keeping this view stable, the color Doppler is switched off, providing the grasping view without color and improving the temporal resolution (B). This view can help to make the relevant assessments of the grasping site. In this example (D), the length of the posterior leaflet can be measured at the exact site of the intended grasp (D).

in single leaflet device attachment (SLDA). The graspable portion of the leaflet stretches from the leaflet tip to the hinge at the base (see Fig. 7.9). Care should be taken to separate the leaflet tip from the primary chords to avoid overestimating its length. This can be facilitated by frame-by-frame search for clear leaflet/chord separation.

Flail width/gap. A combination of a ruptured chord and the excursion of the leaflet tip above the opposing leaflet or the annulus defines a flail leaflet segment.[32] Flails vary in size and location. Large flails were excluded from the pivotal randomized trial of TEER.[32] Although such cases have been treated successfully "off-label,"[33] observational data suggest that TEER of very large flail segments (width ≥15 mm, gap ≥10 mm) may pose a higher risk of reintervention.[34] Flail width can be measured on TTE in a carefully selected parasternal short-axis view.[32] Alternatively, the flail width can be measured in the commissural view (Fig. 7.10). The flail gap, or the maximal height above the opposing leaflet, is best measured in the orthogonal long-axis view and occasionally in the 4-chamber view, depending on the location.[32] 3D MPR provides full control of selecting the optimal plane and can be used for precise measurements, provided that spatial and temporal resolutions are adequate (see Fig 7.10).

Indentations versus clefts. With the advent of the 3D echo, the surgical en-face view of the mitral valve became ubiquitous

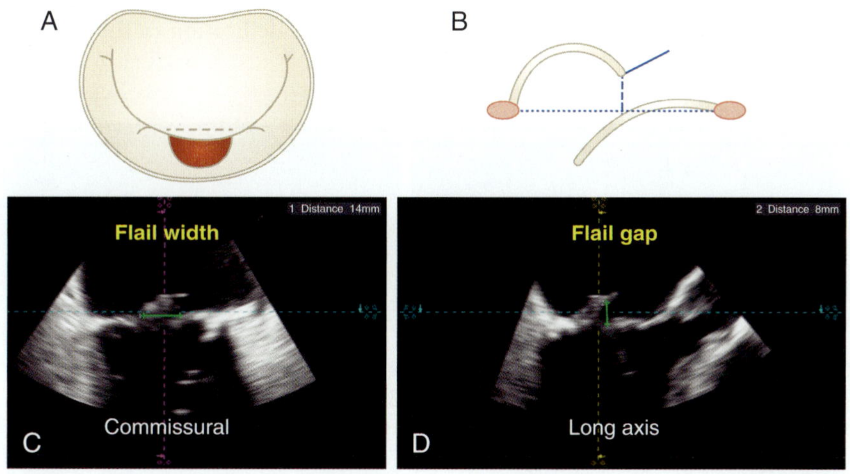

Fig. 7.10 Measuring Flail Width and Gap. The width of the flail can be measured along the coaptation line in the short-axis view and the flail gap in apical 4- and 3-chamber views (A and B). Three-dimensional imaging does not rely on getting the exact 2D plane during acquisition and allows reconstruction of desired views for valid measurements (C and D).

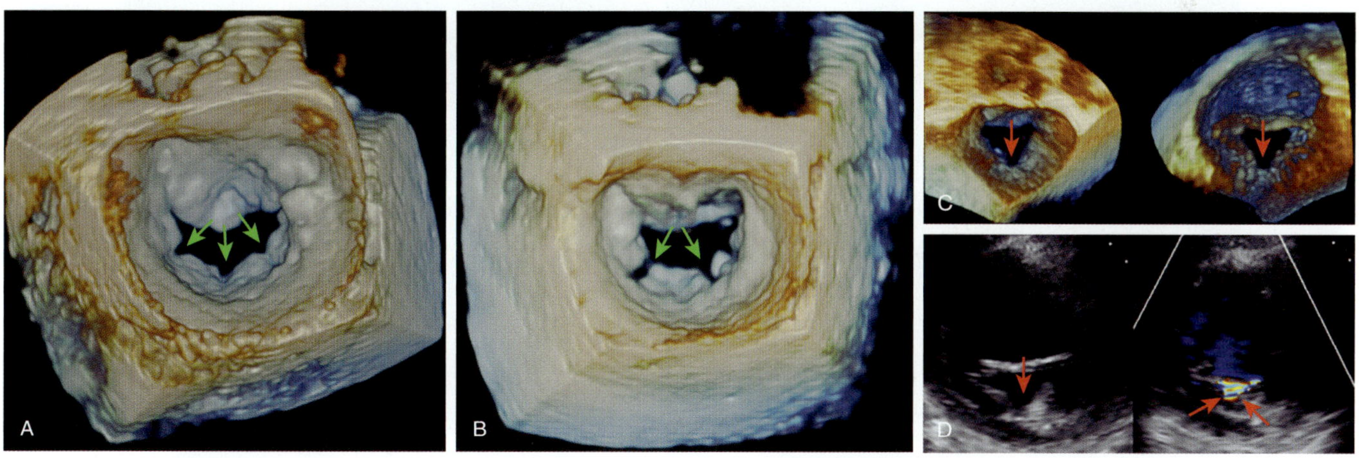

Interscallop indentations Deep/cleft-like indentations Cleft

Fig. 7.11 Indentations and Clefts. The posterior mitral leaflet is naturally divided by interscallop indentations (A, *arrows*). These indentations occasionally are deep (cleft-like), cutting closer to the posterior annulus (B, *arrows*). These are distinct from true clefts, which reach all the way to the annulus and in unexpected locations, such as in this example (C), where the cleft is seen in the middle of the posterior leaflet *(arrows)*. If a true cleft is present, it is important to determine whether it allows the regurgitant flow through it. This is best assessed by color Doppler in short-axis view (D, *arrows*) or reconstructed from 3D color data. In this example, MR is seen originating from within the cleft. Such cases are not easily treated with edge-to-edge repair.

in clinical practice leading to a wider appreciation of mitral anatomy, including normal morphologic variations of the leaflets. The posterior leaflet is naturally subdivided into scallops (P1, P2, and P3) by interscallop indentations (Fig 7.11). The extent or incision of these indentations toward the posterior annulus is variable.[35,36] Prominent or deep indentations have also been referred to as "clefts," inviting controversy due to confusion with the congenital prototype in endocardial cushion defects.[37] The classic congenital clefts commonly involve the anterior leaflet, normally free of indentations. The term—"cleft-like indentation" (CLI)—has also been used to describe deep indentations providing some distinction from clefts associated with congenital syndromes.[38,39]

In the context of TEER, the important question is whether the CLI is causing MR in a particular case. The answer usually lies in short-axis views of the MV from the LV perspective, where the color Doppler may show an extension of the jet origin into the CLI. 3D color imaging can be helpful to visualize this on a volume-rendered image and reconstruct the precise diagnostic short-axis plane. Limited data suggest that CLIs are prevalent in patients referred for TEER (14%) and do not alter procedural outcomes.[39] However, cases involving CLI may be more likely to involve multiple devices and advanced interventional techniques.[39,40]

Calcium in the grasping area. Leaflet calcification in the grasping area is a potential problem for leaflet insertion into the clip and proper engagement of the grippers (Fig. 7.12). Mild calcifications do not usually present a significant problem, particularly if located on the LV surface. The impact of moderate or severe calcification in the grasping area on TEER outcomes

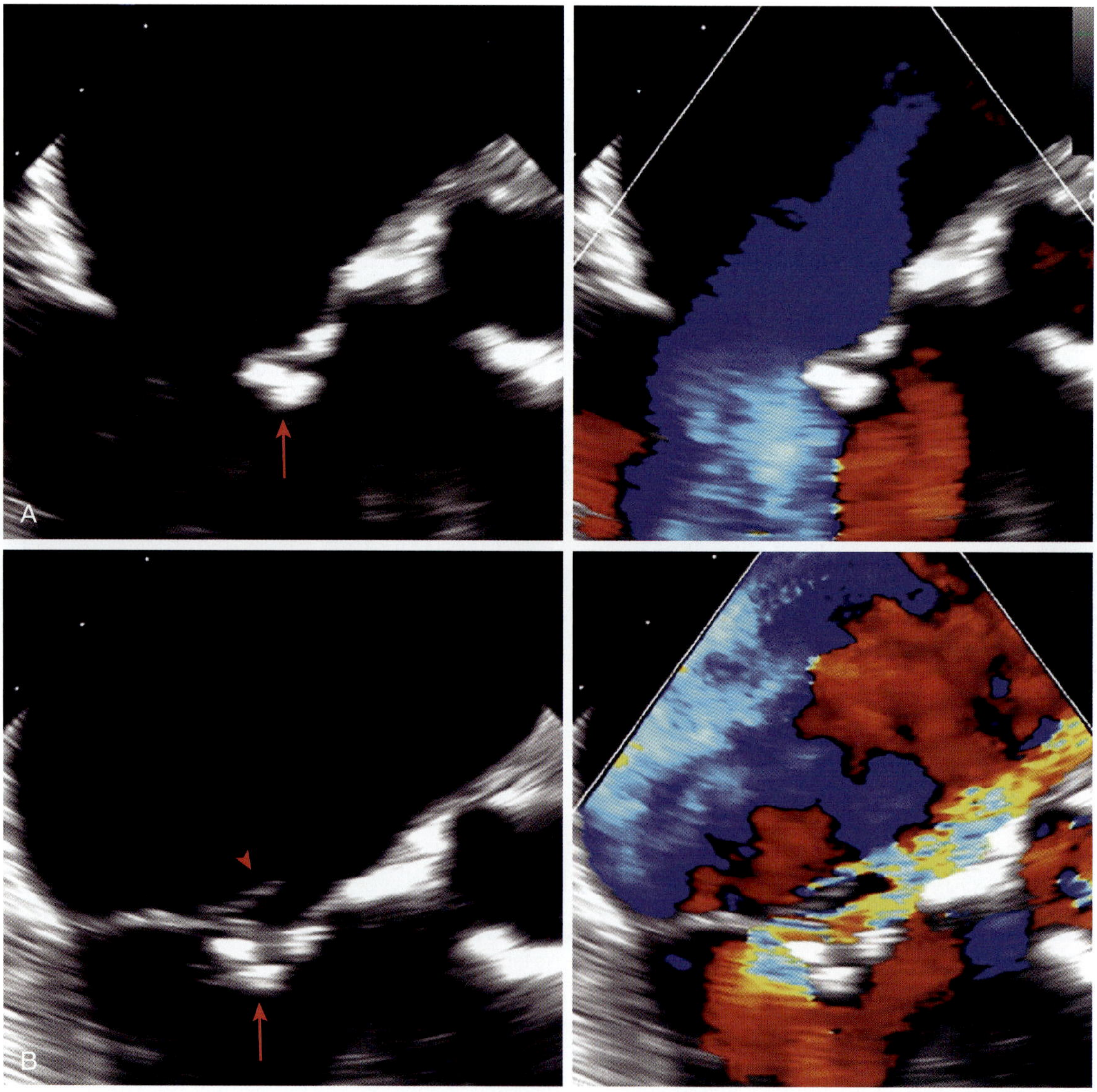

Fig. 7.12 Calcium in the Grasping Area. Calcification in the grasping area presents significant challenges for edge-to-edge because of the potential interference with leaflet insertion and/or leaflet retention. This example shows significant focal calcification at the tip of the anterior leaflet (A, *arrow*), which happens to be in the grasping corresponding to the location of the posterior flail (B, *arrowhead*).

is largely unknown because these patients have been excluded from the randomized trials of TEER repair.[41,42]

Perforations. Leaflet perforations are usually the sequalae of endocarditis.[43,44] Echocardiographically, a perforation is represented by a focal defect within the affected leaflet (Fig. 7.13). The opposing tissue fragments can be identified on 2D and 3D imaging (see Fig 7.13). TEE has superior sensitivity compared to TTE in detecting perforations.[44] On color Doppler perforations present with characteristically turbulent and narrow "lightsaber-like" jets originating away from the coaptation line (see Fig 7.13). Perforations are not feasible for TEER and are best handled surgically.

Commissural jets. True commissural jets can be visualized in their full extent (flow convergence, vena contracta, and the jet area) in the commissural view, directed towards the opposite commissure and nearly parallel to the coaptation line (Fig. 7.14). Accordingly, when imaged in standard long-axis views, commissural jets would only be seen partially, obscured by other jets, or missed altogether. Commissural involvement can also be confirmed by 3D color Doppler (see Fig. 7.14). The commissures are tight spaces criss-crossed with chordae tendineae demanding minimal and precise navigation in order to avoid chordal disruption. Imaging commissural regions is often difficult and involves nonstandard, landmark-poor views and advanced probe manipulations. Registry data suggest that TEER in noncentral (non-A2P2) scallops disease can be performed safely and effectively by experienced operators after a learning curve.[45]

Interatrial septum. The catheter's path to the mitral valve lies through the RA, interatrial septum, and the LA. Right atrial masses, especially near the fossa ovalis—the site of transseptal puncture—are potential sources for embolism during

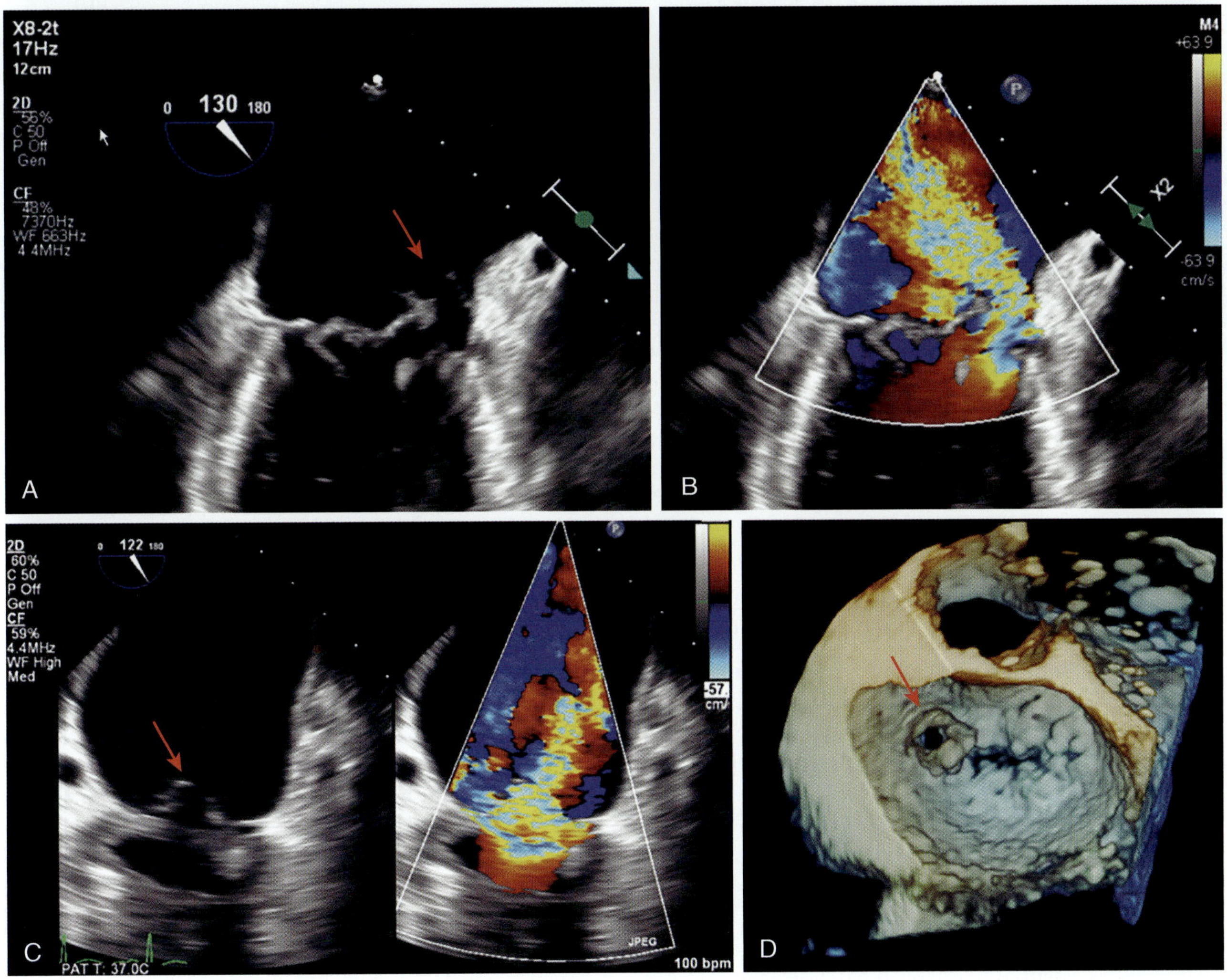

Fig. 7.13 Perforations. Perforations are usually seen in the context of infectious endocarditis. The top row shows a perforation within the A1 scallop as seen on transesophageal echo in a modified 2-chamber view (A and B). Opposing tissue fragments are usually seen (A, *arrow*) corresponding to the origin of a highly turbulent MR jet (B). The bottom row presents images from a different patient with endocarditis and a perforated lateral commissural cusp (C, *arrow*). The perforation can be clearly identified on the 3D volume-rendered image (D, *arrow*).

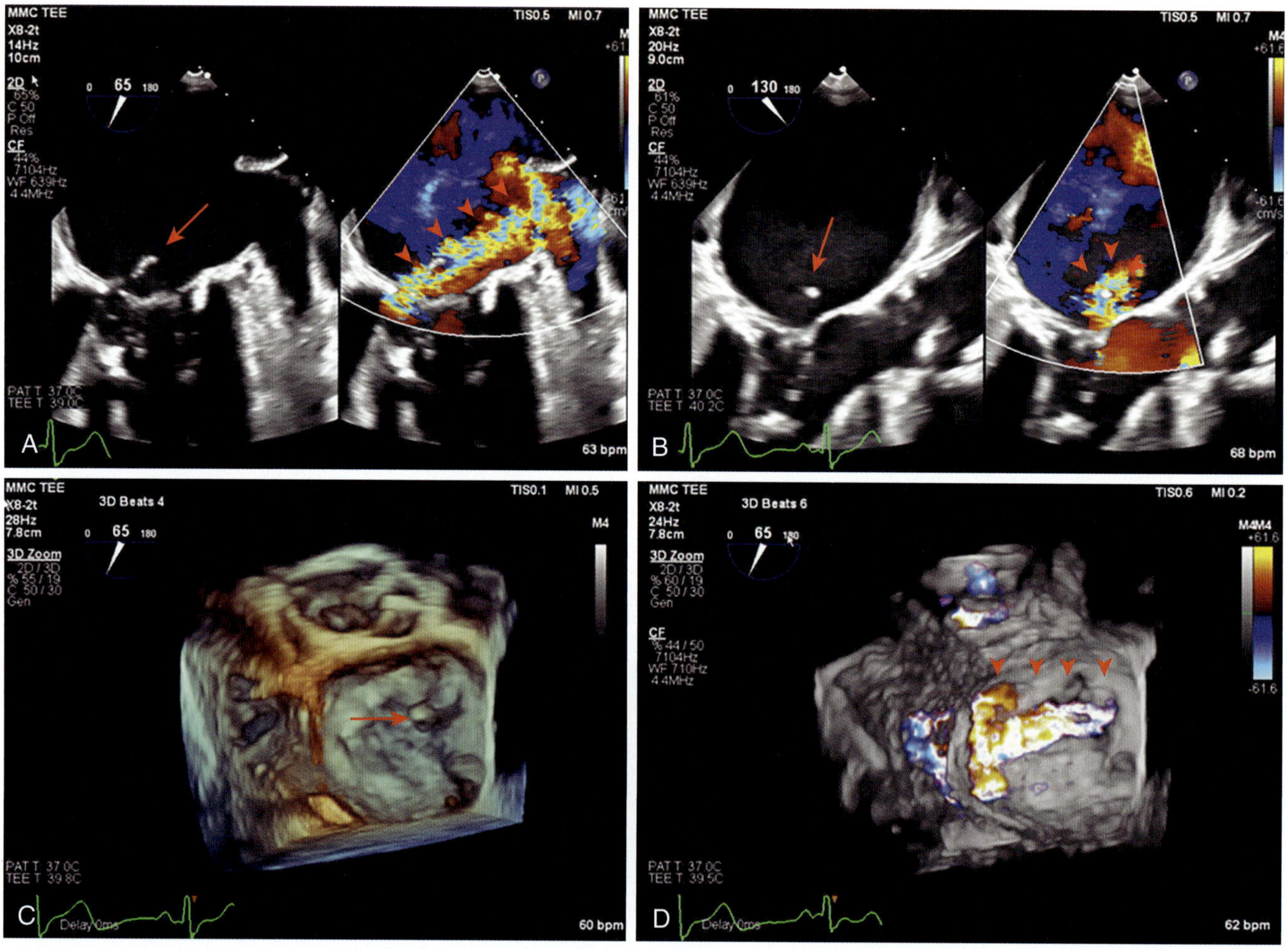

Fig. 7.14 Commissural Disease. This example shows a flail medial commissural cusp (A–C, *arrows*). Because commissural jets are often directed to the opposite commissure, the jet is seen in its entirety in the commissural view (A, *arrowheads*) and en-face in the long-axis view (B, *arrowheads*). 3D volume-rendered with color Doppler shows the commissural jet directed toward the lateral commissure reaching the left atrial appendage (D, *arrowheads*).

or after the procedure as long as the iatrogenic atrial septal defect (ASD) remains open. These should be excluded from screening imaging. Although the patent foramen ovale (PFO) is not a significant problem for TEER, it does provide a path of least resistance to the transseptal needle, which may result in the suboptimal orientation of the delivery system—the "aorta hugger."[46]

PROCEDURAL IMAGING

Baseline Assessment

Baseline imaging is essential to establish baseline anatomic and hemodynamic parameters as a reference for any changes during the procedure. This is also the opportunity for the structural imager to clarify any diagnostic uncertainty lingering from the screening studies.

The initial survey should confirm a safe route for the catheters into the RA, the interatrial septum, and the LA. Thrombi are occasionally discovered on baseline imaging in the left atrial appendage (LAA) or in the RA and may pose an unacceptable risk of systemic embolization. The pericardial space should be imaged and recorded in multiple views to serve as a baseline in case a pericardial effusion is encountered during the procedure, given a small but present risk of perforation. Other important baseline reference parameters include transmitral gradients, MVA by high-quality TEE 3D planimetry (if previously not assessed), and Doppler assessment of systolic flow pulmonary veins as a surrogate of LA pressure. Baseline assessment should confirm the location of target MR jets. It is worth noting that MR severity may be diminished under general anesthesia and hypotension compared to "awake" studies.[19] Finally, leaflet lengths should be confirmed to meet the manufacturer-specified minimal leaflet length required for adequate grasp. Baseline lengths of both leaflets have also been used in the assessment of leaflet insertion—the inserted length being the difference between the baseline leaflet length and the leaflet length that remains outside of the device after grasp.[47]

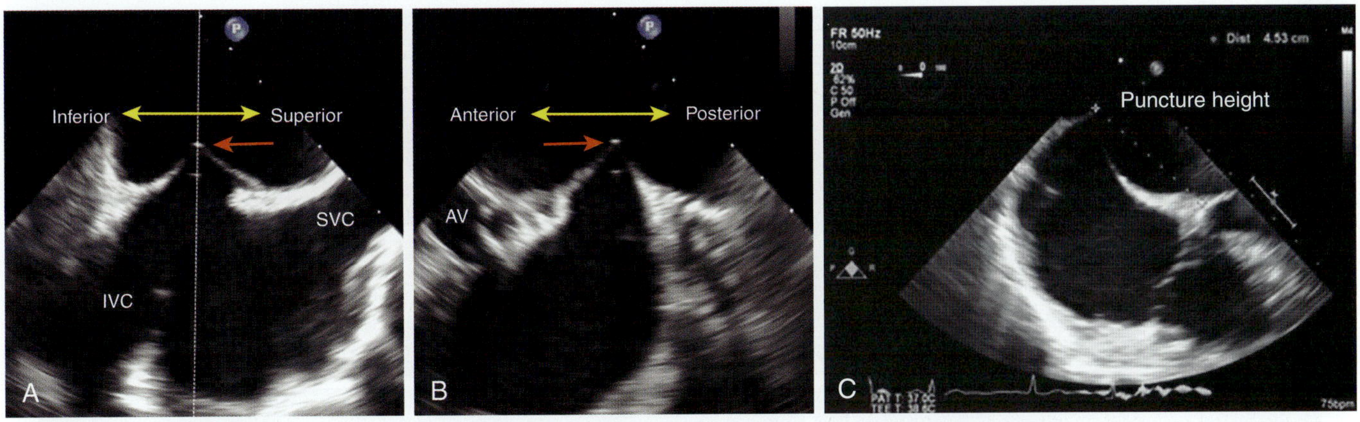

Fig. 7.15 Echo Guidance of the Transseptal Puncture. Standard TEE views for guiding transseptal puncture are the bicaval view (A) and the orthogonal basal short-axis view (B) —both can be viewed simultaneously using biplane mode. The bicaval view shows the septum in the infero-superior plane, while the basal short-axis view shows the septum in the antero-posterior plane. Definitive tenting of the fossa *(arrows)* by the transseptal needle must be visualized before the puncture to ensure the correct location and avoid cardiac perforation. Once adequate tenting has been observed at the intended site, the puncture height can be estimated in the 4-chamber view from the tenting point to the mitral annulus (C). *IVC*, inferior vena cava.

Procedural Steps

Transseptal Puncture

The TS puncture is guided using the two orthogonal views of the interatrial septum: the bicaval, representing the superior-inferior axis, and the AV short-axis view representing the antero-posterior axis (Fig. 7.15). The site of transseptal puncture determines the trajectory of the delivery system and is tailored to the location of pathology. Lateral and central locations are easier to reach with superior punctures, which allow for the shortest route to these targets. Medial locations are best reached using inferior punctures, which also provide height by being anatomically more posterior.[48] The goal is to gain enough height above the mitral leaflets to allow adequate distance range for the device to reach the leaflet tips as well as to achieve coaxiality of the delivery catheter with the mitral inflow.

The true 4-chamber view is used to measure the height of the transseptal puncture above the aortic annulus or the coaptation plane (see Fig. 7.15). If PFO is present, it should not be used as the transseptal conduit because it will direct the system anteriorly and result in suboptimal trajectory in most cases. The moving tip of the transseptal needle, as it descends inferiorly from superior vena cava (SVC), can be tracked with biplane guidance to ensure septal contact. Sharp tenting of the fossa should be clearly demonstrated before proceeding further to ensure that the puncture is performed at the intended location.

Entry of Catheters

After the transseptal access is established, the guidewire is introduced into the LA with its tip positioned within one of the left pulmonary veins, away from the LAA. Color flow Doppler may help detect the wire by its characteristic mosaic sparkly appearance (see Fig 7.16). In the next stage, the coiled dilator followed by the steerable guide will cross into the LA (see Fig. 7.16). The tip of the guide appears as the double line on echo—a reference landmark for guide position (see Fig. 7.16). The guide tip should be clearly visualized in the LA to ensure that it's fully across the septum and not simply stretching the fossa. The imager should also make sure that the guide is not advanced too far so as to touch the LA wall. Risk of perforation aside, there is a potential to introduce air into the system: aspiration through the distal port while the tip is covered will create negative pressure within the system, drawing room air through the valve in the steerable guide subsequently resulting in systemic air embolization as the clip advances through the guide.[49]

Steering

Once the guide is in position, the clip can be introduced into the LAA and steered towards the mitral valve. Safe steering depends on continuous echocardiographic tracking of the tip of the clip and the surrounding LA structures (see Fig. 7.17). In most cases, steering involves negotiating between the advancement of the clip and the retraction of the guide back toward the septum to allow more room to advance the clip further. Biplane imaging may be helpful to exclude the foreshortening of the device (see Fig. 7.17). Steering entirely in 3D is possible, provided that adequate spatial and temporal resolution can be achieved (see Fig. 7.17). Any uncertainty in clip position during steering on 3D should be resolved with dedicated 2D and/or biplane imaging, which provide superior spatial and temporal resolution.

Positioning and Trajectory Setting

After the clip is steered towards the mitral valve, it is positioned over the target jet. The delivery catheter should be as coaxial as possible with the mitral inflow (Fig 7.18). The benefits of coaxiality are twofold: it results in optimal alignment of the clip with the leaflets and minimizes acoustic shadowing of the clip arms by the shaft of the catheter on echo. If "aorta hugger" orientation

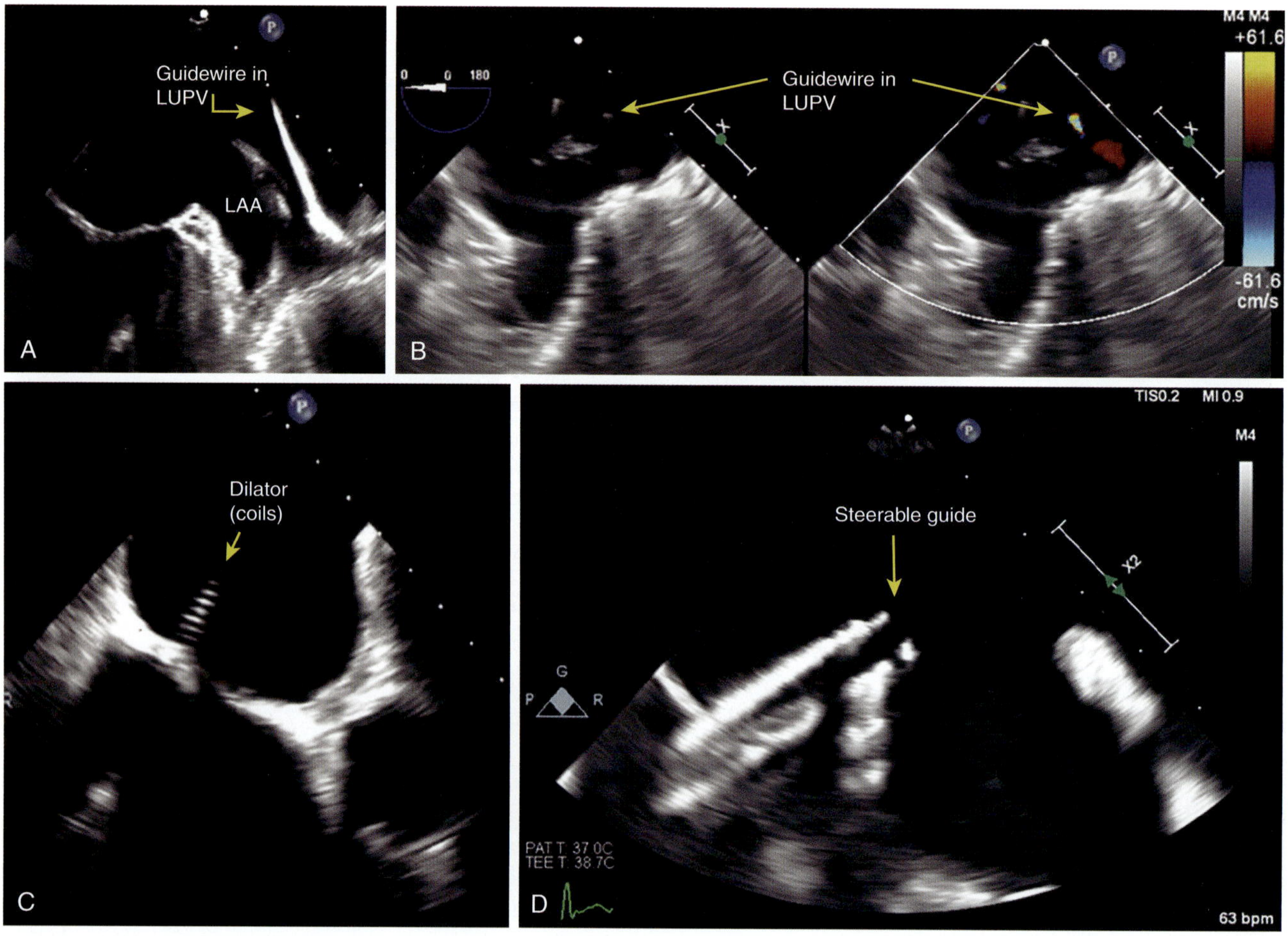

Fig. 7.16 Catheter Entry. After a successful transseptal puncture, the guidewire is introduced and guided into one of the left pulmonary veins, usually the left upper (A). When the guidewire position is uncertain (B), turning on the color flow Doppler may help identify the wire by the characteristic sparkly mosaic artifact *(circled)*. The coils of the dilator can be clearly seen crossing the septum (C). The steerable guide (D) follows the dilator into the left atrium . *LAA,* Left atrial appendage, *LUPV,* left upper pulmonary vein.

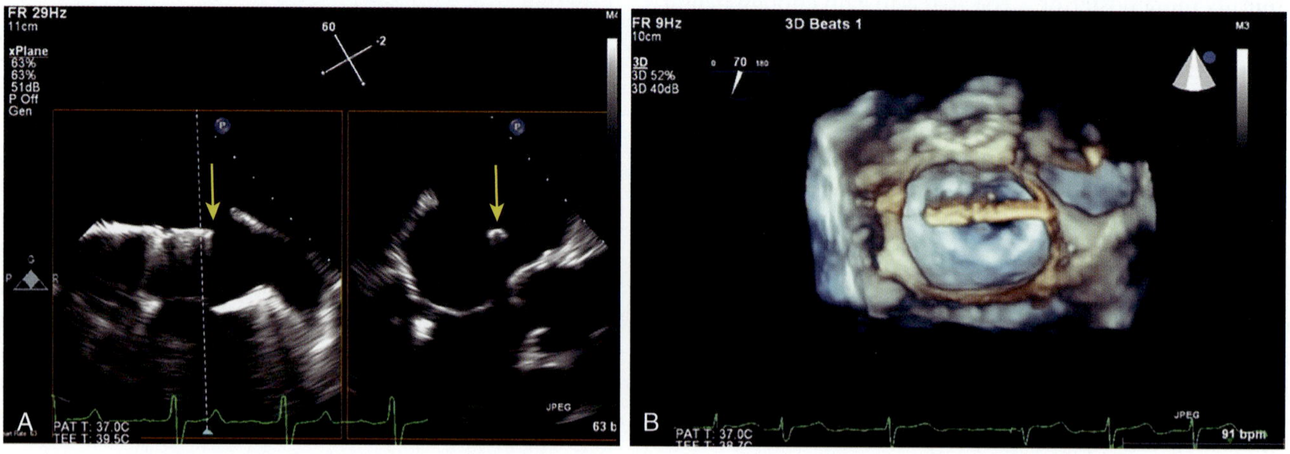

Fig. 7.17 Steering. The device is introduced into the left atrium through the guide catheter and steered to the target under close echocardiographic guidance to avoid injury to the heart. Steering is accomplished by negotiating between pushing the device forward and retracting the guide back to the septum to make more room for the device to advance. (A) Biplane feature can help visualize the tip of the device *(arrows)* in two orthogonal planes to avoid contact with the endocardial surface. (B) Steering can also be guided using 3D volume-rendered imaging, provided that the resolution—both spatial and temporal—is adequate (see text).

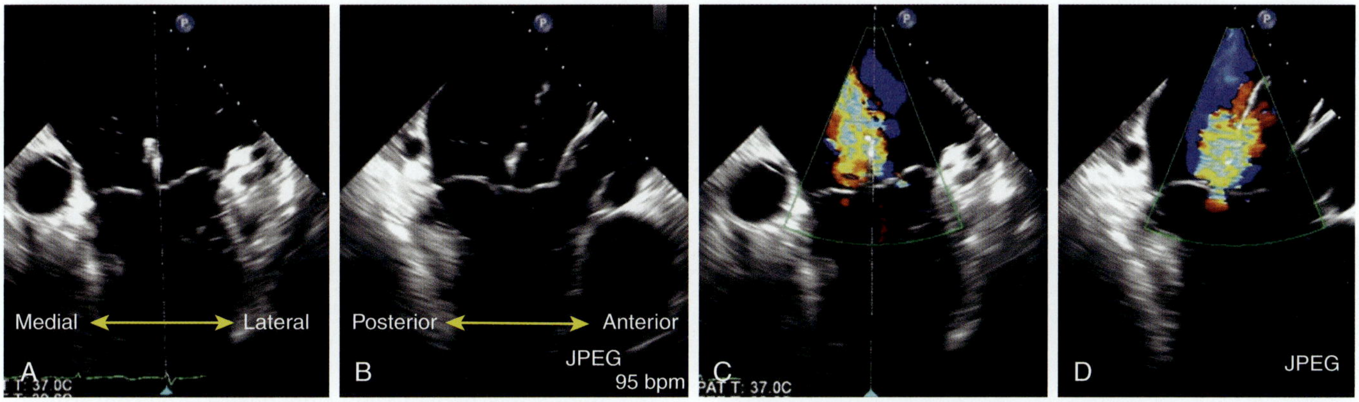

Fig. 7.18 Positioning the Device Above the Target Jet. Once steered toward the mitral valve, the device is positioned above the intended target using the commissural view representing medial-lateral direction and (A and C) and the long-axis view representing antero-posterior direction (B and D). In most cases, the preferred position is in the middle of the target jet (C). The catheter orientation should be as coaxial with mitral inflow as possible.

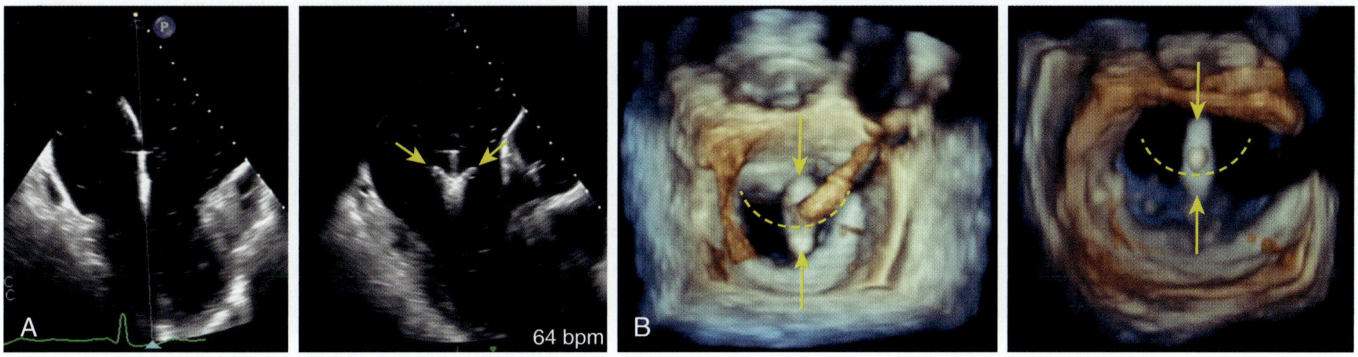

Fig. 7.19 Once in position, the arms of the device *(A, B, arrows)* are oriented perpendicular to the coaptation line (B, curved *yellow line*). This process is guided in the en-face plane: the 3D surgical view (B) or the short-axis shallow transgastric view.

is present, it can be corrected by adjusting the guide and the delivery catheter to improve coaxiality.[46] This precise position of the clip is inferred from the simultaneous (biplane) imaging in commissural (medial-lateral) and long-axis (posterior-anterior) views. In most cases, the optimal position of the device bisects the origin of the target jet (see Fig 7.18), although alternative clip positions may be considered in complex cases involving wide regurgitant areas.[33] Once the position is confirmed, the trajectory of the delivery catheter should also be checked to make sure the device does not "dive" medially or laterally as it is being advanced towards the LV—the position may need to be adjusted to compensate for such deviations. In addition, respirophasic changes in the position of the heart may be important to account for during clip positioning. In some cases, briefly holding mechanical ventilation may help achieve the necessary precision in the positioning of the device and maintaining the desired position during subsequent grasp.

Orientation and Crossing

Once in position, the clip arms should be oriented perpendicular to the segment of the coaptation line below. This is best performed using 3D volume-rendered guidance in the surgical view (Fig. 7.19). A shallow, transgastric, short-axis view of the mitral valve is also adequate for this purpose. Proper surgical view orientation (aortic valve at 12 o'clock and horizontal orientation of the commissural line) is essential to avoid misalignment when using 3D. The open-armed clip should be rotated in either direction (clockwise or counterclockwise) until its arms are perpendicular to the coaptation line (see Fig. 7.19). In the A2P2 region, the orientation will correspond to 12 to 6 o'clock position of the arms while 1 to 7 o'clock and 11 to 5 o'clock orientations are usually the norm for more distant lateral and medial targets, respectively, due to the natural curvature of the coaptation line. Once oriented, the clip's grippers should be tested and clearly identified as anterior or posterior. Clip orientation can inadvertently change with catheter manipulations and should be rechecked after crossing into the LV and frequently thereafter. 3D volume-rendered imaging can still be used for this purpose in the LV, with the 3D gain lowered gradually to remove the leaflet tissue obstructing the full view of the clip arms (see Fig. 7.19).

Grasp

Oriented and in position, the device is ready for grasp. Adequate leaflet insertion is fundamental to procedural success. The goal of imaging is to demonstrate the full insertion of both leaflets into the clip just during the descent of the grippers (Fig. 7.20). Once sandwiched between the arms and the grippers, the leaflets become difficult to visualize. Hence, the descent of the grippers is the focal point of the TEER procedure. Imaging should be optimized for the grasping sequence to simultaneously show the device arms, both leaflets, and the grippers (see Fig. 7.20). A biplane cut across the clip in the commissural view can produce this grasping view in the secondary plane. Alternatively, a dedicated long-axis view can be used for this purpose, and, occasionally, a 4-chamber view can provide the best visualization of the grasp in non-A2P2 cases. The echo view can be magnified for better visualization. It is particularly helpful to record the grasp sequence for an off-line frame-by-frame analysis of leaflet insertion.[50] While simultaneous grasp of both leaflets is desirable, newer devices allow grasping leaflets independently, one at a time, which also provides an opportunity to optimize individual leaflet insertion by briefly lifting the grippers allowing more leaflet tissue to enter the device. Any concerns about the adequacy of the grasp should be voiced and evaluated by the team before releasing the device—the point of no return.[50]

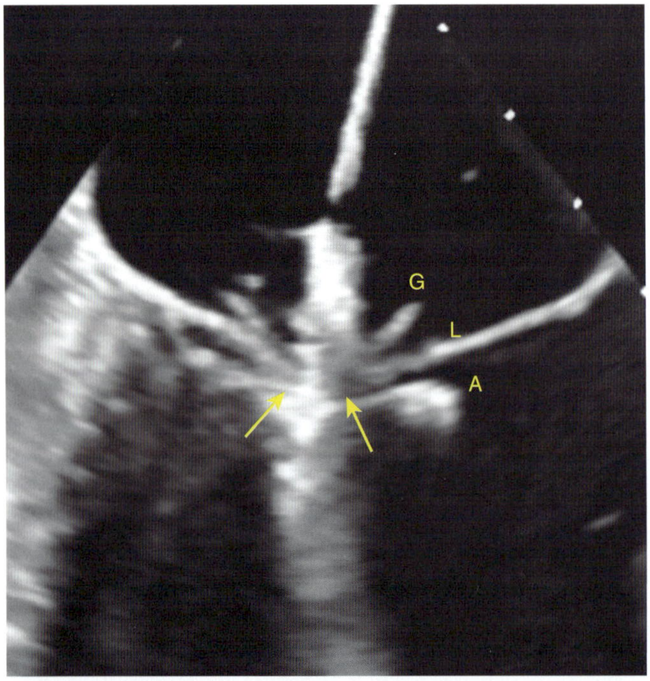

Fig. 7.20 Grasp. Key elements of successful grasp are illustrated here. The goal is to clearly visualize (1) the full wingspan of the device arms (A), (2) leaflets inserting all the way into the device *(arrows)* and resting on the arm (L), and the grippers above (G). The best time to assess leaflet insertion is just before or during (pictured) the descent of the released grippers.

There are supportive signs of adequate leaflet insertion (Fig. 7.21). A tissue bridge between anterior and posterior leaflets should be noted in surgical or 2D transgastric short-axis view. The remaining portion of the leaflet outside of the device can be measured and compared to the leaflet length at baseline, the difference approximating the inserted segment, provided the views are comparable.[47] Leaflet segments just outside the device should look taut and appear to bisect the device in the commissural view, reflecting the depth of insertion (see Fig. 7.21). Sagging of the residual free portion of the leaflet may be a sign of suboptimal insertion.

Several issues may complicate the grasp (Fig. 7.22). Leaflets can get caught on open grippers along the distal portion of the delivery catheter, particularly if they are redundant and hypermobile. Chordal interference may preclude leaflet insertion. As the clip arm is pushing against the chord, the leaflet tip tends to curl inward instead of splaying on the clip arm (see Fig. 7.22). Occasionally the leaflet may be fully captured in diastole but slip away in systole, which may require timing the descent of the grippers to diastole. The manufacturer-recommended minimum amount

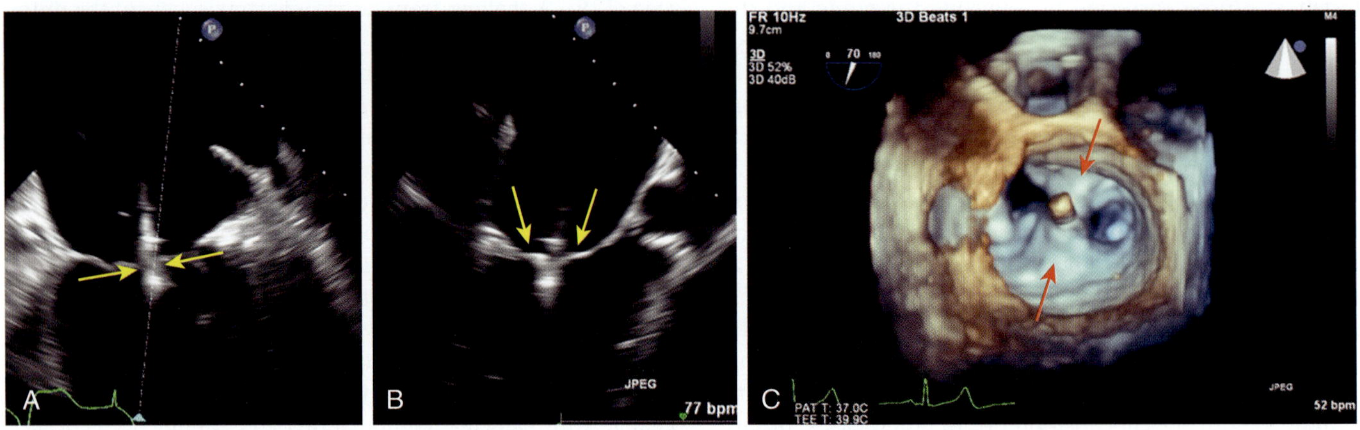

Fig. 7.21 Indirect Assessment of Leaflet Insertion. Confirmation of adequate leaflet insertion is essential to prevent SLDA. Once grasped, leaflets within the device are obscured, and indirect clues to the adequacy of the grasp must be used. Pictured here are echocardiographic signs supporting adequate insertion. (A) Commissural view showing leaflets bisecting the device *(arrows)* as opposed to hanging off the upper edge, if the insertions were insufficient. (B) The long-axis view orthogonal to (A), showing taut segments of the leaflets immediately outside the device *(arrows)*. (C) Tissue bridge *(arrows)* created by the device seen en-face in the surgical view. (The shallow transgastric view can also be used for this purpose.)

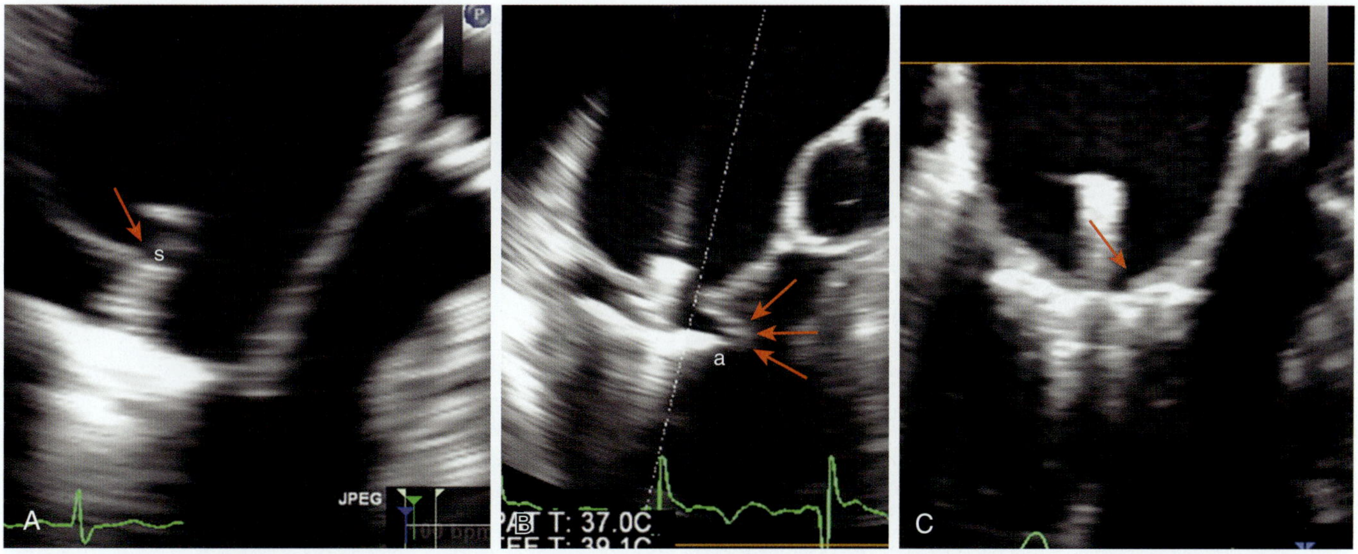

Fig. 7.22 Common Grasp Pitfalls. Examples in which a leaflet tip is prevented from being fully inserted into the arms of the device. (A) The posterior leaflet is caught on the shaft *(s)* of the delivery catheter *(red arrow)*. (B) The anterior leaflet is prevented from entering the device by chordal interference. The anterior arm *(a)* of the device is pushing on the primary chord *(red arrows)*. (C) Anterior leaflet is sliding off the arm in diastole *(red arrow)*.

of tissue for adequate grasp ranges from 6 to 9 mm depending on the size of the device (Abbott training slides).

Post-grasp Assessment

Residual MR assessment. Even suboptimal insertion can sometimes produce significant, albeit not durable, MR reduction. This may tempt the operators to accept a suboptimal grasp along with the increased risk of single leaflet device attachment (SLDA). It may be advisable to defer the assessment of MR reduction until adequate leaflet insertion is confirmed. This may also minimize leaflet injury from repeated clip tightening. Once comfortable with the insertion, the imager can present the view that shows the regurgitation at its worst and observe a reduction of MR in real time as the clip is tightened.

Grading residual MR after TEER is challenging due to often eccentric, multiple jets and a lack of validated, quantitative techniques to assess MR in this setting.[51] Neither VCW nor PISA method are reliable to describe multiple jets. The PISA method also requires angle correction when the flow convergence zone is adjacent to the TEER device—an additional source of error. Current guidelines recommend an integrative approach including visual assessment of color Doppler, pulmonary vein flow, VCW, and 3D VCA, as well as supportive parameters, such as LV size and pulmonary pressures.[51,52]

Planimetry of the 3D VCA using multiplanar reconstruction has had some validation in the setting of TEER (Fig. 7.23).[53,54] It provides a quantitative assessment of total residual EROA (VCA). This method is well suited to handle multiple and eccentric jets but relies on adequate spatial and temporal resolution, as well as expertise in 3D echo and reconstructive techniques. Frame rate, the currency of 3D echo, should be balanced with adequate spatial resolution. There are several ways to improve the quality of 3D color data. Reducing the size of the region of interest during acquisition while not excluding key landmarks to maintain spatial awareness will increase frame rate and temporal resolution. Multibeat acquisition, an overlay of multiple beats to combine frame rate, should avoid misalignment (splicing) artifacts which can be minimized by a respiratory hold. The spatial resolution of 3D color Doppler can be improved by increasing line density, provided that an adequate frame rate (above 10 Hz) can be maintained.

When MR reduction is substantial, a sudden appearance or increase in the spontaneous echo contrast and/or an increase in systemic blood pressure have been observed clinically in some patients. The emergence of antegrade systolic flow in pulmonary veins usually correlates with significant MR reduction (see Fig. 7.23). Newer TEER delivery systems include built-in pressure sensors which can transduce LA pressure directly, which can corroborate reduction in MR. Systemic blood pressure is an important factor in the residual MR assessment. Low blood pressure will reduce the momentum of the regurgitant jets leading to underestimation of regurgitation on color Doppler. If clinically appropriate, blood pressure can be raised pharmacologically to the "awake" levels, and MR is reassessed to make sure reduction has been adequate.

Residual mitral valve area assessment. Prior to deploying the TEER device, pathologic mitral stenosis must be excluded. Transmitral gradients should be assessed using CW Doppler (Fig. 7.24). In general, mean mitral valve gradients less than 5 mm Hg are acceptable provided they are interpreted in the context of cardiac output, i.e., heart rate and stroke volume.[25] If there is uncertainty about how accurately the gradients reflect residual stenosis, the MVA should be planimetered using 3D multiplanar reconstruction (see Fig 7.24). Each residual mitral valve orifice should be reconstructed and measured individually because they rarely lie in the same plane.[25]

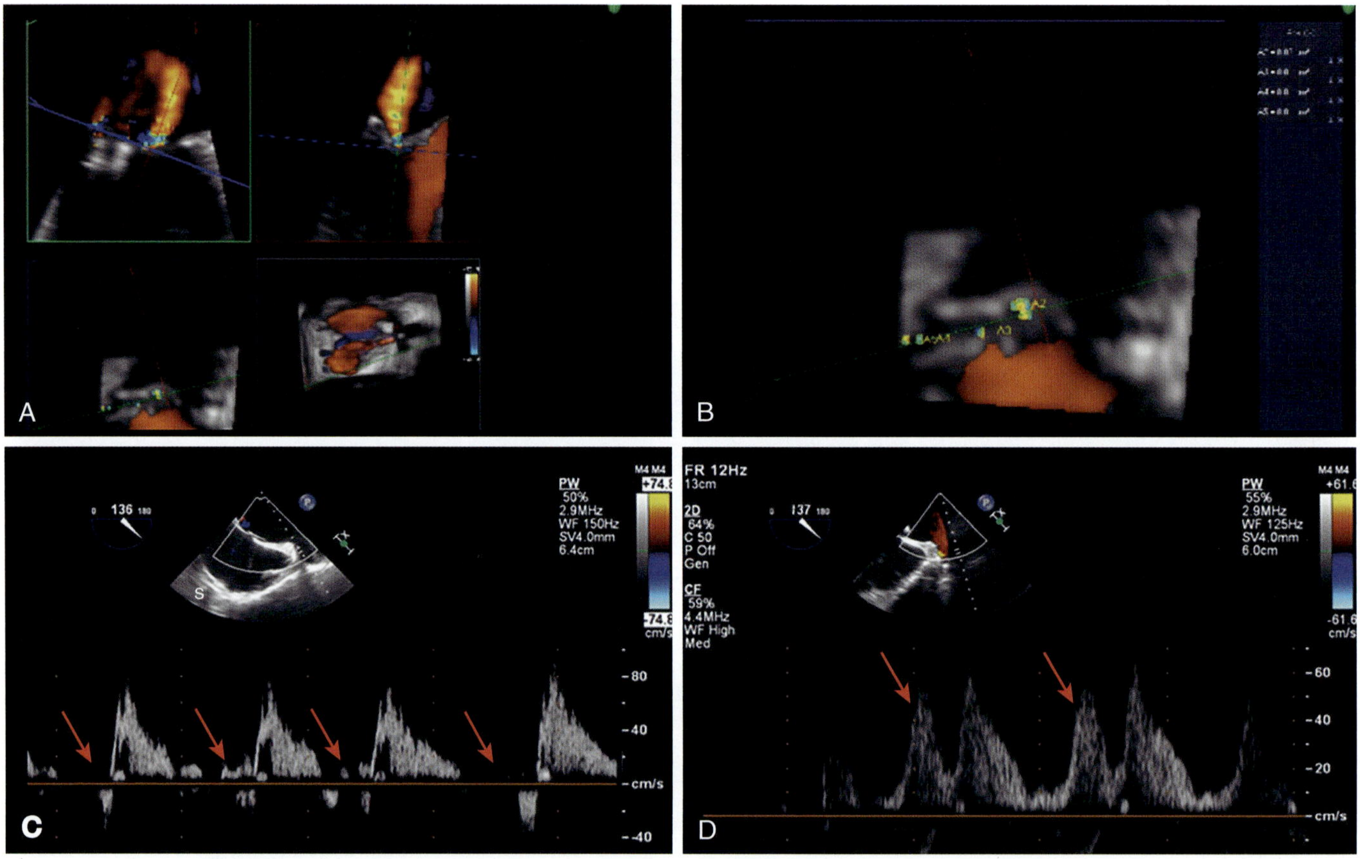

Fig. 7.23 Residual MR assessment. Quantifying residual MR posttranscatheter edge-to-edge repair is difficult due to lack of well-validated methods. 3D multiplanar reconstruction (A) and planimetry (B) of the vena contracta areas of the individual jets has been employed in this setting. In addition, a significant reduction in mitral regurgitation is frequently accompanied by improved forward systolic flow in the pulmonary veins (C, D).

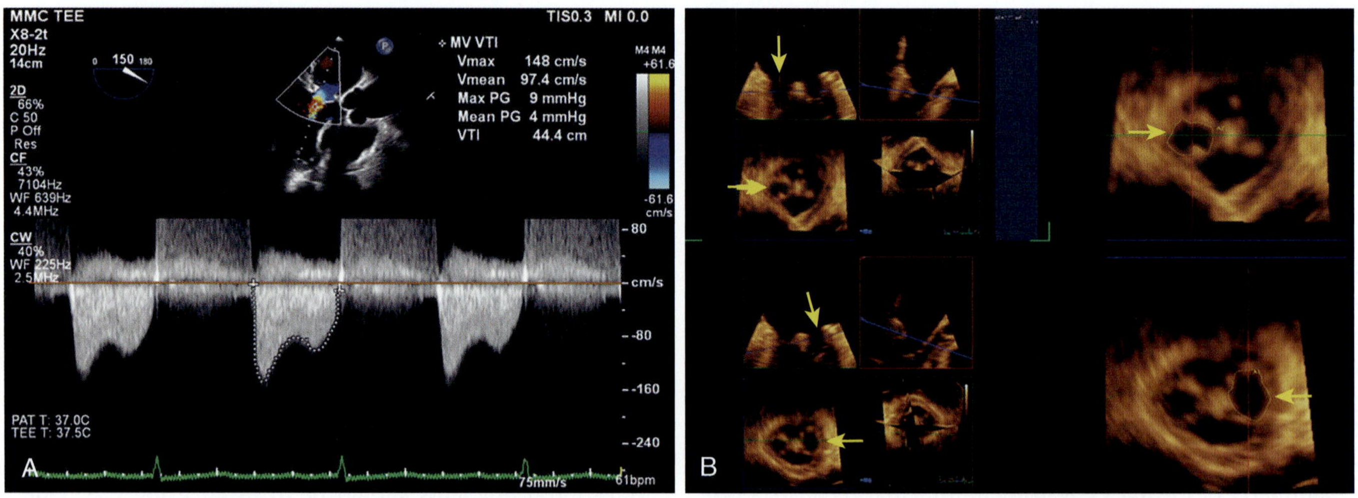

Fig. 7.24 Residual Mitral Stenosis assessment. Transcatheter edge-to-edge repair (TEER) results in reduction of the mitral valve area and increase in transmitral gradients. Accurate assessment of residual stenosis is mandatory prior to releasing any TEER device. Transmitral gradients (A) should be interpreted in the context of heart rate, LV systolic function, and the effects of general anesthesia. Particularly in cases where the gradients are borderline for pathologic stenosis (≥5 mm Hg) or if there is any uncertainty in the accuracy of Doppler assessment, planimetry of the residual mitral valve area should be performed using 3D multiplanar reconstruction (B). Each orifice should be reconstructed and planimetered individually *(arrows)* because they lie in separate imaging planes.

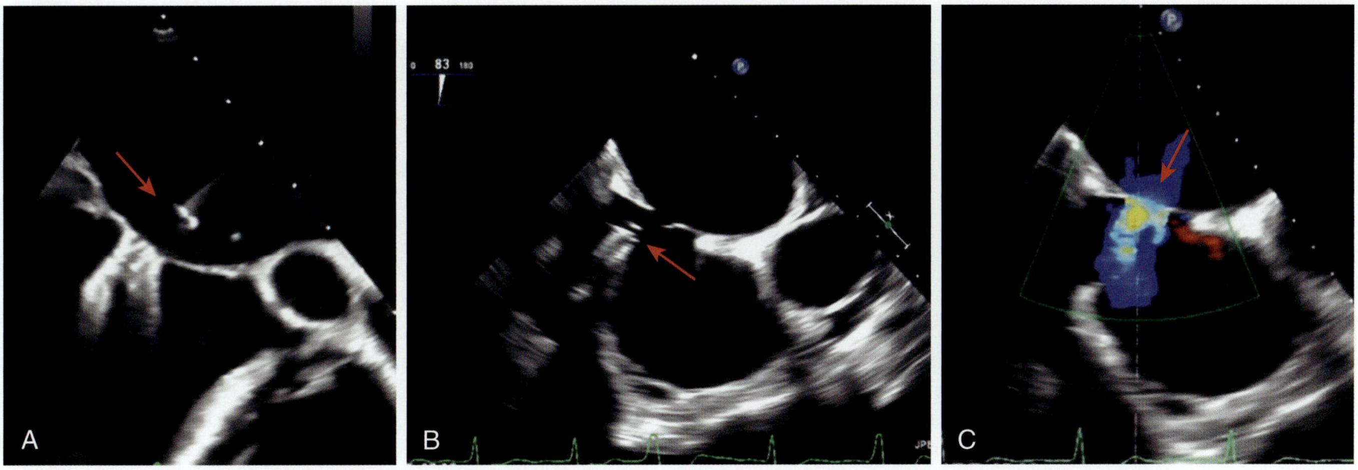

Fig. 7.25 Release and Exit. (A) After confirming adequate insertion, MR reduction, and absence of pathologic stenosis, the device is released from the delivery catheter *(arrow)*—a point of no return in this procedure. (B) The steerable guide exits the LA *(arrow)*, leaving behind an interatrial septal defect. (C) Left to right interatrial shunt seen after the guide exit. Significant right to left shunt can sometimes occur in patients with pre-existing elevated right-sided pressures.

Release and Exit

Upon final confirmation of adequate leaflet insertion, MR reduction, and absence of pathologic stenosis, the device can be deployed (Fig 7.25). It is not unusual to see minor postdeployment changes in MR severity as a result of tension release. Device stability and mitral hemodynamics should be reassessed after full deployment. Final MV gradients are documented to serve as future reference. If no more devices are to be implanted, the system can be steered out of the LA, avoiding contact with intracardiac structures under echo guidance (see Fig. 7.25). The iatrogenic atrial septal defect (ASD) is uniformly present upon exit of the steerable guide—as many as 50% may remain open after 6 months with a largely unknown impact on clinical outcomes.[55,56] While it persists, the left to right shunt may further reduce LA pressures after the MitraClip procedure.[57] On the other hand, right to left shunting may occur in as many as 5% of patients in the setting of elevated right-sided pressures. If the iatrogenic ASD has clinically significant effects on arterial oxygen saturation or hemodynamics, it can usually be closed percutaneously.

FOLLOW-UP IMAGING

Follow-up imaging provides ongoing assessment of device stability, presence of pathologic mitral stenosis, recurrence of significant MR, changes in LV size, and the right heart. The goal of the first postprocedural TTE is to exclude acute complications such as pericardial effusion or right to left shunt and ensure device stability. On this and all subsequent follow-up studies, the device should be assessed in multiple views to confirm attachment to both leaflets. This is best observed in the long-axis views: parasternal long-axis (PLAX), apical 3- and 5-chamber. In addition, biplane imaging of each device in short-axis and apical 2C views can generate the orthogonal long-axis view and facilitate the evaluation of leaflet insertion (Fig. 7.26). If SLDA is present on follow-up TTE, the device is usually highly mobile, although the mobility may not be as pronounced in the setting of severe LV systolic dysfunction. If suspected, a TEE can confirm the presence of SLDA and assess the feasibility of possible reintervention (Table 7.3).

Transmitral gradients are assessed at each follow-up and interpreted in the context of cardiac output: the higher the HR and/or stroke volume, the higher the gradients. Similarly, the gradients may be artificially low in the setting of a low flow state. Dedicated imaging at the leaflet tips level may allow planimetry of the residual area, provided the view and spatial resolution are adequate. Area measurements are relatively flow-independent. Biplane imaging can be used to optimize the short axis for planimetry if the biplane cursor is placed across the leaflet tips (Fig. 7.27). Direct planimetry of the transthoracic 3D reconstructed images can be performed if spatial and temporal resolution are adequate. In cases without significant mitral or aortic regurgitation (mild or less), the continuity equation may be used to derive MVA. The pressure half-time method has not been validated in this setting.[57]

Most of the established quantitative methods of MR assessment have not been validated in patients after TEER repair.[51] Grading residual MR on follow-up transthoracic studies is further complicated by the frequent multiplicity and eccentricity of residual jets as well as the device-generated acoustic shadowing. In the COAPT trial, only color jet area/direction, pulmonary vein flow pattern, and to a lesser extent, VCW were found to be the most reliable parameters.[52] Planimetry of the 3D VCA is a novel quantitative method in clinical use but requires further validation.[53] An integrative approach based on all available qualitative and quantitative data represents the most

TABLE 7.3 Special Imaging Considerations on Follow-Up After Transcatheter Mitral Edge-to-Edge Repair

Clinical Questions	Imaging Considerations
Is there pericardial effusion?	• Important on the immediate postprocedure study.
Is there pathologic mitral stenosis?	• Transmitral gradients are reliably measured by CW Doppler but must be interpreted in the context of cardiac output, particularly the patient's heart rate. Significant stenosis can be masked by bradycardia. On the other hand, gradients can be significantly increased in the setting of rapid heart rate, which may lead to overestimation of the degree of iatrogenic stenosis. Other factors affecting cardiac output will, in turn, affect the gradients and should be taken into account. • Planimetry of the residual valve area is relatively independent of cardiac output and heart rate. The residual valve area is best estimated by planimetry, preferably 3D or biplane.
How much MR remains?	• Quantitation is difficult because conventional methods have not been validated in this setting[51]. In the Cardiovascular Outcomes Assessment of the MitraClip Percutaneous Therapy for Heart Failure Patients with Functional Mitral Regurgitation (COAPT) trial, color Doppler jet area, vena contracta of the dominant jet, and pulmonary vein flow were helpful to assess residual MR after edge-to-edge (E2E)[52]. In general, systolic reversal in pulmonary vein flow on pulsed wave Doppler is associated with significant residual MR; systolic dominant flow indicates milder degree of regurgitation. • Although adequate data are technically difficult to acquire due to limitations of present technology, planimetry of the total vena contracta area (effective regurgitant orifice area [EROA]) on 3D color Doppler multiplanar reconstruction is feasible and may be the best technique at this time (Grayburn editorial and the girl's paper), especially when multiple jets are present. • Pitfalls of color Doppler (see Fig. 7.6) remain relevant after E2E repair: higher blood pressure will augment the appearance of the jets on color Doppler and may lead to overestimation of MR. Low blood pressure may diminish color jet size and lead to underestimation of MR. Color Doppler settings (color gain, Nyquist limit, transducer frequency) may significantly alter the size of the color jet. "Flat and wide" jet appearance should raise concern for a significant eccentric jet.
Has the LV changed in size/function after the intervention?	• Serial assessment of LV size by volumetric measurements (Simpson's biplane) using echo contrast if appropriate. • Significant reduction of chronic severe MR is expected to result in reduction in LV size (reverse remodeling). The end-diastolic volume should decrease following successful transcatheter mitral valve (TMV) repair, and mild reduction in LVEF should be expected as a result. This is later followed by decrease in systolic volume and corresponding increase in LVEF. Lack of a significant decrease in LV size may be a clue indicating insufficient MR reduction.
Is there a significant interatrial shunt across iatrogenic ASD?	• Usually closes spontaneously and is rarely hemodynamically significant. • Shunt direction should be evaluated, particularly in the setting of reduced arterial blood oxygen saturation. If ASD becomes clinically significant, percutaneous closure is currently the first-line option.
What is the state of the right side of the heart (pulmonary artery pressures, RV function, TR)?	• Serial assessments of pulmonary pressures and the right side of the heart are helpful to correlate with changes in MR severity. Significant impediments to forward flow caused by tricuspid regurgitation (TR), RV function, or pulmonary hypertension may result in low flow state on the left side, lower transmitral gradients and potentially mask significant stenosis.

(Modified from Marcoff L, Gillam LD. Role of the imager in transcatheter mitral valve repair. *Curr Cardiol Rep.* 2020;22(10):120.

comprehensive and objective way to grade residual MR after transcatheter repair.[51]

Finally, changes in the LV size after TEER should reflect a reduction in the regurgitant volume. If the MR was reduced significantly (2+ or less), the LV end-diastolic volume decreases given the lower preload. In DMR, the LVEDV reduction is more pronounced than LVESV, but in FMR, both are significantly reduced over time.[58] Absence of reverse remodeling after TEER, especially if MR severity is uncertain, may be a clue to insufficient MR reduction. When indicated, echo contrast should be used to improve LV endocardial definition.[59]

TRANSCATHETER MITRAL VALVE REPLACEMENT

In addition to mitral valve TEER (MitraClip, PASCAL), there are a number of additional transcatheter approaches to the treatment of mitral valve disease. These interventions are varied and include some of the following:

- TMVR: multiple devices in development (Tendyne, Intrepid, Sapien M3, EVOQUE, and others)
- Direct mitral annuloplasty: Cardioband, Millipede Iris
- Indirect mitral annuloplasty: Carillon Mitral Contour System (MCS)

At present, the Tendyne TMVR, Cardioband, and Carillon devices are the only non-TEER therapies that have achieved regulatory approval (CE mark only). Additional transcatheter mitral therapies include transcatheter mitral valve-in-valve replacement (SAPIEN 3 transcatheter heart valve implanted within a degenerated surgical bioprosthesis) and paravalvular mitral regurgitation repair—these are outside the scope of this chapter and discussed separately. There are multiple additional mitral valve investigational therapies in various stages of development that will be discussed in subsequent chapters.

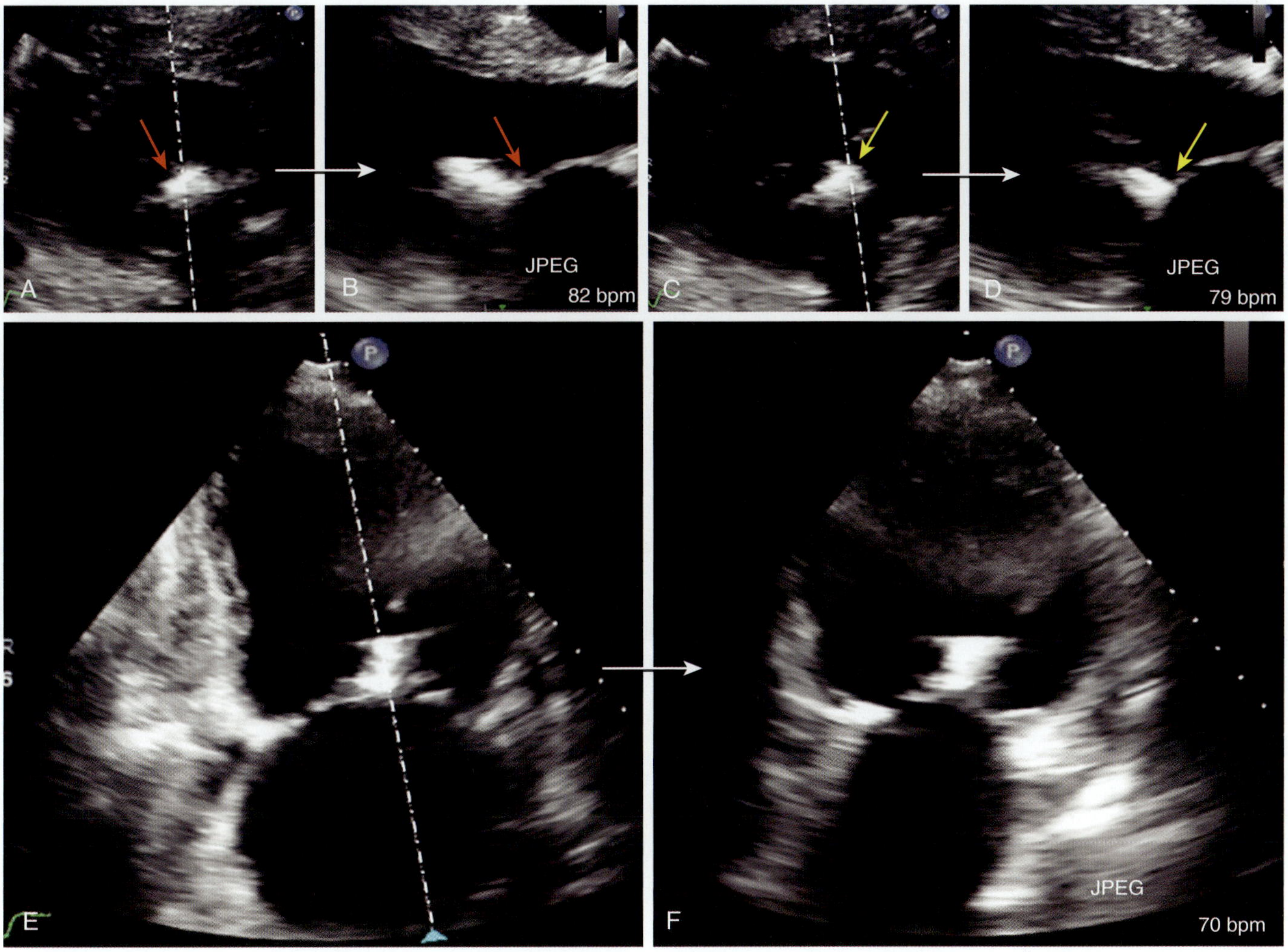

Fig. 7.26 Follow-Up Assessment of the Device Attachment to the Leaflets by Transthoracic Echo. Biplane imaging may help evaluate device attachment to the mitral leaflets. (A) Follow-up transthoracic echo for a patient with two devices implanted close together. The biplane cursor *(dashed line)* is directed across the medial device on the left *(arrow)*, generating the long-axis view (B) where leaflet insertion can be better visualized. The lateral device on the right can be interrogated in a similar manner (C and D). The same principle applies in apical 2-chamber view (E and F).

Many of the imaging principles reviewed previously as part of a mitral TEER evaluation are also relevant to TMVR and transcatheter annuloplasty devices. At baseline, a complete TTE and TEE are necessary to assess mitral valve anatomy and function. In contrast to TEER imaging needs, cardiac multidetector row computed tomography (MDCT) is an indispensable tool when evaluating patients for TMVR and transcatheter annuloplasty. MDCT is the primary imaging modality to assess mitral valve/device suitability (annular sizing, calcification, subvalvular anatomy, predicted neo-LVOT area) and procedural access site selection (transapical, transseptal approaches).[60] The use of dedicated 3D TEE mitral valve quantification software has also been described for the evaluation of mitral annular dimensions and TMVR planning.[61]

TMVR and transcatheter annuloplasty procedural guidance is performed using a combination of both TEE and fluoroscopy. The specific imaging protocols may vary depending on the device being used, the access approach (transapical vs. transseptal), and the anchoring mechanism. Similar to mitral TEER, successful implantation of TMVR and annuloplasty devices relies on a combination of mid-esophageal biplane imaging and real-time 3D imaging views.[62] Device-specific monitoring needs are variable and can include circumflex artery to annulus proximity (Cardioband), LVOT obstruction (TMVR), and presence of competitive transmitral flow (i.e., antegrade diastolic flow paravalvular to a TMVR device). The postimplant evaluation of paravalvular regurgitation can be challenging; an integrative approach that includes qualitative (e.g., pulmonary vein flow pattern, jet appearance), semi-quantitative (e.g., vena contracta width), and quantitative (e.g., 3D VCA) parameters is recommended.[51]

FUTURE DIRECTIONS

Transcatheter mitral valve interventions (TEER, TMVR) are a complex and rapidly evolving field. Continued advances in

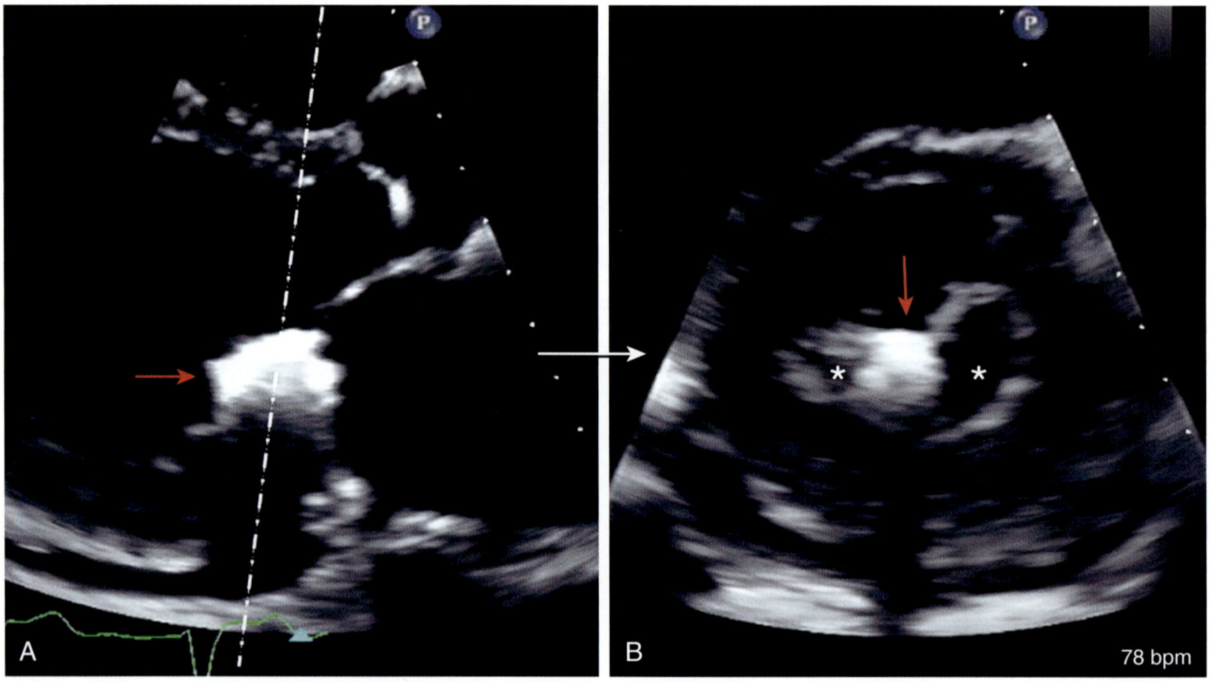

Fig. 7.27 Follow-Up Assessment of the Residual Mitral Valve Area by Transthoracic Echo. Parasternal views showing a single transcatheter edge-to-edge repair device *(red arrows)*. Biplane imaging makes it easier to locate the right plane for planimetry of the mitral valve area. (A) Placing the biplane cursor *(dashed line)* at the leaflet tips will generate the short-axis view (B) showing the residual double-orifice mitral valve, which can be estimated by direct planimetry (*). Note that the temporal resolution of biplane imaging is lower than dedicated 2D imaging.

cardiac imaging have led to significant improvements in the diagnosis and treatment of mitral valve disease. Some of the most significant improvements have come in the field of 3D echocardiography, thereby allowing many of these transcatheter mitral procedures to become feasible, safe, and efficient.

Advances in ultrasound machine processing power and TEE probe technology have resulted in significant improvements in 3D TEE spatial and temporal resolution. The more recent introduction of real-time 3D multiplanar reconstruction (RT-3D MPR, "live MPR") has proven to be a valuable asset within the transcatheter mitral imaging space. RT-3D MPR allows for improved on-axis imaging as well as visualization of any imaging plane within the 3D volume.[63,64] RT-3D MPR results in degradation of image quality; however, when used in concert with 2D and multiplane imaging, this tool can enhance device visualization and greatly facilitate procedural guidance.

TEE-based transcatheter mitral procedural guidance is preferred; however, in certain situations, TEE may be contraindicated or suboptimal quality. 2D intracardiac echocardiography (ICE) and, more recently, real-time 3D ICE have been used successfully to perform mitral TEER.[65] The use of 3D ICE overcomes some of the limitations of single plane 2D ICE imaging; however, compared to TEE, image quality is inferior. Future developments in 3D ICE may allow for its increased utilization as an alternative to TEE.

Fusion imaging (FI) is a relatively novel modality that relies on co-registration of echocardiography and fluoroscopy to generate a hybrid image. FI provides real-time visualization of echocardiographic structures overlayed on a fluoroscopic image and has been used for a variety of structural heart interventions (e.g., paravalvular leak repair, atrial septal defect closure, LAA occlusion). The successful use of FI has also been described during transcatheter mitral interventions.[66] FI may provide incremental efficiency benefits during key procedural steps such as transseptal puncture, device navigation, left atrial steering, and axial alignment.[67,68]

Structural heart disease (SHD) and, in particular, transcatheter mitral valve therapies are a cutting-edge, complex, and a growing field within cardiovascular disease. The subspecialty of the SHD imager is in its relative infancy—it creates new demands and requires the acquisition of new and advanced multi-modality imaging skills (echocardiography, MDCT). The SHD interventional imager is a crucial member of the multidisciplinary heart team, involved in all aspects of the mitral patient's care—baseline diagnosis of disease, procedural planning, device selection, intraprocedural guidance, and postprocedural follow-up. Due to its ubiquity, ease of use, and portability, echocardiography remains the primary imaging tool for the majority of these tasks.

SELF-ASSESSMENT QUESTIONS

1. Which standard TEE view most reliably separates MR into individual jets to select targets for TEER?
   A. Mid-esophageal long-axis (3-chamber view)
   B. Mid-esophageal 2-chamber view
   C. Mid-esophageal mitral commissural view
   D. Mid-esophageal 4-chamber view
2. Which of the following mitral pathologies would be optimal for TEER?
   A. Tethered mitral valve with posterior leaflet length of 5 mm
   B. Rheumatic mitral valve with a single central regurgitant jet and mean antegrade gradient of 5 mmHg at 60 bpm
   C. P2 flail with anterior leaflet measuring 15 mm
   D. P2 flail with complete loss of secondary chordal support
   E. A2 flail, severe MAC, mitral valve area of 2.5 cm^2 by 3D planimetry
3. A 90-year-old woman with severe MR due to P2 flail undergoes TEER. Anterior and posterior leaflets are successfully grasped, and adequate leaflet insertion is confirmed. The device is closed, and trace residual MR is seen medially. Pulmonary vein flow is systolic dominant (reversed at baseline). Which of the following would be the next best procedural step?
   A. Deploy the device, place a second device just lateral to the first to eliminate all of the residual MR
   B. Deploy the device, place a second device just medial to the first to eliminate all of the residual MR
   C. Reposition the device to see if the residual MR gets better
   D. Deploy the device to see if the MR reduction is adequate
   E. Check mitral gradients to assess for pathologic stenosis

See page 316 for the answers.

REFERENCES

1. Wang DD, Geske J, Choi AD, et al. Navigating a career in structural heart disease interventional imaging. *JACC Cardiovasc Imaging*. 2018;11(12):1928–1930.
2. Hahn RT, Feroze M, Kodali S, et al. Core competencies in echocardiography for imaging structural heart disease interventions: an expert consensus statement. *JACC Cardiovasc Imaging*. 2019;12(12):2560–2570.
3. Hahn RT, Abraham T, Adams MS, et al. Guidelines for performing a comprehensive transesophageal echocardiographic examination: recommendations from the American Society of Echocardiography and the Society of Cardiovascular Anesthesiologists. *J Am Soc Echocardiogr*. 2013;26(9):921–964.
4. Lang RM, Badano LP, Tsang W, et al. EAE/ASE recommendations for image acquisition and display using three-dimensional echocardiography. *J Am Soc Echocardiogr*. 2012;25(1):3–46.
5. Mitchell C, Rahko PS, Blauwet LA, et al. Guidelines for performing a comprehensive transthoracic echocardiographic examination in adults: recommendations from the American Society of Echocardiography. *J Am Soc Echocardiogr*. 2019;32(1):1–64.
6. Kupferwasser I, Mohr-Kahaly S, Menzel T, et al. Quantification of mitral valve stenosis by three-dimensional transesophageal echocardiography. *Int J Card Imaging*. 1996;12(4):241–247.
7. Carpentier A. Cardiac valve surgery–the "French correction. *J Thorac Cardiovasc Surg*. 1983;86(3):323–337.
8. Zoghbi WA, Adams D, Bonow RO, et al. Recommendations for noninvasive evaluation of native valvular regurgitation: a report from the American Society of Echocardiography developed in collaboration with the society for cardiovascular magnetic resonance. *J Am Soc Echocardiogr*. 2017;30(4):303–371.
9. Deferm S, Bertrand PB, Verbrugge FH, et al. Atrial functional mitral regurgitation: JACC review topic of the week. *J Am Coll Cardiol*. 2019;73(19):2465–2476.
10. Lancellotti P, Moura L, Pierard LA, et al. European Association of Echocardiography recommendations for the assessment of valvular regurgitation. Part 2: mitral and tricuspid regurgitation (native valve disease). *Eur J Echocardiogr*. 2010;11(4):307–332.
11. Bonow RO, Carabello BA, Chatterjee K, et al. 2008 Focused update incorporated into the ACC/AHA 2006 guidelines for the management of patients with valvular heart disease: a report of the American College of Cardiology/American Heart Association Task Force on Practice Guidelines (Writing Committee to Revise the 1998 Guidelines for the Management of Patients With Valvular Heart Disease): endorsed by the Society of Cardiovascular Anesthesiologists, Society for Cardiovascular Angiography and Interventions, and Society of Thoracic Surgeons. *Circulation*. 2008;118(15):e523–e661.
12. Grayburn PA, Weissman NJ, Zamorano JL. Quantitation of mitral regurgitation. *Circulation*. 2012;126(16):2005–2017.
13. Nishimura RA, Otto CM, Bonow RO, et al. 2014 AHA/ACC guideline for the management of patients with valvular heart disease: a report of the American college of cardiology/American heart association task force on practice guidelines. *J Am Coll Cardiol*. 2014;63(22):e57–e185.
14. Kehl DW, Rader F, Siegel RJ. Echocardiographic features and clinical outcomes of flail mitral leaflet without severe mitral regurgitation. *J Am Soc Echocardiogr*. 2017;30(12):1162–1168.
15. Iwakura K, Ito H, Kawano S, et al. Comparison of orifice area by transthoracic three-dimensional Doppler echocardiography versus proximal isovelocity surface area (PISA) method for assessment of mitral regurgitation. *Am J Cardiol*. 2006;97(11):1630–1637.
16. Kahlert P, Plicht B, Schenk IM, et al. Direct assessment of size and shape of noncircular vena contracta area in functional versus organic mitral regurgitation using real-time three-dimensional echocardiography. *J Am Soc Echocardiogr*. 2008;21(8):912–921.
17. Zeng X, Levine RA, Hua L, et al. Diagnostic value of vena contracta area in the quantification of mitral regurgitation severity by color Doppler 3D echocardiography. *Circ Cardiovasc Imaging*. 2011;4(5):506–513.
18. Klein AL, Stewart WJ, Bartlett J, et al. Effects of mitral regurgitation on pulmonary venous flow and left atrial pressure: an intraoperative transesophageal echocardiographic study. *J Am Coll Cardiol*. 1992;20(6):1345–1352.
19. Mihalatos DG, Gopal AS, Kates R, et al. Intraoperative assessment of mitral regurgitation: role of phenylephrine challenge. *J Am Soc Echocardiogr*. 2006;19(9):1158–1164.
20. Hung J, Otsuji Y, Handschumacher MD, et al. Mechanism of dynamic regurgitant orifice area variation in functional mitral regurgitation: physiologic insights from the proximal flow convergence technique. *J Am Coll Cardiol*. 1999;33(2):538–545.
21. Enriquez-Sarano M, Sinak LJ, Tajik AJ, et al. Changes in effective regurgitant orifice throughout systole in patients with mitral valve

prolapse. A clinical study using the proximal isovelocity surface area method. *Circulation*. 1995;92(10):2951–2958.
22. Schwammenthal E, Chen C, Benning F, et al. Dynamics of mitral regurgitant flow and orifice area. Physiologic application of the proximal flow convergence method: clinical data and experimental testing. *Circulation*. 1994;90(1):307–322.
23. Wiener PC, Friend EJ, Bhargav R, et al. Color doppler splay: a clue to the presence of significant mitral regurgitation. *J Am Soc Echocardiogr*. 2020;33(10):1212–1219 e1.
24. Neuss M, Schau T, Isotani A, et al. Elevated mitral valve pressure gradient after mitraclip implantation deteriorates long-term outcome in patients with severe mitral regurgitation and severe heart failure. *JACC Cardiovasc Interv*. 2017;10(9):931–939.
25. Biaggi P, Felix C, Gruner C, et al. Assessment of mitral valve area during percutaneous mitral valve repair using the MitraClip system: comparison of different echocardiographic methods. *Circ Cardiovasc Imaging*. 2013;6(6):1032–1040.
26. Baumgartner H, Hung J, Bermejo J, et al. Echocardiographic assessment of valve stenosis: EAE/ASE recommendations for clinical practice. *J Am Soc Echocardiogr*. 2009;22(1):1–23 quiz 101–102.
27. Zamorano J, Cordeiro P, Sugeng L, et al. Real-time three-dimensional echocardiography for rheumatic mitral valve stenosis evaluation: an accurate and novel approach. *J Am Coll Cardiol*. 2004;43(11):2091–2096.
28. Zamorano J, de Isla LP, Sugeng L, et al. Non-invasive assessment of mitral valve area during percutaneous balloon mitral valvuloplasty: role of real-time 3D echocardiography. *Eur Heart J*. 2004;25(23):2086–2091.
29. Mannaerts HF, Kamp O, Visser CA. Should mitral valve area assessment in patients with mitral stenosis be based on anatomical or on functional evaluation? A plea for 3D echocardiography as the new clinical standard. *Eur Heart J*. 2004;25(23):2073–2074.
30. Sugeng L, Weinert L, Lammertin G, et al. Accuracy of mitral valve area measurements using transthoracic rapid freehand 3-dimensional scanning: comparison with noninvasive and invasive methods. *J Am Soc Echocardiogr*. 2003;16(12):1292–1300.
31. Min SY, Song J-M, Kim Y-G, et al. Discrepancy between mitral valve areas measured by two-dimensional planimetry and three-dimensional transoesophageal echocardiography in patients with mitral stenosis. *Heart*. 2013;99(4):253–258.
32. Feldman T, Foster E, Glower DD, et al. Percutaneous repair or surgery for mitral regurgitation. *N Engl J Med*. 2011;364(15):1395–1406.
33. Singh GD, Smith TW, Rogers JH. Multi-MitraClip therapy for severe degenerative mitral regurgitation: "anchor" technique for extremely flail segments. *Catheter Cardiovasc Interv*. 2015;86(2):339–346.
34. Lesevic H, Karl M, Braun D, et al. Long-term outcomes after mitraclip implantation according to the presence or absence of EVEREST inclusion criteria. *Am J Cardiol*. 2017;119(8):1255–1261.
35. La Canna G, Arendar I, Maisano F, et al. Real-time three-dimensional transesophageal echocardiography for assessment of mitral valve functional anatomy in patients with prolapse-related regurgitation. *Am J Cardiol*. 2011;107(9):1365–1374.
36. Tsang W, Lang RM. Three-dimensional echocardiography is essential for intraoperative assessment of mitral regurgitation. *Circulation*. 2013;128(6):643–652 discussion 652.
37. Nii M. Editorial: What is this cleavage of mitral valve—Commissure, indentation, cleft, or cleft-like indentation?. *J Cardiol Cases*. 2016;13(2):40–41.
38. Mantovani F, Clavel M-A, Vatury O, et al. Cleft-like indentations in myxomatous mitral valves by three-dimensional echocardiographic imaging. *Heart*. 2015;101(14):1111–1117.
39. Korber MI, Friedrichs KP, Aydin F, et al. Impact of cleft-like indentations on procedural outcome of percutaneous edge-to-edge mitral valve repair. *Catheter Cardiovasc Interv*. 2020;97(6):1236–1243.
40. Taramasso M, Maisano F. Challenging mitral clefts with MitraClip: the convergent clips strategy. *EuroIntervention*. 2016;12(8):e1071.
41. Feldman T, Kar S, Elmariah S, et al. Randomized comparison of percutaneous repair and surgery for mitral regurgitation: 5-Year Results of EVEREST II. *J Am Coll Cardiol*. 2015;66(25):2844–2854.
42. Stone GW, Lindenfeld J, Abraham WT, et al. Transcatheter mitral-valve repair in patients with heart failure. *N Engl J Med*. 2018;379(24):2307–2318.
43. Cziner DG, Rosenzweig BP, Katz ES, et al. Transesophageal versus transthoracic echocardiography for diagnosing mitral valve perforation. *Am J Cardiol*. 1992;69(17):1495–1497.
44. De Castro S, Cartoni D, d'Amati G, et al. Diagnostic accuracy of transthoracic and multiplane transesophageal echocardiography for valvular perforation in acute infective endocarditis: correlation with anatomic findings. *Clin Infect Dis*. 2000;30(5):825–826.
45. Estevez-Loureiro R, Franzen O, Winter R, et al. Echocardiographic and clinical outcomes of central versus noncentral percutaneous edge-to-edge repair of degenerative mitral regurgitation. *J Am Coll Cardiol*. 2013;62(25):2370–2377.
46. Sorajja P, Kanda B, Bae R, et al. Maneuvers for technical success with transcatheter mitral valve repair. *Catheter Cardiovasc Interv*. 2018;92(3):617–626.
47. Kreidel F, Frerker C, Schlüter M, et al. Repeat MitraClip therapy for significant recurrent mitral regurgitation in high surgical risk patients: impact of loss of leaflet insertion. *JACC Cardiovasc Interv*. 2015;8(11):1480–1489.
48. Singh GD, Smith TW, Rogers JH. Targeted transseptal access for mitraclip percutaneous mitral valve repair. *Interv Cardiol Clin*. 2016;5(1):55–69.
49. Nielsen NE, Boano G, Nylander E, et al. Massive air embolism during mitraclip insertion. In: Feldman FO., Franzen O., Low R. et al, eds. *Atlas of Percutaneous Edge-to-Edge Mitral Valve Repair*. London: Springer; 2013.
50. Rogers JH, Smith T. Repeat MitraClip procedures: in search of the perfect grasp. *JACC Cardiovasc Interv*. 2015;8(11):1490–1492.
51. Zoghbi WA, Asch FM, Bruce C, et al. Guidelines for the Evaluation of valvular regurgitation after percutaneous valve repair or replacement: a report from the American society of echocardiography developed in collaboration with the society for cardiovascular angiography and interventions, Japanese society of echocardiography, and society for cardiovascular magnetic resonance. *J Am Soc Echocardiogr*. 2019;32(4):431–475.
52. Asch FM, Grayburn PA, Siegel RJ, et al. Echocardiographic Outcomes After Transcatheter Leaflet Approximation in Patients With Secondary Mitral Regurgitation: The COAPT Trial. *J Am Coll Cardiol*. 2019;74(24):2969–2979.
53. Avenatti E, Mackensen GB, El-Tallawi KC, et al. Diagnostic value of 3-dimensional vena contracta area for the quantification of residual mitral regurgitation after MitraClip procedure. *JACC Cardiovasc Interv*. 2019;12(6):582–591.
54. Grayburn PA. The Challenge of Assessing Residual Mitral Regurgitation During MitraClip Procedures: Is 3-Dimensional Vena Contracta Area the Answer?. *JACC Cardiovasc Interv*. 2019;12(6):592–594.

55. Smith T, McGinty P, Bommer W, et al. Prevalence and echocardiographic features of iatrogenic atrial septal defect after catheter-based mitral valve repair with the MitraClip system. *Catheter Cardiovasc Interv*. 2012;80(4):678–685.
56. Schueler R, Öztürk C, Wedekind JA, et al. Persistence of iatrogenic atrial septal defect after interventional mitral valve repair with the MitraClip system: a note of caution. *JACC Cardiovasc Interv*. 2015;8(3):450–459.
57. Hoffmann R, Altiok E, Reith S, et al. Functional effect of new atrial septal defect after percutaneous mitral valve repair using the MitraClip device. *Am J Cardiol*. 2014;113(7):1228–1233.
58. Grayburn PA, Foster E, Sangli C, et al. Relationship between the magnitude of reduction in mitral regurgitation severity and left ventricular and left atrial reverse remodeling after MitraClip therapy. *Circulation*. 2013;128(15):1667–1674.
59. Lang RM, Badano LP, Mor-Avi V, et al. Recommendations for cardiac chamber quantification by echocardiography in adults: an update from the American Society of Echocardiography and the European Association of Cardiovascular Imaging. *J Am Soc Echocardiogr*. 2015;28(1):1–39.
60. Bax JJ, Debonnaire P, Lancellotti P, et al. Transcatheter Interventions for Mitral Regurgitation. *JACC: Cardiovas Imag*. 2019;12(10):2029–2048.
61. Mak GJ, Blanke P, Ong K, et al. Three-dimensional echocardiography compared with computed tomography to determine mitral annulus size before transcatheter mitral valve implantation. *Circ Cardiovasc Imaging*. 2016;9(6):e004176.
62. Gheorghe LL, Mobasseri S, Agricola E, et al. Imaging for Native Mitral Valve Surgical and Transcatheter Interventions. *JACC: Cardiovascular Imaging*. 2021;14(1):112–127.
63. Harb SC, Krishnaswamy A, Kapadia SR, et al. The added value of 3D real-time multiplanar reconstruction for intraprocedural guidance of challenging mitraclip cases. *JACC: Cardiovas Imaging*. 2020;13(8):1809–1814.
64. Geyer M, Sotiriou E, Tamm AR, et al. Advanced protocol for three-dimensional transesophageal echocardiography guidance implementing real-time multiplanar reconstruction for transcatheter mitral valve repair by direct annuloplasty. *J Am Soc Echocardiogr*. 2019;32(10):1359–1365.
65. Sanchez CE, Yakubov SJ, Singh G, et al. 4-Dimensional intracardiac echocardiography in transcatheter mitral valve repair with the mitraclip system. *JACC: Cardiovasc Imaging*. 2021 S1936-878X(20)31030-5.
66. Faletra FF, Pozzoli A, Agricola E, et al. Echocardiographic-fluoroscopic fusion imaging for transcatheter mitral valve repair guidance. *Eur Heart J Cardiovasc Imaging*. 2018;19(7):715–726.
67. Melillo F, Fisicaro A, Stella S, et al. Systematic fluoroscopic-echocardiographic fusion imaging protocol for transcatheter edge-to-edge mitral valve repair intraprocedural monitoring. *J Am Soc Echocardiogr*. 2021;34(6):604–613.
68. Afzal S, Veulemans V, Piayda K, et al. Real-time echocardiographic-fluoroscopic fusion imaging for transcatheter edge-to-edge mitral valve repair. *J Am Soc Echocardiogr*. 2020;33(5):635–636.

8

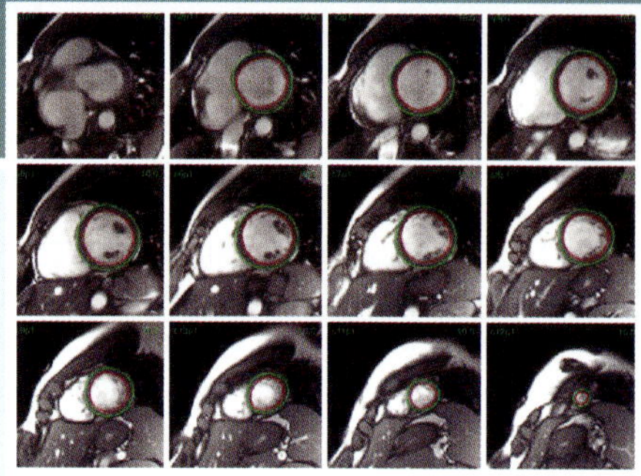

Cardiac Magnetic Resonance Imaging for Mitral Regurgitation

Katie M. Hawthorne

CHAPTER OUTLINE

LEARNING OBJECTIVES

1. Review how valvular regurgitation can be quantified with cardiac magnetic resonance imaging.
2. Discuss the role of cardiac magnetic resonance imaging for mitral valve disease.
3. Review the advantages/disadvantages of cardiac magnetic resonance imaging.

INTRODUCTION

Over the last several decades, cardiac magnetic resonance (CMR) has emerged as an invaluable tool in cardiovascular imaging. CMR is a comprehensive noninvasive imaging modality that offers high spatial and temporal resolution without ionizing radiation. Images can be acquired in any imaging plane without limitation by body habitus, chest wall anatomy, or lung interference. CMR is considered the gold standard for noninvasive assessment of left ventricular volumes and ejection fraction with high accuracy and reproducibility.[1–4] Functional cardiac assessment can be obtained without contrast. Myocardial tissue characteristics such as myocardial infarction, fibrosis, or infiltration can be assessed using gadolinium-based contrast.

MITRAL REGURGITATION

CMR is particularly useful in the evaluation of mitral regurgitation with the ability to accurately quantify severity of regurgitation, further delineate pathophysiology and mechanism of mitral regurgitation, and assess hemodynamic effects of volume overload as the gold standard for assessment of left atrial and ventricular size.[2,3]

Severity of mitral regurgitation is the basis of management recommendations within the American College of Cardiology/American Heart Association valvular guidelines; therefore, accurate determination of severity is critical.[5,6] Symptoms of mitral regurgitation such as fatigue, dyspnea, and decreased exercise tolerance can also be seen in many common disease states and ensuring accurate diagnosis is key. Even more, when considering early surgery for asymptomatic patients, we must ensure an accurate quantification of mitral regurgitation severity. There is also significant importance placed on left ventricular ejection fraction and end-systolic dimension, which can often be better assessed with CMR.

CARDIAC MAGNETIC RESONANCE TECHNIQUES USED FOR ASSESSMENT OF MITRAL REGURGITATION

Cardiac Morphology and Ventricular Volumes

Steady state free precession (SSFP) sequences are the backbone of CMR and are used to calculate left and right ventricular volumes, ejection fraction, and ventricular mass. SSFP sequences have excellent contrast between myocardium and blood pool with high temporal resolution, which is why CMR has become the gold standard for calculating ventricular volumes and ejection fractions.[2,3] Gated SSFP sequences are obtained using a series of short breath holds acquired over multiple phases of the cardiac cycle and reconstructed into a cine movie (see Video 8.1). Left ventricular (LV) volumes are calculated using the Simpson method of disks using short-axis SSFP sequences through the entire left ventricle (Fig. 8.1; Video 8.1). Left ventricular end-diastolic (EDV) and end-systolic volumes (ESV) are calculated to determine stroke volume (SV) (SV = EDV − ESV) and ejection fraction (EF% = SV/EDV). In addition, left atrial volume can be calculated using multiple short-axis slices or by utilizing the biplane area-length method as in echocardiography.

Phase Contrast

Phase contrast imaging or velocity encoded gradient echo imaging (VENC) is a CMR technique for quantifying blood flow.[7] A plane perpendicular to the path of flowing blood is selected. A velocity encoded image is created for multiple phases of the cardiac cycle. Quantification of blood flow is performed by software after the reader outlines the vessel of interest for each phase (Fig. 8.2). For quantification of mitral regurgitation, a plane perpendicular to the ascending aorta is selected and quantification of aortic flow (aortic stroke volume) is determined. CMR flow measurements have extensive validation and represent a unique capability of considerable value.[6,8,9]

Determining Severity of Mitral Regurgitation

Mitral regurgitant volume (MRV) is determined by subtracting aortic stroke volume (obtained by phase contrast) from left ventricular stroke volume (calculated from short-axis SSFP). Mitral valve RV = LV SV − aortic SV regurgitant fraction (%) = MRV/LV SV (Fig. 8.3). RVs and fraction are calculated without hemodynamic or shape assumptions and are not affected by the eccentricity of the MR jet or orifice geometry. CMR is generally more accurate and reproducible for quantitating RV, regurgitant fraction, and well as left atrial and ventricular volumes and ejection fraction.[6,8,9]

Thresholds for severity generally follow those for echocardiography and the guidelines from the American College of Cardiology/American Heart Association.[5] Mitral regurgitation is considered severe with a RV is greater than or equal to 60 mL or regurgitant fraction of greater than or equal to 50%, although a cutoff of 48% for severe has previously been recommended.[6,10]

WHEN TO USE GADOLINIUM

Gadolinium with **d**iethylene**t**riamine**p**ent**a**cetate (Gd-DTPA) is an extracellular contrast agent this is distributed in the interstitial fluid space and plasma, very little enhancement occurs during their steady state distribution in compact myocardium, where most of the volume is composed of intracellular fluid within myocytes. When the cell membrane becomes permeable during acute or chronic injury, the distribution volume of extracellular gadolinium agents increases dramatically, which shortens relaxation times of the atoms and alters appearance on magnetic resonance. Gd-DTPA can be seen immediately within blood vessels as used in MRI angiography, early in areas of cellular disruption such as interstitial edema, and late in areas of scar, infiltration, or fibrosis. Gadolinium should be used to characterize myocardial tissue. In regard to mitral regurgitation, gadolinium could be used to differential normal verus abnormal myocardium for functional mitral regurgitation as well as assess for malignant mitral valve prolapse (MVP) in primary mitral regurgitation (discussed later).

ECHOCARDIOGRAPHY VERSUS CARDIAC MAGNETIC RESONANCE

Echocardiography will always serve as the first-line modality for assessment of mitral regurgitation. Echocardiography has many advantages, including wide availability, portability, ability to assess supportive signs of severity, such as dilated left atrial and ventricular dilation or pulmonary hypertension and excellent special resolution. The American Society of Echocardiography guidelines recommend integrating numerous parameters for full assessment of mitral regurgitation severity: color flow jet, density of mitral regurgitation signal on continuous-wave Doppler, vena contracta width, pulmonary vein flow reversal, peak velocity of E-wave with pulsed Doppler, regurgitant index, effective regurgitant orifice area (EROA) using proximal isovelocity surface area (PISA), and RV.[5,6,11] Historically, area of color flow jet has been used to assign a degree of mitral regurgitation. This is often inaccurate, and use of this parameter alone is not recommended.[6,12] Interrogation of multiple parameters is required, however the guidelines do not suggest a weight for each component or how to reconcile if there are inconsistencies. Quantitative methods (PISA, EROA, RV) improve accuracy of mitral regurgitation assessment and must be incorporated whenever possible; however, it is important to acknowledge limitations and consider alternative imaging to aid in valvular assessment if needed. PISA, EROA, RV are limited by orifice morphology, geometric assumptions, or multiple jets. PISA formulation assumes a hemispheric geometry, which is of course not always the case and loses accuracy with eccentric jets. Caution must also be used when using these parameters in non-holosystolic mitral regurgitation as severity will be overestimated. Interobserver variability in these commonly used parameters and lack of a single reproducible echocardiographic parameter for severity of mitral regurgitation are significant limitations.[13]

ADVANTAGES OF CARDIAC MAGNETIC RESONANCE

CMR has several advantages over echocardiography. CMR provides a view of the heart without limitations of body habitus or imaging window. As discussed previously, CMR is considered the gold standard for assessing ventricular volumes and ejection fraction. Reproducibility of left ventricular volumes, ejection fraction, regurgitant fraction, and RVs is superior with CMR.[14] Quantification of mitral regurgitation does not rely upon the characteristics of the regurgitant jet. Volumes and regurgitant fraction can be quantified without contrast. CMR can also provide insight into the underlying mechanism of regurgitation.

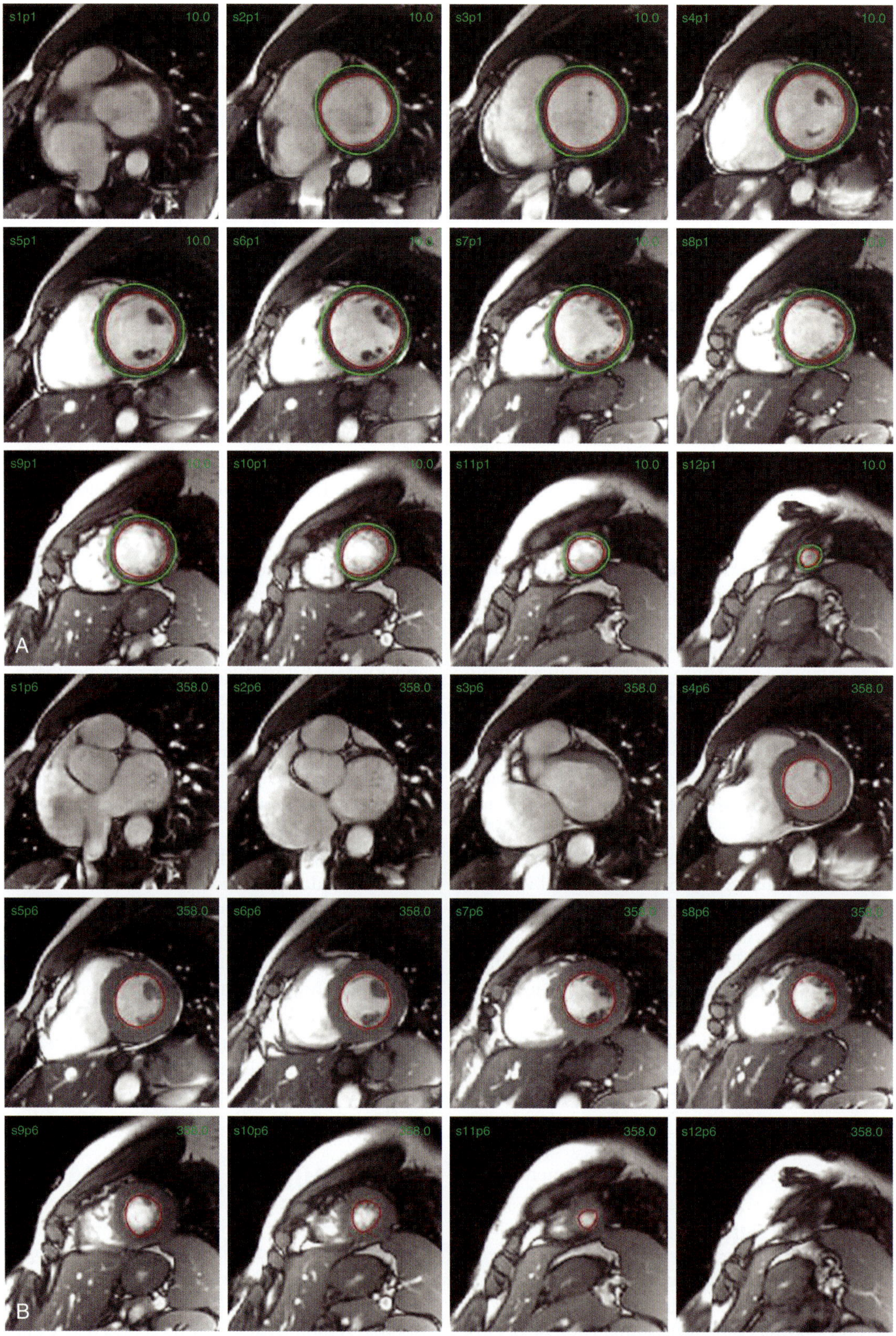

Fig. 8.1 Short-Axis Steady State Free Precession. Left ventricular volumes are obtained from sequential short-axis slices acquired from the mitral annulus to the apex with a fixed thickness. Endocardial contours are traced at end-diastole and end-systole to obtain an area. (A) Left ventricular end-diastolic volume (LVEDV) and (B) end-systolic volume (LVESV) are calculated by summation of the volumes (area × thickness) of each short-axis slice. No geometric assumptions are made. Stroke volume = LVEDV − LVESV. In this case, LVEDV measured 244 mL, LVESV 88 mL. SV = 244 − 88 = 156 mL.

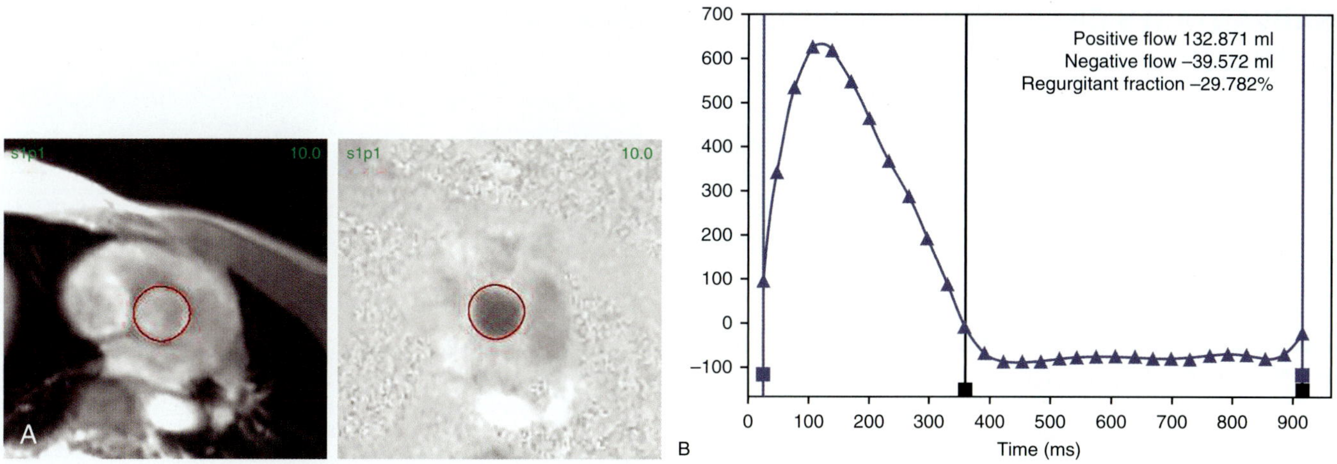

Fig. 8.2 Phase Contrast of the Aortic Root to Assess Forward and Retrograde Flow. Phase contrast (A) produces two sets of cine images: a magnitude image which is the anatomic reference (A) and a velocity map (B) that has pixel values related to velocity and direction of flow. These maps are postprocessed by drawing an area of interest around the aortic root (A, red circle) producing a flow versus time graph (B). This example has a forward flow of 132.9 mL and negative (regurgitant) flow of 39.6 mL with a regurgitant fraction of 29.8%.

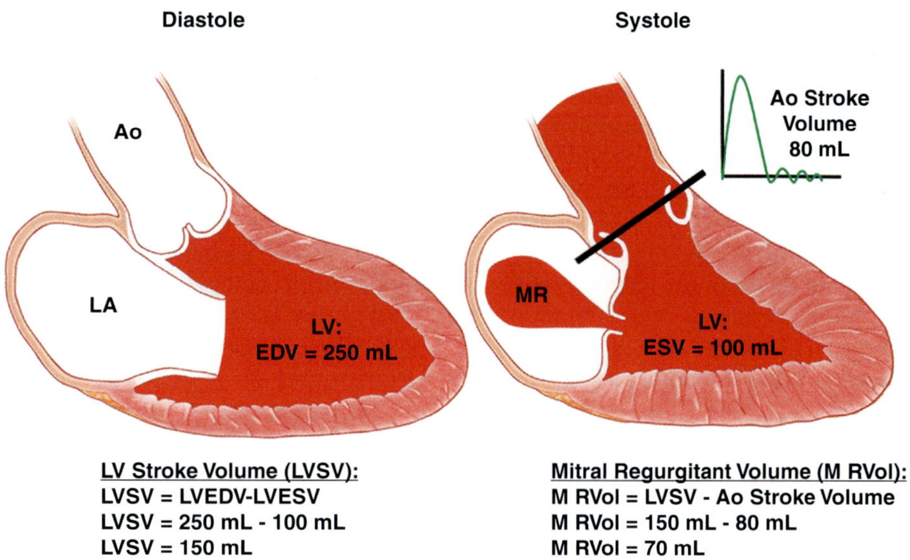

Fig. 8.3 Example Cardiac Magnetic Resonance Method for Quantification of Mitral Regurgitation (MR). As described in Fig. 8.1, left ventricular volumes are calculated at end-diastole (LVEDP) and during end-systole (LVESV). Stroke volume (SV) is computed as the difference between LVEDP and LVESV; in this example, LV SV is 150 mL. The volume of blood crossing the aortic (AO) valve is measured by performance of a phase-contrast acquisition in the aorta (as detailed in Fig. 8.2); in this example, 80 mL. The mitral RVol (M RVol) is computed as the difference between the LV SV and aortic forward SV; in this example, 70 mL. (From Zoghbi WA, et al. Recommendations for noninvasive evaluation of native valvular regurgitation: a report from the American society of echocardiography developed in collaboration with the society for cardiovascular magnetic resonance. *J Am Soc Echocardiogr*. 2017;30(4):303–371.)

DISADVANTAGES OF CARDIAC MAGNETIC RESONANCE

One major disadvantage of cardiac MRI is claustrophobia. Patients must also lie flat and cooperate with breath holding commands and holding still. Several implantable devices remain incompatible, although most contemporary cardiac devices are safe. Availability and expertise are growing, although remains more limited than echocardiography.

DISCORDANCE BETWEEN ECHO AND CARDIAC MAGNETIC RESONANCE

Quantification of mitral regurgitation is often discordant between echocardiogram and CMR.[15,16] In one multicenter study,[15] 34% of patients with severe mitral regurgitation by echocardiography had mild MR on CMR and 78% with severe by echocardiography had nonsevere by CMR. In this same study, the authors found that there was a stronger correlation between MR severity by CMR and postsurgical left ventricular remodeling. Although not yet conclusive, data suggest that CMR is more accurate and several authors recommend considering CMR when the MR severity is influencing clinical decisions, such as surgery.[4,15]

MALIGNANT MITRAL VALVE PROLAPSE

No CMR discussion about mitral valve disease would be complete without mentioning malignant MVP. MVP, which is the most common valvular disease, is an infrequent but likely underestimated cause of sudden cardiac death. CMR may help identify patients at increased risk. The hallmark of arrhythmogenic MVP is evidence of late gadolinium enhancement (fibrosis/scar) in the inferobasal left ventricle or associated papillary muscles which can only be evaluated using CMR (Fig. 8.4). Late gadolinium enhancement has been associated with complex ventricular arrhythmias in MVP patients.[17,18] It is hypothesized that endomyocardial stretch and subsequent fibrosis is the arrhythmic mechanism in patients with MVP.

Mitral annular disjunction (MAD) is defined as the atrial displacement of the mitral valve hinge from the ventricular myocardium and is closely linked to MVP (Fig. 8.5, Video 8.2).[19] MAD has been independently associated with malignant ventricular arrhythmias, including sudden cardiac death. Further studies are needed on this finding and clinical significance.

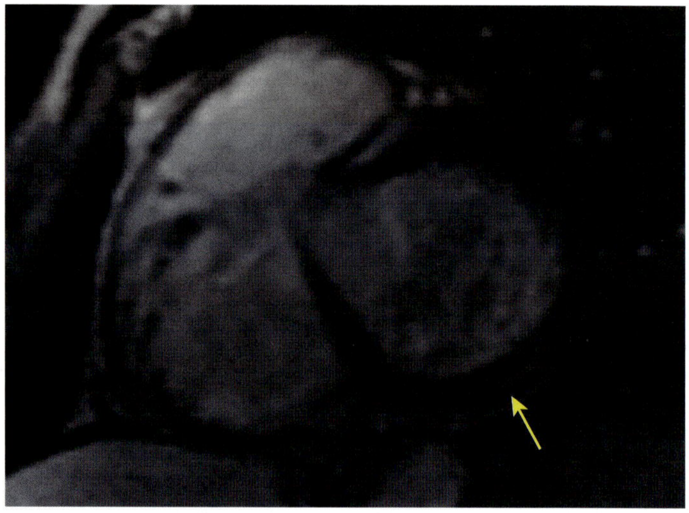

Fig. 8.4 Malignant Mitral Valve Prolapse. This patient has mitral valve prolapse and presented with sustained ventricular tachycardia. Cardiac magnetic resonance revealed mid-myocardial late gadolinium enhancement (scar) in the basal inferolateral wall *(yellow arrow)*.

SUMMARY: WHEN TO CONSIDER CARDIAC MAGNETIC RESONANCE FOR MITRAL REGURGITATION

CMR is currently indicated in patients with mitral regurgitation to assess left and right ventricular volumes, function, or mitral regurgitation severity when these issues are not satisfactorily addressed by echocardiography—a Class I indication.[5] CMR should be highly considered for:

- Poor acoustic windows on echocardiogram
- Discrepancy between echocardiogram and physical examination/clinical history
- Discrepancies on severity using the multiple echocardiographic parameters
- Eccentric mitral regurgitation jets
- Nonholosystolic MR
- Multiple MR jets
- Multiple valvular abnormalities

SELF-ASSESSMENT QUESTIONS

1. Which of the following is an indication for cardiac MRI in mitral regurgitation?
   a. Poor acoustic windows on echocardiogram
   b. Discrepancy between echocardiogram and physical examination/clinical history
   c. Eccentric mitral regurgitation jets, nonholosystolic MR
   d. Multiple MR jets
   e. All of the above
2. Cardiac MRI is considered the gold standard for ventricular volumes and ejection fraction.
   a. True
   b. False
3. Which are findings suggestive of malignant mitral valve prolapse? (select all that apply)
   A. Mitral annular disjunction
   B. Greater than 2 mm of mitral valve prolapse
   C. Late gadolinium enhancement
   D. Severe mitral regurgitation
   E. All of the above

See page 316 for the answers.

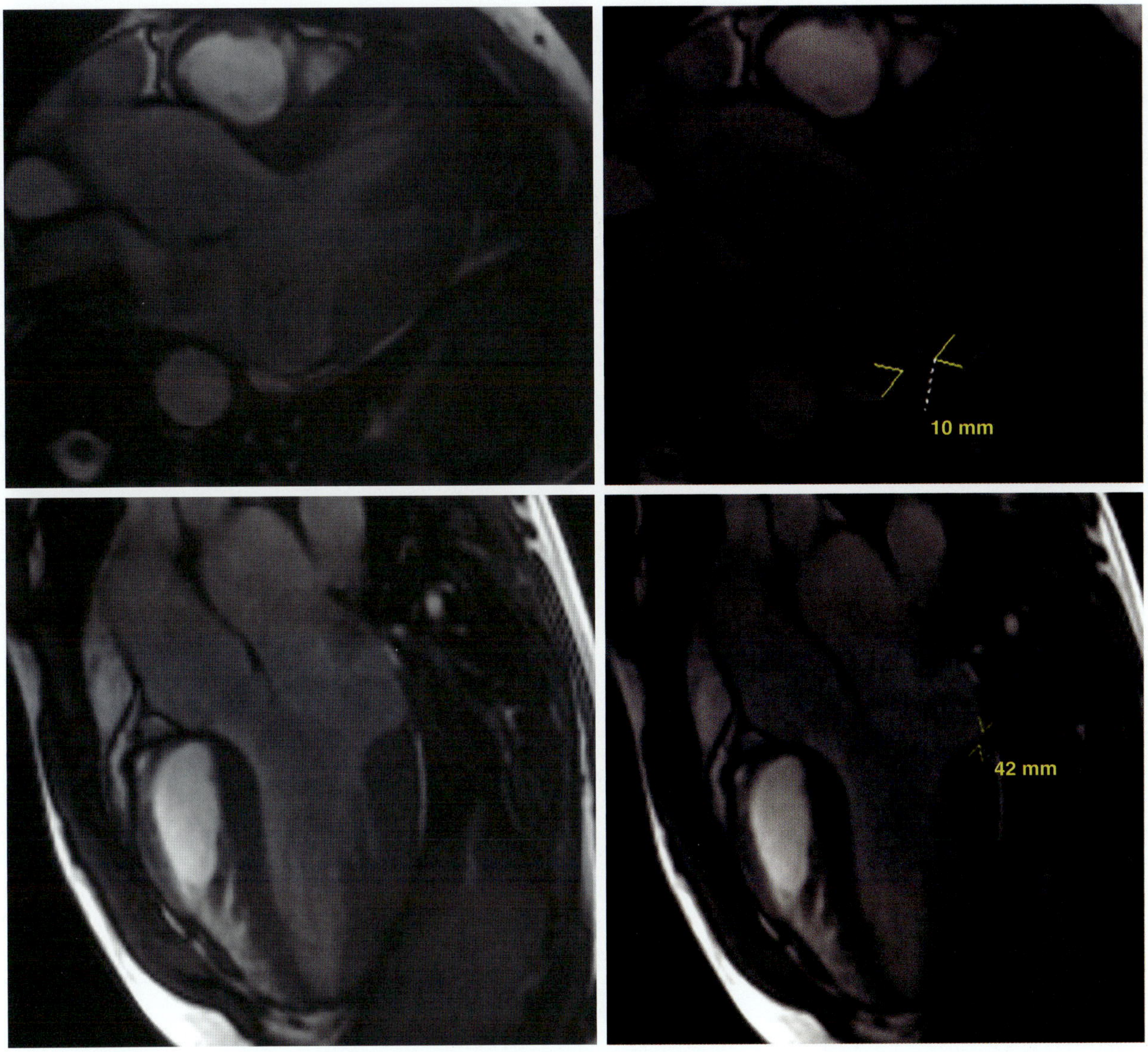

Fig. 8.5 End-systolic image in 3-chamber view of two patients with mitral valve prolapse and mitral annular disjunction (MAD), left still image at end-systole with corresponding image measuring MAD on right. Both patients underwent CMR for frequent premature ventricular beats. The (top) patient had evidence of late gadolinium enhancement as seen in Fig. 8.4.

REFERENCES

1. Rehr RB, Malloy CR, Flipchuk NG, et al. Left ventricular volumes measured by MR imaging. *Radiology*. 1985;156:717–719.
2. Bellenger NG, Burgess MI, Ray SG, et al. Comparison of left ventricular ejection fraction and volumes in heart failure by echocardiography, radionuclide ventriculography and cardiovascular magnetic resonance; are they interchangeable? *Eur Heart J*. 2000;21:1387–1396.
3. Grothues F, Smith GC, Moon JC, et al. Comparison of interstudy reproducibility of cardiovascular magnetic resonance with two-dimensional echocardiography in normal subjects and in patients with heart failure or left ventricular hypertrophy. *Am J Cardiol*. 2002;90:29–34.
4. Uretsky S, Supariwala A, Nidadovolu P, et al. Quantification of left ventricular remodeling in response to isolated aortic or mitral regurgitation. *J Cardiovasc Magn Res*. 2010;12:32.
5. Nishimura RA, Otto CM, Bonow RO, et al. 2014 AHA/ACC guideline for the management of patients with valvular heart disease: a report of the American College of Cardiology/American Heart Association Task Force on Practice Guidelines. *J Am Coll Cardiol*. 2014;63:e57–185.
6. Zoghbi WA, Adams D, Bonow RO, et al. Recommendations for noninvasive evaluation of native valvular regurgitation: a report from the American Society of Echocardiography developed in collaboration with the Society for Cardiac Magnetic Resonance. *J Am Soc Echocardiogr*. 2017;30(4):303–371.
7. Beerbaum P, Korperick H, Barth P, et al. Noninvasive quantification of left-to-right shunt in pediatric patients. *Circulation*. 2001;103:2476–2482.
8. Gatehouse PD, Rolf MP, Graves MJ, et al. Flow measurement by cardiovascular magnetic resonance: a multi-centre multi-vendor study of background phase offset errors that can compromise

the accuracy of derived regurgitant or shunt flow measurements. *J Cardiovasc Magn Reson*. 2010;12:5.

9. Fujita N, Chazouilleres AF, Hartiala JJ, et al. Quantification of mitral regurgitation by velocity encoded cine nuclear magnetic resonance imaging. *J Am Coll Cardiol*. 1994;23:951–958.
10. Gelfand EV, Hughes S, Hauser TH, et al. Severity of mitral and aortic regurgitation as assessed by cardiovascular magnetic resonance: optimizing correlation with Doppler echocardiography. *J Cardiovasc Magn Reson*. 2006;8:503–507.
11. Bonow RO, O'Gara PT, Adams DH, et al. Focused update of the 2017 ACC expert consensus decision pathway on the management of mitral regurgitation. *J Am Coll Cardiol*. 2020;75:2236–2270.
12. Lancellotti P, Moura L, Pierard LA, et al. European Association of Echocardiography. European Association of Echocardiography recommendations for the assessment of valvular regurgitation. Part 2: mitral and tricuspid regurgitation (native valve disease). *Eur J Echocardiogr*. 2010;11:307–332.
13. Uretsky S, Argulian E, Narula J, et al. Use of cardiac magnetic resonance imaging in assessing mitral regurgitation current evidence. *J Am Coll Cardiol*. 2018;71:547–563.
14. Harris AW, Krieger EV, Kim M, et al. Cardiac magnetic resonance imaging versus transthoracic echocardiography for prediction of outcomes in chronic aortic or mitral regurgitation. *Am J Cardiol*. 2017;119:1074–1081.
15. Uretsky S, Gillam L, Lang R, et al. Discordance between echocardiography and MRI in the assessment of mitral regurgitation severity a prospective multicenter trial. *J Am Coll Cardiol*. 2014;65:1078–1088.
16. Lopez-Mattei JC, Ibrahim H, Shaikh KA, et al. Comparative assessment of mitral regurgitation severity by transthoracic echocardiography and cardiac magnetic resonance using an integrative and quantitative approach. *Am J Cardiol*. 2016;117:264–270.
17. Basso C, Perazzolo Marra M, Rizzo S, et al. Arrhythmic mitral valve prolapse and sudden cardiac death. *Circulation*. 2015;132:556–566.
18. Han Y, Peters DC, Salton CJ, et al. Cardiovascular magnetic resonance characterization of mitral valve prolapse. *JACC Cardiovasc Imaging*. 2008;1:294–303.
19. Dejgaard LA, SKjolsvik ET, Lie ØH, et al. The mitral annulus disjunction arrhythmic syndrome. *J Am Coll Cardiol*. 2018;72:1600–1609.

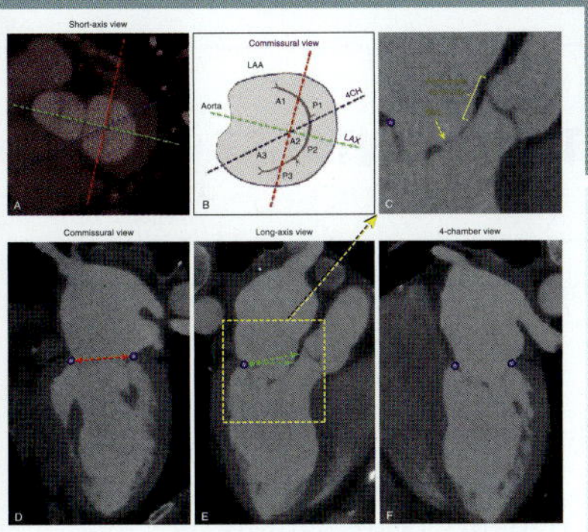

9

Computed Tomography Scan in Mitral Valve Disease and Its Treatments

Elina Khasanova, Andrew Chatfield, Philipp Blanke, Jonathon Leipsic

CHAPTER OUTLINE

LEARNING OBJECTIVES

1. Understand the methodology of mitral annular segmentation by computed tomography (CT) prior to transcatheter mitral valve replacement.
2. Learn about CT reformats and reconstruction planes in the assessment of mitral valve pathology.
3. Conceptualize mitral annular dynamism and factors affecting annular measurement on cardiac CT angiography with whole cardiac cycle coverage.
4. Utilize CT data for pre-procedural planning: identification of fluoroscopic angles, localization of left ventricle apex, navigation prior to transseptal puncture.
5. Familiarize with the concept of neo-left ventricular outflow tract (LVOT) and risks regarding LVOT obstruction.

INTRODUCTION

Anatomic and functional evaluation prior to transcatheter mitral valve (TMV) repair and TMV replacement (TMVR) by multidetector computed tomography angiography (CTA) has emerged as an essential part of pre-procedural planning, complimenting the significant amount of information obtained from transesophageal echocardiogram (TEE).[1–4] The role of CTA has evolved, mimicking its use in TAVR with a focus on reproducible annular measurement, evaluation of landing zone, neo-left ventricular outflow tract assessment, and pattern of mitral annular calcification.[5,6] Computer tomography (CT) provides three-dimensional (3D) sets of data of cardiac morphology with a larger field of view compared to echocardiography, excellent image quality owing to millimetric spatial resolution, isotropic image quality throughout the data set, and good temporal resolution. Multiplanar reconstruction capabilities and functional data sets are additional benefits of the modality that can help provide information on the morphology and function of the mitral valve.[3,7]

CT ANATOMY OF THE MITRAL VALVE

The mitral valve structure is complex; it comprises non-planar non-circular annulus, leaflets, and subvalvular apparatus. The adjacent anatomical structures, notably the left ventricular outflow tract (LVOT) and circumflex artery, contribute to its complexity.

The Leaflets

CT anatomy of mitral valve leaflets and segmentation according to Carpentier's nomenclature is depicted by Fig. 9.1A and

Fig. 9.1C.[8] The most lateral scallop (labeled as P1) is adjacent to the anterolateral commissure, P2 (middle) is centrally located, and the most medial (P3 scallop) is adjacent to posteromedial commissure. Similarly, the anterior scallops are labeled as A1, A2, and A3. The leaflets converge at the anterolateral and posteromedial commissures. The coaptation zone, or line, is a semilunar arc conformation with the leaflets converging at the commissures. Despite better visualization of the mitral valve scallops by echocardiography, which is proven to have better temporal resolution than CT, post-processing techniques such as minimum intensity projection (MIP) may improve visualization of the thin low-attenuation leaflets.[2]

Mitral Annulus

Mitral annulus (MA) (from Latin "small ring") gives attachment to the mitral valve formed by a junction of the left atrium, left ventricle (LV), and the leaflets. It is a non-rigid fibromuscular structure changing shape throughout the cardiac cycle and incorporating several structures along the hinge points. The MA 3D configuration is saddle-shaped with anterior and posterior peaks or horns. The anterior horn, more fibrous and less prone to dilatation, extends between the trigones to the aortic root ("aortomitral continuity" or "intervalvular fibrosa") (Fig. 9.1B and Fig. 9.1D).[2,9] The continuity between the aortic and mitral valve is a cardiac CT anatomical landmark for identifying the LV. Its relationship with LVOT is crucial for consideration of suitability for TMVR due to potential risk of LVOT obstruction (refer to further discussion in the Left Ventricular Outflow Tract Obstruction Assessment section).

In healthy individuals, the posterior horn is located at the junction of the atrial and ventricular myocardium and formed by insertion of the posterior mitral leaflet (PML), and the nadir of the annulus is located close to the fibrous trigones. The fibrous trigones represent the anatomic junction between the anterior and posterior annulus and can be identified on CT scan as focal areas of triangular thickening of the medial and later ends of the fibrous annulus (Fig. 9.1E). This part of the annulus is mainly muscular and, therefore, susceptible to dilatation (seen in mitral regurgitation [MR]) and calcification.

Subvalvular Apparatus

The subvalvular apparatus has a dual role in maintaining valvular competence and enhancing LV systolic pump function. It consists of papillary muscles and the chordae tendineae.

The papillary muscles are positioned along the mid to apical segments of the LV. The papillary muscles are comprised of one to three muscular bundles that extend from the myocardium and attach to the mitral leaflets through the chordae tendineae. The papillary muscles are named based on their location and the commissures they relate to (i.e., anterolateral and posteromedial).

Fibrous string-like chords of the chordae tendineae are highly variable in their number and configuration. Chordae can be distinguished based on their leaflet insertion (Fig. 9.1F). The primary chordae attach to the free edges of the mitral valve leaflets; the second-order chordae insert to the bodies of the leaflets. Finally, tertiary chordae are only found in the posterior leaflet and attach directly to the ventricular wall.[10–12]

TECHNIQUE OF ACQUISITION, CONTRAST INJECTION PROTOCOL

ECG-gated contrast-enhanced multiphasic CTA covering the entire cardiac cycle is required for mitral valve and annulus assessment.

Data acquisition is either synchronized by retrospective or prospective electrocardiography (ECG)—gating, tube voltage, and current set according to the patient's body habitus. For example, tube voltage varies from 100 to 120 kV in our institution and current from 400 to 600 mA to ensure optimal image quality. Gantry rotation time is one of the adjustable parameters and may be set to 0.24 to 0.33 second. However, some of the aforementioned settings are vendor-specific. Tube current modulation is avoided to ensure high image quality throughout the cardiac cycle.

Image acquisition initiates when the region of interest attenuation reaches the 150 HU threshold within the LV. The acquisition starts at the level of carina and covers the heart to its base. In the case of transapical access, the acquisition should cover the entire thoracic cage to better assess the intercostal space.

Contrast material injection protocol requires a single breath-hold following biphasic injection of 60 to 70 mL of intravenous contrast media (320 mg I/mL) at the rate of 4.5 to 6.5 mL/s and 50 mL saline chaser via an 18-gauge needle in an antecubital vein. Other recommended parameters include slice thickness of 0.5 mm, increment 0.5, and iterative reconstruction for noise reduction.

IMAGES POST-PROCESSING

Reconstruction Planes

Mitral apparatus is best evaluated using standard two-chamber (2ch) or commissural, four-chamber (4ch), three-chamber (3ch), and short-axis views (Fig. 9.2).[5]

The short-axis stack is the set of images covering atria to apex orthogonal to the interventricular septum on the 4ch view and parallel to atria-ventricular valves. Mitral valve anatomy can be defined by using this plane (Fig. 9.2A).

The 2ch view is achieved by rotating the images perpendicularly to the mitral valve and parallel to the cardiac septum. This axis gives an overview of the left atrium, ventricle, and mitral valve (Fig. 9.2D).

When the border between the mitral and aortic valves is localized on the axial slices, and the images are rotated from this point, a 3ch view can be reconstructed. Using a true commissural (2ch) view on cardiac CTA transecting at P1-P3 scallops, major or intercommissural (IC) MA diameter can be assessed. Perpendicular on-axis long-axis or 3ch view depicts A2-P2 scallops, but lacking distinct MA landmark at A2 secondary to aortomitral continuity (see Fig. 9.2B–E) results in variable measurement of minor septal-lateral (SL) diameter.

4ch view is achieved by rotating upwards from the apex of the heart on the axial slices, is aligned along intrinsic axes of the heart, and provides accurate anatomical representations of the cardiac structures. The mitral valve comes into view, and the apex of the heart is well demarcated (Fig. 9.2F).

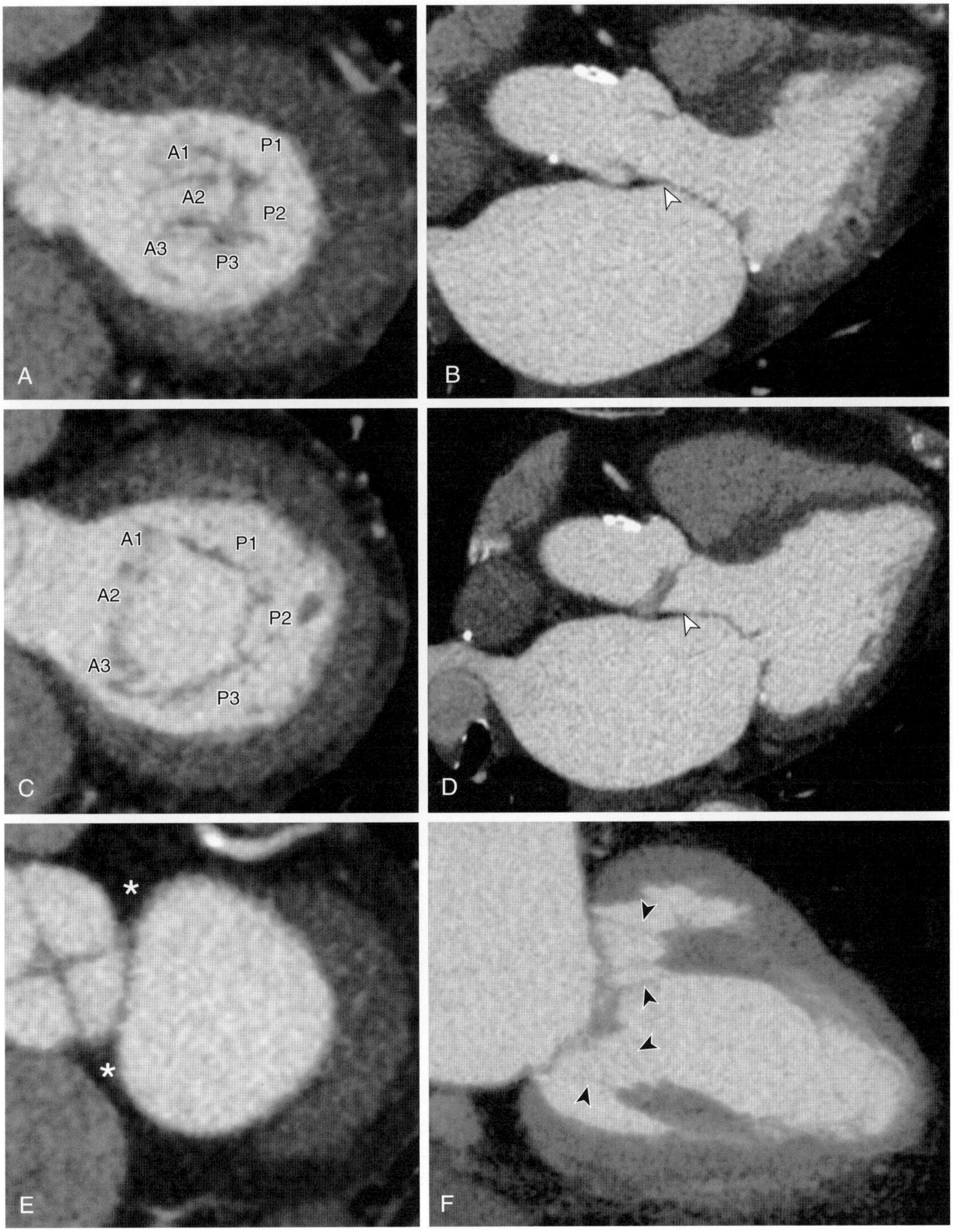

Fig. 9.1 CT Anatomy of the Mitral Valve. (A and B) Mitral valve is closed at end-systole. (C and D) Images show the opened valve at end-diastole, (C) with the division of the anterior (A1–A3) and posterior (P1–P3) mitral valve leaflet. (B and D) highlight the aortomitral continuity forming the anterior horn of the annulus remaining fixed in position throughout the cycle *(arrowwheads)*. (E) Image shows mitral annulus and fibrous trigones *(stars)*. (F) Minimum intensity projection at end-systole highlights the complex fan-like radiation of fine tendineae running from the papillary muscles to the mitral leaflets *(arrowheads)*. (From Weir-McCall JR, Blanke P, Naoum C, et al. Mitral valve imaging with CT: relationship with transcatheter mitral valve interventions. *Radiology*. 2018;288[3]:638–655.)

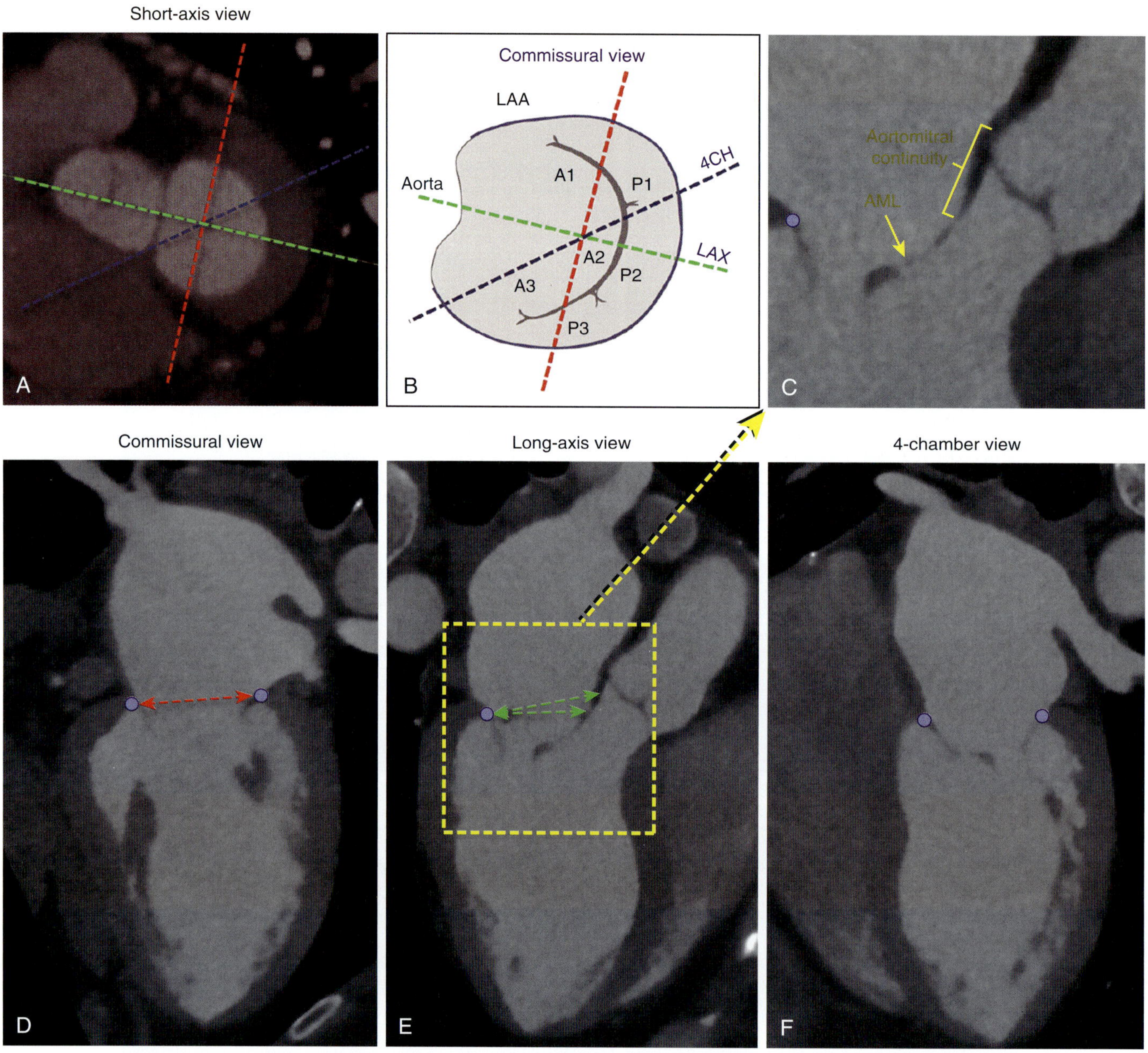

Fig. 9.2 Short-axis view of the mitral annulus (MA) region (A) and schematic of the leaflet scallops (B) with dashed lines indicating the orientation of the views in D to F. (D) Commissural view transecting at P1–P3 (major MA diameter) (B). (E) Long-axis *(LAX)* view transecting through A2–P2, oriented perpendicularly to the commissural view. The long-axis view lacks a distinct MA landmark at A2 (C, *inset*). (F) Four-chamber view with a diagonal orientation. *LAA*, left atrial appendage; *MA*, mitral annulus (From Blanke P, Naoum C, Webb J, et al. Multimodality imaging in the context of transcatheter mitral valve replacement: establishing consensus among modalities and disciplines. *JACC Cardiovasc Imaging*. 2015;8[10]:1191–1208.)

Annular segmentation is performed using long- and short-axis reformats aligned with the LV long axis by the principle of stepwise rotation; the techniques will be described in the following paragraph.[2,9]

Two- and 3-chamber reconstructions yielded higher diagnostic accuracy in evaluating mitral prolapse than echocardiography; this will be discussed in one of the following paragraphs.[13]

Phases of the Cycle

Mitral annular conformation changes in shape and in size throughout the cycle, and multiphase images allow for the evaluation of the annulus and the landing zone across the cardiac cycle. These multiphase data sets allow for CT to complement echocardiography in evaluating mitral pathologic conditions and dynamic leaflet motion. CT features of pathological conditions involving mitral valve will be further discussed in the

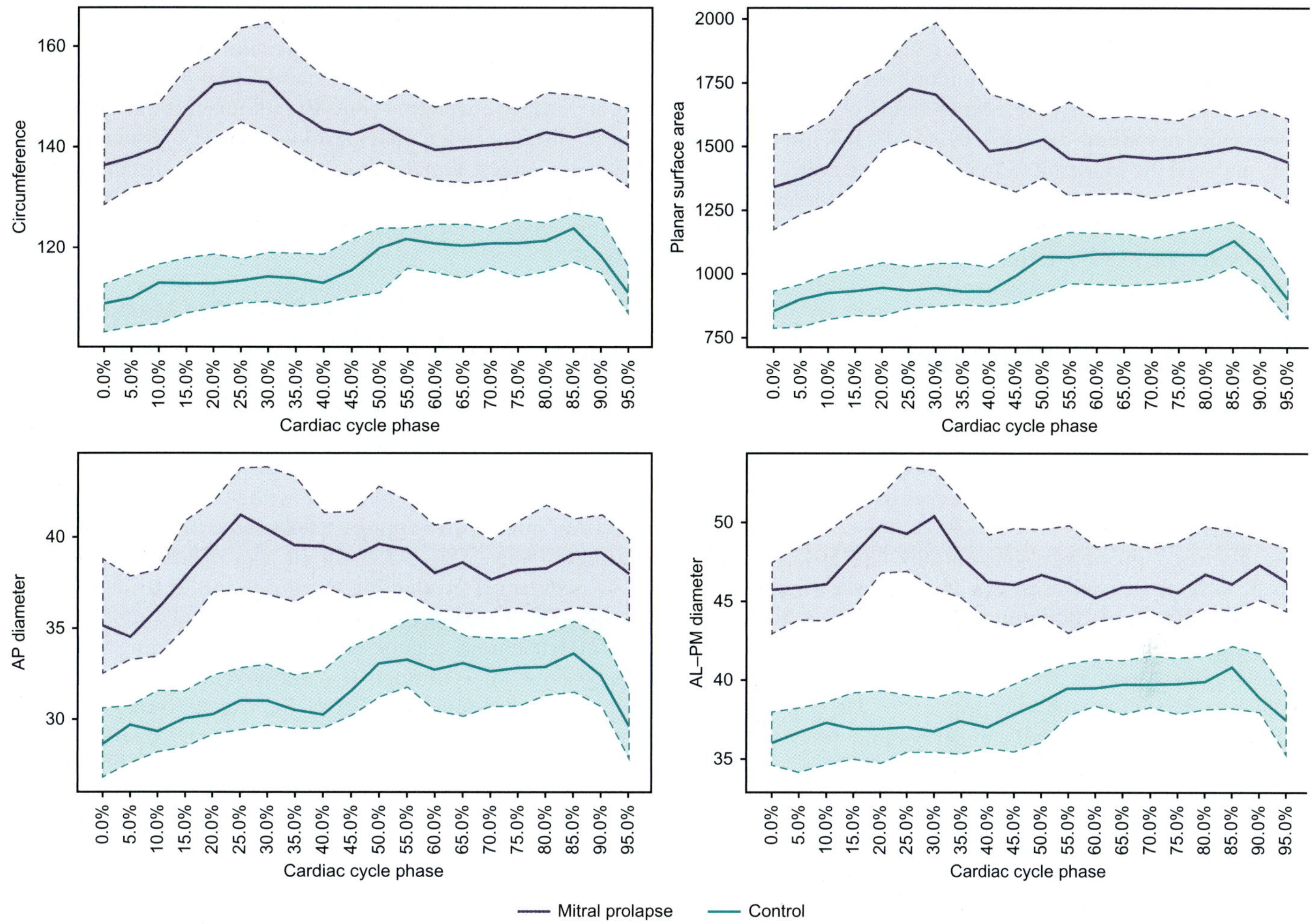

Fig. 9.3 Mitral annular dimensions (mean, standard deviation) throughout the cardiac cycle for patients with surgically proven mitral prolapse *(blue line)* and control group without mitral prolapse *(green line)*. A–P distance, annular distance measured between the anterior and posterior horn; AL–PM distance, annular diameter measured between the anterolateral and posteromedial annulus. (From Rizvi A, Marcus RP, Guo Y, et al. Dynamic computed tomographic assessment of the mitral annulus in patients with and without mitral prolapse. *J Cardiovasc Comput Tomogr.* 2020;14[6]:502–509.)

CT paragraph in the evaluation of mitral valve disease. Multiphase image data-sets are reconstructed at a minimum of 10% R-R interval using a medium soft-tissue convolution kernel in the axial plane. Smaller increments, 5% of R-R intervals (i.e., 20 phases), are preferential to allow a detailed assessment of the leaflets during systole.[14]

Mitral valve opening is the most reliable factor to define end-systole and end-diastole rather than phase reconstruction designation from the CT scanner, which can be compromised by severe arrhythmia or faster heart rates. The absolute millisecond reconstruction at 50 msec intervals available from specific vendors can improve image quality affected by irregular heart rate.[15]

MITRAL ANNULAR DYNAMISM

MA dynamism is one of the challenges for TMVR. Importantly, mitral annular dimensions differ between normal state and mitral valve pathologies. In the absence of MR, due to early systolic contraction annulus demonstrates a more pronounced saddle shape and minimal annular dimension, which increases toward late systole.[16] The diastolic shape of the annulus is more circular and increases in size by more than 20%.[17] Abnormal mitral annular dynamism due to mitral incompetence is observed in primary MR patients with diffuse myxomatous mitral valve degeneration. Flattening of saddle-shape annulus, higher variability in mitral annular circumference, planar area, and increased intercommissural diameter were detected in the patients with primary MR compared to normal subjects. Mitral valve prolapse (MVP) patients tend to have maximal annular area measurements during systole secondary to annular disjunction and protrusion towards the left atrium (Fig. 9.3).[18,19] In patients with secondary MR, the extent of annular dimension changes are diminished.[9,20] The presence of MA calcification also leads to loss of annular contraction and loss of early systolic folding along the IC diameter.[21] Therefore, annular dynamism highly dependent on underlying mitral valve pathology emphasizes the importance of multiphasic CTA acquisition for TMVR planning.[5,18] Hence, segmentation of the MA could be performed in the end-diastole (70% to 90% R-R interval) and in the end-systolic phase (30% to 40% R-R interval) to ensure accurate annular segmentation and determine the largest annular area.[3,18,22] Ultimately, the evaluation of atrial contraction (typically at 85% to 95% of the cardiac cycle) and dimensions might be helpful in annular assessment.[9]

3D ANNULAR SEGMENTATION

Accurate measurement of the MA is imperative to determine the appropriate size of the TMVR device. Inaccurate sizing of the landing zone has devastating consequences—undersizing can lead to device embolization, whereas oversizing can result in annular rupture.

As discussed previously, anatomically, the MA is saddle-shaped, with an anterior horn extending between the trigones along the aortomitral continuity. In a healthy state, the maximum height of the saddle is in the middle of the anterior part of the annulus, another rise along the posterior leaflet, and the deepest part is at the fibrous trigones.[5,23] Decreased saddle height and more planar mitral annular contour are observed in the patients with secondary MR; however, this does not affect already planar D-shaped annular segmentation.[9]

Typically, pre-TMVR, 3D segmentation of the MA is performed in end-systole by measuring the intersection of the left atrium and left ventricular blood flow, commonly identified by the basal insertion points of the anterior and PMLs. The MA geometric assessment can be achieved by using standard post-processing CTA software or a manual approach.[2,5] Several parameters are integrated into annular sizing reports and help inform device selection. These include the projected two-dimensional area, perimeter, IC, SL, and intertrigonal distances.

Saddle-Shaped Annulus

True saddle-shaped area and perimeter measurements can be obtained by utilizing specialized software. In this approach, a variable number of segmentation points are manually placed along the insertion of the PML and along the insertion of the non-coronary and right coronary aortic cusp into the intervalvular fibrosa by stepwise rotation of a long-axis view aligned to the LV long axis (Fig. 9.4A–C).[5]

D-shaped Annulus

Blanke et al. have proposed a simplified D-shaped model for mitral annular sizing based on the observation that the anterior horn of the saddle-shaped contour would otherwise project into the LVOT.[9] The resulting D-shaped MA is more planar and does not project onto the LVOT. In this approach, the anterior horn is excluded by drawing a virtual line between the medial and lateral trigones to form the D shape of the annulus (Fig. 9.4D–F). Post-processing provides the annular area and perimeter and major and minor dimensions. The perimeter consists of the posterior annulus (PML insertion) and the trigone-trigone (TT) distance. Furthermore, annular geometry is characterized by measurement of the SL distance (minor diameter) and the IC distance (major diameter). For standardization and because of the arc-shaped coaptation zone, the authors recommend assessing IC distance in a parallel fashion to the TT distance, which yields the largest dimension. Similarly, the SL distance should be assessed perpendicularly to TT and IC (see Fig. 9.4E).

This approach facilitates and standardizes annular sizing for TMVR.

Manual Technique for Mitral Annulus Measurement

An alternative approach to MA evaluation is a manual technique following a similar technique to that used for obtaining the aortic valve annular plane.[24] Fig. 9.5 provides a detailed description of the manual technique of MA measurement proposed by Weir-McCall et al.[2] This involves sequential identification of the two fibrous trigones followed by the free edge annular ring insertion point. After approximately centering the cursor over the mitral valve (Fig. 9.5A–C), an approximate mitral planar view is obtained by aligning the image to the atrioventricular groove (Fig. 9.5E–G).

The left fibrous trigone is identified by panning the short-axis oblique view through the upper ventricle (Fig. 9.5E–G) until the well-defined triangle of the trigone comes into view (H, *arrowhead*). The image should then be centered on the left trigone, and the vertical axis rotated so that it aligns with the approximate location of the right trigone (Fig. 9.5G). The right fibrous trigone is then obtained by rotating the vertical axis (Fig. 9.5I–K) until the second well-defined triangular trigone comes into view (Fig. 9.5L, *arrowhead*). Finally, the free edge of the annulus *(dashed yellow line)* is obtained by rotating the horizontal axis (Fig. 9.5M–O) until its insertion in the ventricle (Fig. 9.5P). From this segmentation, the annular area and perimeter (Fig. 9.5Q) and TT, SL, and IC distances can be measured (R).

CT IN EVALUATION OF MITRAL VALVE DISEASE

CT plays an important role in defining the landing zone for TMV procedures and complements echocardiography evaluation of mitral pathologic conditions such as leaflet thickening and calcification.

Mitral Annular Calcification

CT provides inherent advantages in evaluating mitral annular calcification (MAC) by providing a detailed and clear definition of the pattern of annular calcium, which can help determine device suitability.

Blooming from MAC complicates a clear definition of the boundary between the blood pool and calcified annular segments. However, annular segmentation by CT can be reproducible and consistent if "harmonious smoothly marginated" annular contouring excluding protuberant calcification is maintained. This allows prevention of individualized nonstandardized segmentation and, therefore, prevents the reader specific impact on complex underlying MA anatomy, despite the absence of defined segmentation methodology correlated with downstream procedural outcome.[2]

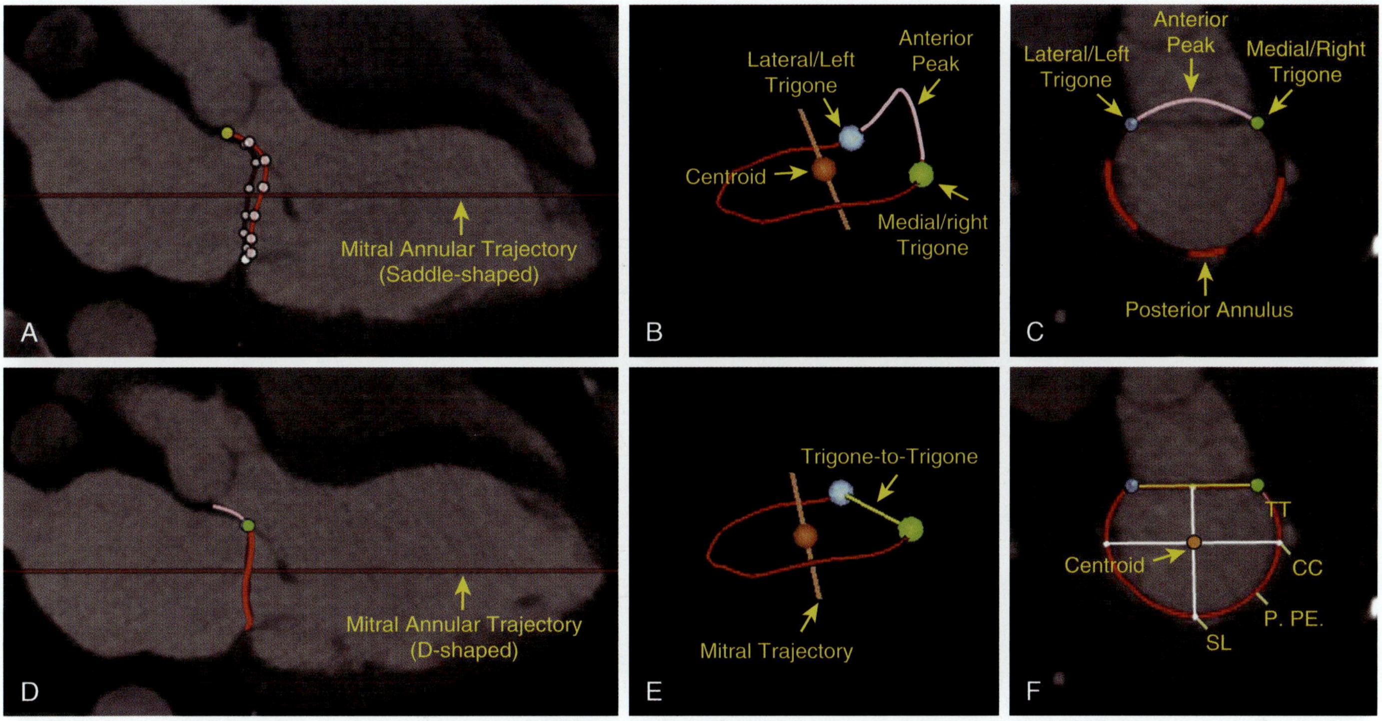

Fig. 9.4 Saddle-shaped mitral annulus (MA) segmentation as a cubic spline interpolation (A) Saddle-shaped annulus. (B) Pink line, anterior peak; red line, posterior peak (PML insertion); green and blue dots, fibrous trigones. Importantly, the anterior peak projects into the LVOT (short-axis view [C] and long-axis view [D]). The more planar D-shaped annular contour is created by truncating the saddle-shaped contour at the trigone-to-trigone distance (*yellow lines* [E and F]). Important measurements are the projected area septal-lateral (SL) and intercommissural (IC) distances; the latter is oriented perpendicularly to SL while transecting through the centroid (F). (From Blanke P, Naoum C, Webb J, et al. Multimodality imaging in the context of transcatheter mitral valve replacement: establishing consensus among modalities and disciplines. *JACC Cardiovasc Imaging*. 2015;8[10]:1191–1208.)

Balloon-expandable aortic transcatheter heart valves require extensive MAC involving at least 75% of the circumference of all four quadrants of the annulus heart valves for adequate anchoring based on radial force and friction.[25] Only qualitative MAC classification was available before Guerrero et al. proposed MAC scoring system predicting anchoring and risk of embolization and migration of a Sapien valve in valve-in-MAC procedures.[26] This score is based on average calcium thickness (<5 mm = score 1; 5–9.99 mm = score 2; ≥10 mm = score 3), degree of annulus circumference involved (<180° = score 1; 180°–270° = score 2; ≥270° = score 3), calcification at one or both trigones (one trigone = score 1; both trigones = score 2), and calcification of one or both leaflets (one leaflet = score 1; two leaflets = score 2) (Fig. 9.6). Severity grade is assigned based on total points accumulated with 3 points or less considered mild, 4 to 6 points moderate, greater than or equal to 7 considered severe MAC. Fig. 9.7 illustrates an example of MAC scoring according to the classification system. Patients with a MAC score less than or equal to 6 have a 60% embolization and/or migration rate versus 9.7% in patients with MAC greater than or equal to 7.[26]

Caseous annular calcification is a form of MAC with a core of liquefactive necrosis that forms through an incompletely understood process and predominantly occurs in the perianular area adjacent to PML.[27] Caseous MAC is homogeneously hyperattenuating similar to the blood pool on contrast-enhanced CT. Fig. 9.8 provides an example of non-contrast CT utilization in differentiating caseous MAC from a granuloma, abscess or, rarely, a neoplasm. It is also important to distinguish caseous calcium from a solid non-caseous MAC, as the latter provides more anchoring for TMVR devices.[3]

Leaflet Thickening and Vegetations

Mitral vegetation from infective endocarditis is the second most common mass of mitral apparatus after idiopathic MAC.[28] Patients with rheumatic disease, MVP, or a mitral valve prosthesis are predisposed to this pathology. ECG-gated cardiac CT has a sensitivity of 97% and specificity of 88% for detection of valvular abnormalities associated with infective endocarditis. Additionally, CT is useful to search for secondary findings associated with endocarditis, such as pseudoaneurysm and septic infarction, in a situation when echocardiography is negative for detection of major features (leaflet thickening, oscillating valvular mass, abscess) of infective endocarditis.[29] Fig. 9.9 illustrates nodular thickening of This allows prevention of individualized non the anterior mitral valve leafler (AML) predominantly at A1 (Fig. 9.9C) in keeping with vegetation in the context of infective endocarditis, additional vegetation is identified adjacent to the posterior leaflet of the tricuspid valve (Fig. 9.9D).

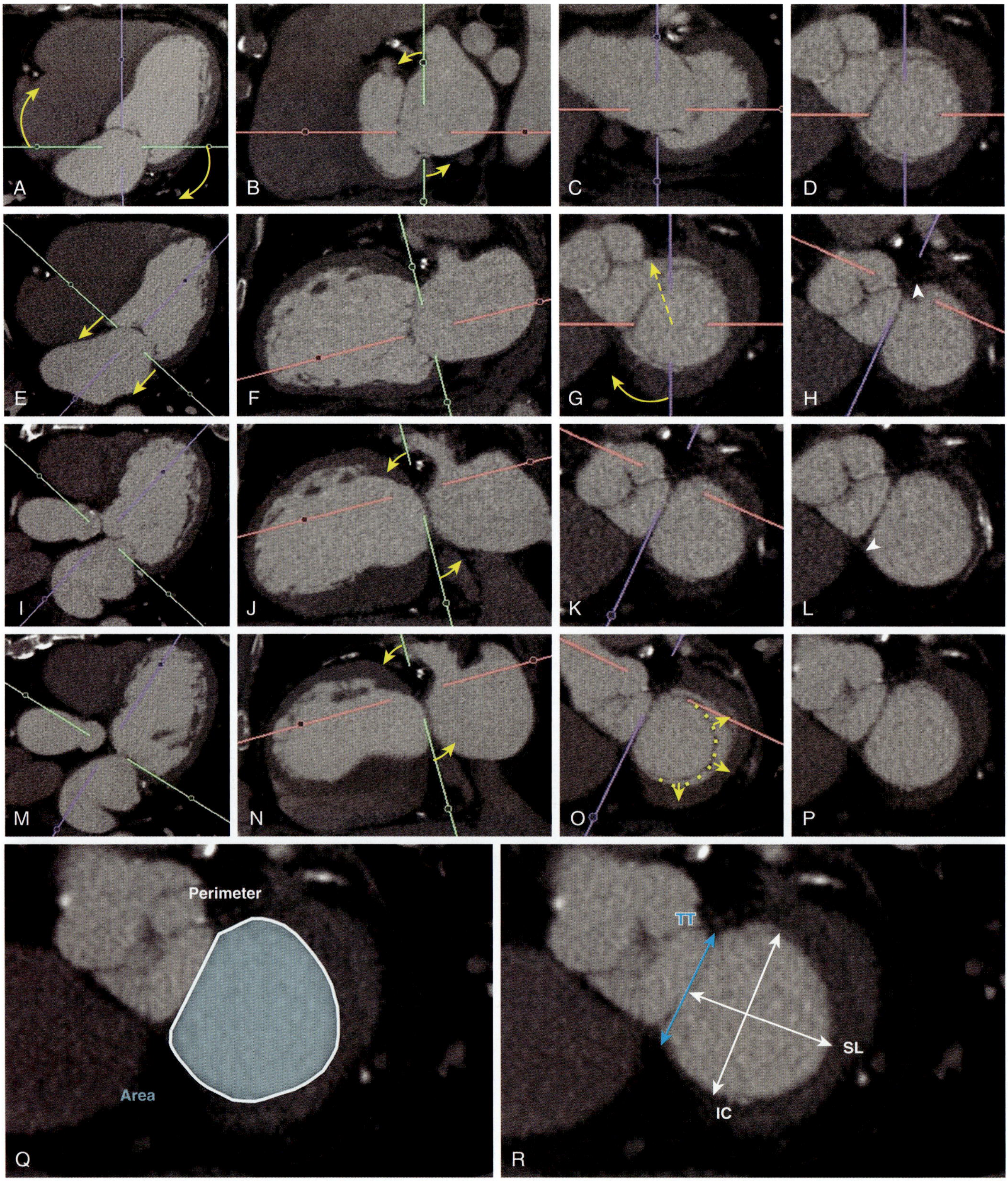

Fig. 9.5 Manual technique for obtaining a planar view through the mitral annulus from which the annular area, TT, and SL distances can be obtained. Please refer to the description of the technique in the text. Curved arrows indicate rotating the image, and straight arrows indicate moving the plane without altering its angulation. The right-hand images (D, H, L, P) are the approximate appearance the annulus should assume at each step of the process. *IC,* Intercommissural; *SL,* septal-lateral; *TT,* trigone-trigone. (From Weir-McCall JR, Blanke P, Naoum C, et al. Mitral Valve Imaging with CT: relationship with transcatheter mitral valve interventions. *Radiology.* 2018;288[3]:638–655.)

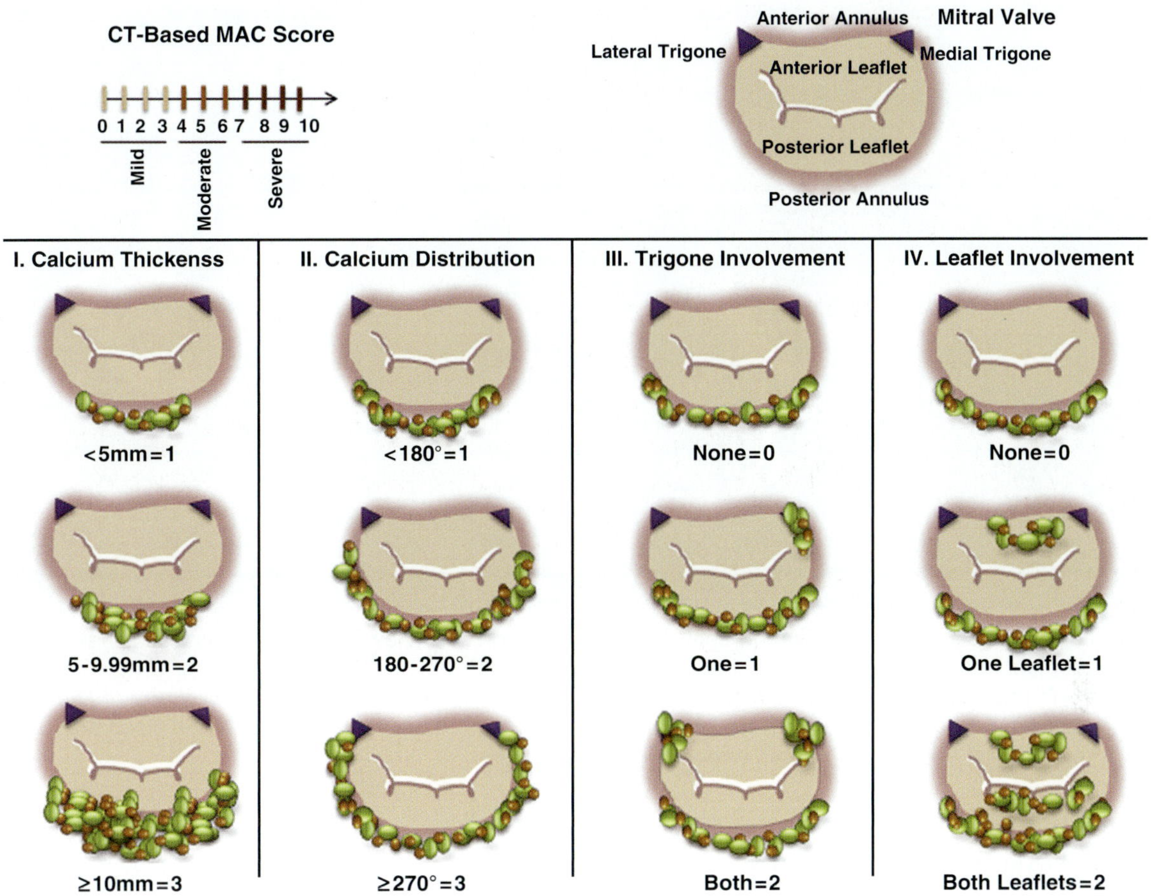

Fig. 9.6 *CT*-based mitral annular calcification *(MAC)* score varies from mild to severe and accounts for the thickness of the mitral annulus calcium, its distribution, involvement of the trigones and leaflets. *CT*, computed tomography; *MAC*, mitral annular calcification (From Guerrero M, Wang DD, Pursnani A, et al. A Cardiac computed tomography-based score to categorize mitral annular calcification severity and predict valve embolization. *JACC Cardiovasc Imaging*. 2020;13[9]:1945–1957.)

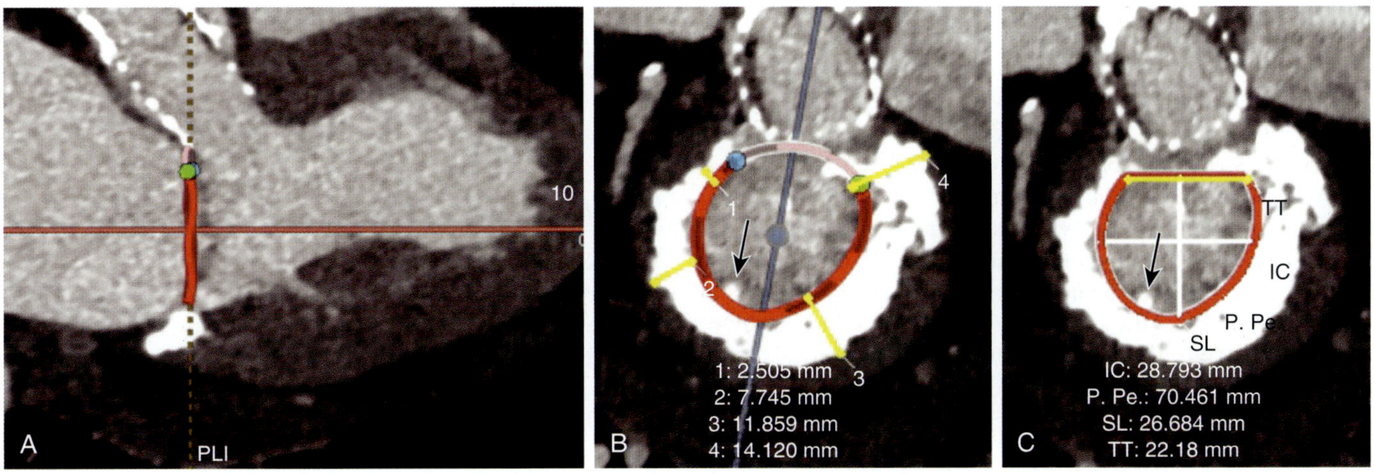

Fig. 9.7 Annular Segmentation in Mitral Annular Calcification Using D-Shaped Method. (A) Mitral annulus (B and C) Annular contouring was performed by excluding protruding spiculated calcium *(arrows)*. (B) Calcium thickness (>10 mm) is measured in short-axis view, calcification is distributed along nearly entire annular circumference and involves trigones; therefore, mitral annular calcification score according to classification system is equal to 8.

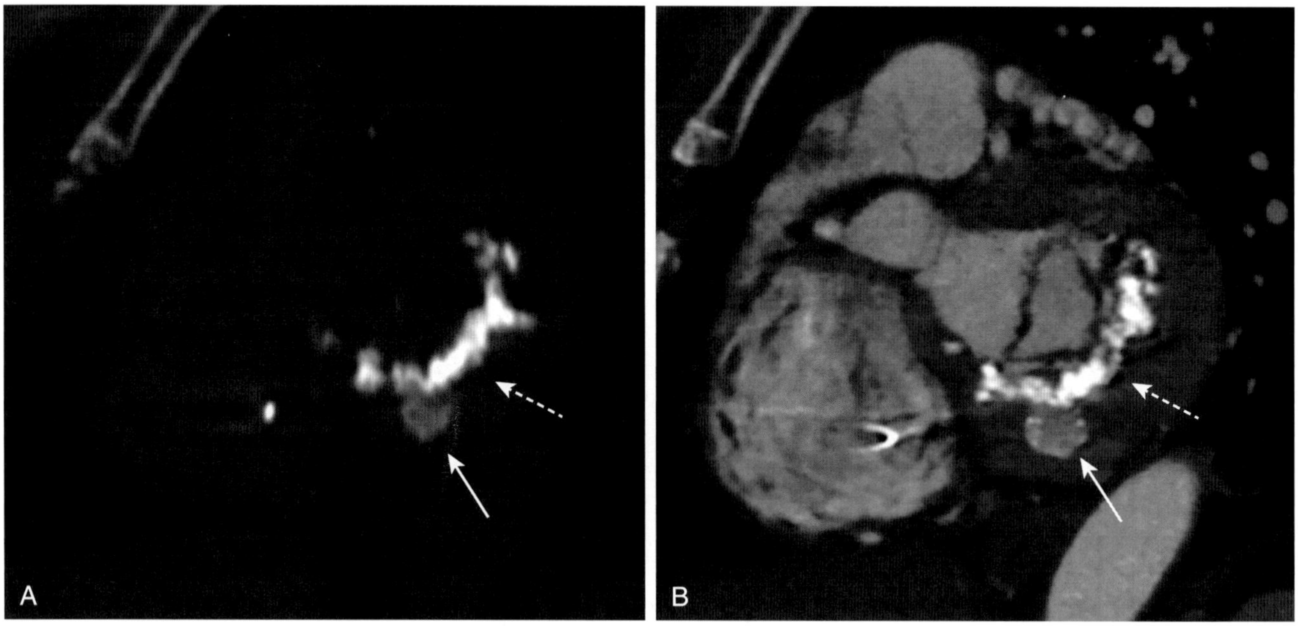

Fig. 9.8 Cardiac Computed Tomography Angiography Short-Axis View. (A) Non-contrast acquisition depicts nodular caseous mitral annular calcification (MAC) below P3 scallop *(solid arrow); note,* high attenuation of the solid MAC extends along posterior mitral annulus *(dashed arrow)* and involves lateral trigone. (B) the attenuation of caseous MAC is similar to the one of the blood pool on contrast-enhanced CT *(solid arrow).*

CT IN EVALUATION OF MITRAL VALVE PROLAPSE

MVP is defined as the systolic displacement of the mitral valve leaflets toward the left atrium of ≥2mm.[30,31] Echocardiography is considered the gold standard imaging modality for assessing the mitral valve and its pathology, including MVP.[32] In some instances, echocardiographic assessment of MVP is diminished. CT offers superior spatial resolution when assessing MVP, as well as simultaneous assessment of the coronary arteries.[33] Feuchtner et al. showed that the combined use of the 3ch and 2ch views allowed for the accurate (sensitivity 96% and specificity 93%) diagnosis of MVP at coronary CT angiography.[13] The best quality images for analyzing MVP are obtained during the phases 25% to 35% of the cardiac cycle.[33] Mitral annular disjunction is a structural abnormality of the MA fibrosus associated with mitral valve prolapse. It occurs under the posterior mitral valve (MV) leaflets, whereas disjunction is prevented anteriorly due to the adjacent fibrous trigones.[34] The resultant disjunction can be difficult to diagnose but ultimately causes atrial displacement of the annulus away from the LV at the level of the atrio–mitral valve junction.[35] It is a dynamic process that cannot be seen in diastole but instead in systole when the separation is at its largest (Fig. 9.10).

APEX LOCALIZATION

In peri-procedural planning, the use of multidetector cardiac CT further enhances the physician's knowledge of the planned procedure by accurately defining the ideal LV access point. In transapical (TA) TMVR systems, success of the procedure can be greatly improved by traversing the valve coaxially. The location of the LV access point orthogonal to the true MA plane varies among individuals and is most often not at the true apex but frequently localized at the anterolateral or anterior ventricular segments.[32] From the MA plane, an orthogonal line can be projected antero-apically beyond the epicardium on post-processing, identifying the ideal LV access point, commonly located laterally or anteriorly to the true apex (Fig 9.11). The proposed coaxial path can then be examined regarding its relationship to the skeletal chest wall (to plan the ideal intercostal space to enter the chest cavity, papillary muscles, or coronary arteries, and the true distance from the chest wall to the MA plane) (Fig 9.12).[5]

SEPTAL PUNCTURE

Many currently available transcatheter mitral valve repair systems are accessed via a transseptal puncture (TSP). The expanding use of CT to further define the anatomy of the interatrial septum is beneficial. During acquisition, a prolonged injection to ensure that there is adequate contrast opacification of the right heart to allow assessment of the interatrial septum if a transseptal approach is being considered.[2] CT can be used as a guiding tool to anticipate the puncture site, minimize complications such as aortic injury, and detect abnormalities of the septum such as a patent foramen ovale (PFO) or an aneurysmal septum, which can make the interventional procedure more challenging.[33]

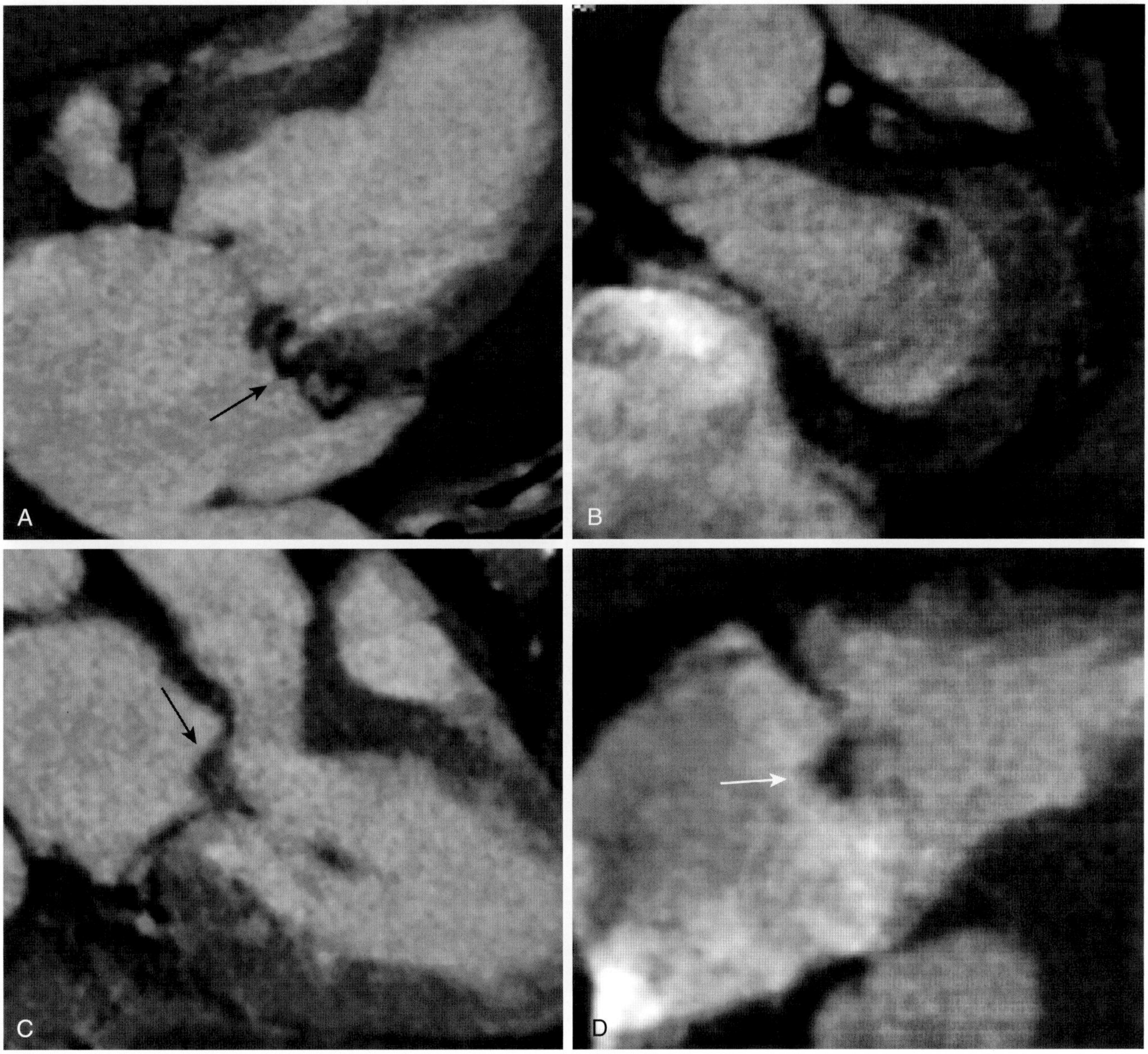

Fig. 9.9 Cardiac computed tomography angiography, end-systole: nodular thickening of anterior mitral valve leafler (AML) adjacent to A1-P1 scallops *(black arrow)* visualized on (A) 2 chamber, (B) short-axis, and (C) three chamber views. (D) Additional focal thickening of the anterior leaflet of the tricuspid valve in the context of methicillin-resistant *Staphylococcus aureus* (MRSA) bacteremia and infective endocarditis

FLUOROSCOPIC ANGLE PREDICTION

Similar to the application of multidetector computerized tomography (MDCT) in transcatheter aortic valve replacement (TAVR) planning, the MDCT can accurately predict fluoroscopic coplanar angles in advance to increase the chances of successful coaxial TMVR deployment. [34] During MDCT planning, this requires a detailed assessment of the MA plane and the alignment of the SL and IC lines to ensure coaxial deployment (Fig 9.13).[2] There are many TMVR systems in development, and they may require different coplanar angles for successful implantation; therefore, knowledge of the proposed valve is essential. Additionally, the use of centerline mapping, relevant to adjacent anatomy, such as the location of the coronary sinus and the left circumflex artery, can be defined either transmitted to the hybrid or can provide a roadmap during the procedure to define patient-specific risk.[2]

LEFT VENTRICULAR OUTFLOW TRACT OBSTRUCTION ASSESSMENT

Regarding TMVR therapies, currently, the most feared complication is LVOT obstruction. LVOT is the anatomic structure through which the left ventricular stroke volume exits into the aorta, which lies between the anterior leaflet of the mitral valve and the ventricular septum (Fig 9.14).[15] After implantation, the

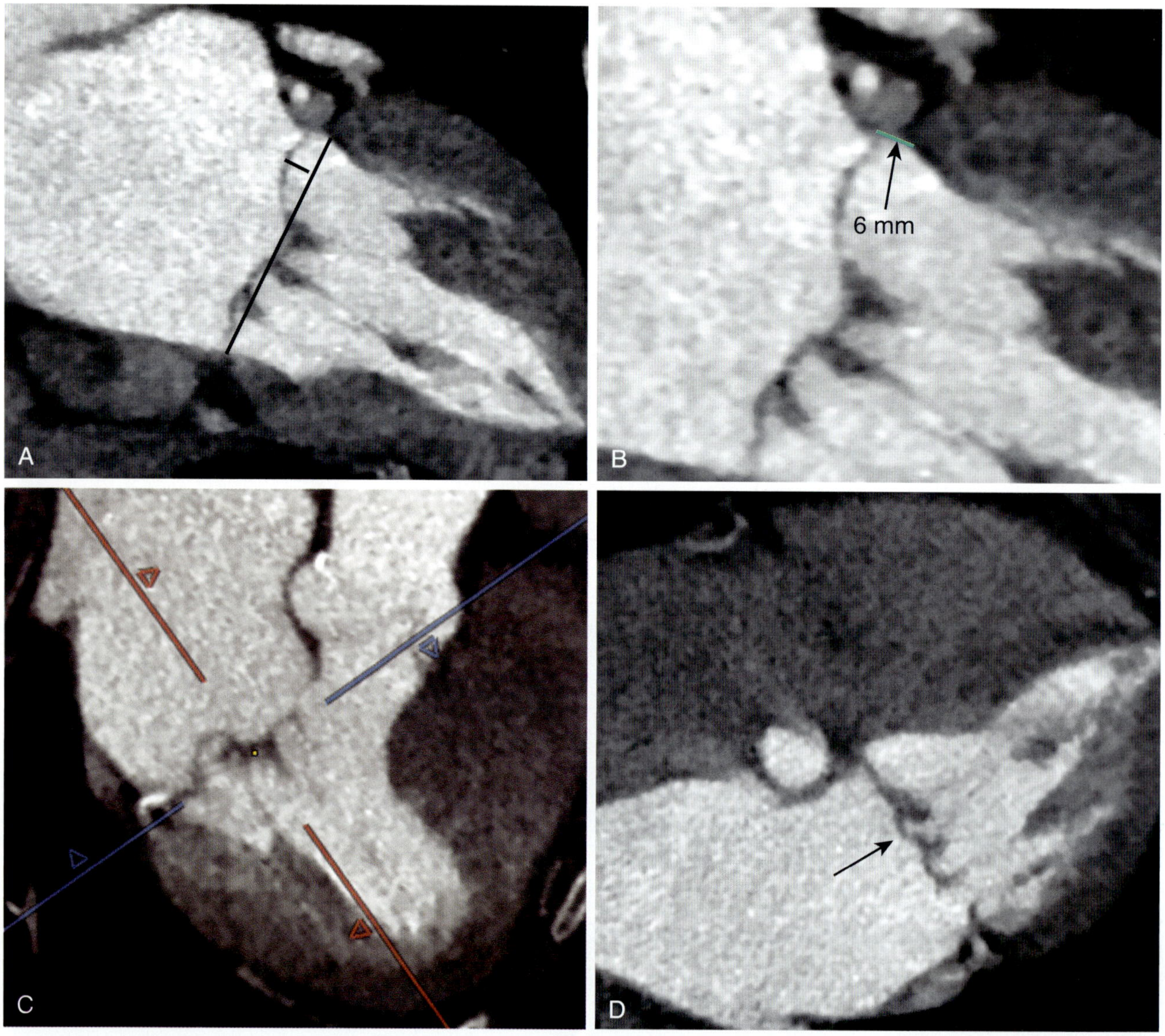

Fig 9.10 Cardiac computed tomography angiography in an 82-year-old male depicting bileaflet mitral valve prolapse at A2–P2 in (A) 2ch, (C) 3 ch, and (D) 4 ch views. (B) magnified inset from (A), arrow indicates mitral annular disjunction.

TMVR elongates the outflow tract into the LV; it pins the native AML open, displacing it toward the septum, thereby creating a "neo-LVOT."[15,35] Tracing a centerline through the middle of the residual space between the septum and the simulated implanted transcatheter heart valve (THV defines the neo-LOVT.[2] Advanced software can simulate a THV using a stereolithographic file in the mitral position by embedding a cylinder into the CT data set. Subsequent segmentation and planimetric assessment of the neo-LVOT cross-sectional area can now be performed at different periods of the cardiac cycle.[15] Risks of LVOT obstruction post TMVR are many, including the size and shape of the LV, septal hypertrophy, LVOT-mitral angle, anterior mitral leaflet size, and overall THV type/size and positioning (Fig 9.15).[35,36] In a recent study of patients undergoing TMVR due to failed mitral bioprosthetic valves (valve-in-valve), annuloplasty rings (valve-in-ring) and mitral annular calcification (valve-in-MAC) were demonstrated in the neo-LVOT area $\leq$1.7cm^2 predicted LVOT obstruction with a sensitivity of 96.2% and specificity of 92.3% with high mortality approaching 35%.[36] Recent evidence suggests that the thresholds may need to be procedure and device-specific. Analysis of the Intrepid feasibility experience suggested that for that device, early systole may yield more appropriate and predictive measurements of the post-implant neo-LVOT reflecting the A2–P2 constraint of the device. While a provocative analysis, it is important to recognize that these findings do not apply to a traditional aortic THV in MAC nor necessarily to other TMVR devices;[37] measurements taken throughout the cardiac cycle may offer a more comprehensive assessment of the risk of obstruction. Unsurprisingly, a neo-LVOT will measure smaller at end-systole; however, as the LV volume has been ejected, it may be of more use to measure the neo-LVOT at either early or midsystole.[1]

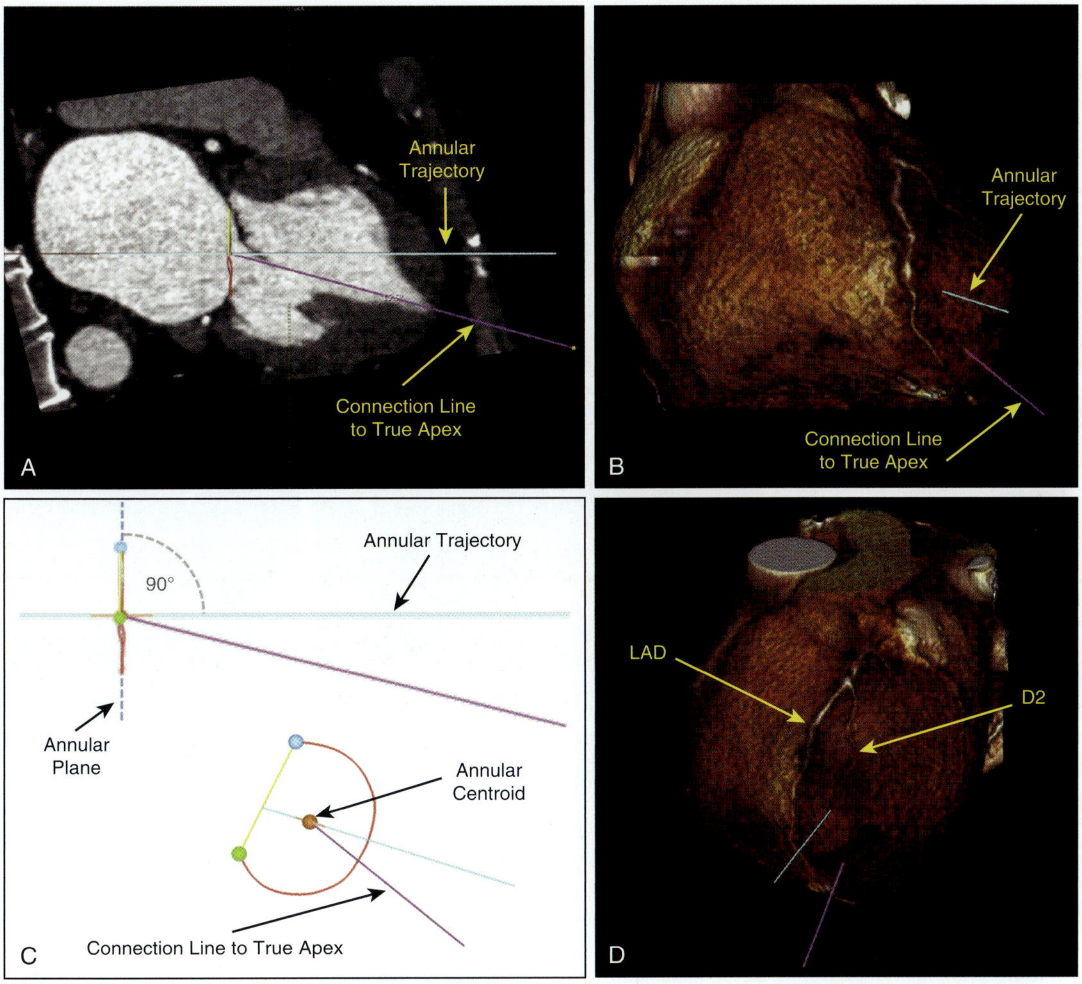

Fig 9.11 Trans apical Access. (A) The true annular trajectory *(light blue)* is perpendicular to the mitral annulus plane, offset from the line connecting the centroid to true left ventricle apex *(purple line)*. Volume rendered images to assess ideal access point, (A) long axis, (B) true anterior posterior (AP) orientation. (C) Schematic view. (D) Access point at left anterior oblique 45, CRA 25. (From Blanke P, Naoum C, Webb J, et al. Multimodality imaging in the context of transcatheter mitral valve replacement: establishing consensus among modalities and disciplines. *JACC Cardiovasc Imaging.* 2015;8[10]:1191–1208.)

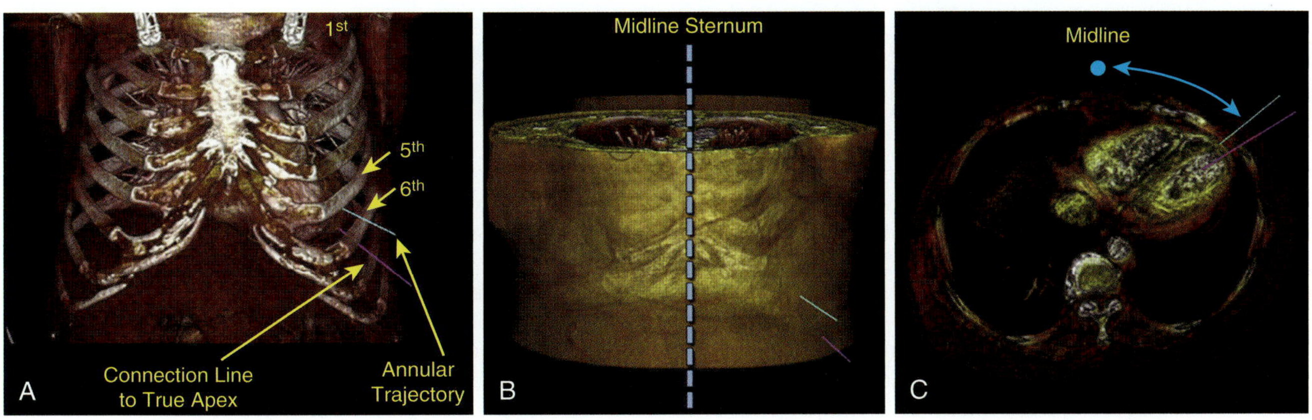

Fig 9.12 (A) The annular trajectory *(light blue)* and the line to the true left ventricle (LV) apex *(purple line)* are assessed in relation to the ribs, intercostal spaces, midline, and sternum. (B and C) Depict the relationship of the sternum to the midline and therefore the distance to the best spot for the line coaxial with the true LV apex. (From Blanke P, Naoum C, Webb J, et al. Multimodality imaging in the context of transcatheter mitral valve replacement: establishing consensus among modalities and disciplines. *JACC Cardiovasc Imaging.* 2015;8[10]:1191–1208.)

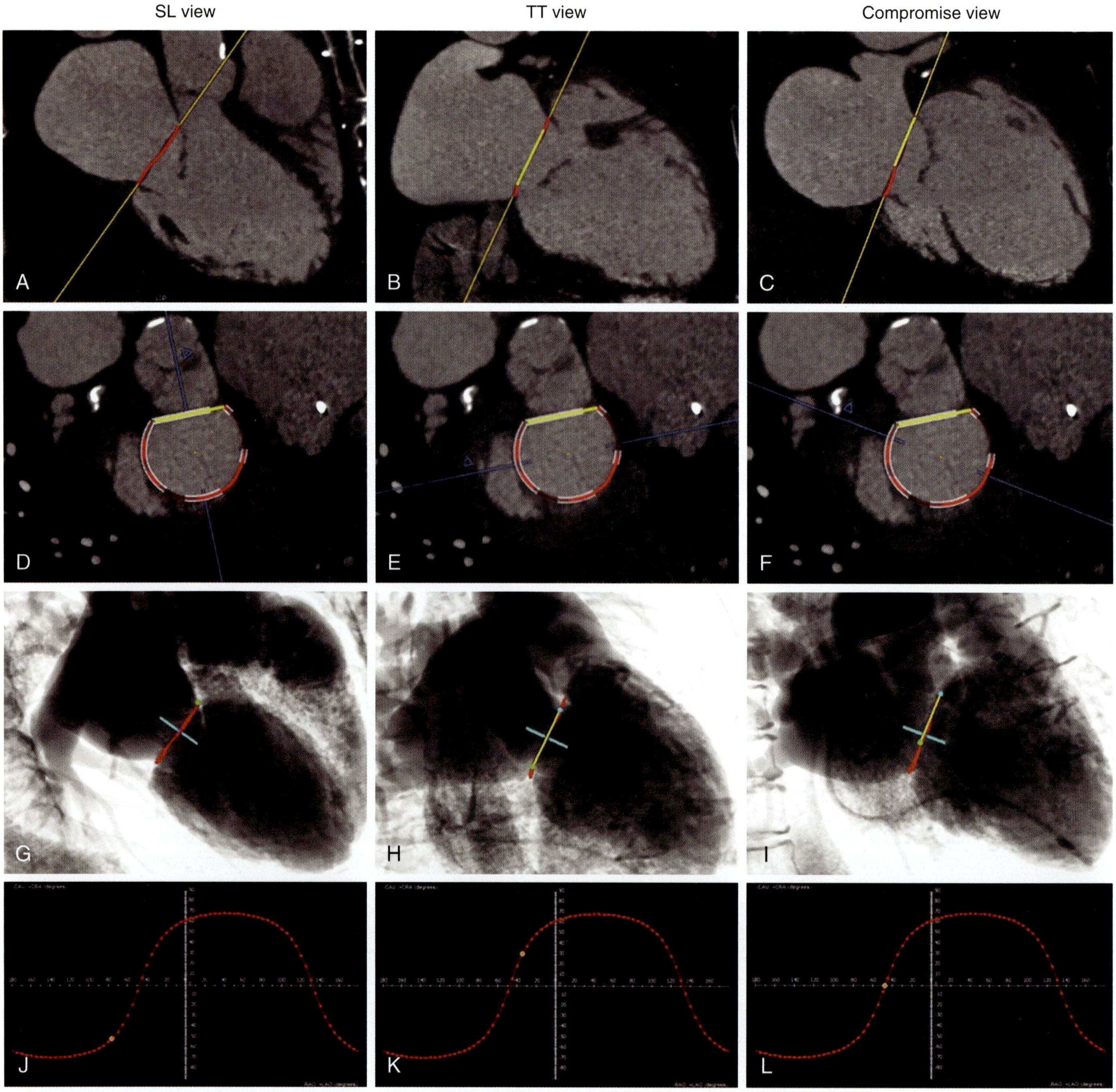

Fig. 9.13 Prediction of Fluoroscopic Angulation for Coplanar Deployment. (A–C) long-axis views of the MV obtained aligned to the septal-lateral line *(SL)*, trigone-to-trigone line *(TT)*, and the commonly used compromise view. (D–E) Annular views, with the blue line demonstrating how A–C views intersect the annulus, (G–I) images show how these views would appear on invasive angiogram based on the 3D CT data. (J and K) images demonstrate the sinusoidal path the c-arm would follow as it rotates around the patient to continuously provide a tangential valvular view, with the x-axis describing the LAO-RAO tilt required and the y-axis describing the CRA-CAU tilt required. The yellow dots demonstrate where each of the (A–C) views lie on this axis. *CRA,* Cranial; *CAU,* caudal; *LAO,* left anterior oblique; *RAO,* right anterior oblique. (From Weir-McCall JR, Blanke P, Naoum C, et al. Mitral valve imaging with ct: relationship with transcatheter mitral valve interventions. *Radiology*. 2018;288[3]:638–655.)

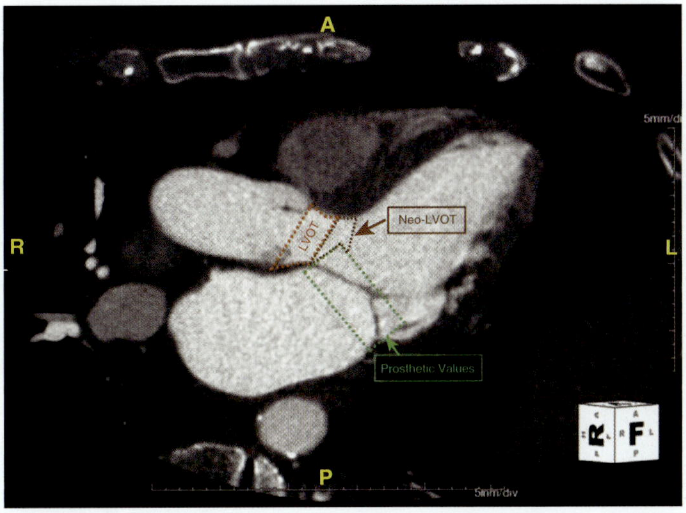

Fig 9.14 Computed Tomography Angiography 3-chamber View Defining the Anatomical Neo-LVOT. The left ventricular outflow tract (LVOT) is defined by the basal mid anteroseptal wall and the mitral intervalvular fibrosa *(orange dotted line)*. Following valve placement, the prosthetic valve protrudes into the basal left ventricular cavity *(green dotted line)* to produce the neo-LVOT *(red dotted line)*. (From Reid A, Ben Zekry S, Turaga M, et al. Neo-LVOT and transcatheter mitral valve replacement: expert recommendations. *JACC Cardiovasc Imaging.* 2021 Apr;14[4]:854–866.)

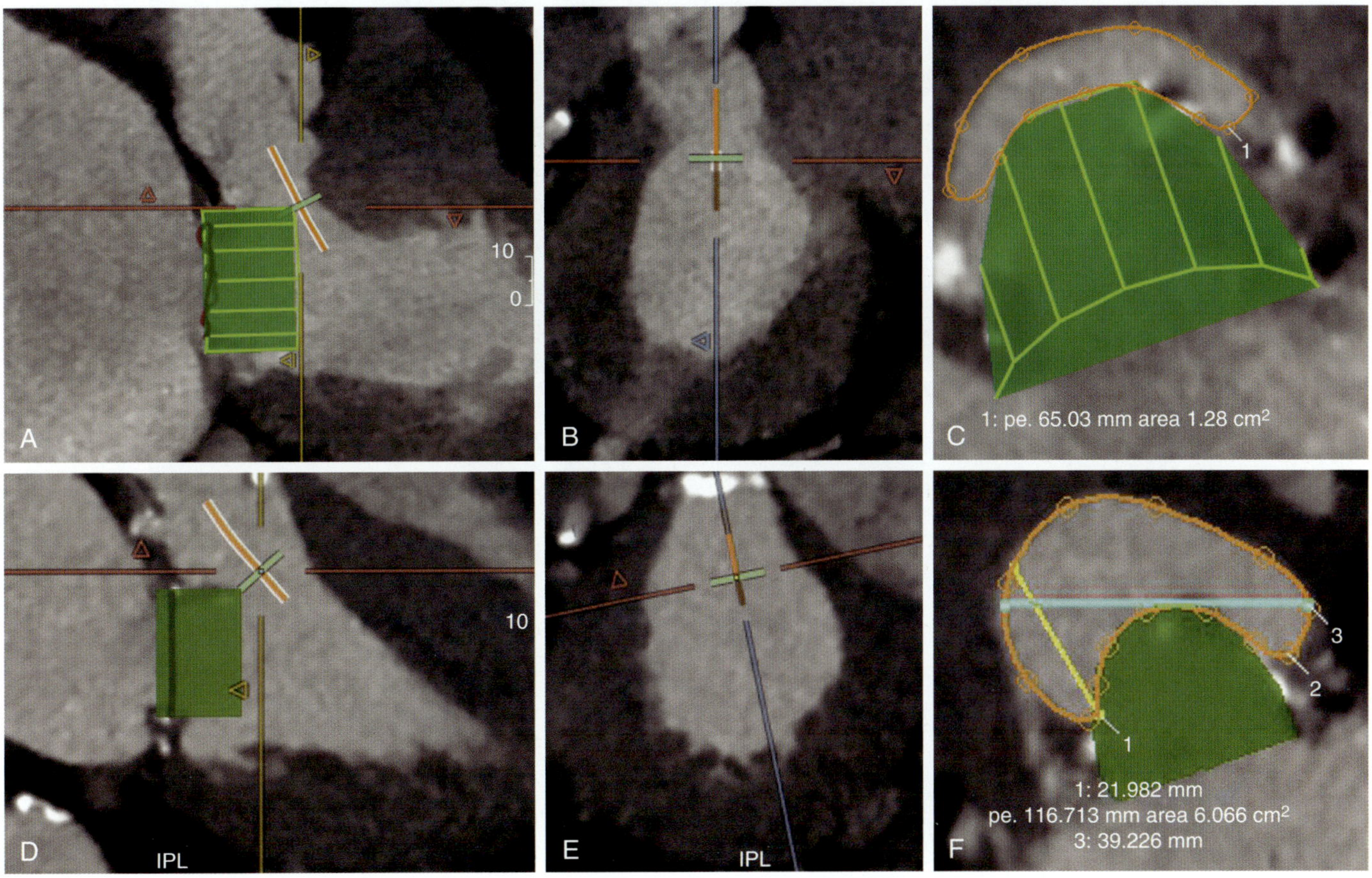

Fig 9.15 Neo-LVOT Assessment by Cardiac CT. (A and D) Segmentation of neo-left ventricular outflow tract (LVOT) using manually drawn centerline that follows LVOT trajectory. Neo-LVOT area is interrogated by using green slider. (B and E) Cross-sectional short-axis views. (C and F) The smallest Neo-LVOT areas *(curved orange dotted line)*. (C) Neo-LVOT area measured 1.3 cm^2 suggestive of high-risk LVOT obstruction. (D) Neo-LVOT area 6 cm^2, low risk of LVOT obstruction.

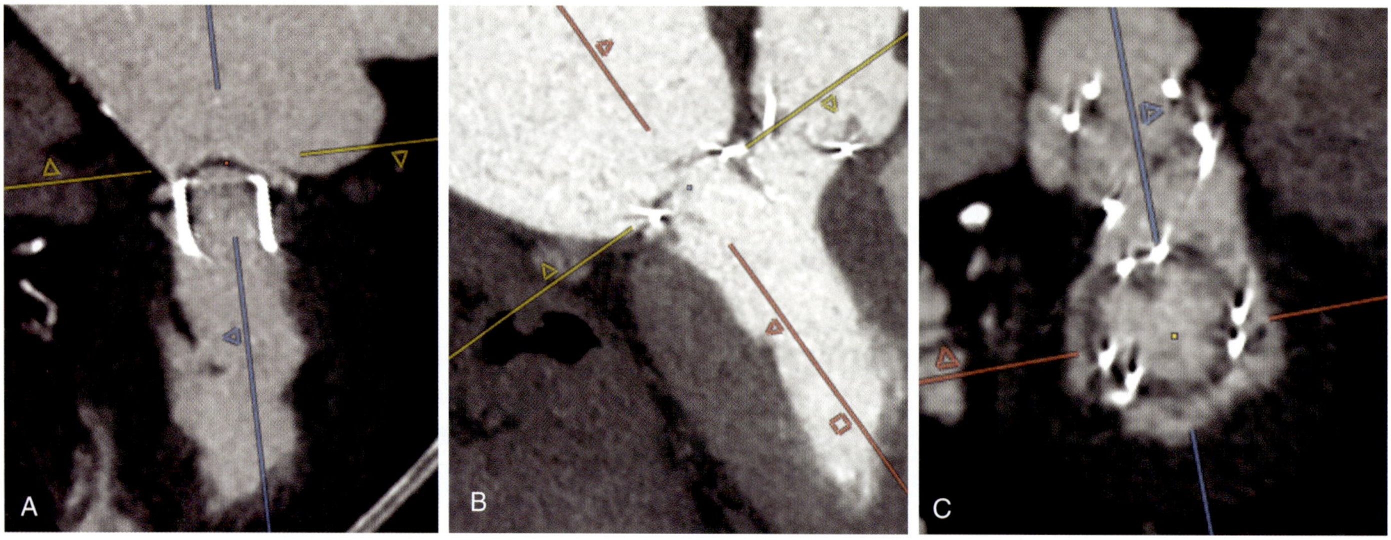

Fig. 9.16 Cardiac computed tomography angiography, systole for mitral valve-in-valve procedural planning. Left-to-right: 2-, 3-chamber, and short-axis views.

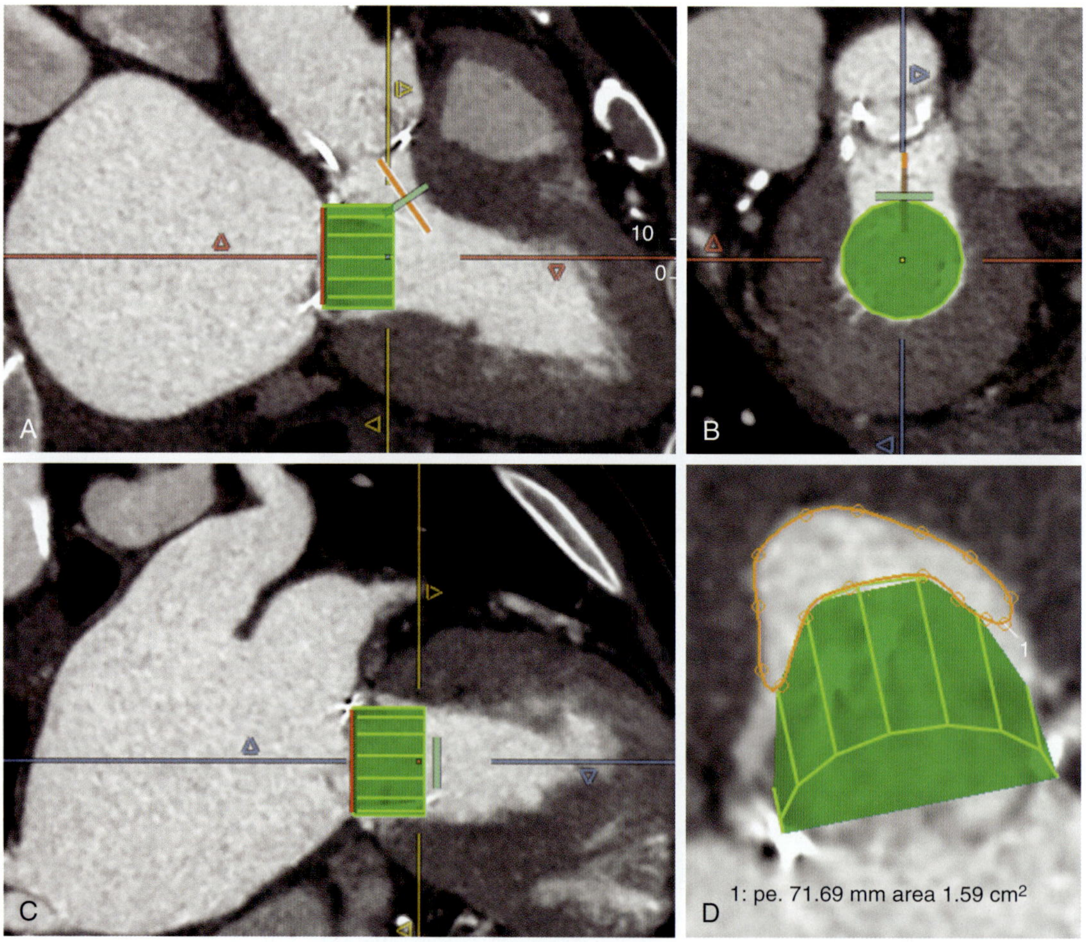

Fig. 9.17 Simulation of a 26 mm transcatheter mitral valve insertion using specialized software embedding a cylinder into the CT data set. The anticipated neo-LVOT (left ventricular outflow tract) area measures 1.6 cm^2 (end systole).

CASE-BASED ASSESSMENT

A 77-year-old man with severe MR and a history of AVR and MVR in China underwent IV contrast-enhanced ECG-gated cardiac CT with full cardiac cycle coverage for mitral valve-in-valve assessment.

1. Please evaluate Fig. 9.16 and identify the findings:
   A. Circumferential thickening along bioprosthetic mitral valve leaflet consistent with HALT
   B. Prolapse of the bioprosthetic mitral valve leaflet
   C. Vegetation of the bioprosthetic mitral valve leaflet
   D. B and C
   E. A and B
2. What is the risk of LVOT obstruction in this patient undergoing evaluation for TMVR (valve-in-valve procedure) with neo-LVOT area of 1.6 cm^2? (Fig. 9.17)
   A. High risk
   B. Low risk
   C. No risk
   D. Risk does not depend on area but is procedure and device-specific.

See page 316 for the answer.

REFERENCES

1. Naoum C, Blanke P, Cavalcante JL, Leipsic J. Cardiac computed tomography and magnetic resonance imaging in the evaluation of mitral and tricuspid valve disease: implications for transcatheter interventions. *Circ Cardiovasc Imaging*. 2017;10(3):e005331.
2. Weir-McCall JR, Blanke P, Naoum C, et al. Mitral valve imaging with CT: relationship with transcatheter mitral valve interventions. *Radiology*. 2018;288(3):638–655.
3. Ranganath P, Moore A, Guerrero M, et al. CT for Pre- and Post-procedural Evaluation of Transcatheter Mitral Valve Replacement. *Radiographics*. 2020;40(6):1528–1553.
4. Kim JH, Kim EY, Jin GY, Choi JB. A review of the use of cardiac computed tomography for evaluating the mitral valve before and after mitral valve repair. *Korean J Radiol*. 2017;18(5):773–785.
5. Blanke P, Naoum C, Webb J, et al. Multimodality imaging in the context of transcatheter mitral valve replacement: establishing consensus among modalities and disciplines. *JACC Cardiovasc Imaging*. 2015;8(10):1191–1208.
6. Abdelghani M, Spitzer E, Soliman II O, et al. A simplified and reproducible method to size the mitral annulus: implications for transcatheter mitral valve replacement. *Eur Heart J Cardiovasc Imaging*. 2017;18(6):697–706.
7. Flachskampf FA, Ropers D. Computed tomography to analyze mitral valve: an answer in search of a question. *JACC Cardiovasc Imaging*. 2009;2(5):566–568.
8. Carpentier AF, Lessana A, Relland JY, et al. The "physio-ring": an advanced concept in mitral valve annuloplasty. *Ann Thorac Surg*. 1995;60(5):1177–1185 discussion 1185–1176.
9. Blanke P, Dvir D, Cheung A, et al. A simplified D-shaped model of the mitral annulus to facilitate CT-based sizing before transcatheter mitral valve implantation. *J Cardiovasc Comput Tomogr*. 2014;8(6):459–467.
10. Ho SY. Anatomy of the mitral valve. *Heart*. 2002;88(suppl 4):iv5–10.
11. Rodriguez F, Langer F, Harrington KB, et al. Importance of mitral valve second-order chordae for left ventricular geometry, wall thickening mechanics, and global systolic function. *Circulation*. 2004;110(11 suppl 1):II115–122.
12. Lam JH, Ranganathan N, Wigle ED, Silver MD. Morphology of the human mitral valve. I. Chordae tendineae: a new classification. *Circulation*. 1970;41(3):449–458.
13. Feuchtner GM, Alkadhi H, Karlo C, et al. Cardiac CT angiography for the diagnosis of mitral valve prolapse: comparison with echocardiography1. *Radiology*. 2010;254(2):374–383.
14. Ewe SH, Klautz RJ, Schalij MJ, Delgado V. Role of computed tomography imaging for transcatheter valvular repair/insertion. *Int J Cardiovasc Imaging*. 2011;27(8):1179–1193.
15. Reid A, Ben Zekry S, Turaga M, et al. Neo-LVOT and Transcatheter mitral valve replacement: expert recommendations 14(4):854-866. Published online November 25, 2020. PMID: 33248959. *JACC Cardiovasc Imaging*. 2020; 14(4):854–866. doi:10.1016/j.jcmg.2020.09.027
16. Levack MM, Jassar AS, Shang EK, et al. Three-dimensional echocardiographic analysis of mitral annular dynamics: implication for annuloplasty selection. *Circulation*. 2012;126(11 suppl 1):S183–S188.
17. Flachskampf FA, Chandra S, Gaddipatti A, et al. Analysis of shape and motion of the mitral annulus in subjects with and without cardiomyopathy by echocardiographic 3-dimensional reconstruction. *J Am Soc Echocardiogr*. 2000;13(4):277–287.
18. Rizvi A, Marcus RP, Guo Y, et al. Dynamic computed tomographic assessment of the mitral annulus in patients with and without mitral prolapse. *J Cardiovasc Comput Tomogr*. 2020;14(6):502–509.
19. Clavel MA, Mantovani F, Malouf J, et al. Dynamic phenotypes of degenerative myxomatous mitral valve disease: quantitative 3-dimensional echocardiographic study. *Circ Cardiovasc Imaging*. 2015;8(5).
20. Kaplan SR, Bashein G, Sheehan FH, et al. Three-dimensional echocardiographic assessment of annular shape changes in the normal and regurgitant mitral valve. *Am Heart J*. 2000;139(3):378–387.
21. Pressman GS, Movva R, Topilsky Y, et al. Mitral annular dynamics in mitral annular calcification: a three-dimensional imaging study. *J Am Soc Echocardiogr*. 2015;28(7):786–794.
22. Alkadhi H, Desbiolles L, Stolzmann P, et al. Mitral annular shape, size, and motion in normals and in patients with cardiomyopathy: evaluation with computed tomography. *Invest Radiol*. 2009;44(4):218–225.
23. Asgar AW. Sizing the mitral annulus: is CT the future? *JACC Cardiovasc Imaging*. 2016;9(3):281–282.
24. Blanke P, Weir-McCall JR, Achenbach S, et al. Computed tomography imaging in the context of transcatheter aortic valve implantation (TAVI)/transcatheter aortic valve replacement (TAVR): an expert consensus document of the society of cardiovascular computed tomography. *JACC Cardiovasc Imaging*. 2019;12(1):1–24.
25. Eleid MF, Cabalka AK, Williams MR, et al. Percutaneous transvenous transseptal transcatheter valve implantation in failed bioprosthetic mitral valves, ring annuloplasty, and severe mitral annular calcification. *JACC Cardiovasc Interv*. 2016;9(11):1161–1174.
26. Guerrero M, Wang DD, Pursnani A, et al. A cardiac computed tomography-based score to categorize mitral annular calcification severity and predict valve embolization. *JACC Cardiovasc Imaging*. 2020;13(9):1945–1957.

27. Izgi C, Cevik C, Basbayraktar F. Caseous calcification and liquefaction of the mitral annulus: a diagnostic confounder. *Int J Cardiovasc Imaging*. 2006;22(3-4):543–545.
28. Kohsaka S, Jin Z, Rundek T, et al. Impact of mitral annular calcification on cardiovascular events in a multiethnic community: the Northern Manhattan Study. *JACC Cardiovasc Imaging*. 2008;1(5):617–623.
29. Feuchtner GM, Stolzmann P, Dichtl W, et al. Multislice computed tomography in infective endocarditis: comparison with transesophageal echocardiography and intraoperative findings. *J Am Coll Cardiol*. 2009;53(5):436–444.
30. Criley JM, Lewis KB, Humphries JO, et al. Prolapse of the mitral valve: clinical and cine-angiocardiographic findings. *Br Heart J*. 1966;28(4):488–496.
31. Freed LA, Benjamin EJ, Levy D, et al. Mitral valve prolapse in the general population: the benign nature of echocardiographic features in the Framingham Heart Study. *J Am Coll Cardiol*. 2002;40(7):1298–1304.
32. Blanke P, Park JK, Grayburn P, et al. Left ventricular access point determination for a coaxial approach to the mitral annular landing zone in transcatheter mitral valve replacement. *J Cardiovasc Comput Tomogr*. 2017;11(4):281–287.
33. Wunderlich NC, Beigel R, Siegel RJ. The role of echocardiography during mitral valve percutaneous interventions. *Cardiol Clin*. 2013;31(2):237–270.
34. Blanke P, Dvir D, Naoum C, et al. Prediction of fluoroscopic angulation and coronary sinus location by CT in the context of transcatheter mitral valve implantation. *J Cardiovasc Comput Tomogr*. 2015;9(3):183–192.
35. Blanke P, Naoum C, Dvir D, et al. Predicting LVOT Obstruction in Transcatheter Mitral Valve Implantation: Concept of the Neo-LVOT. *JACC Cardiovasc Imaging*. 2017;10(4):482–485.
36. Yoon SH, Bleiziffer S, Latib A, et al. Predictors of Left Ventricular Outflow Tract Obstruction After Transcatheter Mitral Valve Replacement. *JACC Cardiovasc Interv*. 2019;12(2):182–193.
37. Meduri CU, Reardon MJ, Lim DS, et al. Novel Multiphase Assessment for Predicting Left Ventricular Outflow Tract Obstruction Before Transcatheter Mitral Valve Replacement. *JACC Cardiovasc Interv*. 2019;12(23):2402–2412.

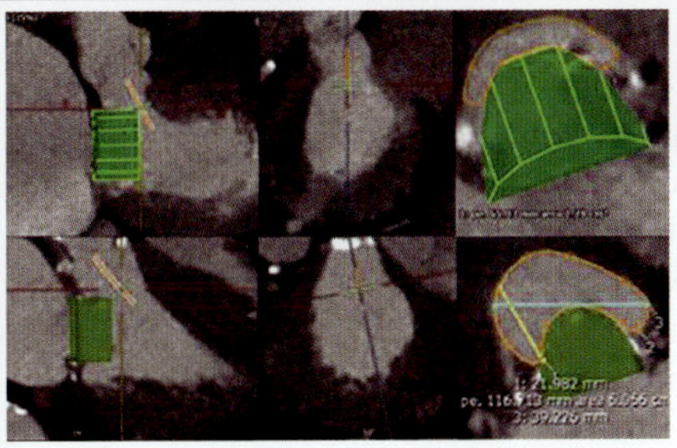

10

Cardiac Catheterization

Eric M. Gnall, Manju Bengaluru Jayanna

CHAPTER OUTLINE

LEARNING OBJECTIVES

1. Understand the role of cardiac catheterization and its limitation in estimation of stenotic valve area and assessment of severity of mitral regurgitation.
2. Know the critical technical procedural aspects of performing cardiac catheterization as it pertains to assessment of mitral valve disease.
3. The components of Gorlin formula, and their effects on transmitral gradient and application of the formula to assess mitral valve stenosis.
4. Role of cardiac catheterization in assessment of concomitant cardiovascular diseases in patients undergoing intervention for mitral valve disease.

TECHNICAL ASPECTS OF CARDIAC CATHETERIZATION

Assessment of hemodynamics and gradients in mitral valve disease often necessitates simultaneous measurement of intracardiac pressures. This is even more important in the presence of concomitant pathological conditions that affect left heart hemodynamics such as aortic valve disease, hypertrophic cardiomyopathy, and precapillary pulmonary hypertension. Choice of access is based on the roadmap for planned assessment in a particular patient. For venous access, internal jugular or brachial access is necessary if exercise hemodynamics are to be assessed. Transseptal access for direct measurement of left atrial pressure requires transfemoral venous access. Simultaneous aortic and left ventricular measurements could be performed with a dual lumen such as Langston Pigtail Catheter (Teleflex, Wayne, PA, USA) or simultaneous placement of pigtail catheters in aorta and left ventricle from two arterial access points. Smaller sized 4F and 5F diagnostic catheters reduce vascular complications, however larger diameter catheters should be used if hemodynamic tracings are of inadequate quality. Left ventricle pressures should be measured with catheters with side holes. Specifically, we recommend only using side-hole pigtail catheters for performing ventriculogram and left ventricular pressure measurements. All hemodynamic measurements should be performed prior to contrast administration. Fluid-filled catheters used to obtain hemodynamic tracings should not be of excessive length because the natural frequency falls below the physiologic range, causing an overamplification of signal, leading to falsely elevated hemodynamic readings. The opposite effect, damping, a loss of physiologic signal occurs most often due to air trapped in the circuit and rarely due to formation of small thrombi in smaller diameter systems. Mean pulmonary artery wedge pressure reflects mean left atrial pressure, however the severity may be overestimated due to delay in transmission of pressure contour through the pulmonary circulation resulting in a phase shift compared to left ventricular end-diastolic tracing.[1] Other potential causes such as under wedging could be corrected my checking oxygen saturation in wedge position.[2]

A transseptal puncture may be necessary on rare occasions when wedge tracings are inadequate or unreliable to guide therapeutic decisions. Intracardiac echocardiography (ICE) or transesophageal echocardiography (TEE) use enhances safety of transseptal approach. Use of ICE obviates the need for additional operators and general anesthesia during the procedure. The puncture should be performed using left anterior oblique (LAO) projections, and a Brockenbrough needle is passed through the fossa ovalis, until a jump across the septum into the left atrium is noticed and confirmed by change in the pressure waveform. The dilator and sheath are advanced over the needle. The dilator and needle are then withdrawn. We use an NRG RF transseptal needle (Baylis Medical, Montreal, Quebec, Canada) which uses radio frequency (RF) energy, delivered through a closed-tip device. The manufacturer recommends a single 10W pulse delivered over a period of 2 seconds. The main advantage is eliminating the need for mechanical pressure, and hence reducing excessive "jump" and possible complications of catheter exit. Other alternative approaches include the SafeSept transseptal device (Pressure Products, San Pedro, CA, USA), which uses J-shaped terminal nitinol wire with a sharpened end, and the TransLas catheter (LasCor GmbH, Taufkirchen, Germany), which uses laser energy.[3]

When performing left ventriculogram for assessing mitral regurgitation, large bore side-hole catheters should be used and it is necessary to use large enough contrast amount to completely opacify the cardiac chambers, to avoid underestimation of lesion severity. Contrast injection should be timed to avoid ventricular ectopy. The injection should be fast enough to quickly opacify the chambers but slow enough to avoid stimulating the ventricle causing ectopy. To avoid contrast being superimposed on a background of spine or descending aorta, high right anterior oblique views are often required.

HEMODYNAMICS

Estimation of Stenotic Valve Area

The Gorlin formula published in a seminal paper in 1951 by Dr. Richard Gorlin, a cardiologist, and his father S. G. Gorlin, ME, an engineer, is still utilized today in its modified form to estimate valve orifice area based on flow and pressure gradient across the valve.[4,5] It utilizes two basic principles of hydraulics. The first formula relates flow across a round orifice to velocity and area of the orifice as $F = AVC_c$, where F is the flow rate, A is the orifice area, V is velocity of flow, and C_c is the coefficient of orifice contraction. The second formula relates velocity across the orifice and pressure gradient across the orifice as $V^2 = (C_v)^2$ 2 gh, where V is velocity of flow; C_v is the coefficient of velocity, correcting for energy loss due to friction. Combining these two equations, the Gorlins developed the formula for estimating valve area by measurement of pressure gradient across the valve.

The Gorlin formula in its general form states $\boldsymbol{A = F/(C \times \sqrt{2gh})}$ where:

A = cross-sectional area in cm^2 of the orifice,
F = flow rate in cm^3 per second,
C = empirical constant,
g = gravity acceleration (980 cm/s^2), and
h = pressure gradient across the orifice in mm Hg.

The empirical constant C includes two components, $C = C_c \times C_v$. The coefficient of orifice contraction C_c accounts for the fact that fluids through an orifice tend to flow through its middle, hence the physiological orifice is smaller than the measured physical orifice. The velocity coefficient C_v accounts for the fact that some of the pressure gradient is not converted to flow and lost in the form of heat because of friction within the valve. Both these coefficients have never been determined. For the mitral valve, the Gorlins used an empirical constant of 0.7 and found the calculated and measured values to be within 0.2 cm^2 in six patients postmortem and in five patients at the time of surgery.[5] Initial transmitral valve gradients were based on hemodynamic measurements by right heart catheterization only, where the pulmonary capillary wedge pressure was assumed to reflect the left atrial pressure and left ventricular end-diastolic pressure was assumed to be 5 mm Hg. Subsequently, with the development of transseptal and retrograde arterial techniques, direct measurement of transmitral gradient was possible and the constant for the mitral position was revised to 0.85 in 1971.[4] Constants for the other valve positions have not been estimated and a perfect, practically impossible empirical value of 1 is still utilized.[1]

The antegrade flow across the mitral valve occurs only in diastole. The number of seconds in a minute during which there is diastolic flow is calculated by multiplying the diastolic filling period (DFP) (seconds per beat) by the heart rate (HR) (beats per minute) (Fig. 10.1A and B; Fig. 10.2). Then the diastolic flow in cm^3 per second is calculated by dividing the estimated or measured cardiac output (CO) (cm^3/min) by the seconds per minute during which there is diastolic flow. Thus, the Gorlins formula for mitral position for calculating the valve area A is

$$A = \frac{CO/(DFP \times HR)}{0.85 \times 44.3 \times \sqrt{h}}$$

Cardiac Output

Assessment of CO is integral to estimating valve area by Gorlin formula and an essential component of hemodynamic evaluation. CO is measured by the Fick principle or an indicator dilution technique. The reference method for measuring CO is utilizing the Fick principle in which CO is measured O_2 consumption divided by the difference between arterial and venous O_2. In practice, direct measurement of oxygen consumption is rarely, if ever performed, due to the cumbersome nature of the technique and expense. Rather, standard tables for an assumed value of oxygen consumption based on body surface area, with or without a correction for age and sex are used. Thermodilution based on an indicator dilution methodology is a more accurate measurement of CO. The method is unreliable when there is significant intracardiac shunt, low CO states, significant tricuspid regurgitation, or irregular rhythm.[1] This results in wide variations between calculated CO by different methodologies.[7]

The Gorlin formula provides insight into some aspects of the dynamic nature of transmitral gradient during rest and exercise in patients with mitral valvular stenosis. For example, doubling CO will lead to a four time increase in the gradient across the valve, if HR and DFP remain constant. Similarly, increases in HR and reduction in diastolic filling time lead to exponential increase in transmitral gradient. Hence, a patient with near normal transmitral gradient may experience significant symptoms during exercise due to increase in CO and HR with simultaneous reduction in diastolic filling time, all leading to exponential increase in left atrial pressure.

Understanding the assumptions and derivation of the Gorlin formula is important to appreciate its limitations. The formula is less accurate than color flow Doppler, valve area by planimetry, and tends to underestimate the valve area, especially in low flow

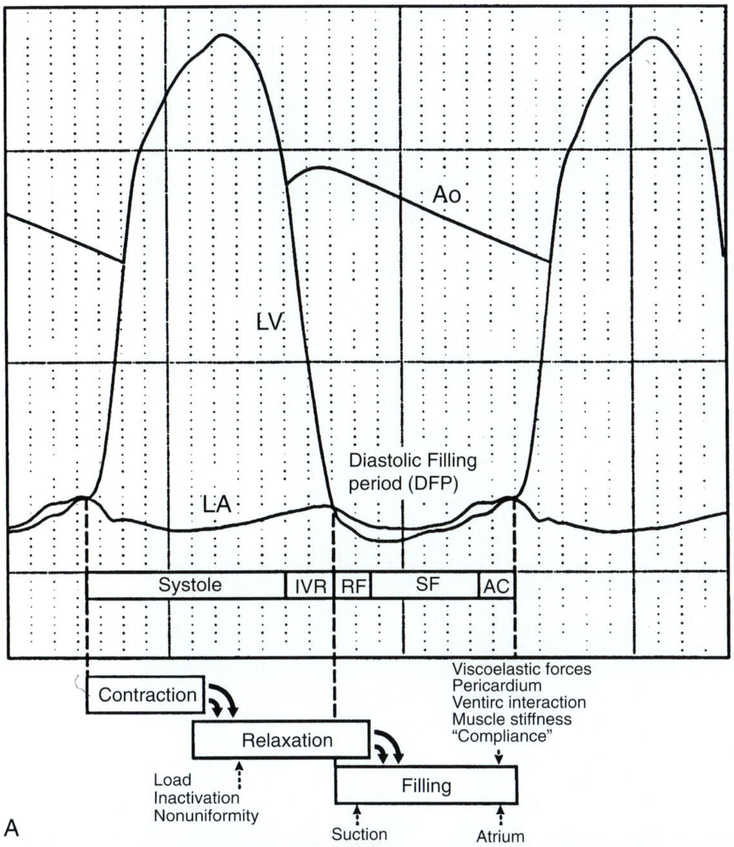

Fig. 10.1 (A) Measurement of diastolic filling period. The high-fidelity left ventricular *(LV)* and left atrial *(LA)* pressures are shown with a schematic representation of ascending aortic pressure *(Ao)*. In the classic system, the cardiac cycle is divided into systole and four phases of diastole: isovolumetric relaxation *(IVR)*, rapid filling *(RF)*, slow filling *(SF)*, and atrial contraction *(AC)*. In a more practical and simplified system, the cardiac cycle is divided into contraction, relaxation, and diastolic filling. The diastolic filling period begins at mitral valve opening and continues until end-diastole, hence includes RF, SF, and AC. (Modified from Nishimura RA, Tajik AJ. Evaluation of diastolic filling of left ventricle in health and disease: Doppler echocardiography is the clinician's Rosetta Stone. *J Am Coll Cardiol*. 1997;30[1]:8–18.)[6] (B) Hemodynamic assessment in a patient with mitral stenosis showing simultaneous LV and Ao tracing. Diastolic filling period begins with the opening of the mitral valve and ends with the closure of the mitral valve.
EDP, End diastolic pressure.

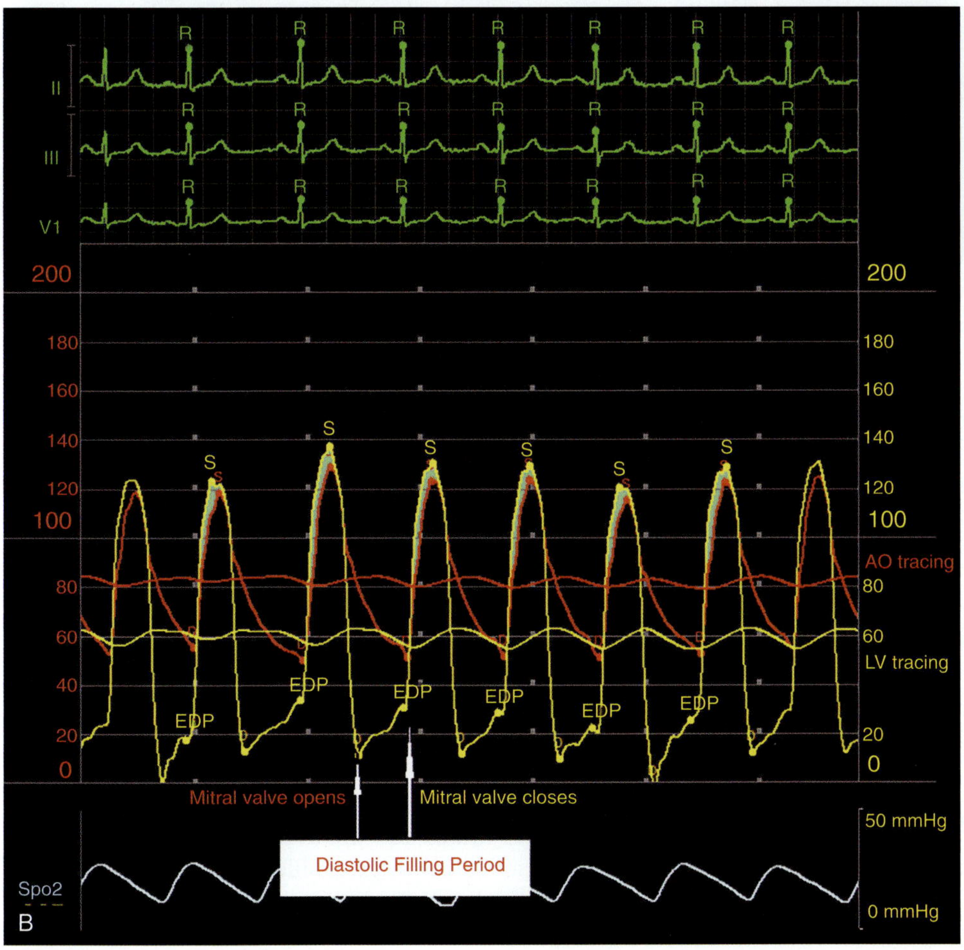

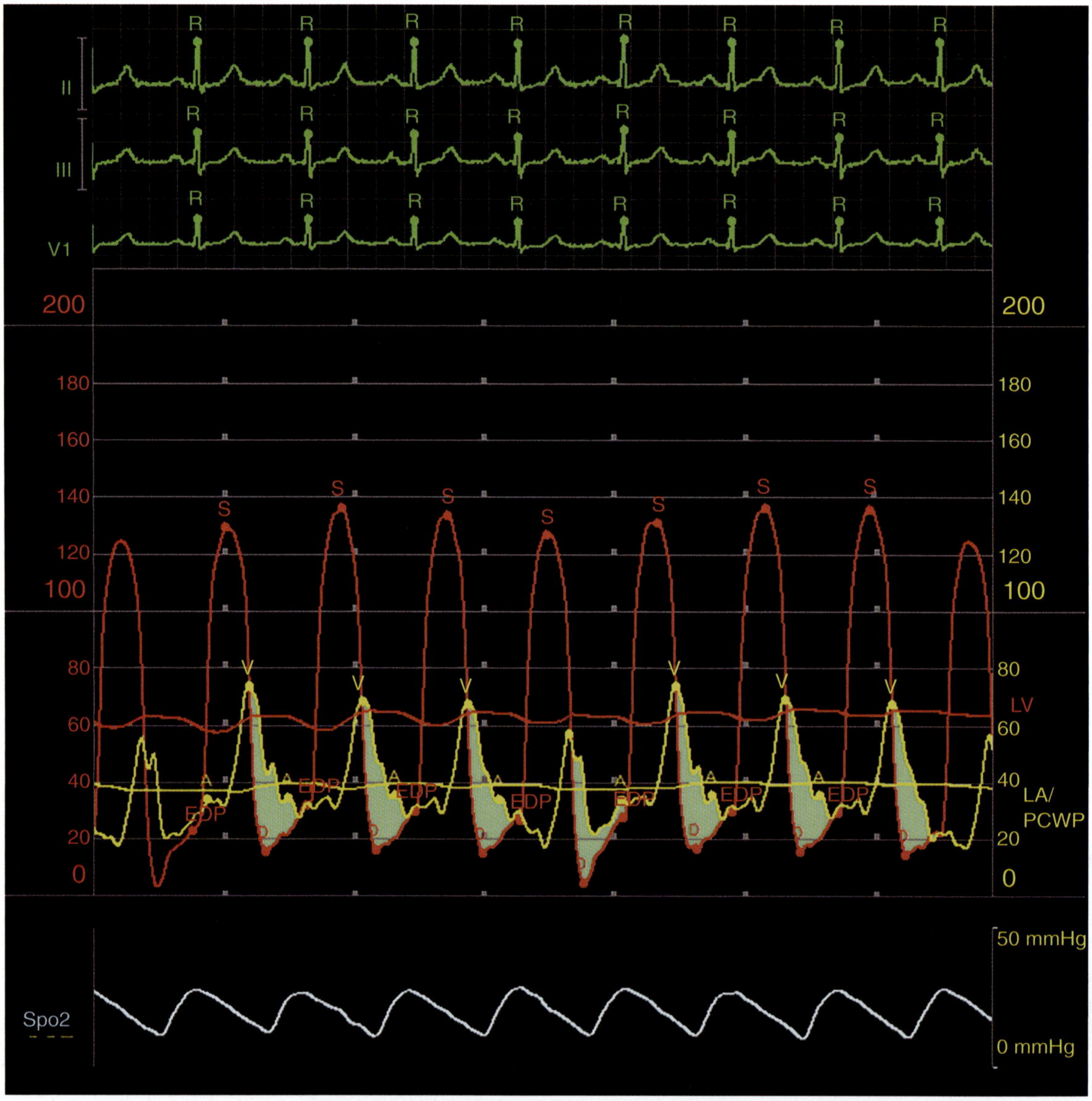

Fig. 10.2 Assessment of transmitral gradient in a patient with mitral stenosis. Pulmonary capillary wedge pressure and LV mean gradient were assessed. Mean gradient, 15 mm Hg. *LA*, Left atrial; *LV*, left ventricular; *PCWP*, Pulmonary capillary wedge pressure.

states.[8] This is likely because the value of the empirical constant does not hold true across the range of CO. Hence, valve area measurements have largely been supplanted by other modalities discussed in other chapters in this book. However, the guidelines continue to recommend hemodynamic assessment in symptomatic patients when noninvasive tests are inconclusive or when there is a discrepancy between the findings on noninvasive testing and physical examination regarding severity of the valve lesion. This is less of a concern in mitral valvular heart disease since Doppler beam is easily directed parallel to the valvular jet velocities in apical windows (Chapters 5 and 6).[9]

Other Aspects of Hemodynamic Assessment in Mitral Disease

Assessment of pulmonary vascular hypertension is an important component of hemodynamic assessment. Cardiac catheterization is the reference standard for diagnosis of pulmonary hypertension. Cause of elevated pulmonary arterial pressures (PAP) must be delineated as secondary to left-sided filling pressures (post capillary pulmonary hypertension), secondary to intrinsic pulmonary vascular disease (precapillary pulmonary hypertension), or a combination of both. In presence of elevated left heart fillings pressures, diastolic pressure gradient ≥7 mm Hg indicates presence of concomitant intrinsic pulmonary vascular disease. Diastolic pressure gradient is defined as diastolic PAP minus mean pulmonary capillary wedge pressure.

Furthermore, 2014 ACC/AHA guideline for management of valvular heart disease recommends additional diagnostic interventions as indicated—dobutamine for low flow states, pulmonary vasodilators in precapillary pulmonary hypertension, and exercise hemodynamics in patients with ambiguous symptoms.[9]

TABLE 10.1 Seller Criteria for Semiquantitative Assessment of Mitral Regurgitation

Grade	Angiographic Assessment	Regurgitant Fraction Estimate
1+ Mild	Regurgitation that clears with each beat and never opacifies the entire left atrium.	<20%
2+ Moderate	Regurgitation that does not clear with one beat and generally does opacify the entire left atrium, but faintly, with several beats.	20%–40%
3+ Moderately severe	Regurgitation in which the left atrium is completely opacified and achieves equal opacification with the left ventricle but requires more than one beat.	40%–60%
4+ Severe	Regurgitation that results in opacification of the entire left atrium within one beat.	>60%

Assessment of Mitral Regurgitation

Echocardiography and magnetic resonance imaging have largely supplanted routine use of left ventricular angiography for assessing severity of mitral regurgitation. However, there are instances when assessment of severity by echocardiography may be technically challenging, incomplete, and there is discrepancy between the patient's symptoms and findings on noninvasive assessment. A semi-quantitative assessment based on degree of opacification of the left atrium with left ventricular angiography may be utilized (Table 10.1). As expected, the assessment is subject to interobserver variability and lack of standardization of technique for performing and interpretation.

A more quantitative but cumbersome process used to estimate regurgitant stroke volume is by calculation of total ventricular stroke volume from left ventriculogram and subtracting forward stroke volume (calculated by Fick or thermodilution methods). Regurgitant fraction is then calculated by dividing regurgitant stroke volume by total stroke volume. As one can surmise, although theoretically a more accurate measurement, each of these steps has a number of assumptions, is cumbersome, and the final estimate is likely to be unreliable. Hence, this is rarely used in modern day practice. A more reliable measurement of quantification of regurgitant volume using magnetic resonance imaging has been described elsewhere (Chapter 8).

Coronary Angiography

Coronary angiography is indicated prior to any major cardiac surgery including mitral valve surgery in patients who are at risk for coronary artery disease (CAD). In addition, it helps evaluate ischemic heart disease as a possible etiology of mitral regurgitation. It is reasonable to perform computed tomography (CT) coronary angiogram as the first initial step instead to evaluate for presence of obstructive CAD in patients who are considered to be low-risk for CAD. A follow-up invasive angiogram may be performed if CT angiogram shows evidence of CAD and viable myocardium by noninvasive testing to better define anatomy and possible revascularization (Chapter 9).[9] Even in young patients who are at low risk for CAD, the risks of proceeding with major cardiac surgery without defining coronary anatomy, potentially increasing surgical time, needs to be balanced against the extremely low risk of a diagnostic coronary angiogram.

ASSESSMENT QUESTIONS

1. What is the gold standard for assessing pulmonary arterial pressures in patients with mitral valve disease?
   A. Right ventricular outflow tract Doppler profile and peak velocity
   B. Cardiac MRI regression model that includes right ventricle dimension measurements and the extent of black blood slow flow
   C. Right heart catheterization
   D. Computed tomography angiography
2. The safest method to perform left ventriculogram to assess mitral regurgitation is using
   A. End hole catheter
   B. Any side-hole catheter such as a Tiger catheter
   C. Pigtail catheter
   D. Multipurpose guide catheter
3. Applying the Gorlin formula, transmitral gradient across a stenotic valve,
   A. Increases linearly with increase in HR
   B. Increases in proportion to the inverse of square root of the HR
   C. Increases exponentially with both increases in HR and CO
   D. Does not change and is constant across a wide range of CO and is minimally affected by HR

See page 316 for the answers.

REFERENCES

1. Nishimura RA, Carabello BA. Hemodynamics in the cardiac catheterization laboratory of the 21st century. *Circulation.* 2012;125(17):2138–2150.
2. Lange RA, Moore JR DM, Cigarroa RG, Hillis LD. Use of pulmonary capillary wedge pressure to assess severity of mitral stenosis: is true left atrial pressure needed in this condition? *J Am Coll Cardiol.* 1989;13(4):825–831.
3. O'Brien B, Zafar H, De Freitas S, et al. Transseptal puncture—review of anatomy, techniques, complications and challenges. *Int J Cardiol.* 2017;233:12–22.
4. Cohen MV, Gorlin R. Modified orifice equation for the calculation of mitral valve area. *Am Heart J.* 1972;84(6):839–840.
5. Gorlin R, Gorlin SG. Hydraulic formula for calculation of the area of the stenotic mitral valve, other cardiac valves, and central circulatory shunts. I. *Am Heart J.* 1951;41(1):1–29.

6. Nishimura RA, Tajik AJ. Evaluation of diastolic filling of left ventricle in health and disease: Doppler echocardiography is the clinician's Rosetta Stone. *J Am Coll Cardiol.* 1997;30(1):8–18.
7. Hillis LD, Firth BG, Winniford MD. Analysis of factors affecting the variability of Fick versus indicator dilution measurements of cardiac output. *Am J Cardiol.* 1985;56(12):764–768.
8. Segal J, Lerner DJ, Miller DC, et al. When should Doppler-determined valve area be better than the Gorlin formula?: Variation in hydraulic constants in low flow states. *J Am Coll Cardiol.* 1987;9(6):1294–1305.
9. Nishimura RA, Otto CM, Bonow RO, et al. 2014 AHA/ACC Guideline for the Management of Patients With Valvular Heart Disease: executive summary: a report of the American College of Cardiology/American Heart Association Task Force on Practice Guidelines. *Circulation.* 2014;129(23):2440–2492.

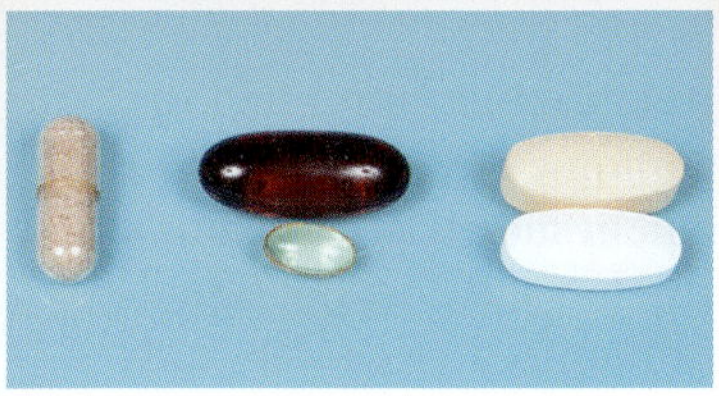

11 Diuretics and Neurohormonal Medications

Benjamin I. Horn, Steven M. Domsky

CHAPTER OUTLINE

LEARNING OBJECTIVES

1. Understand the benefits of medical treatment in mitral stenosis and regurgitation.
2. Know which medications are indicated and their function in management of mitral stenosis and regurgitation.
3. Gain insight into the preoperative management in patients with severe mitral stenosis and regurgitation.

INTRODUCTION

In this chapter we review the medical management for mitral stenosis and mitral regurgitation. We go over the pathophysiology of the disease process to understand which medications may be most useful. We will review the medications that are helpful for use in both valve diseases and indications for initiation. The main medications we will discuss are β-blockers, angiotensin-converting enzyme inhibitors (ACEIs) and angiotensin II receptor blockers, nitrates and other after load reducers, as well as diuretics. We will review the preoperative treatment course for patients and medications that can be used to delay surgery or stabilize patients preoperatively. We hope this will be a valuable resource for understanding how to medically manage patients who have severe mitral valve disease.

MITRAL STENOSIS

Narrowing of the mitral valve impairs left atrial emptying which causes increased left atrial volume and pressure. This relationship between flow and pressure is quite profound when we consider that the pressure gradient for a given flow rate is a function of the square of the transvalvular flow rate. A doubling of flow rate would quadruple the pressure gradient. A 50% increase in flow would result in a 125% increase in pressure gradient. This causes increased back pressure into the pulmonary veins and ultimately pulmonary congestion. Given the relationship between heart rate and flow to the mitral valve gradient, reversible causes of increased heart rate and flow should be considered and treated if appropriate such as anemia, arrythmias, hyperthyroidism, or infection.

While medical therapy cannot relieve or alter the obstruction, it can help with decongestion to relieve symptoms. Narrowing of the mitral valve decreases left ventricular filling resulting in reduced cardiac output despite preserved left ventricular function. This increased back pressure causes elevation in pulmonary artery pressures which over time can be worsened by pulmonary artery vasoconstriction and changes of pulmonary artery hypertension that further elevate pulmonary pressures even out of proportion to left atrial pressure and results in right ventricular dysfunction.

Although pulmonary vasodilators address the pulmonary vasoconstriction and right ventricular dysfunction, increased flow to the left heart in advanced mitral stenosis can increase left atrial pressure and precipitate pulmonary edema. Thus, pulmonary vasodilators are contraindicated in the setting of significant mitral stenosis. Fortunately, pulmonary hypertension appears to improve over time at least partially after mechanical correction of mitral stenosis, with one study of 60 patients undergoing balloon valvuloplasty or surgical commissurotomy having an average decrease for pulmonary artery systolic pressure of 55 mm Hg preoperatively to 32 mm Hg 3-years postoperatively.[1] Additionally, in contrast to mitral regurgitation, left ventricular (LV) filling is impaired, thus there is no role for afterload reduction as this can precipitate hypotension in an already underfilled ventricle.

Diuretics

Diuretics can help relieve symptoms when pulmonary congestion occurs from increased left atrial pressure. Salt and fluid restriction are advisable as well. In more advanced and severe mitral stenosis, pulmonary hypertension and right ventricular overload can also occur which may respond to diuretics as well. However, it is notable that a retrospective propensity matched study of 494 rheumatic heart disease patients did find patients with chronic diuretic use (versus intermittent diuretic use) was associated with increased risks of all-cause mortality (adjusted hazard ratio [HR] = 2.47, 95% confidence interval (CI): 1.54 to 3.97, $P < .001$) and cardiovascular death (adjusted HR = 3.67, 95% CI: 1.95 to 6.89, $P < .001$).[2] This is a notable association but in a retrospective propensity match study does not prove causation.

β-Blockers and Nondihydropyridine Calcium Channel Blockers

Left ventricular filling occurs in diastole and is impaired in mitral stenosis. While time in systole is relatively fixed, diastolic filling time is variable based on heart rate. Thus, by slowing the heart rate and increasing diastolic filling time, left ventricular filling is improved. Also, by slowing diastolic filling time the gradient across the mitral valve is decreased and left atrial pressure is lowered. β-blockers and nondihydropyridine calcium channel blockers help by slowing heart rate and therefore increasing diastolic filling time and lowering flow rate. This results in reducing the transmitral gradient and secondarily reducing pulmonary congestion and pulmonary hypertension.[3] β-blockers and nondihydropyridine calcium channel blockers can also blunt the increase in heart rate associated with exertion and thus may have a role in reducing exertional symptoms.

Ivabradine

Although β-blockers are the standard of care in mitral stenosis, they are not always well tolerated. Ivabradine slows the heart rate by regulating the funny channel current in sinoatrial cells, thus it is only effective for patients in sinus rhythm and does not significantly lower blood pressure. In a randomized crossover study of 33 patients with mild-moderate mitral stenosis, they found ivabradine and metoprolol to be equally efficacious in reducing symptoms and improving hemodynamics compared with baseline. Mean gradient decreased 42% and 37%, respectively. Pulmonary artery systolic pressure was reduced by 23% and 27%, respectively. Exercise duration increased from 7.9 minutes at baseline to 10.6 and 10.3 minutes, respectively.[4] A recent meta-analysis of five randomized trials of ivabradine versus β-blockers in mitral stenosis concluded ivabradine was comparable to β-blockers in relevant endpoints. They concluded ivabradine was better compared to β-blockers in total exercise duration (mean difference: 32.73 s [95% CI: 12.19, 53.27]; $P = .002$), maximum HR achieved after exercise (mean difference: −3.87 beats/min (95% CI: −5.88, −1.860; $P = .0002$), and work capacity (mean difference: 0.56 metabolic equivalents [METs] (95% CI: 0.33, 0.80; $P < .00001$); inferior to β-blockers in resting HR achieved (mean difference: 1.83 s (95% CI: 0.39, 3.28; $P = .01$); and comparable to β-blockers in terms of mean gradient (mean difference: −0.52 mm Hg (95% CI: −1.20, 0.16; $P = .13$).[5]

Digoxin

With a narrow therapeutic window of efficacy and potential of toxicity, digoxin is not a first-line therapy but may have a role for heart rate lowering when blood pressure does not allow other heart rate lowering medications, especially in the presence of atrial fibrillation or atrial flutter which are common with mitral stenosis.

ACUTE MITRAL REGURGITATION

In acute mitral regurgitation, the left atrium has not had time to compensate with dilation or increasing pressure like in chronic mitral regurgitation. The sudden increase in left atrial pressures can lead to rapid pulmonary congestion causing shortness of breath. Additionally, the usual volume of left ventricular loading is increased with the addition of regurgitated blood into the left atrium resulting in left ventricular volume overload. Because the unprepared left ventricle has not yet dilated to compensate with a substantial percentage of blood volume going backward into the atrium, stroke volume drops acutely (i.e., if a 100 mL ventricle has an ejection fraction of 60%, stroke volume is 60 mL if no regurgitation and 30 mL if half is regurgitated into the left atrium).

Without leaflet coaptation, blood flows directly back into the left atrium at the beginning of systole meaning there is no isovolumetric contraction. There is also no isovolumetric relaxation as blood continues to flow into the left atrium even after the aortic valve closes. Because the left atrium has increased pressure from the additional flow this causes a rise in left ventricular end-diastolic pressure. The left ventricle maintains its ejection fraction by using its preload reserve, but there may be a decrease in forward stroke volume.[6]

In patients where the acute mitral regurgitation is due to ischemia or infarct the most important treatment is restoring blood flow to the affected territory.[7] As in the setting of acute mitral regurgitation with developing or worsening cardiomyopathy, the treatment of the underlying heart failure is crucial to improve the mitral regurgitation. While acute mitral regurgitation due to papillary muscle rupture is best treated with emergency surgery, in the preoperative setting medical therapy is important to relieve symptoms and stabilize patients.[8] In this time, negative inotropes should be avoided and there should be consideration of hemodynamic monitoring with pulmonary artery catheter with inotropes such as milrinone, dobutamine, or levosimendan in addition to diuretics.[9] Therefore, medical therapy and the addition of mechanical support if needed are crucial components in the treatment of acute mitral regurgitation as a bridge to surgical correction.

Afterload Reduction

Nitrates are the vasodilator of choice in acute mitral regurgitation, especially intravenous nitrates like nitroprusside, but angiotensin-converting enzyme (ACE) inhibitors and angiotensin receptor blockers (ARBs) are also used.[10] As described earlier, the stroke volume acutely drops with acute mitral regurgitation. Vasodilators can improve the situation by reducing the outflow pressure gradient and makes conditions more favorable for forward flow into the left ventricle. This is accomplished by a decrease in systemic vascular resistance or the decreased resistance to the left ventricular ejection. There will be a decrease in left atrial pressure and left ventricular filling pressure, which will decrease the volume in the left ventricle. A decreased left ventricular volume will decrease the effective regurgitant orifice. By decreasing the left ventricular end diastolic and systolic volume, nitrates reduce ventricular dilation and affect remodeling.[11]

ACEIs and ARBs are also used in the setting of acute mitral regurgitation. In a study of 23 adults with moderate chronic mitral regurgitation lisinopril was shown to decrease the mitral regurgitant fraction by 6.4% ± 3.5% as compared to placebo 3.7% ± 3.2%.[12] Furthermore, a decrease in mitral regurgitant fraction means a reduced regurgitant flow, regurgitant volume, left ventricular end-diastolic volume, and increased stroke volume. They are used mostly in asymptomatic, hypertensive patients or those with left ventricular dysfunction. Of note, these medications should be used with caution in patients with renal dysfunction.

Diuretics

Diuretics are the key to treatment in the setting of pulmonary edema specifically in symptom management in the setting of acute mitral regurgitation. Diuretics maintain a negative sodium and water balance to decreased cardiac filling pressures. This causes decreased left ventricular dilation, reducing left ventricular end-diastolic and systolic volume, which will decrease function mitral regurgitation and improve myocardial function.[13] By decreasing the left ventricular end-diastolic volume this will improve the regurgitant orifice, thus decreasing the regurgitant volume.

β-Blockers

β-blockers are typically reserved for treatment in patients with left ventricular systolic dysfunction as they have a positive effect on remodeling and ejection fraction. They work by reducing the volume of mitral regurgitation in patients with heart failure and with functional (secondary) mitral regurgitation. β-blockers can improve forward stroke volume with little effect on cardiac output. In a study of 895 patients, the use of β-blockers showed a decreased mortality hazard of 0.62 (95% CI 0.46 to 0.83, $P = .002$).[14] Also, patients being treated with β-blockers had less mitral valve surgery (19% vs. 37%; $P = .0001$) in the 11-year follow-up of the study.[14] Of note, β-blocker initiation should be withheld in the setting of possible cardiogenic shock.

CHRONIC PRIMARY MITRAL REGURGITATION

Chronic primary mitral regurgitation is due to dysfunction of the valve structure, which can include the leaflets, chordae tendineae, papillary muscles, or annulus. Typically, the left ventricle and left atrium dilate to accommodate increased volume. Dilation of the left atrium leads to pulmonary hypertension and elevated pressure in the right ventricle. Also, when mitral regurgitation is severe, there can be left ventricular dysfunction. In chronic severe primary mitral regurgitation, primarily leaflet dysfunction, surgical therapy is the treatment of choice and medical management is often used as a bridge to surgery. The main treatment benefits are seen with β-blockers and ACEIs and angiotensin II receptor blockers as they reduce afterload, lessen mitral regurgitation, and prevent left ventricular remodeling. Diuretics are added to these therapies in the preoperative and postoperative setting of primary mitral regurgitation. The main effect of treatment is to attenuate the effects of left ventricular volume overload in the presurgical intervention period. However, large trials are needed to further clarify the benefits of medical therapy.

There are two groups of patients with chronic primary mitral regurgitation, compensated and decompensated. In chronic compensated mitral regurgitation, the left ventricle becomes dilated from increased volume and preload returns to near normal. The left ventricular end-diastolic volume and afterload will increase, and the large left atrium maintains lower pulmonary venous pressure.[15] In chronic decompensated mitral regurgitation, there is often a decreased ejection fraction so as the left ventricle dilates with increased volume and increased afterload there is an increase in pulmonary venous pressure leading to symptomatic heart failure. Even in the setting of a "normal" ejection fraction the forward flow may be sub-normal as much of this "normal" stroke volume is regurgitated backward.

Diuretics

Diuretics are known to reduce the volume in the left ventricle, which helps to alter the regurgitant volume. This is more beneficial in chronic secondary mitral regurgitation (MR), which will be discussed later but is key to helping reverse symptoms of volume overload such as pulmonary edema and optimize before surgery. In the preoperative setting, the use of pulmonary artery catheter in combination with diuresis and afterload reduction and/or inotropes has been beneficial to patients with severe congestive heart failure due to systolic dysfunction. Using a pulmonary artery catheter to help guide diuresis ensures patients are hemodynamically optimized preoperatively. In the postoperative setting, diuretics can help to prevent future fluid accumulation to keep patients euvolemic and maximize cardiac performance.

β-Blockers

β-blockers block the effect of the adrenergic nervous system on the heart that is upregulated in congestive heart failure. By blocking the effects of catecholamines on the heart, stroke volume is increased but with reduced stroke work.[16] In chronic primary MR there is a heightened β-adrenergic state leading to effects similar to that in systolic heart failure with decreased myocyte protein synthesis and extracellular matrix degradation. Therefore, with β-blockade there is improved function of cardiomyocytes and increased contractility. In an observational study of 895 patients, there was an improved mortality HR of 0.62 (P = .002) in patients who received β-blockers compared to those that did not before surgery.[14]

Afterload Reduction

Afterload reduction is theoretically useful by decreasing the impedance to ejection of blood into the aorta therefore decreasing the regurgitant volume. Afterload reducers can be used in three scenarios for primary chronic MR but should not replace surgical treatment.[17]

1. Patients with symptoms or LV dysfunction who are poor candidates for surgery
2. Improves hemodynamic profile before procedure
3. Systemic hypertension

By decreasing LV and left atrial (LA) volume thereby decreasing the size of the mitral annulus this could improve chronic secondary mitral regurgitation.[18] For the most part, studies have not shown significant benefit of ACEIs in the treatment of patients with chronic primary MR,[19] with only modest improvement in right and left ventricular size.[20] However, some studies have shown the use of ACEIs have decreased regurgitant fraction, regurgitant volume, and regurgitant orifice area with treatment up to 1 year.[21,22]

CHRONIC SECONDARY MITRAL REGURGITATION

Secondary (also called functional) mitral regurgitation is caused by dilatation of the left ventricle, wall motion abnormalities, or both. This is due to tethering of one or both leaflets, annular dilatation, and/or papillary muscle dysfunction. In contrast to primary mitral regurgitation that is a disease of the valve, secondary mitral regurgitation is a disease of the left heart.

In patients with reduced ejection fraction, mitral regurgitation portends a worse prognosis. In a retrospective analysis of 2057 symptomatic patients with ejection fraction less than 40%, those with moderately severe or severe mitral regurgitation had a 5-year survival of 40%, compared with 54% for those who did not.[23] Similarly, in a chart review of 1421 consecutive patients with ejection fraction (EF) 35% or less, severe mitral regurgitation was an independent predictor of mortality (relative risk [RR] 1.84).[24] Specifically looking at 303 patients with a Q-wave myocardial infarction, the 194 patients with ischemic mitral regurgitation had a higher mortality rate of 62% versus 39% at 5 years ($P < .001$).[25] Medical management has been accepted as an initial and sometimes effective approach for secondary mitral regurgitation, thus mandated as a first step by modern valve trials and guidelines.

Given that left ventricular dilatation and/or dysfunction is a key factor in secondary mitral regurgitation, pharmacologic therapy is similar to evidence-based therapies for left ventricular dysfunction. Intuitively, lowering blood pressure should lessen the amount of regurgitation with reduced afterload. Fortunately, there are multiple therapies that impact survival in LV dysfunction (Fig. 11.1).[26] MitraClip (Abbott, Abbott Park, IL, USA) became Food and Drug Administration (FDA) approved in March 2019 for moderate-to-severe or severe symptomatic mitral regurgitation despite optimal medical therapy. In a subanalysis of the Cardiovascular Outcomes Assessment of the MitraClip Percutaneous Therapy for Heart Failure Patients with Functional Mitral Regurgitation (COAPT) trial of 614 patients who initially had 3+ or 4+ MR, 34% improved to less than 2+ MR with goal-directed medical therapy alone.[27] In the AHA/ACC 2014 valve guidelines and reaffirmed in the 2017 focused update, medical therapy and resynchronization therapy is the only treatment of secondary mitral regurgitation given the highest Class I recommendation.[17] This includes diuretics for symptomatic relief, β-blockers, afterload reduction with ACEI or angiotensin II receptor antagonist or angiotensin receptor II antagonist with neprilysin inhibition (sacubitril-valsartan) and mineralocorticoid antagonists. There is rapidly emerging evidence for the sodium-glucose cotransporter 2 (SGLT2) inhibitor class for LV dysfunction as well but not yet specifically looked at in secondary mitral regurgitation.

Diuretics

Certainly, diuretics may provide symptomatic relief from pulmonary congestion as detailed above. Additionally, in secondary mitral regurgitation, reducing volume overload can reduce the mitral regurgitation. In 21 dialysis patients with cardiomegaly without manifest heart failure but with coexisting mitral and tricuspid regurgitation, ultrafiltration was intensified in place of their antihypertensive drugs. Mitral regurgitation became undetectable in 13 patients and improved in 7 others. Left ventricular systolic and diastolic dimensions decreased by a mean of 4 mm/m^2 each.[28]

β-Blockers

There are numerous large, randomized trials showing efficacy of β-blockers in systolic dysfunction, with smaller studies looking specifically at mitral regurgitation. In 59 patients with left ventricular dysfunction and mitral regurgitation randomized to carvedilol versus placebo, carvedilol reduced mitral regurgitation at 4 months and maintained at 12 months compared with placebo.[29] In a study of 45 patients with EF less than 30% given carvedilol for 6 months at maximally tolerated doses, EF

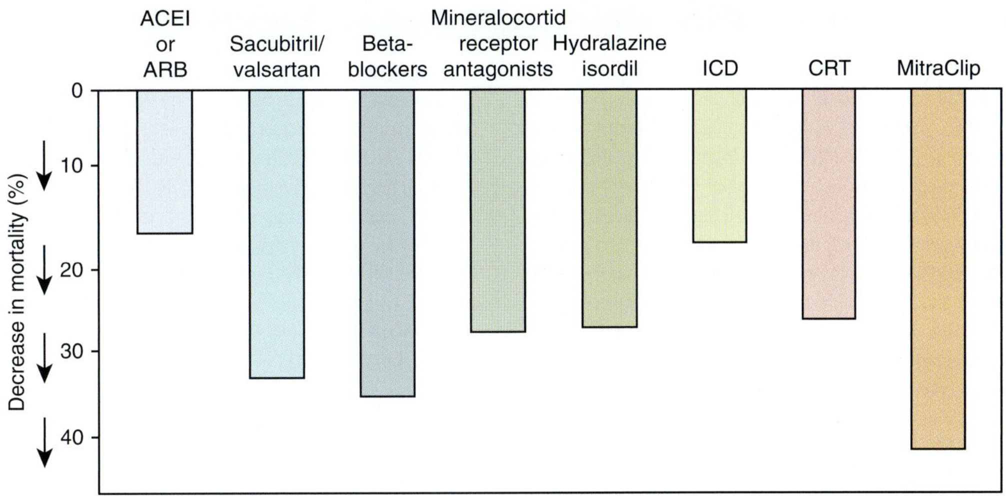

Fig. 11.1 Mortality effects of various interventions for systolic dysfunction. *ACEI*, Angiotensin-converting enzyme inhibitor; *ARB*, angiotensin receptor blocker; *CRT*, cardiac resynchronization therapy; *ICD*, implantable cardioverter defibrillator. (From Goel K, et al. Contemporary management of secondary mitral regurgitation. Eur Cardiol. 2020;15:e22, *Republished with permission* by ©Radcliffe Medical Media 2021.)

improved from 24% to 29% ($P < .0001$), end systolic volume index improved from 106 to 93 mL/m^2 ($P < .0001$), and mitral regurgitation stroke volume improved from 50 to 16 mL ($P < .0001$). Significant improvements were not seen in a matched control group.[30] β-blockers proven to reduce mortality in heart failure with reduced ejection fraction (HFrEF) include metoprolol succinate, carvedilol, and bisoprolol.[31]

Afterload Reduction

As in other forms of mitral regurgitation, afterload reduction results in more favorable conditions for forward flow and potentially reduced regurgitant flow. Decreased left ventricular dilatation and thus decreased mitral annular dilatation can reduce the mitral regurgitation as well, key in initial management of secondary mitral regurgitation.

ACEIs and angiotensin II receptor blockers have long been a staple of treating systolic dysfunction. However, the Prospective Comparason of ARNI with ACEI to Determine Impact on Global Mortality and Morbidity in Heart Failure (PARADIGM-HF) trial showed valsartan-neprilysin combination to be superior to enalapril in reducing all-cause mortality by 16%, cardiovascular death by 20%, and hospitalizations for heart failure by 20% ($P < .001$ for each).[32] A recent study suggests sacubitril-valsartan may be superior to valsartan in reducing secondary mitral regurgitation, where they randomized 118 patients to either of these therapies in addition to standard medical therapy. The decrease in effective regurgitant orifice area was significantly greater in the sacubitril-valsartan group than in the valsartan group (–0.058 vs.–0.018 cm^2; $P = .032$).[33] Additional add-on agents for the treatment of systolic heart failure if blood pressure allows include aldosterone blockers (spironolactone, eplerenone), hydralazine/isosorbide dinitrate in addition to the above or those intolerant of. Ivabradine is a novel agent that received FDA approval in 2015 to reduce the risk of hospitalization for worsening heart failure in patients with stable, symptomatic chronic heart failure with a left ventricular ejection fraction (LVEF) of 35% or lower, who are in sinus rhythm with a resting heart rate of 70 beats/min or higher, and who are either on maximally tolerated doses of β-blockers or have a contraindication to β-blocker use. We are not aware of any studies that look at this medication directly for secondary mitral regurgitation.

SGLT2 inhibitors are a newer class of diabetic medications that are quickly becoming cardiovascular and heart failure medications due to efficacy in these patients. Two recent trials showed efficacy in patients with reduced EF regardless of diabetes status. The Dapagliflozin in Patients with Heart Failure and Reduced Ejection Fraction (DAPA-HF) trial showed a 26% reduction in cardiovascular death, hospitalization or need for intravenous diuretics for heart failure in patients with EF 40% or less with dapagliflozin.[34] Similarly, the Empagliflozin Outcome Trial in Patients with Chronic Heart Failure and a Reduced Ejection Fraction (EMPEROR-Reduced) trial showed a 25% reduction in cardiovascular death or heart failure hospitalization in patients with EF of 40% or less regardless of diabetes status for patients randomized to empagliflozin versus placebo.[35]

SUMMARY

In this chapter we discussed the medical management of mitral valve disease. For mitral stenosis we detail how medical therapy can help relieve symptoms, especially the use of diuretics. We also discussed the indications and utility of ivabradine and digoxin for mitral stenosis. For acute mitral regurgitation we reviewed the treatment course and each medication class for severe disease in the preoperative course. In chronic primary and secondary mitral regurgitation, we discussed the disease process, progression, and how medications are used. The medications not only treat symptoms, but also can delay the need for surgery and stabilize patients. We discuss how each medication is used and how it improves the underlying mitral valve disease process.

CASE-BASED ASSESSMENT

An 81-year-old female presents to the emergency department with worsening dyspnea on exertion. She has a past medical history of persistent atrial fibrillation, coronary artery disease, heart failure with mildly reduced ejection fraction, history of moderate mitral regurgitation, stroke, stage 3 chronic kidney disease, and hypothyroidism. Home medications include apixaban 2.5 mg bid, clopidogrel 75 mg daily, digoxin 0.125 mcg daily, furosemide 20 mg daily, levothyroxine 150 mcg daily, metoprolol succinate 100 mg bid, and rosuvastatin 20 mg nightly. She states that for the last couple of months her ability to exercise has declined. She was previously able to climb up a flight of stairs without having to rest to catch her breath. She also was able to walk over a mile straight, now she can only walk two to three blocks before having to stop due to dyspnea. She does not notice any lower extremity edema or orthopnea, no chest pain, palpitations, or syncopal/presyncopal symptoms. Her vitals reveal blood pressure 132/84, heart rate 80 to 100 (atrial fibrillation), 16 respirations per minute, and 98% on room air. Physical exam reveals a harsh grade III/VI holosystolic murmur loudest at the apex and an irregular rate. Patient has slight bilateral edema and crackles at bilateral bases. Her jugular venous pressure is elevated. The rest of the physical exam is within normal limits. Labs reveal a BNP of 2000 pg/mL, troponin 0.04 ng/mL, creatinine at baseline of 1.4 mg/dL, and a mildly elevated lactate. Electrocardiogram shows atrial fibrillation with ventricular response at 88 beats/min. The remainder of her labs were unremarkable. Chest x-ray shows bibasilar interstitial edema.

1. What is the next best test to help make the diagnosis?
   A. Transesophageal echocardiography
   B. Transthoracic echocardiography
   C. Right heart catheterization
   D. CT pulmonary embolism protocol
   E. Left heart catheterization

She has a transthoracic echo which showed reduced ejection fraction to 35% with a moderately dilated left ventricle and severe functional mitral regurgitation due to failure of leaflet coaptation. The left atrium is severely dilated. Her inferior vena cava is dilated and poorly collapsing. A cardiac catheterization reveals no obstructive coronary disease.

2. What is the next best step in the management of this patient?
   A. Enalapril
   B. Lasix
   C. Nitroglycerine
   D. Milrinone
   E. Norepinephrine

By hospital day 3 she is feeling better with 7 pounds of weight loss. She feels improved but not back to baseline. She has been continued on her home medications in addition to IV Lasix and enalapril 2.5 mg daily. Her murmur is unchanged, and labs are stable. Representative vital signs are heart rate 68 beats/min and her blood pressure is averaging 132/84.

3. After initiation of Lasix what is the next best step in the management?
   A. Switch metoprolol succinate to carvedilol 12.5 mg twice daily
   B. Switch enalapril to valsartan 80 mg Daily
   C. CT surgery consult for consideration of MV surgery versus MitraClip
   D. Switch enalapril to sacubitril-valsartan 24/26 twice daily
   E. Ivabradine

She is discharged on the above regimen and follows up in the office 2 months later on the medications above which now also include Lasix 40 mg daily and sacubitril-valsartan 97 to 103 mg twice daily. She is feeling improved since her hospitalization but has not returned to her prior baseline. Her heart rate is 72 beats/min, and her blood pressure is 110/60. Her murmur is still estimated to be III/VI. Labs show creatinine unchanged at 1.4 mg/dL, potassium is 5.4 mEq/L, and glucose is 130 mg/dL. EKG shows atrial fibrillation with a ventricular response at 72 beats/min. She has a right bundle branch block with QRS duration of 124 ms.

4. What is the best next step in therapy?
   A. Add empagliflozin
   B. Add spironolactone
   C. Repeat echocardiogram
   D. Refer for cardiac resynchronization therapy ± implantable cardioverter defibrillator (ICD)
   E. Refer for surgical intervention

Three months later she returns to the office on all the medications above and is tolerating them well. She still has a loud murmur of mitral regurgitation and feels slightly better but not back to baseline. She is still dyspneic walking a few blocks or a full flight of stairs. Labs, vitals, exam, and EKG are unchanged.

5. What is the most appropriate next step for her?
   A. Add digoxin
   B. Repeat echocardiogram
   C. Refer for MitraClip
   D. Refer for surgical mitral valve repair
   E. Given her suboptimal functional status, offer palliative home inotropes

See page 316 for the answer.

REFERENCES

1. Reyes VP, Raju RS, Wynne J, et al. Percutaneous balloon valvuloplasty compared with open surgical commissurotomy for mitral stenosis. *N Engl J Med.* 1994;331:961–967.
2. Liu C, Lai Y, Guan T, et al. Outcomes of diuretics in rheumatic heart disease with compensated chronic heart failure: a retrospective study. *ESC Heart Fail.* 2020;7(6):3929–3941.
3. Otto CM. *The Clinical Practice of Echocardiography.* 4th ed. Philadelphia: Saunders; 2012:389–407.
4. Saggu DK, Narsin VS, Dwivedi SK, et al. Effect of Ivabradine on heart rate and duration of exercise in patients with mild-moderate mitral stenosis: a randomized comparison with metoprolol. *J Cardiovasc Pharmacol.* 2015;65(6):552–554.
5. Ramos JD, Cunanan EL, Abrahan LL, et al. Ivabradine versus beta-blockers in mitral stenosis in sinus rhythm: An updated meta-analysis of randomized controlled trials. *Cardiol Res.* 2018;9(4):224–230.
6. Slipczuk L, Rafique AM, Davila CD, et al. The role of medical therapy in moderate to severe degenerative mitral regurgitation. *Rev Cardiovasc Med.* 2016;17(1–2):28–39.
7. Watanabe N. Acute mitral regurgitation. *Heart.* 2019;105(9):671–677.
8. Grigioni F, Enriquez-Sarano M, Ling LH, et al. Sudden death in mitral regurgitation due to flail leaflet. *J Am Coll Cardiol.* 1999;34(7):2078–2085.
9. Looney Y, Quinton P. Mitral valve surgery. *Contin Educ Anaesth Crit Care Pain.* 2005;5:199–202.
10. Rengin CG, Tolga SG. Clinical presentation, diagnosis and management of acute mitral regurgitation following acute myocardial infarction. *J Acute Dis.* 2016;5(2):96–101.
11. Yoran C, Yellin EL, Becker RM, et al. Mechanism of reduction of mitral regurgitation with vasodilator therapy. *Am J Cardiol.* 1979;43:773–777.
12. Marcotte F, Honos GN, Walling AD, et al. Effect of angiotensin-converting enzyme inhibitor therapy in mitral regurgitation with normal left ventricular function. *Can J Cardiol.* 1997;13:479–485.

13. Boon NA, Bloomfield P. The medical management of valvar heart disease. *Heart.* 2002;87(4):395–400.
14. Varadarajan P, Joshi N, Appel D, et al. Effect of beta-blocker therapy on survival in patients with severe mitral regurgitation and normal left ventricular ejection fraction. *Am J Cardiol.* 2008;102:611–615.
15. Carabello BA. The relationship of left ventricular geometry and hypertrophy to left ventricular function in valvular heart disease. *J Heart Valve Dis.* 1995;4(suppl 2):S132–S138.
16. Stewart RA, Raffel OC, Kerr AJ, et al. Pilot study to assess the influence of beta-blockers on mitral regurgitant volume and left ventricular work in degenerative mitral valve disease. *Circulation.* 2008;118(10):1041–1046.
17. Nishimura RA, Otto CM, Bonow RO, et al. 2017 AHA/ACC Focused Update of the 2014 AHA/ACC Guideline for the Management of Patients With Valvular Heart Disease: A Report of the American College of Cardiology/American Heart Association Task Force on Clinical Practice Guidelines. *Circulation.* 2017;135(25):e1159–e1195.
18. Evangelista A, Tornos P, Sambola A, Permayer-Miralda G. Role of vasodilators in regurgitant valve disease. *Curr Treat Options Cardiovasc Med.* 2006;8(6):428–434.
19. Borer JS, Sharma A. Drug therapy for heart valve disease. *Circulation.* 2015;132:1038–1045.
20. Strauss CE, Duval S, Pastorius D, et al. Pharmacotherapy in the treatment of mitral regurgitation: a systematic review. *J Heart Valve Dis.* 2012;21:275–285.
21. Tischler MD, Rowan M, LeWinter MM. Effect of enalapril therapy on left ventricular mass and volumes in asymptomatic chronic, severe mitral regurgitation secondary to mitral valve prolapse. *Am J Cardiol.* 1998;82:242–245.
22. Sampaio RO, Grinberg M, Leite JJ, et al. Effect of enalapril on left ventricular diameters and exercise capacity in asymptomatic or mildly symptomatic patients with regurgitation secondary to mitral valve prolapse or rheumatic heart disease. *Am J Cardiol.* 2005;96:117–121.
23. Trichon BH, Felker GM, Shaw LK, et al. Relation of frequency and severity of mitral regurgitation to survival among patients with left ventricular systolic dysfunction and heart failure. *Am J Cardiol.* 2003;91(5):538–543.
24. Koelling TM, Aaronson KD, Cody RJ, et al. Prognostic significance of mitral regurgitation and tricuspid regurgitation in patients with left ventricular systolic dysfunction. *Am Heart J.* 2002;144(3):524.
25. Grigioni F, Enriquez-Sarano M, Zehr KJ, et al. Ischemic mitral regurgitation: long-term outcome and prognostic implications with quantitative Doppler assessment. *Circulation.* 2001;103(13):1759.
26. Goel K, Barker CM, Lindenfeld J. Contemporary management of secondary mitral regurgitation. *Eur Cardiol.* 2020;15:e22 Published 2020 May 12.
27. Kar S, Mack MJ, Lindenfeld JA. Relationship between residual mitral regurgitation and clinical and functional outcomes in the COAPT trial. *Presented at EuroPCR,* Paris, France; 21 May 2019.
28. Cirit M, Ozkahya M, Cinar CS, et al. Disappearance of mitral and tricuspid regurgitation in haemodialysis patients after ultrafiltration. *Nephrol Dial Transplant.* 1998;13(2):389.
29. Lowes BD, Gill EA, Abraham WT, et al. Effects of carvedilol on left ventricular mass, chamber geometry, and mitral regurgitation in chronic heart failure. *Am J Cardiol.* 1999;83(8):1201–1205.
30. Capomolla S, Febo O, Gnemmi M, et al. Beta-blockade therapy in chronic heart failure: diastolic function and mitral regurgitation improvement by carvedilol. *Am Heart J.* 2000;139(4):596.
31. Yancy CW, Jessup M, Bozkurt B, et al. 2017 ACC/AHA/HFSA Focused Update of the 2013 ACCF/AHA Guideline for the Management of Heart Failure: A Report of the American College of Cardiology/American Heart Association Task Force on Clinical Practice Guidelines and the Heart Failure Society of America. *J Am Coll Cardiol.* 2017;70(6):776–803.
32. McMurray JJV, Packer M, Desai AS, et al. Sacubitril-valsartan versus enalapril in heart failure. *New Engl J Med.* 2014;371:993–1004.
33. Kang DH, Park SJ, Shin SH, et al. Angiotensin receptor neprilysin inhibitor for functional mitral regurgitation. *Circulation.* 2019;139:1354–1365.
34. McMurray JJV, Solomon SD, Inzucchi SE, et al. Dapagliflozin in patients with heart failure and reduced ejection fraction. *N Engl J Med.* 2019;381:1995–2008.
35. Packer M, Anker SD, Butler J, et al. Cardiovascular and renal outcomes with Empagliflozin in heart failure. *N Engl J Med.* 2020;383:1413–1424.

12

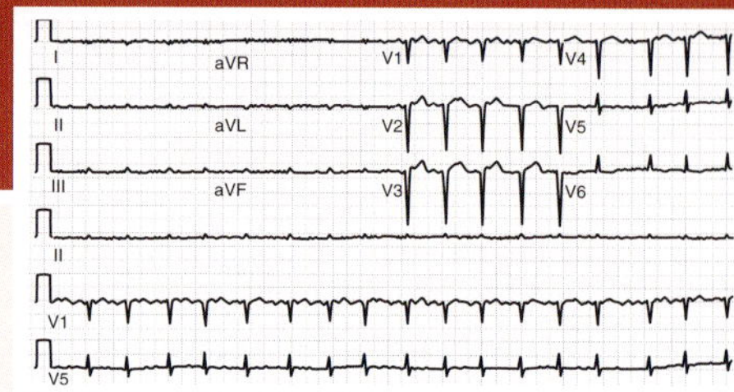

Cardiac Rhythm Management Implantable Devices

Yinn Shaung Ooi, Douglas B. Esberg

CHAPTER OUTLINE

LEARNING OBJECTIVES

- Understand when permanent pacemaker implantation is indicated and when permanent pacemaker implantation is NOT indicated after mitral valve surgery.
- Be able to evaluate the choice of a pacing device, including implantable cardioverter defibrillator (ICD) and the various lead placement options.
- Understand the proper techniques for effective and durable left atrial appendage exclusion. This includes the understanding that left atrial appendage (LAA) exclusion can be difficult to achieve and should only be performed if complete and durable exclusion is possible.
- Understand different management options for atrial fibrillation that occurs both early and later after mitral valve intervention.

INTRODUCTION

Of the four heart valves, diseases of the mitral valve are the most intimately linked with electrical disturbances of the heart. Chronic stable, acute decompensated, stenotic, or regurgitant diseases of the mitral valve are frequently associated with both atrial and ventricular arrhythmias. Pathophysiologically, they arise as a downstream consequence of the mechanical and hemodynamic strains to the cardiac chambers, but they may also occur as a result of a genuine electrocellular aberration that is associated with the disease. Moreover, the medical, transcatheter, and surgical therapies for mitral valve diseases are commonly associated with arrhythmic complications. This chapter aims to review the pathogenesis and management of the various brady- and tachyarrhythmias associated with mitral valve diseases.

CARDIAC IMPLANTABLE ELECTRICAL DEVICES

Pacemakers

Sinus Node Dysfunction

Sinus node dysfunction, which broadly encompasses sinus bradycardia, sinus pauses, and sinoatrial blocks, is commonly associated with mitral valve diseases. There are several explanations that account for this association.

1. Atrial remodeling with fibrosis and scar formation is a common endpoint in untreated mitral valve diseases due to chronic exposure to high pressure and volume in the left atrium. Protein fibril deposition replaces normal myocardial architecture and disrupts cell-cell coupling, such that fibrosis around the sinus node can hamper or block the exit of sinus node impulses or directly disrupt intrinsic pacemaker function.
2. While it is known that atrial arrhythmias, even those manifesting in paroxysms, are associated with sinus node remodeling and dysfunction,[1–3] it comes without surprise that chronic mitral valve diseases which are often associated with persistent long-standing atrial fibrillation (AF) are closely linked to sinus node disease. Persistent AF can directly influence sinus node function by affecting ion channels (calcium clock) responsible for its function, leading to reduced sinus node reserve and dysfunction, or contribute to further atrial anatomical remodeling.
3. Additionally, coexisting tachyarrhythmias requiring treatment may indirectly contribute to further disruption in sinus node function when rate or rhythm controlling medications are administered for their management.

Conduction Disease Following Mitral Valve Surgery

Conduction diseases requiring permanent pacemaker implantation (PPI) following cardiac surgery has been reported to occur in 0.8% to 34% of cases and is more frequent after mitral valve surgery than isolated coronary artery bypass graft (CABG). The association of postoperative conduction disorders with mitral valve surgery is well recognized and presents a significant clinical concern as postoperative conduction disorders requiring permanent pacemaker are associated with increased morbidity, in-hospital length of stay, and cost.

Sinus Node Dysfunction

Sinus node dysfunction is a well-recognized complication of the procedure with a wide reported incidence, ranging from 2% to 21%. While most cases are asymptomatic and transient, a small portion persist and lead to more prominent bradycardia, necessitating implantation of a permanent pacemaker. Aside from an acute increase in sinus node recovery time (SNRT), mitral valve surgery with or without maze has also been shown to attenuate chronotropic response, heart rate variability (HRV), and vagal modulation of sinus node function. Documented mechanisms include injury of the nodal tissue by mechanical trauma due to atrial incisions, surgical interruption of nodal arterial supply, and inadequate atrial preservation during cardiopulmonary bypass.[4]

Atrioventricular Block

Conduction disease involving the atrioventricular node can also occur as a complication of surgical ablation of AF, although at a lower incidence compared to sinus node dysfunction. Additionally, atrioventricular block is usually confined to the early postoperative period, while sinus node dysfunction is dominant in the late postoperative period. The risk of atrial and ventricular (AV) block after mitral valve surgery stems from the proximity of the mitral valve apparatus to the atrioventricular node and bundle of His, where trauma or ischemic injury of the conduction system may occur. As compared to aortic valve surgery, mitral surgery has a lower risk of causing complete and permanent AV block. This comes from the fact that the mitral annulus is relatively distant from the His bundle and the predominance of the compact AV node sits closer to the right side of the heart than the left. The most common cause of AV block in mitral surgery is local tissue edema leading to transient AV node dysfunction.

Risk Factors for Permanent Pacemaker Implantation

Several known preoperative and operative risk factors that predict PPI postoperative to mitral valve surgery have been identified across large-scale databases, spanning from baseline patient characteristics, including echocardiographic features as well as type of surgery, as outlined below:

1. Older age and baseline conduction disturbances, namely sinus node dysfunction, fascicular blocks, and all degrees of atrioventricular block, are associated with increased incidence of PPI during the index hospitalization of the valve surgery, the time period at which the risk for PPI is the greatest, while comorbidities, such as peripheral arterial disease, congestive heart failure, and chronic kidney disease, predict increased risk for PPI in the late postoperative period (beyond 30 days and up to 1 year).[5]
2. Preoperative echocardiographic determinants of the risk of PPI after mitral valve surgery are less vigorously examined in the literature. Nonetheless, left atrial size, specifically left atrial volume index (LAVI), has been found to be an independent predictor of postoperative sinus node dysfunction after mitral valve surgery with concomitant surgical AF ablation.[6] As left atrial size has been found to reflect atrial fibrosis, this association could perhaps come from the function of LAVI as a surrogate marker of right atrial fibrosis, thus indirectly reflecting the functional status of the right atrium, and susceptibility for sinus node dysfunction. Of note, AF recurrence is also found to be higher, conferring lower efficacy of surgical ablation in these patients.
3. Complexity of the surgical procedure carries a substantial impact on the risk of postoperative PPI.[7,8] Multivalvular surgery as opposed to isolated mitral valve surgery poses a significantly higher risk of clinically significant postoperative conduction disease. Combined mitral and aortic valve surgeries, in particular, present the highest risk for PPI. Among isolated surgeries, PPI rates are higher in mitral valve replacement compared to repair. Additionally, concomitant performance of surgical AF ablation either by maze or pulmonary vein isolation (PVI) further increases the risk of PPI,

while interestingly the addition of CABG does not pose the same additive risk.

With specific regard to surgical AF ablation, there are several factors that bear weighting in its influence on the risk of postoperative PPI[5], that include:

1. The type of ablation device used, namely radiofrequency ablation compared to cryoablation alone, has been shown to contribute to a higher incidence of PPI.
2. The type of surgical approach, i.e., bi-atrial maze, a more elaborate approach that requires right and left atrial atriotomies, more time on cardiopulmonary bypass, and creation of extensive endocardial ablation extending to the mitral and tricuspid annuli, as compared to the less complex PVI or left-sided ablation only.[6]

Indication and Appropriate Timing of Permanent Pacemaker Implantation

As aforementioned, the majority of postoperative sinus node dysfunction is mild and transient, while only a small portion of cases are significant enough to necessitate PPI. Sinus node function recovery is common with long-term follow-up. It is most prominent in the first 6 months, and can continuously improve thereafter, with normal sinus nodal function attained in most patients usually at the 1-year mark after surgery.[9] Therefore, PPI for sinus node dysfunction after mitral valve surgery, especially in only mildly symptomatic patients should be restrictively applied because of the transient nature of this disorder.

In patients with clinically significant and persistent bradycardia in the acute postoperative setting either from sinus node dysfunction or atrioventricular block, it should be determined whether to continue hospitalization with temporary pacing or to place a permanent pacemaker (PPM). While the late disease course of conduction disturbances (1 month to a year following mitral valve surgery) is well examined in the literature, there remains a paucity of data with regard to the immediate or acute postoperative course, thus limiting our ability to reliably predict patients who are at risk for persistent dysfunction, versus patients with a high likelihood of recovery who may benefit from a longer observation period before committing to PPI. This is evident at follow-up, where it has been shown that only 30% to 40% of those implanted for sinus node dysfunction and 65% to 100% of those implanted for atrioventricular block actually require pacing.[10,11]

The heterogeneity in the reporting of PPM implantation after cardiac surgery makes it difficult to set standards for the optimal timing for implanting a PPM in a post cardiac surgical patient. The guidelines of the American College of Cardiology, American Heart Association, and Heart Rhythm Society (ACC/AHA/HRS) recommend PPM placement prior to discharge in patients with significant postoperative conduction disease, while the European Society of Cardiology (ESC) recommends 7 days of observation prior to PPM placement for complete AV block and 5 days up to several weeks for sinoatrial dysfunction.[12] In clinical practice, an observation period of up to 7 days is usually applied before implanting a PPM to allow regression of transient bradyarrhythmias. While there remain no conclusive recommendations about the optimal timing of PPI, a waiting period of 7 days is a reasonable approach that is supported by emerging data in the literature.[13,14]

Specific for complete atrioventricular block, a low rate of escape rhythm reflects more extensive injury incurred toward the conduction tree and predicts a lower likelihood of recovery. Hence, in such cases earlier implantation of a pacemaker can be considered to reduce postoperative length of stay. Additionally, while the proportion of atrioventricular block cases that recover is comparatively lower than sinus node dysfunction, and while recovery tends to occur earlier in the postoperative course, in a case of complete atrioventricular block occurring in the first 24 hours and persisting for greater than 48 hours, resolution within the next 1 to 2 weeks is unlikely, and earlier implantation of a pacemaker can be considered.[15]

Device Selection (Single, Dual, Bi-V, His Bundle, Left Bundle, Leadless)

In patients with mitral valve disease requiring cardiac implantable electrical devices (CIEDs), careful consideration of the type of implantable device, lead configuration, and device mode is crucial to ensure best clinical outcome. This is of particular importance in patients with mitral valve disease as various pacing configurations have been linked with worsened mitral regurgitation, as well as increased risk of AF, which as highlighted before, is present in high prevalence in this patient population.

Problems With Right Ventricular Pacing and Atrial Fibrillation

It is well recognized that right ventricular (RV) pacing is associated with issues related to AF, with studies demonstrating a linear relationship between RV pacing percentage and risk of AF. This problem spans not only from a resultant heightened risk of developing new onset AF in patients who were prior naïve, but also to worsened AF burden and increased progression from paroxysmal to persistent AF in patients with preexisting diagnosis of AF.[16]

Appropriate Pacing Configuration to Prevent Atrial Fibrillation

To appreciate the role of optimal pacing for the prevention of AF, it is important to first understand the underlying mechanism by which right ventricular pacing promotes AF. Isolated right ventricular pacing disrupts the normal sequence of activation of atria to ventricles, in other words, induces atrioventricular dyssynchrony, which in turn leads to increased atrial pressure and size, thereby producing a proarrhythmic substrate. It is on this premise that dual-chamber pacing was compared against single-chamber right ventricular pacing in patients with a prior history of AF and was found to reduce the risk of AF by 50%.[17] However, achieving AV synchronous pacing which was historically regarded as "physiologic pacing" does not resolve the entirety of the problem, as a pacing site in the right ventricle apex, in itself, is independently associated with AF. Pacing from the right ventricular apex causes the right ventricle to contract before the left ventricle and the septum to contract before the lateral wall of the left ventricle, simulating effects of left bundle branch block (LBBB). This phenomenon is referred to as ventricular dyssynchrony and can also lead to AF. This is evident with long-term follow-up trials demonstrating increased risk of atrial tachyarrhythmia in patients with dual-chamber pacing compared to atrial only pacing.

Thus, an optimal pacing strategy is one that prioritizes intrinsic atrioventricular conduction and minimizes unnecessary right ventricular pacing, therefore tackling both AV dyssynchrony and ventricular dyssynchrony that beget the risk for AF. This can be achieved with several pacing strategies that are either designed to maximize the AV interval or offer true atrial demand pacing (AAI[R]) with backup ventricular pacing.

To further mitigate the deleterious effects of right ventricular apical pacing, alternative pacing sites to promote more direct engagement of the ventricular conduction system, such as the bundle of His, have been examined in this context. A recent study showed that Hisian area (HA) pacing is associated with lower risk of persistent AF compared to right ventricular apical and septal pacing, both of which carry similar risks for AF.[18] On similar grounds, cardiac resynchronization therapy (CRT) via implantation of a left ventricular pacing lead has been suggested in an observational study to reduce AF burden in patients with left ventricular systolic dysfunction meeting criteria for CRT,[19] although this finding has not been validated in larger scale trials, nonetheless, AF was not a specified end point in those trials.[20] There is also more recent interest in pacing selectively from the left bundle. The effect on AF in these implants remains an area of active study.

An alternative strategy for managing AF in patients requiring atrial pacing is overdrive (antitachycardia) atrial pacing, with pacing algorithms designed both to prevent AF and to pace-terminate AF. A pacing rate that predominates over intrinsic atrial activity suppresses atrial premature beats and affects the pattern of atrial depolarization, thus reducing the triggering of AF. Studies have shown a positive impact of overdrive atrial pacing on AF burden; however, this effect is clinically small, and often leads to symptoms such as palpitations related to pacing.

Problems With Right Ventricular Pacing and Mitral Regurgitation

Abnormal atrioventricular and intraventricular electrical activation sequence during right ventricular apical pacing can also lead to complications related to mitral regurgitation. Loss of mechanical synchrony of the septal and lateral left ventricular walls during systole can result in altered papillary muscle function, interpapillary muscle dyssynchrony leading to tethering of mitral leaflets and distortion of mitral valve apparatus, and ultimately to incomplete valve closure. Abnormal atrioventricular timing can provoke diastolic mitral regurgitation because of the appearance of a diastolic ventriculoatrial gradient. In time, right ventricular pacing can also lead to pacing-induced cardiomyopathy with left ventricular modeling and annular dilation, culminating in further progression or development of mitral regurgitation. It is a complication that can occur as early as immediately post implantation of pacemaker,[21] but more commonly a late complication from chronic high pacing percentage in the right ventricle.

Appropriate Pacing Configuration to Prevent Mitral Regurgitation

While they mechanistically share a common pathway, strategies to tackle pacing-associated mitral regurgitation are similar to that of AF reviewed previously, namely prioritizing atrial pacing to allow intrinsic ventricular conduction while minimizing unnecessary right ventricular pacing, and alternative pacing sites that facilitate "physiologic" intraventricular activation sequence, such as HA, left bundle, or CRT pacing.

The therapeutic role of CRT in functional mitral regurgitation will be reviewed in the next section.

Cardiac Resynchronization Therapy in Functional Mitral Regurgitation

Functional (or secondary) mitral regurgitation is mitral valve incompetency that results from mitral annular dilation, papillary muscle displacement, or abnormal left ventricular geometry or function without an organic defect of the mitral valve apparatus. It is a common complication of both ischemic and dilated cardiomyopathy (DCM), presenting in about 25% to 65% of heart failure patients. There is ample evidence proving its association with unfavorable outcomes, including increased rehospitalization and mortality, up to fourfold, in cases of severe mitral regurgitation.[22]

In the presence of ventricular conduction abnormalities, such as LBBB, the proportion of heart failure patients with mitral regurgitation substantially increases, and its severity correlates with QRS duration. The explanatory mechanism to this association is similar to that of pacing-induced ventricular conduction abnormality and mitral regurgitation as outlined in the previous section. LBBB is likewise associated with adverse outcomes in patients with heart failure, independently and in a compounded effect in the presence of concurrent functional mitral regurgitation.

CRT accomplished by biventricular pacing (simultaneous right and left ventricular pacing with the addition of an additional pacing lead in a lateral cardiac vein via the coronary sinus) has emerged as a useful therapeutic tool in patients with heart failure with reduced ejection fraction (HFrEF). Current AHA/ACC and ESC guidelines recommend CRT in HFrEF patients with significant spontaneous intraventricular conduction disease and in those with anticipated high pacing needs (>40% of the time) to circumvent pacing-induced conduction abnormality.

Up to 85% of patients undergoing CRT have concurrent mitral regurgitation, being of moderate to severe degree in approximately 40% of cases. Its therapeutic role in functional mitral regurgitation is well established. In addition to overcoming the aberrant ventricular activation sequence of conduction abnormalities, which exacerbate mitral regurgitation, CRT is capable of directly offsetting some of the pathophysiologic mechanisms of functional mitral regurgitation (MR).

In functional MR, the progressive loss of mitral valve coaptation reserve stems from an imbalance in tethering forces and closing forces on the mitral valve leaflets in favor of the former. Synchronous biventricular electrical stimulation in CRT leads to more organized contraction of the left ventricle resulting in increased closing forces, and reinforces papillary muscle function leading to decreased tethering forces, thereby reversing this process. Furthermore, increased left ventricular contraction efficiency and unloading in time leads to restoration of left ventricular and mitral annular size (reverse remodeling), further ameliorating functional mitral regurgitation MR.[23]

In summary, CRT has a two fold effect on functional MR, an initial rapid improvement mediated by interpapillary and intraventricular resynchronization, and a later effect attributed to reverse/positive remodeling of the left ventricle. Its effectiveness has been validated by multiple clinical trials demonstrating significant improvement in mitral regurgitation (>1 grade) in more than 30% to 50% of CRT recipients.[24]

Implantable Cardiac Defibrillators

Mitral valve diseases on their own and in isolation are rarely associated with sudden cardiac death, thus implantable cardioverter defibrillator (ICD) implantation is generally not indicated. When performed, it is usually on account of a coexisting condition such as severe cardiomyopathy for the purpose of primary prevention. Mitral valve diseases are rarely the primary or sole indication for ICD implantation.

Arrhythmic Mitral Valve Prolapse

One exception to this is malignant arrhythmic mitral valve prolapse. While sudden cardiac death owing to fatal ventricular arrhythmia related to mitral valve prolapse was historically believed to be an exceedingly rare entity, more contemporary data suggest that its incidence may not be as low as formerly described. The true annual risk of sudden cardiac death in an individual with mitral valve prolapse remains unknown but is estimated to be at 0.9% to 1.9% per year in recent observational studies, a figure substantially greater than previously reported in older literature.[25,26]

Established high-risk features for sudden cardiac arrest in mitral valve prolapse include[25,27]:

- biphasic or inverted T waves in the inferior leads on an electrocardiogram (ECG);
- ventricular arrhythmias or frequent complex ventricular ectopy;
- bileaflet prolapse;
- mitral annular disjunction;
- "Pickelhaube sign" (a spiked high velocity signal across the lateral mitral annulus on echocardiography tissue Doppler); and
- presence of late gadolinium enhancement (LGE) suggesting myocardial scar on cardiac magnetic resonance imaging (MRI).

Careful attention to identify high-risk patients upon initial evaluation is crucial in the management of patients with mitral valve prolapse. In accordance with current AHA and ESC guidelines for ventricular arrhythmias and prevention of sudden cardiac death, implantation of an ICD for secondary prevention is indicated after a resuscitated sudden cardiac arrest deemed attributable to mitral valve prolapse. However, with specific regard to primary prevention in patients with mitral valve prolapse, at present there remains no guideline recommendations to assist in the prospective identification of high-risk patients that will benefit from prophylactic ICD implantation. More randomized data is needed to guide a proactive, risk stratification-based approach for the management of this unique disease entity.[28]

Choice of Implantable Cardioverter Defibrillator

As with pacemakers, ICDs have multiple lead configurations that each may benefit certain patient populations. In general, it is preferable to place only a single RV lead for defibrillation,[29] however if there is a concomitant need for pacing, leads should be chosen that are appropriate for that indication (i.e., dual chamber or CRT). There are also certain specific ICD technologies that can be considered. For patients with known or suspected AF, there are technologies that allow for monitoring of AF without the need for a separate atrial lead. There is an RV ICD lead with a separate proximal dipole that sits in the atrium and can give an atrial electrogram similar to what is seen with a separate atrial lead. This dipole cannot deliver reliable pacing in the atrium but is useful for diagnostics. There are also algorithms that look at rhythm irregularity as a surrogate for AF and can be helpful in long-term management.

Another ICD choice is an entirely extravascular system. The only currently available system consists of a pulse generator placed subcutaneously in the mid-axillary line at the level of the ventricular apex and a single lead tunneled subcutaneously to the parasternal area. This device has the advantage of remaining outside the vascular space, which decreases the likelihood of device-related endocarditis. It is also more easily extracted and is expected to be more durable. This device would not be indicated in a patient that has a need for pacing, since it does not have that capability. Other types of extravascular ICDs are currently under development.

Implantable Loop Recorders

Implantable loop recorders (ILRs) can be a helpful tool for tracking AF after mitral valve surgery. These devices can be implanted quickly and easily at the bedside and provide 3 to 5 years of continuous monitoring. LRs are frequently used for tracking arrhythmias after catheter-based ablation of AF and can serve a similar purpose for mitral surgery.

Management After Surgical Atrial Fibrillation Ablation

As highlighted before, while AF is intimately associated with mitral valve disease, a considerably high proportion of patients undergoing mitral valve surgery are likely to have concomitant surgical ablation of AF. The Cox-Maze procedure with or without PVI has been the gold standard for the surgical treatment of AF. The reported AF cure rate after a "full-maze procedure" (combination of standard atrial incisions with PVI) ranges widely from 70% to 90%.[30] Recurrence of AF after surgical ablation is not uncommon and presents a clinical challenge with regard to decisions relating to antiarrhythmic and anticoagulation therapy, as well as cardiac monitoring.

To reflect upon AF recurrence after surgical ablation, one should make a clear distinction between early recurrence and late failure, as they do differ fundamentally from a mechanistic level, as well as approach to management. Early recurrence referred to as recurrent AF within 30 days to 3 months postoperation is exceedingly common (especially within the first 10 days), with an incidence rate of 43% to 59%, the majority of which are transient and do not necessarily represent treatment failure per se.

There are two distinct circumstances related to early recurrence of AF after Cox-Maze ablation:

1. Inflammatory response and atrial myocardial edema in the burn areas, as well as postoperative pericarditis, both of which tend to resolve when inflammation and edema resides. This constitutes the bulk of cases.
2. A small proportion are due to early reconnection or reconstitution of conduction across ablation lines, which tends to persist after months following surgery, reflecting late failure.[31]

Management of Early Recurrence

The routine use of antiarrhythmic agents postoperatively in the first few months (and withdrawn around 6 to 12 months if no recurrence is detected) is common practice and is effective in preventing early recurrence of arrhythmia. In the event that a recurrent episode occurs early postoperatively, timely treatment with electrical cardioversion and an extended course of antiarrhythmic therapy should be considered. While the effectiveness of early antiarrhythmic therapy on long-term recurrence is less clear, the role of early electrical cardioversion in preventing late recurrence is better substantiated by evidence, with studies showing that cardioversion within 1 month of recurrence after catheter ablation portends to superior long-term maintenance of sinus rhythm, which can be reasonably extrapolated to the surgical ablation population.[32]

Management of Late or Persistent Atrial Fibrillation

As discussed above, late failure, generally defined as recurrence occurring after or persisting beyond the post ablation blanking period (first 3 months after ablation), is caused by reconnection of conduction across lines of electrical block with incompletely (or non transmurally) ablated tissue, or simply due to gaps in ablation lines. Less frequently, a nonpulmonary vein trigger, most commonly in the coronary sinus, left atrial appendage, or both, can lead to late occurrence independent of pulmonary vein reconnection, manifesting typically as atypical atrial flutter.

Predictors of late failure of surgical AF ablation have been examined in several studies and the following determinants have been identified:

- Advanced age[33]
- Large preoperative left atrial dimension (LAD) ≥58 to 60 mm[30,34]
- A large cardiothoracic ratio[30]
- Early postoperative atrial tachycarrhythmias[34,35]
- Procedural aspects—ablation lesion sets, "cut and sew" method versus energy-based ablation techniques, and the respective energy source used[31]

Antiarrhythmic therapy may be useful in the treatment of late recurrence of AF. However, extrapolating data derived from patients of failed initial catheter ablation, a repeat ablation from a percutaneous approach is likely to be a more effective long-term strategy to maintain sinus rhythm compared to antiarrhythmic therapy.[36]

Stroke Prevention and Anticoagulation Therapy After Surgical Ablation of Atrial Fibrillation and Left Atrial Appendage Exclusion

The issue of stroke risk and the need for anticoagulation therapy after Cox-maze procedure remains unresolved. In clinical practice, patients are commonly restarted on anticoagulation therapy postoperatively and continued for at least 3 months, taking into account individual clinical determinants of stroke risk, namely CHA_2DS_2 VASc scores. Omission of anticoagulation therapy is considered after 3 months in patients free of AF, particularly in those with increased risk of bleeding. This is a reasonable strategy especially in cases of concomitant left atrial appendage excision/ligation and is supported by emerging evidence in the literature.[37] In patients with AF recurrence, the decision to continue anticoagulation therapy can present a challenge and should be highly individualized. A case-based approach weighing the risk of bleeding with chronic anticoagulation against stroke risk considering clinical risk factors as well as AF burden is paramount to ensure best outcomes. In this context, extended monitoring by means of an ILR is reasonable to better define AF burden to guide decision about anticoagulation therapy.

Concomitant surgical left atrial appendage exclusion adds an additional layer of complexity to this conundrum. Despite the long existence of surgical left atrial appandage (LAA) ligation, with its first description published over a century ago, its efficacy for preventing stroke remains poorly defined.[38–40]

In this day and age, various surgical techniques to achieve LAA exclusion exists, as listed below:

- Over-sew technique with or without excision of the appendage either via an endocardial or epicardial approach.
- Device-enabled techniques
  - Non cutting stapler (e.g., Endo GIA II, Medtronic, Minneapolis, MN, USA or EZ45, Ethicon Inc., Cincinnati, OH, USA)
  - Cutting stapler (e.g., Echelon Flex, Ethicon Inc., New Brunswick, NJ, USA)
  - Snaring systems which only gain marginal attention in the cardiothoracic community
  - Clip Systems (e.g., AtriClip, AtriCure Inc, West Chester, OH, USA)

A major limitation of surgical LAA ligation is recanalization or incomplete closure of the orifice, or occlusion involving only a partial length of the appendage resulting in a residual "stump." Early studies evaluating the success rates of LAA closure revealed surprisingly poor results. The incidence of failure of LAA exclusion, ubiquitously defined by echocardiographic assessment as the presence of residual flow between the left atrium and appendage or a persistent stump greater than 1 cm in length, was demonstrated to be as high as 60% of cases.[41,42] This led to traditional techniques, particularly simple over-sewing without LAA excision and non cutting stapler devices which were found to have the highest failure rates to fall out of favor, and the advent of modern techniques with superior success rates. The most robust clinical experience currently available involves the AtriClip device, a parallel clamp with cloth covering that exerts uniform pressure at the base of the LAA, which aims to achieve atrophy of the LAA. Success rates using this device were reported to be as high as 94%.[43,44]

While the efficacy of stroke prevention in percutaneously delivered LAA occlusion devices is well substantiated by data, the case is different in its surgical counterpart, and extrapolation demands caution as although they are conceptually similar, the differences in technique of deliverance may translate to a significant difference in clinical outcomes. An eagerly anticipated large, randomized surgical-controlled trial, the LAAOS III trial, assessing concomitant LAA exclusion in patients with AF undergoing cardiac surgery is currently enrolling patients to deliver the long needed robust data for surgical LAA closure.

Confirmation of completeness of surgical LAA closure by imaging is crucial prior to making a decision about the need for long-term oral anticoagulation. Considering the present lack of concrete clinical efficacy data for stroke prevention, discontinuation of anticoagulation should be all the more avoided if closure is inadequate, whereas it may be considered in cases of successful closure and high clinical risk of bleeding. Intraoperative surveillance for complete closure is done routinely with transesophageal echocardiogram (TEE). Conversely, routine performance of further follow-up postoperative imaging, typically beyond 3 months, either by TEE or computerized tomography angiography (CTA) remains in question. At least in the post-AtriClip population, there is respectable data to justify against this, with studies showing lasting complete closure in all cases wherein intraoperative TEE demonstrated satisfactory device placement and complete closure.[44–46] That said, the decision to pursue follow-up imaging should be considered if other techniques were used and individualized based on whether or not it will impact decision about long-term oral anticoagulation.

SUMMARY

A significant overlap exists between mitral valve diseases and a wide array of electrical disturbances of the heart, occurring as epiphenomena or direct sequelae of one another. Mitral valve interventions are not uncommonly faced with postoperative conduction disturbances or arrhythmia that may warrant placement of cardiac implantable electrical devices. Advancement in device technologies has opened doors to unique therapeutic approaches for the various arrhythmic complications of this patient population and is deserving of further exploration. Needless to say, comprehensive management of mitral valve diseases demands special attention to the electrical system of the heart, and the same can be said in reverse. Hence, a complete mitral valve heart team is one that is built upon a collaborative partnership between cardiology, cardiothoracic surgery, and electrophysiology.

CASE-BASED ASSESSMENT

1. A 76-year-old man underwent mitral valve repair with an annuloplasty ring and neochords via lateral thoracotomy. At the time of surgery, two epicardial atrial pacing wires were placed. It is now POD #1 and the patient is awake, extubated, and hemodynamically stable. The electrocardiogram (ECG) is shown in Fig. 12.1.
   What is the next best step?

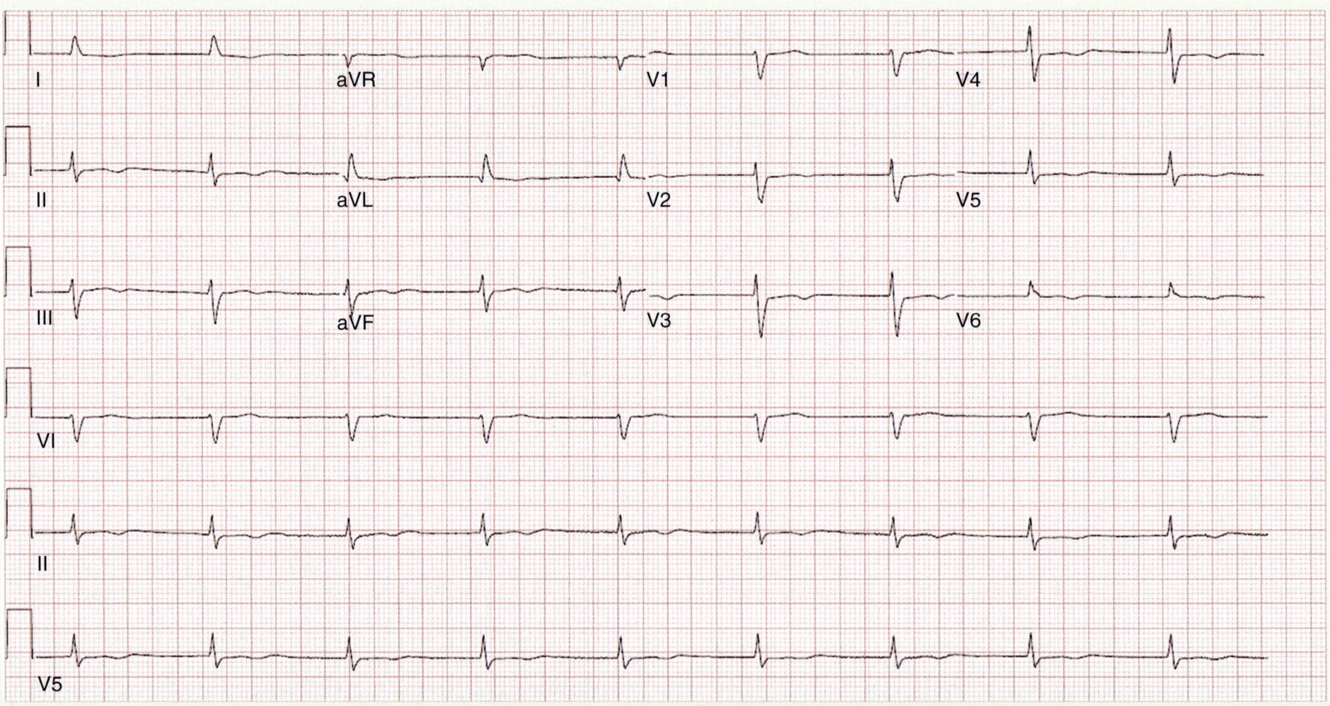

Fig. 12.1 The ECG of a 76-old-man discussed in question 1 of the Case-Based Assessment.

A. Start a dobutamine infusion.
B. Begin pacing at 70 bpm from the epicardial atrial wires.
C. Place a transvenous RV temporary pacemaker and monitor for recovery.
D. Place a permanent dual-chamber pacemaker.

2. A 63-year-old woman with symptomatic mitral regurgitation due to mitral valve prolapse (MVP) and a 3-year history of persistent atrial fibrillation undergoes mitral valve repair with pulmonary vein isolation and mitral isthmus ablation with radiofrequency energy and left atrial appendage closure with an atrial clip device. She leaves the OR in a paced atrial rhythm with intact AV conduction at 80 bpm and is placed on amiodarone and low-dose metoprolol. She recovers well but is 100% atrial paced for 3 days in the ICU. Every time the atrial pacing cable is disconnected to evaluate for underlying rhythm there is a pause for several seconds and the cable is reconnected. The next step in her care should be:
A. Placing a permanent dual-chamber pacemaker.
B. Stoping amiodarone and metoprolol and reassess.
C. Adjusting the rate of the temporary pacemaker.
D. Starting a dobutamine infusion.

3. A 38-year-old man is resuscitated from an out-of-hospital cardiac arrest due to ventricular fibrillation. Coronary angiography showed no significant coronary artery disease. An echocardiogram showed mildly dilated LV with normal LV systolic function, bileaflet mitral valve prolapse, and moderate to severe MR. Telemetry showed sinus rhythm with occasional PVCs, and MRI revealed areas of LGE in the basal lateral LV. He is diagnosed with malignant MVP and undergoes successful MV repair. His echo on post-op day 3 showed a normally functioning mitral valve with no MVP and trace MR. The LV systolic function remains normal. Prior to discharge, this patient should:
A. Undergo placement of a dual-chamber ICD.
B. Undergo placement of an entirely subcutaneous ICD system.
C. Have a wearable vest defibrillator for 3 months and then repeat an echocardiogram.
D. None of the above. He had definitive surgery and he is no longer at risk for sudden cardiac arrest.

See page 316 for the answers.

REFERENCES

1. John RM, Kumar S. Sinus node and atrial arrhythmias. *Circulation*. 2016;133(19):1892–1900. doi:10.1161/CIRCULATIONAHA.116.018011.
2. Jackson LR, Rathakrishnan B, Campbell K, et al. Sinus node dysfunction and atrial fibrillation: a reversible phenomenon? *Pacing Clin Electrophysiol*. 2017;40(4):442–450. doi:10.1111/pace.13030.
3. van den Berg MP, van Gelder IC. Atrial fibrillation and sinus node dysfunction. *J Am Coll Cardiol*. 2001;38(5):1585. doi:10.1016/s0735-1097(01)01546-7.
4. Kulikov AA, Bokeria LA. Assessment of sinoatrial node function in patients with persistent and long-standing persistent forms of atrial fibrillation after Maze III procedure combined with mitral valve operation. *J Atr Fibrillation*. 2016;9(1):1408. doi:10.4022/jafib.1408.
5. Moskowitz G, Hong KN, Giustino G, et al. Incidence and risk factors for permanent pacemaker implantation following mitral or aortic valve surgery. *J Am Coll Cardiol*. 2019;74(21):2607–2620. doi:10.1016/j.jacc.2019.08.1064.
6. Kim D, Shim CY, Hong GR, et al. Sinus node dysfunction after surgical atrial fibrillation ablation with concomitant mitral valve surgery: determinants and clinical outcomes. *PLoS One*. 2018;13(9):1–13. doi:10.1371/journal.pone.0203828.
7. Dagenais F, Ailawadi G, Perrault LP, et al. Pacemaker implantation after mitral valve surgery with atrial fibrillation ablation. *J Am Coll Cardiol*. 2019;73(19):2427–2435.
8. Lee JMS, Kalman JM. Sinus node dysfunction and atrial fibrillation: two sides of the same coin? *Europace*. 2013;15(2):161–162. doi:10.1093/europace/eus223.
9. Pasic M, Musci M, Siniawski H, et al. Transient sinus node dysfunction after the Cox-maze III procedure in patients with organic heart disease and chronic fixed atrial fibrillation. *J Am Coll Cardiol*. 1998;32(4):1040–1047. doi:10.1016/S0735-1097(98)00358-1.
10. Chung MK. Cardiac surgery: postoperative arrhythmias. *Crit Care Med*. 2000;28(10 Suppl.):N136–N144. doi:10.1097/00003246-200010001-00005.
11. Merin O, Ilan M, Oren A, et al. Permanent pacemaker implantation following cardiac surgery: indications and long-term follow-up. *Pacing Clin Electrophysiol*. 2009 Jan;32(1):7–12. doi: 10.1111/j.1540-8159.2009.02170.x. PMID: 19140907.
12. Brignole M, Auricchio A, Baron-Esquivias G, et al. 2013 ESC guidelines on cardiac pacing and cardiac resynchronization therapy. *Eur Heart J*. 2013;34(29):2281–2329. doi:10.1093/eurheartj/eht150.
13. Socie P, Nicot F, Baudinaud P, et al. Frequency of recovery from complete atrioventricular block after cardiac surgery. *Am J Cardiol*. 2017;120(10):1841–1846. doi:10.1016/j.amjcard.2017.07.090.
14. Bis J, Go K. Permanent pacemaker implantation after cardiac surgery: optimization of the decision making process. *J Thorac Cardiovasc Surg*. 2021;162(3):816–824. doi:10.1016/j.jtcvs.2020.01.082 e3.
15. Kim MH, Deeb GM, Eagle KA, et al. Complete atrioventricular block after valvular surgery and the timing of pacemaker implantation. *Am J Cardiol*. 2001;87(5):649–651.
16. Veasey RA, Arya A, Silberbauer J, et al. The relationship between right ventricular pacing and atrial fibrillation burden and disease progression in patients with paroxysmal atrial fibrillation: the long-MinVPACE study. *Europace*. 2011;13(6):815–820. doi:10.1093/europace/euq463.
17. Lamas GA, Lee KL, Sweeney MO, et al. Ventricular pacing or dual-chamber pacing for sinus-node dysfunction. *N Engl J Med*. 2002;346(24):1854–1862.
18. Pastore G, Zanon F, Baracca E, et al. The risk of atrial fibrillation during right ventricular pacing. *Europace*. 2016;18(3):353–358. doi:10.1093/europace/euv268.
19. Fung JWH, Yu CM, Chan JYS, et al. Effects of cardiac resynchronization therapy on incidence of atrial fibrillation in patients with poor left ventricular systolic function. 2005;96(5):728–731. doi:10.1016/j.amjcard.2005.04.053.
20. Sharma AK, Heist EK. The utility of cardiac resynchronization therapy in patients with atrial fibrillation. *J Innov Card Rhythm Manag*. 2012;3(January):621–626. doi:10.19102/icrm.2012.030104.
21. Miranda R, Almeida S, Brandão L, et al. Acute severe mitral regurgitation as an early complication of pacemaker implantation. *Europace*. 2010;12(12):1791–1792. doi:10.1093/europace/euq191.
22. Khatib M, Tolosana JM, Trucco E, et al. EAARN score, a predictive score for mortality in patients receiving cardiac resynchronization therapy based on pre-implantation risk factors. *Eur J Heart Fail*. 2014;16(7):802–809.
23. Spartera M, Galderisi M, Mele D, et al. Role of cardiac dyssynchrony and resynchronization therapy in functional mitral regurgitation. *Eur Heart J Cardiovasc Imaging*. 2016;17(5):471–480. doi:10.1093/ehjci/jev352.

24. Cabrera-bueno F, Molina-mora MJ, Alzueta J, et al. Persistence of secondary mitral regurgitation and response to cardiac resynchronization therapy. *Eur J Echocardiogr.* 2010;11(2):131–137. doi:10.1093/ejechocard/jep184.
25. Miller MA, Dukkipati SR, Turagam M, et al. Arrhythmic mitral valve prolapse. *J Am Coll Cardiol.* 2018;72(23):2904–2914. doi:10.1016/j.jacc.2018.09.048.
26. Spartalis M, Tzatzaki E, Spartalis E, et al. Mitral valve prolapse: An underestimated cause of sudden cardiac death—a current review of the literature. *J Thorac Dis.* 2017;9(12):5390–5398. doi:10.21037/jtd.2017.11.14.
27. Han HC, Ha FJ, Teh AW, et al. Mitral valve prolapse and sudden cardiac death: a systematic review. *J Am Heart Assoc.* 2018;7(23):e010584. doi:10.1161/JAHA.118.010584.
28. Basso C, Iliceto S, Thiene G, et al. Mitral valve prolapse, ventricular arrhythmias, and sudden death. *Circulation.* 2019;140(11):952–964. doi:10.1161/CIRCULATIONAHA.118.034075.
29. Hohnloser S, Heinz K, Dorian P, et al. Prophylactic use of an implantable cardioverter-defibrillator after acute myocardial infarction. *N Engl J Med.* 2004;351(24):2481–2488.
30. Yosuke DX. Risk Factors of recurrence of atrial fibrillation (AF) after AF surgery in patients with AF and mitral valve disease. *Semin Thorac Cardiovasc Surg.* 2018;30(3):271–278. doi:10.1053/j.semtcvs.2018.01.004.
31. Altman RK, Proietti R, Barrett CD, et al. Management of refractory atrial fibrillation post surgical ablation. *Ann Cardiothorac Surg.* 2014;3(1):91–97. doi:10.3978/j.issn.2225-319X.2013.12.08.
32. Baman TS, Gupta SK, Billakanty SR, et al. Time to cardioversion of recurrent atrial arrhythmias after catheter ablation of atrial fibrillation and long-term clinical outcome. *J Cardiovasc Electrophysiol.* 2009;20(12):1321–1325. doi:10.1111/j.1540-8167.2009.01553.x.
33. Lee SH, Kim JB, Cho WC, et al. The influence of age on atrial fibrillation recurrence after the maze procedure in patients with giant left atrium. *J Thorac Cardiovasc Surg.* 2006;141(4):1015–1019. doi:10.1016/j.jtcvs.2010.08.036.
34. Damiano RJ, Schwartz FH, Bailey MS, et al. The Cox maze IV procedure: Predictors of late recurrence. *J Thorac Cardiovasc Surg.* 2009;141(1):113–121. doi:10.1016/j.jtcvs.2010.08.067.
35. Maroto LC, Carnero M, Silva JA, et al. Early recurrence is a predictor of late failure in surgical ablation of atrial fibrillation. *Interact CardioVasc Thorac Surg.* 2011;12(5):681–686. doi:10.1510/icvts.2010.261842.
36. Pokushalov E, Romanov A, De Melis M, et al. Progression of atrial fibrillation after a failed initial ablation procedure in patients with paroxysmal atrial fibrillation. *Circ Arrhythm Electrophysiol.* 2013;6(4):754–760. doi:10.1161/CIRCEP.113.000495.
37. Hwang SK, Yoo JS, Kim JB, et al. Long-term outcomes of the maze procedure combined with mitral valve repair: risk of thromboembolism without anticoagulation therapy. *Ann Thorac Surg.* 2015;100(3):840–844. doi:10.1016/j.athoracsur.2015.02.073.
38. Hanke T. Surgical management of the left atrial appendage: a must or a myth? *Eur J Cardiothorac Surg.* 2018;53(1):i33–i38. doi:10.1093/ejcts/ezy088.
39. Caliskan E, Emmert MY. Surgical occlusion of the left atrial appendage: it is time to adopt newer techniques! *Eur Heart J.* 2018;39(45):3993–3995. doi:10.1093/eurheartj/ehy704.
40. Squiers JJ, Edgerton JR. Surgical closure of the left atrial appendage: the past, the present, the future. *J Atr Fibrillation.* 2018;10(5):1–5. doi:10.4022/jafib.1642.
41. Kanderian AS, Gillinov AM, Pettersson GB, et al. Success of surgical left atrial appendage closure. Assessment by transesophageal echocardiography. *J Am Coll Cardiol.* 2008;52(11):924–929. doi:10.1016/j.jacc.2008.03.067.
42. Dawson AG, Asopa S, Dunning J. Should patients undergoing cardiac surgery with atrial fibrillation have left atrial appendage exclusion?. *Interact Cardiovasc Thorac Surg.* 2010;10(2):306–311. doi:10.1510/icvts.2009.227991.
43. Ellis CR, Aznaurov SG, Patel NJ, et al. Angiographic efficacy of the atriclip left atrial appendage exclusion device placed by minimally invasive thoracoscopic approach. *JACC Clin Electrophysiol.* 2017;3(12):1356–1365. doi:10.1016/j.jacep.2017.03.008.
44. Ailawadi G, Gerdisch MW, Harvey RL, et al. Exclusion of the left atrial appendage with a novel device: early results of a multicenter trial. *J Thorac Cardiovasc Surg.* 2011;142(5):1002–1009. doi:10.1016/j.jtcvs.2011.07.052 e1.
45. Emmert MY, Puippe G, Baumüller S, et al. Safe, effective and durable epicardial left atrial appendage clip occlusion in patients with atrial fibrillation undergoing cardiac surgery: First long-term results from a prospective device trial. *Eur J Cardio-thoracic Surg.* 2014;45(1):126–131. doi:10.1093/ejcts/ezt204.
46. Kurfirst V, Mokraaék A, Aänádyová J, et al. Epicardial clip occlusion of the left atrial appendage during cardiac surgery provides optimal surgical results and long-term stability. *Interact Cardiovasc Thorac Surg.* 2017;25(1):37–40. doi:10.1093/icvts/ivx065.

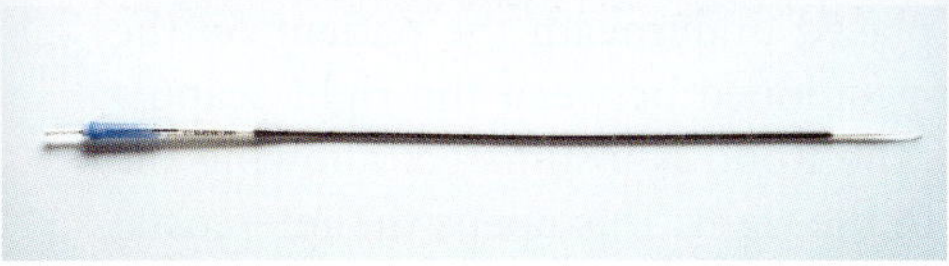

13

Medical Devices and Instruments

K. Marco Rodriguez, Chidinma Tiko-Okoye, Shaylyn C. Bennett, Roberto Rodriguez

CHAPTER OUTLINE

LEARNING OBJECTIVES

- Basic knowledge of sternotomy instruments
- Basic knowledge of thoracotomy and mini-thoracotomy instruments
- Review of available catheters and cannulas
- Tips and pitfalls of the devices and instruments

MITRAL APPROACHES

Median Sternotomy

The approach to the mitral valve, through a median sternotomy, requires the same basic principles required for open heart surgery and cardiopulmonary bypass. For cardiopulmonary bypass, the ascending aorta is cannulated directly; venous drainage can be accomplished by direct bi-caval cannulation or percutaneous bi-caval cannulation. The percutaneous bi-caval cannulation can be done with a single venous cannula or two venous cannulas (right internal jugular vein and common femoral vein), under transesophageal echocardiogram (TEE) guidance. If using a single venous cannula, a 25 Fr will suffice. In patients requiring more than 5 L/min, a 28 Fr or a 26 Fr cannula can be used. The ALPINE family of femoral venous cannulas, manufactured by Surge Medical, have multiple reinforced drainage baskets to provide optimal drainage from the superior vena cava (SVC), right atrium, and inferior vena cava (IVC), simultaneously (Fig. 13.1). The bi-caval view must confirm placement of the guidewire into the SVC from the common femoral vein. Once the guidewire is in place, TEE Transesophageal echocardiogram must confirm placement of the cannula as far up the SVC as possible. This TEE guidance is critical in mini-thoracotomy approaches. During full sternotomy, manual confirmation of cannula placement is recommended along with TEE.

In case of two cannulas needed for venous drainage, a second cannula can be placed from the right internal jugular vein into the SVC. A 15 Fr or a 17 Fr cannula can be used. We prefer to use a stiff or extra stiff guidewire when placing the 26 Fr, 28 Fr, and any internal jugular cannula placement. This facilitates placement and prevents wire bending and false tracking of the cannulas. The use of serial dilators at the delivery site is recommended. Any dilators can work, but we recommend using the Maquet Avalon Elite vascular access kits (Fig. 13.2) (Getinge, Wayne, NJ). It contains a 210 cm guidewire, along with 10, 12, 16, 20, 24, 26, and 30 Fr dilators. They enable access by the Seldinger technique with an extended dilator tip, designed for smooth vessel insertion and guidewire tracking.

Antegrade and retrograde catheters are placed for cardioplegia delivery and de-airing of the heart. Once cardiopulmonary bypass is initiated, aortic cross-clamp is performed and arrest is initiated. We then proceed with exposure of the left atrium. Several pericardial sutures are placed at the level of the SVC and IVC. With proper retraction and opening of the left pleural space, the interatrial groove is exposed. The atrium is opened at the level of the right superior pulmonary vein; the atriotomy is extended down towards the IVC. Once the atriotomy is performed, the sternal retractors with mitral valve exposure extensions are placed. Several full sternotomy retractors are available: the McCarthy/Kapp surgical retractor (Kapp Surgical Instrument Inc, Cleveland, Ohio), the Cosgrove sternal retractor (Kapp Surgical Instrument Inc, Cleveland, Ohio), and the Morse sternal retractor (Teleflex Inc, Morrisville, NC) (Fig. 13.3). These retractors have adaptable mitral valve

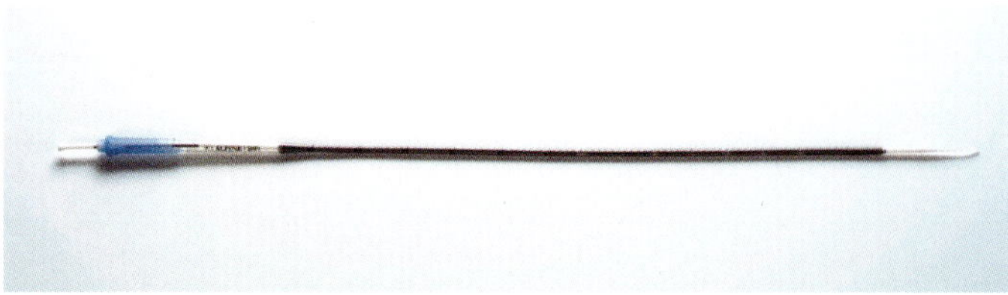

Fig. 13.1 The ALPINE FVC is designed with a tapered distal tip and mating extended introducer to provide insertion into the femoral vein and navigation up to the SVC. Multiple reinforced drainage baskets have been placed at strategic locations to provide optimal drainage from the SVC, right atrium, and IVC. The femoral venous catheters are available in five diameters, from 20 Fr through 28 Fr, to accommodate various patient sizes and surgical preferences. *IVC, Inferior vena cava; SVC, superior vena cava.* (From Surge Cardiovascular, Grand Rapids, MI.)

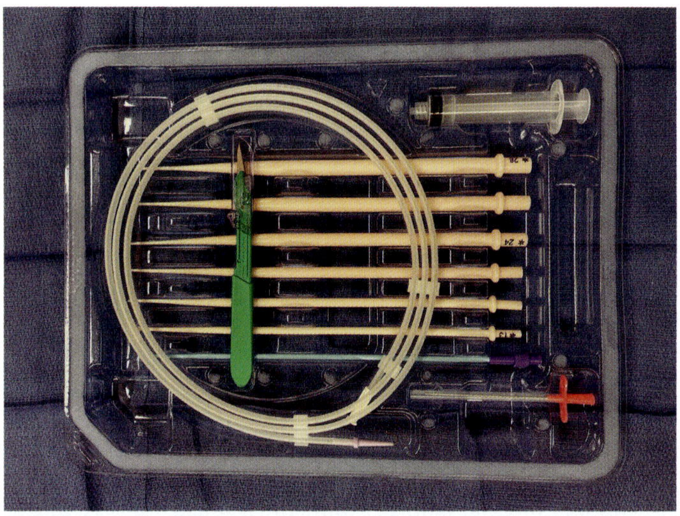

Fig. 13.2 Maquet Avalon Elite vascular access kits. These dilators support vascular cannulation procedures to ensure safe vascular access. They enable vascular access by Seldinger technique. The extended dilator tip is designed for smooth vessel insertion and guidewire tracking. They have a large range of dilator sizes for standard 0.038 inch guidewires. (Getinge, Wayne, NJ.)

extensions, designed to withdraw the left atrium and expose the mitral valve.

Instrumentation for manipulation, repair, or replacement of the mitral valve can be achieved with standard instrumentation. We prefer to use the minimally invasive instruments (telescopic instruments) to facilitate mitral valve surgery. In the minimally invasive section, a brief description of the instrumentation will be done.

Minimally Invasive (Mini-Thoracotomy) Approach

There are many options for cannulation, instrumentation, and approach for mitral valve repairs or replacements via right thoracotomy. In this section, our approach to the mitral valve, through a right thoracotomy approach, is described. Some consider this to be a minimally invasive approach. The right thoracotomy incision is no larger than 4 cm, with a femoral cutdown and direct cannulation of the femoral vessels. The mitral valve repair or replacement is visualized with a 5-mm camera.

The patient is placed supine in the operating table, and a Roho Thyroid Pillow is placed underneath the patient on the right side. The pillow is positioned between the right scapula and the right iliac crest. The Roho is insufflated, allowing the patient to slightly rotate to the right. This opens the intercostal spaces and the right femoral area.

Once the patient is positioned, they are prepped and draped in the usual manner. A right femoral cutdown is performed, exposing the common femoral vein and artery. A 3 to 4 cm incision is made on the right antero lateral aspect of the chest wall (Fig. 13.4). The pectoralis major should be retracted cephalad, and the third intercostal space should be identified.[1]

The third intercostal space is dissected, and the chest wall is entered. The lungs are deflated, and the pulmonary trunk is visualized. The trunk must be easily accessed from the incision site. At this point, a soft tissue retractor is placed. We prefer the ThruPort soft tissue retractor, which is used to allow visualization of intrathoracic structures and provide entry for the instruments into the thoracic cavity during specific cardiac surgical procedures (Fig. 13.5). To increase adhesion, the Compound Benzoin Tincture may be applied to the skin. In morbidly obese patients, the Alexis wound retractor facilitates exposure and access to the chest cavity (see Fig. 13.5).

Then, the chest wall retractor is placed, the diaphragm is visualized, and a 3-0 Vicryl or Ethibond (Ethicon, Raritan, NJ) suture is placed at the dome. A 14 gauge IV is then used to pass the suture through the chest wall, with the help of any crochet suture hook (Fig. 13.6). The diaphragm is then retracted in a caudal direction. At this point in time, heparin is given and cannulation is initiated.

The femoral venous cannula is placed with echocardiographic guidance. The wire is placed, and evidence of wire positioning from the IVC to the SVC must be identified. The bi-caval view will facilitate wire positioning. If the procedure is being performed in a hybrid room or a room with fluoroscopic imaging, one can easily confirm proper wire placement. Venous cannulas can be placed with a 0.035 guidewire with a J-tip. Most cannulas contain an insertion kit with the 0.035 guidewire. In case the required flow for cardiopulmonary bypass is greater than 5 L/min, a venous cannula greater than 25 Fr is recommended. For all cannulas greater than 25 Fr we recommend using a stiffer wire for placement. A 180 or 260 cm Amplatz extra- or super-stiff guidewire with a J-tip (Fig. 13.7) is recommended to avoid false tracking in the iliacs and IVC. This wire is also recommended for any right internal jugular venous cannula placement.

We recommend a second venous drainage. In the right internal jugular vein, a 15 to 17 Fr venous cannula can be placed for further drainage. Another option is the use of an endo pulmonary vent (EPV), placed by anesthesia. The vent is placed by anesthesia, and placement in the pulmonary artery can be confirmed by echocardiogram or fluoroscopy. The patient setup can be seen in Fig. 13.8.

The arterial cannula should be placed with some echocardiographic guidance. The Seldinger technique must be used to place all cannulas. The wire placement, in the descending

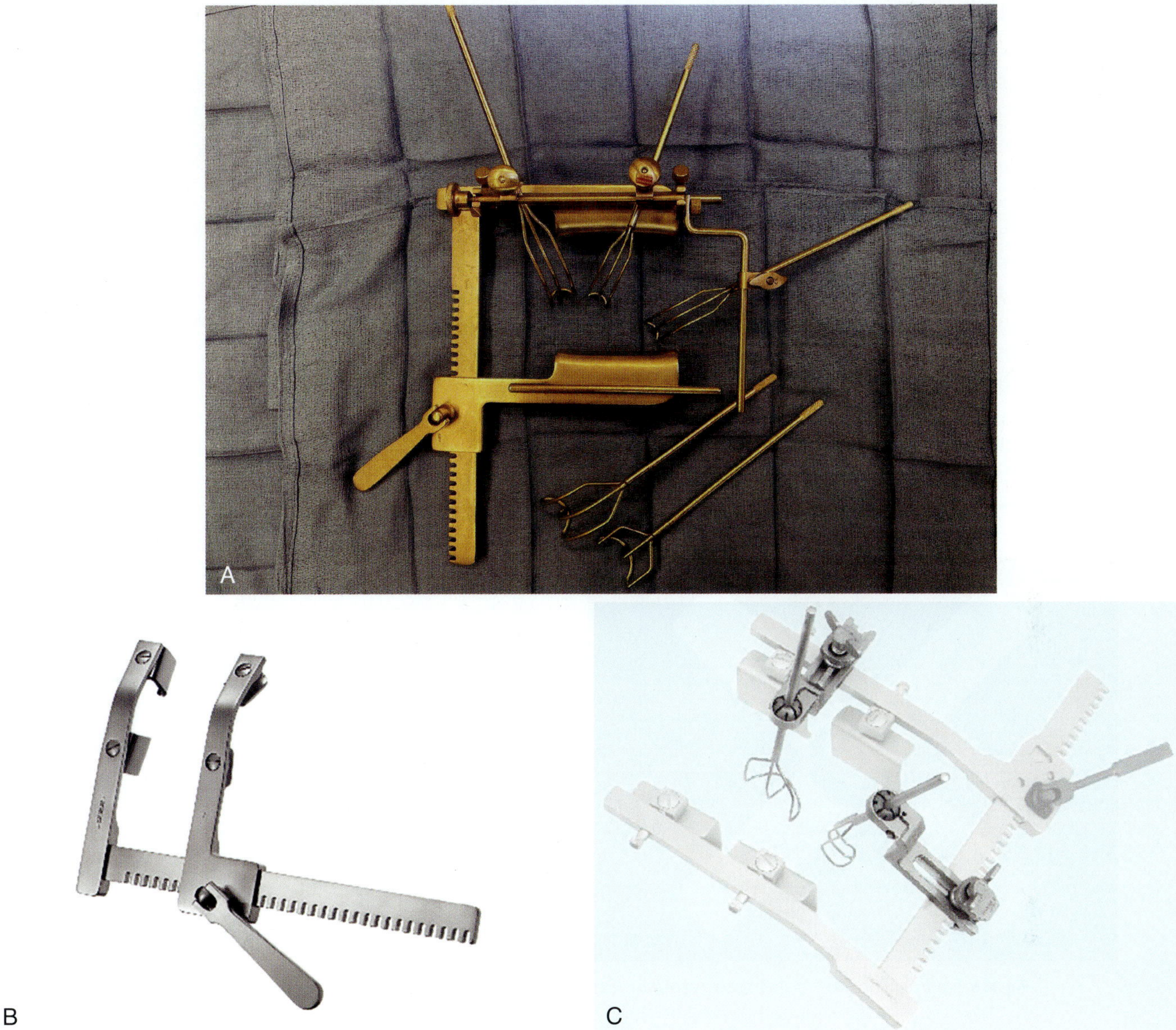

Fig. 13.3 (A) Mitral valve retractor. This instrument is mounted in a sternal retractor. It provides exceptional and consistent exposure of the right and left atrium, tricuspid and mitral valve for surgical repair or replacement, while reducing the need for surgical assistance. (B and C) Morse sternal retractor. This retractor has multiple ball joint adapter bayonets designed to hold malleable atrial retractors. (B, C, Permission granted by Integra LifeSciences Corporation, Princeton, New Jersey, USA.)

thoracic aorta, must be confirmed by echocardiogram before placing the arterial cannula. The cannula size is dependent on the size of the common femoral artery and the required flows. Sizes are available from 15 to 23 Fr.

Cardiopulmonary bypass is initiated, and ventilation is terminated.

Once extracorporeal circulation is established, the pericardium is opened 2 cm anterior to the phrenic nerve on the right. Three stay sutures are placed on each margin of the opened pericardium, allowing for visualization and exposure of the aorta and the interatrial groove.

Cardioplegia delivery can be accomplished in an antegrade or retrograde fashion. Retrograde cardioplegia delivery can be distributed with the ProPlege peripheral cardioplegia device. This can be placed by the anesthesia team, with echocardiographic and fluoroscopic guidance (Fig. 13.9). We commonly use an extended-length antegrade cardioplegia cannula. A 3-0 Ethibond pledget suture is placed in the ascending aorta, and the antegrade catheter is placed and anchored. The antegrade cardioplegia cannula has been designed with a sharp beveled introducer needle for insertion, and cannula side ports have been designed for enhanced cardioplegia solution flow. The placement

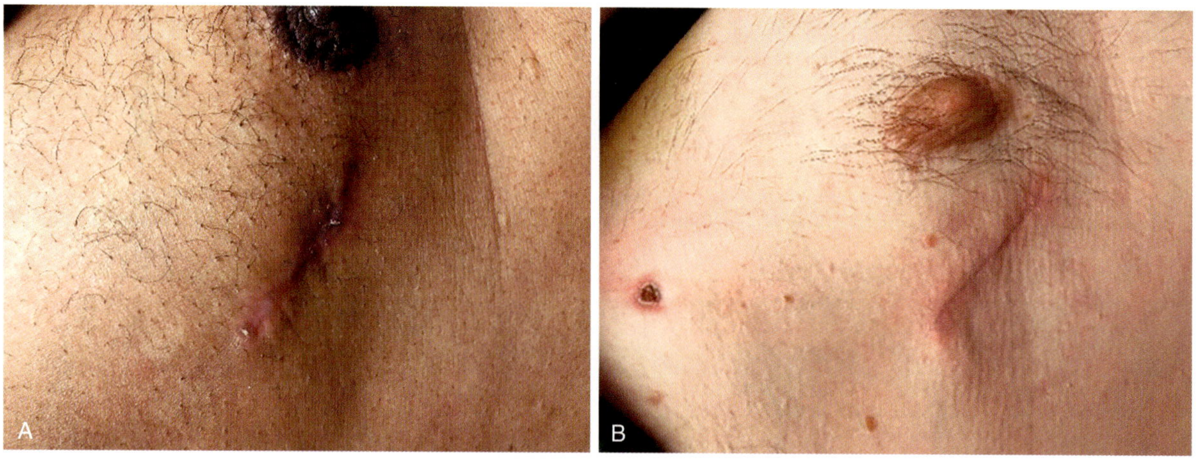

Fig. 13.4 Incision Location and Size. Incision at the anterior axillary line at the inferior border of the pectoralis major. This corresponds to the 3rd interconstal space (A and B). The camera port site can be seen in B, this site is also used for chest tube insertion at the end of the procedure.

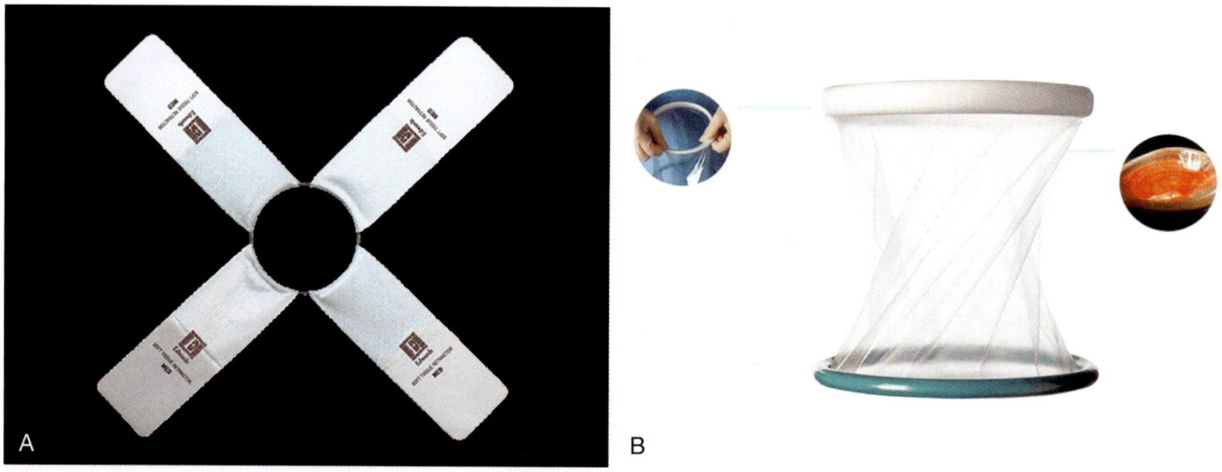

Fig. 13.5 (A) The ThruPort soft tissue retractor (Edwards Lifesciences Corporation, Irvine, CA) is used to allow visualization of intrathoracic structures and provide entry for the instruments into the thoracic cavity during specific cardiac surgical procedures. The ThruPort soft tissue retractor is designed to be inserted into an intercostal incision and retract tissue to form a port. (B) Alexis wound protectors/retractors (Applied Medical Resources Corporation, Rancho Santa Margarita, CA) provide 360 degrees of circumferential, atraumatic retraction. Alexis wound protector/retractors maintain moisture at the incision site and reduce superficial surgical site infections following colorectal surgeries.

is similar to the open sternotomy cases. The 3-0 pledgeted suture will facilitate closure with the Cor-Knot device, once removed.

At this point in time, a 5 mm, zero-degree camera is placed at the mid axillary line, approximately at 8 o'clock. The CO_2 is initiated through the camera port, and light source is started. Passive or active camera holders can be used to facilitate viewing. An extensive variety of passive camera holders (Fig. 13.10) (some active) are available in the market. We currently use an old AESOP.[2] Aortic clamping can be performed with the IntraClude intra-aortic occlusion balloon or the Chitwood Clamp (Fig. 13.11). If the occlusion balloon is used, the EndoReturn arterial cannula must be used for femoral access. The EndoReturn has the capability of delivering antegrade cardioplegia, and the use of the antegrade cannula is not necessary (Fig. 13.12).

A standard dose of cardioplegia is delivered to the root, and cardiac arrest is started. We use 1250 mm of cold del Nido solution. After cardioplegia delivery, dissection along the interatrial groove is done, and the left atrium is entered. The atriotomy is then extended to expose the mitral valve. We utilize the Obadia 3D atrial retractor (Fig. 13.13), which is inserted in the third intercostal space, close to the sternal edge. The valve is evaluated, and the approach to repair or replacement is determined. The annuloplasty or replacement is then carried out in a standard fashion.

There are some key instruments that facilitate the repair or replacement of the valve. The minimally invasive cardiac

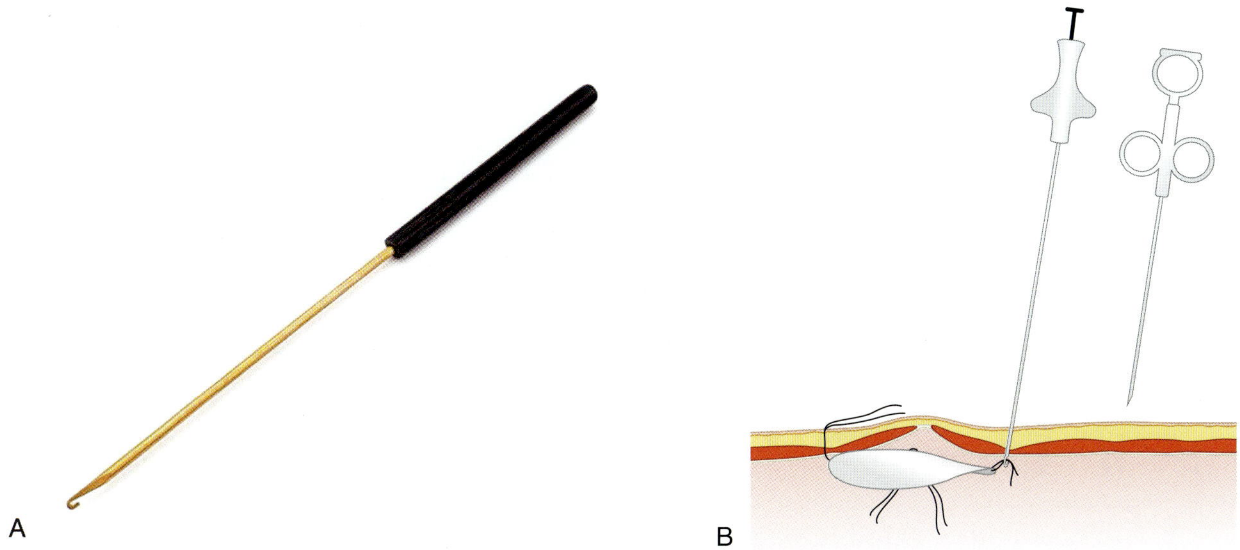

Fig. 13.6 (A) Any crochet suture hook can be utilized along with a 14 gauge IV. (B) The use of laparoscopic suture passers can offer the precise control of a rigid needle that can easily pass through subcutaneous tissue. (Re-drawn from CooperSurgical Inc., Trumbull, CT.)

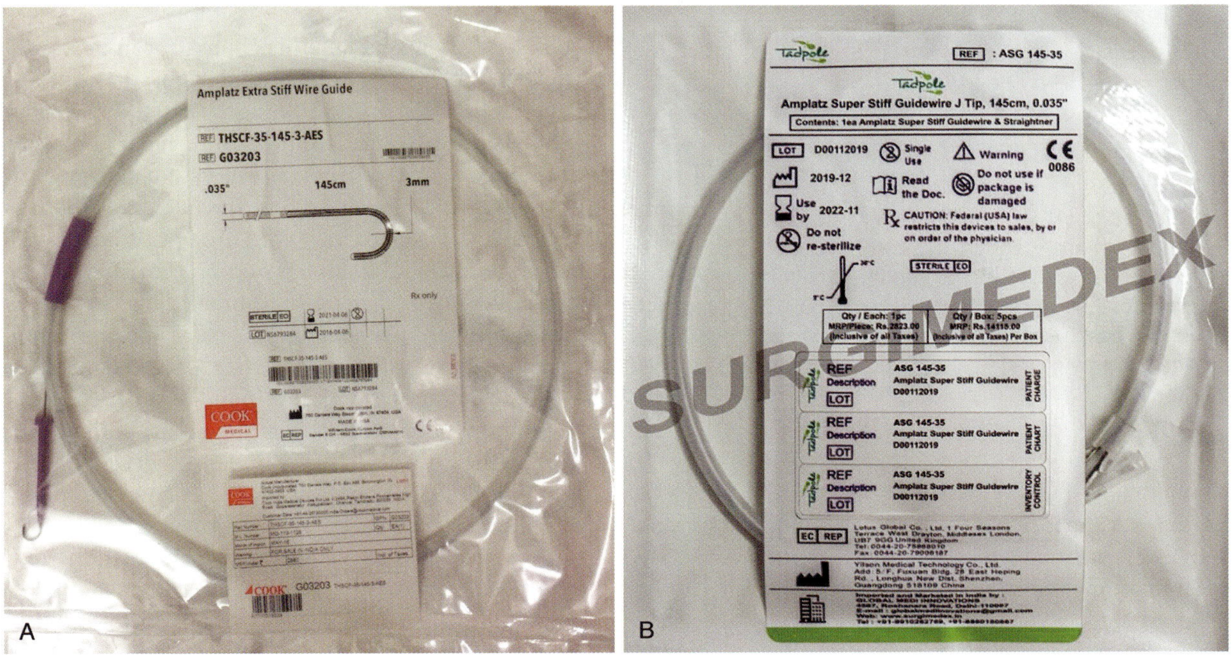

Fig. 13.7 Amplatz Extra-Stiff Guide wire for Femoral and Jugular Venous Cannula Placement. (A, From Cook Medical, Bloomington, IN; B, from Surgimedex, Delhi, India.)

instruments, also known as video-assisted thoracoscopic surgery (VATS) instruments, are available in a variety of lengths and types. The minimally invasive cardiac surgery (MICS) Debakey forceps, the Resano forceps, curved scissors, and needle holders can be accessible in 11.75 inch, 14 inch, and 16 inch of total length (Wexler Surgical, Houston, TX).[3] These instruments are necessary and facilitate access to the mitral valve for repairs and replacements (Fig. 13.14). The laparoscopic or VATS knot pusher can also facilitate closure of the left atrium, as well as repair of the mitral valve. Finally, the LSI Solutions Cor-Knot device is an automated suture fastening system that provides a strong, secure, and safe alternative to hand-tied knots. It has also shown to significantly reduce the operating times and cardiopulmonary bypass times.[4,5]

The left atrium is closed with continuous 4-0 polypropylene sutures. The heart is de-aired, which is confirmed using transesophageal echo. The aortic cross-clamp is then removed. A period is allowed for cardiac recovery, and the patient is re-warmed.

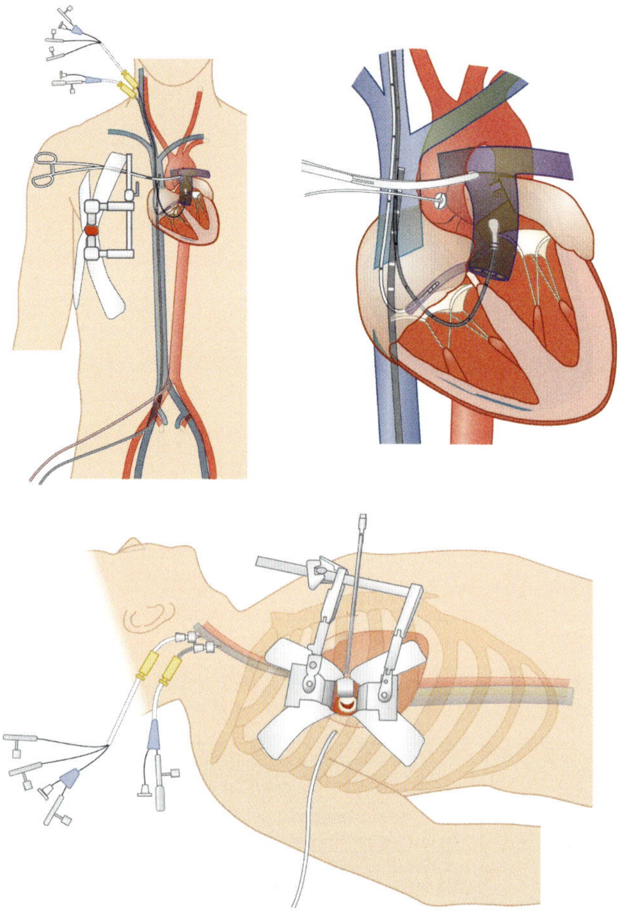

A

B

Fig. 13.8 Patient Setup. (A) Venous and arterial femoral cannulas in place. The endopulmonary vent (EPV) can be placed by anesthesia in the right internal jugular and guided into the pulmonary artery under echocardiographic guidance. The EPV can be substituted with a 15-17 Fr venous cannula in the superior vena cava. (B) The retractor is place in the 3rd intercostal space. (Redrawn from Javadikasgari H, Suri RM, Tappuni B, et al. Minimally invasive mitral valve repair. *Heart.* 2018;104:861–867.)

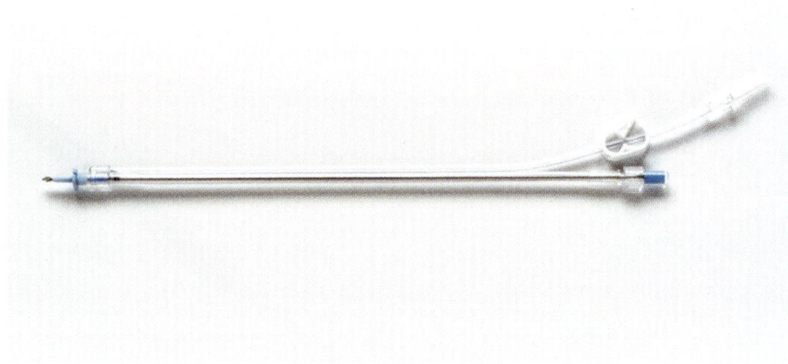

Fig. 13.9 Antegrade cannulae are designed to deliver cardioplegia solution to the heart via the coronary ostia in the normal direction of blood flow (antegrade perfusion). Aortic root cannulas are intended to infuse cardioplegia directly into the aortic root near the aortic valve. The Surge Cardiovascular line of Antegrade Cardioplegia Cannulae have been designed with a sharp beveled introducer needle for insertion and cannula side ports for enhanced cardioplegia solution flow. These antegrade cannulae are offered in two diameters, both with and without vent lines to match surgical preference. An extended length option is available to accommodate minimally invasive approaches. (From Surge Cardiovascular, Gran Rapids, MI.)

The aortic cross-clamp is removed, and cardiopulmonary bypass is discontinued. Protamine is then given for heparin reversal. The femoral cannulas are removed, and the femoral vessels are repaired. Intercostal blocks are performed with a cryoprobe. Blake drains (Ethicon, Sommerville, NJ) are placed for mediastinal and right chest drainage. The ribs are re-approximated with a double-stranded #1 PDS (polydioxanone) suture. The chest wound is closed in anatomic layers, with Vicryl in the subcutaneous tissue and Vicryl and Dermabond in the skin. The groin wound is closed in anatomic layers, using Vicryl in the subcutaneous tissue and Monocryl and Dermabond skin. Following completion of the case, post operative TEE is utilized to review ventricular function and assess functionality of the mitral valve.

Left Thoracotomy

The left posterior thoracotomy approach to the mitral valve in not commonly used. It was first described in 1960 by Nichols et al.[6] and Clowes et al.[7] This approach can be used in patients with multiple sternotomies and right thoracotomies. These patients have extensive adhesions, and a "new" approach can facilitate the exposure and procedure. It has also been described in patients with severe pectus excavatum deformity.[8]

The patient is brought into the operating room and placed supine in the operating table. Adequate anesthesia is established, and a double-lumen endotracheal tube is required. At this point in time, the left common femoral vein is accessed through a percutaneous approach. Using the Seldinger technique, an extra-stiff Amplatz wire (Marlborough, MA) is placed from the common femoral vein to the superior vena cava, with either fluoroscopic or echocardiographic guidance. The wire is kept sterile at this point, with plans to access once the patient is prepped and draped. The patient is now placed in a right lateral decubitus position. The chest is then opened using a left posterior lateral incision, through the fourth intercostal space. Standard thoracotomy retractors are used (Fig. 13.15). We use the Maquet off-pump (Getinge, Wayne, NJ) sternal retractor; it facilitates pericardial suture anchoring. With intermittent ventilation, the inferior pulmonary ligament is divided, and the descending thoracic aorta is exposed.

The patient is then fully heparinized, and the 20 Fr aortic cannula is used to cannulate the descending thoracic aorta in the usual manner. At this point in time, the wire and the left common femoral vein are exposed, and a femoral venous cannula 25 to 28 Fr is inserted under echocardiographic guidance. Cardiopulmonary bypass is initiated, and the patient is cooled down to 28°C, at which point ventricular fibrillation is initiated. The pericardium is then opened approximately 1 to 2 cm anterior to the phrenic nerve and retracted with retention sutures (Fig. 13.16). The left superior pulmonary vein is identified, as

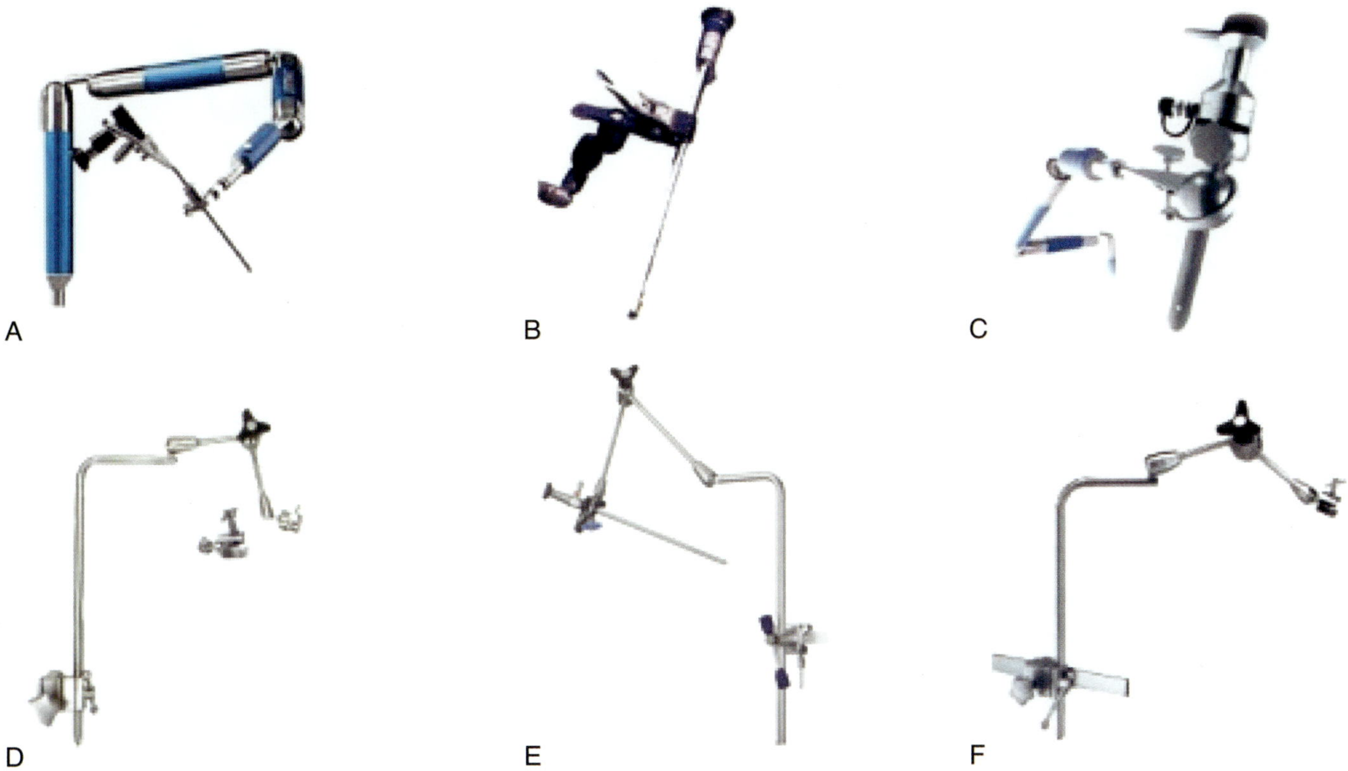

Fig. 13.10 Passive Camera Holders. They can be subdivided into products that facilitate single-handed repositioning (A–C) and the products that do not (D–F). (A) Unitrac (AESCULAP, Tuttlingen, Germany © B. Braun Melsungen AG.); (B) Endofreeze (AESCULAP, Tuttlingen, Germany © B. Braun Melsungen AG.); (C) Laparostat (CIVCO Medical Solutions, Coralville, IA); (D) Martin arm (Courtesy by KLS Martin Group); (E) Karl Storz holding system (© KARL STORZ SE & Co. KG, Germany); (F) Assisto (GEOMED Medizin-Technik, Tuttlingen, Germany.)

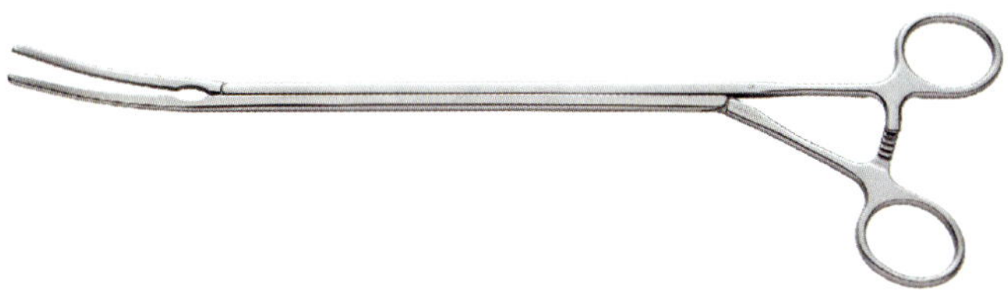

Fig. 13.11 The Thoracoscopic Chitwood DeBakey Clamp (Scanlan International, St. Paul, MN) was developed around 1996 for the repair and replacement of diseased heart valves using minimally invasive surgical procedures. It has a dual pivot point with a sliding shaft and traditional ring-style handles. This instrument can be used for both video-assisted thoracoscopic surgery (VATS) and minimally invasive surgery (MIS).

well as the left atrial appendage. The left atrium is entered at the level of the left superior pulmonary vein, and the incision is extended toward the base of the left atrial appendage.[9] A handheld retractor is then used to open the left atrium and retract anteriorly; the valve is visualized, and it is inverted, compared to the standard surgeon's view. The valve can then be replaced in the standard fashion. The left atrium is closed, re-warming and de-airing maneuvers are performed. The patient is then weaned from cardiopulmonary bypass. The left thoracotomy approach is reserved for patients with a history of multiple cardiac procedures with severe hostile chests. This approach can facilitate exposure and replacement of the mitral valve in such cases. This approach does have some disadvantages and contraindications. There is no access to the ascending aorta for direct aortic cross-camping and or cannulation, especially in these re-operative patients. During fibrillatory arrest, the aortic valve must remain competent to avoid any air embolus. Patients with moderate or severe aortic insufficiency (AI) would not be candidates, since there is limited access to the aortic valve and the risk of air embolus is considerable. AI also impedes visualization of the mitral valve with flooding of blood in the surgical field. Compared to median sternotomy, patients are more likely to experience post-thoracotomy pain syndrome. Placement of epidural anesthesia can improve postoperative pain management, allowing for the patient to have improved pulmonary toilet and early extubation. This also leads to early ambulation and therefore decreases the likelihood of postoperative pulmonary complications.

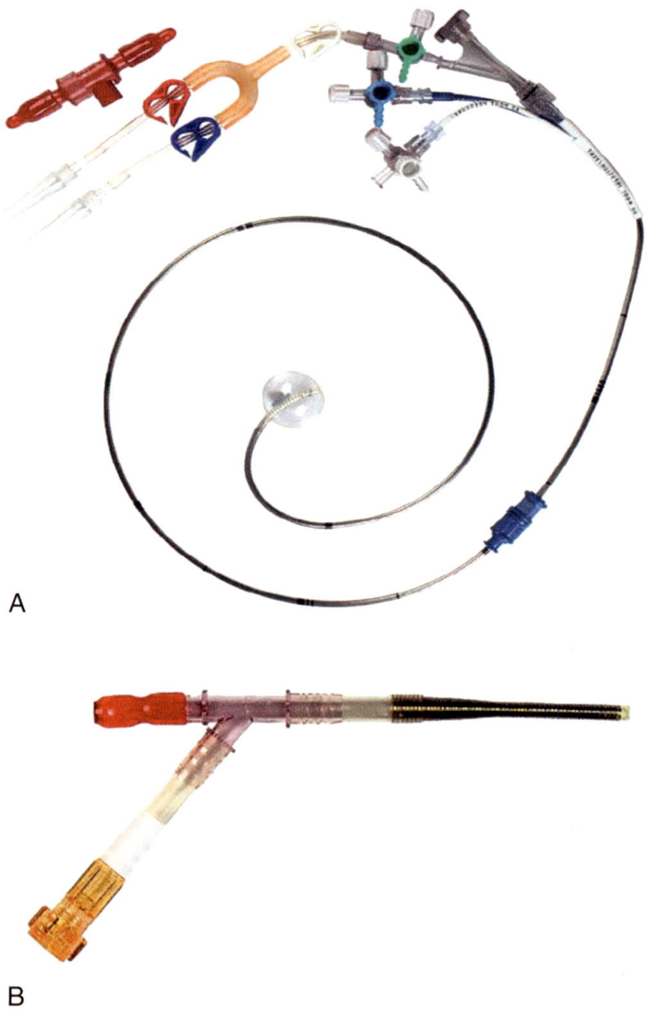

Fig. 13.12 The EndoReturn arterial cannula and 19 Fr (6.3 mm) arterial cannula (Edwards Lifesciences, Irvine, CA) are indicated for patients undergoing cardiopulmonary bypass. They are intended to deliver oxygenated blood for cardiopulmonary bypass during surgery. The EndoReturn arterial cannula with hemostasis valve also allows the hemostatic introduction and removal of vascular catheters such as the EndoClamp aortic catheter. The IntraClude intra-aortic occlusion device (Edwards Lifesciences) is indicated for use in patients undergoing cardiopulmonary bypass. The IntraClude intra-aortic occlusion device occludes and vents the ascending aorta when the balloon is inflated. The device's central lumen allows delivery of cardioplegia to arrest the heart. The pressure lumen allows monitoring of the aortic root pressure.

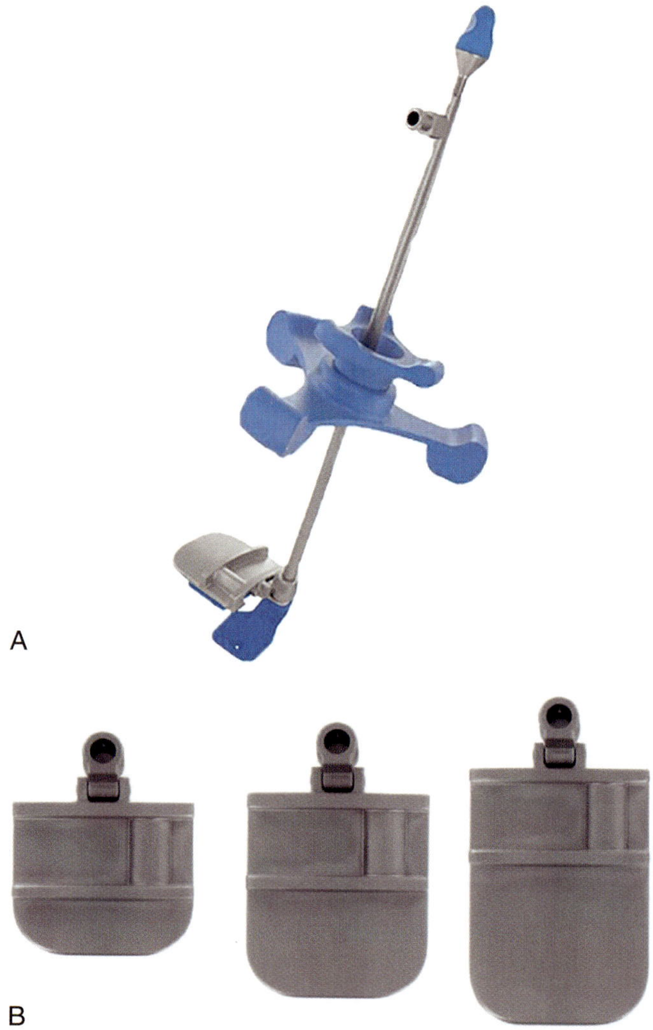

Fig. 13.13 (A) The Obadia 3D Atrial Retractor with Flexible Blade (Delacroix-Chevalier, Paris, France) for mitral valve exposure. (B) Variable size and depth retractors for atrial exposure.

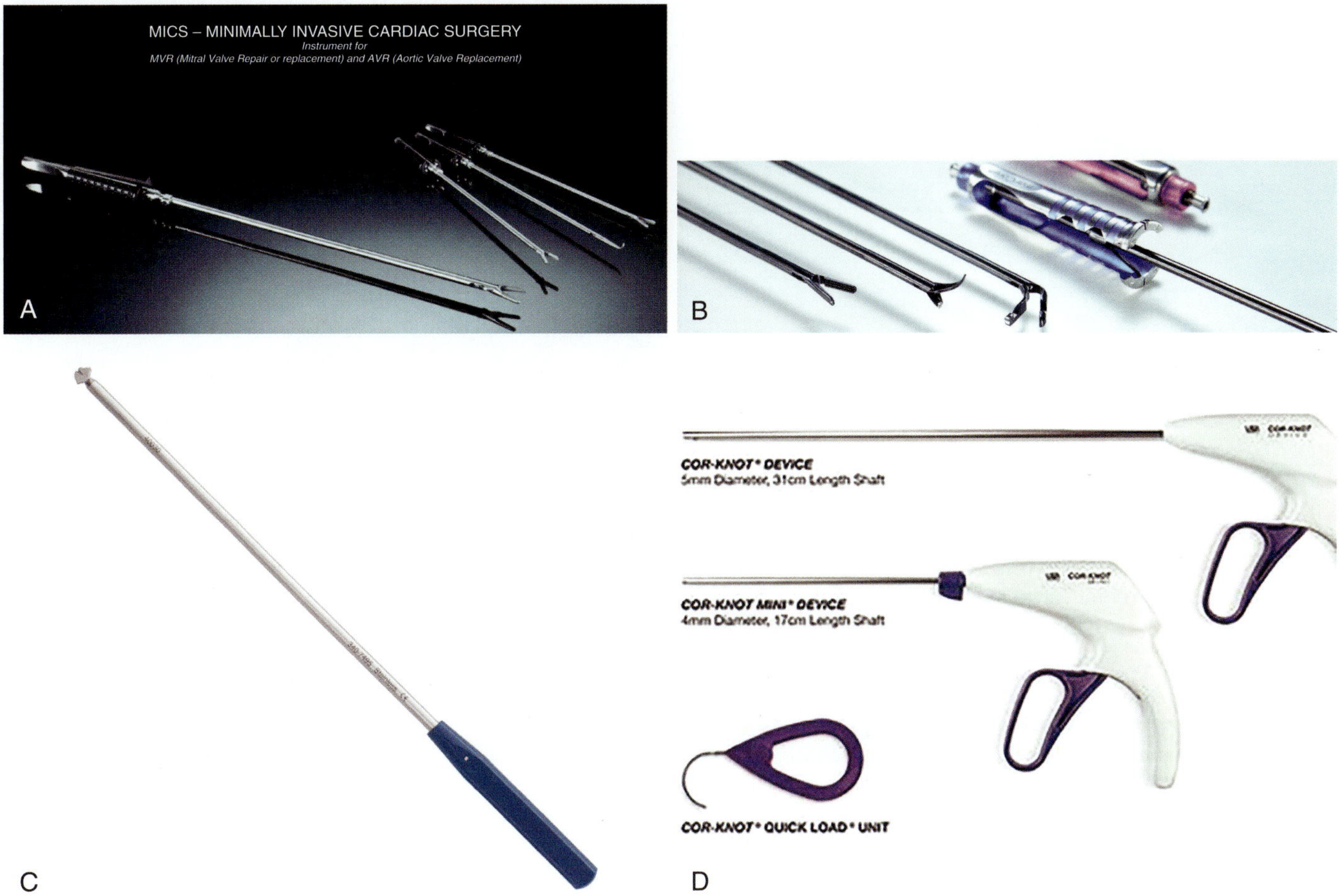

Fig. 13.14 A & B, Video-Assisted Minimally Invasive Cardiac Surgery Instruments. (A and B, Courtesy by KLS Martin Group). C, The laparoscopic knot pusher is intended for use in thoracic surgery in advancing throws of extracorporeal knots to a surface or object into the thoracic cavity (Atricure, OH, USA). D, The Cor-Knot device is faster than hand-tying and offers strength, security, and reliability in cardiac valve replacement and repair (LSI Solutions LLC, Victor, NY.)

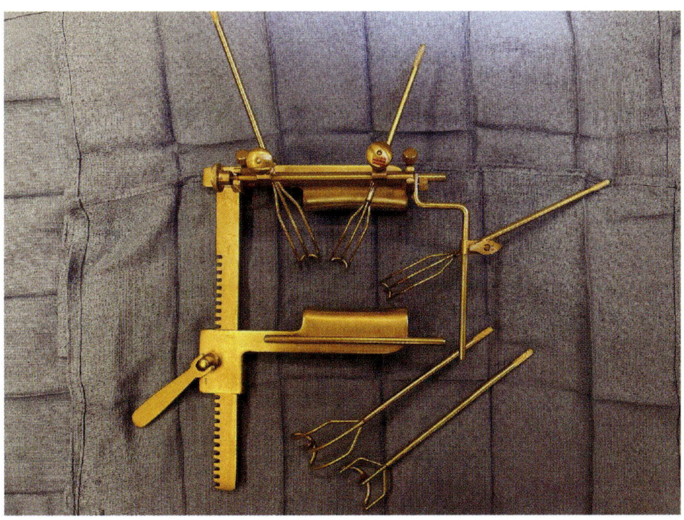

Fig. 13.15 Off-Pump Stabilizer/Positioner for off-pump coronary artery bypass (OPCAB).

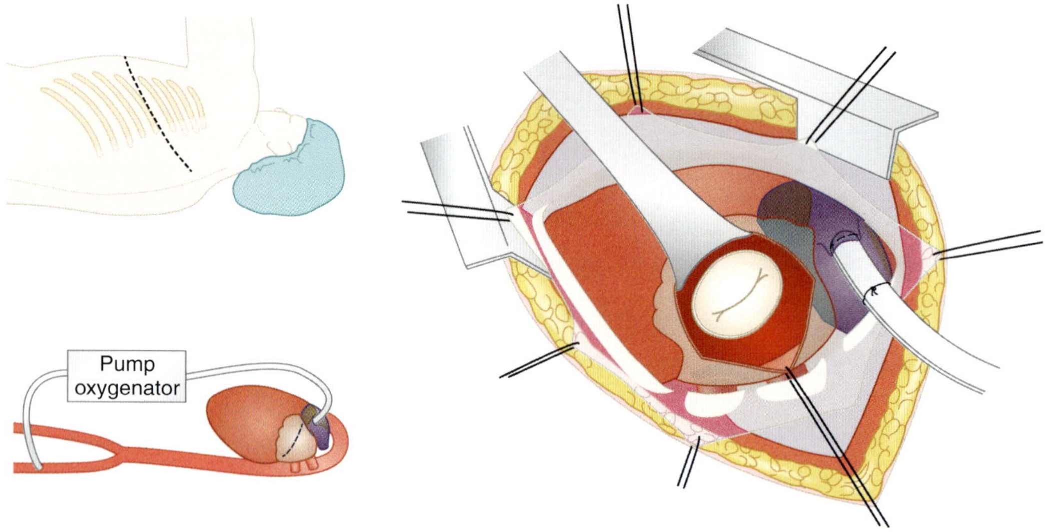

Fig. 13.16 Nichols et al.[6] and Clowes et al.[7] described using a left thoracotomy to approach the mitral valve. (From Pezzella AT, Utley JR, Vander Salm TJ. Operative approaches to the left atrium and mitral valve: an update. *Oper Tech Thorac Cardiovasc Surg.* 1998;3[2]:74–94.)

SELF-ASSESSMENT QUESTIONS

1. Instrumentation can facilitate the surgical approach to the mitral valve. Essential anatomy and instrument design are needed to provide alternative options for mitral valve surgery. Exposure to mitral valve is essential for all approaches. Name two key steps or instruments required for great exposure of the valve for all three approaches.
2. What instruments do we consider to be essential for all approaches to the mitral valve?
3. The left thoracotomy approach is not commonly used. It is reserved for patients who have had multiple thoracic surgeries and/mediastinal surgeries. What is a true contraindication for the left thoracotomy approach?

See page 317 for the answers.

REFERENCES

1. Javadikasgari H, Suri RM, Tappuni B, et al. Minimally invasive mitral valve repair. *Heart.* 2018;104:861–867.
2. Kim SJ, Lee SC. Technical and instrumental prerequisites for single-port laparoscopic solo surgery: state of the art. *World J Gastroenterol.* 2015;21(15):4440–4446.
3. Wexler Surgical VATS MICS V6 Catalog, 2021. https://www.wexlersurgical.com/flip/VATS_MICS_Catalog_V6/mobile/index.html.
4. Rodriguez R, Sutter FP, Samules LE, et al. Clinical outcomes of patients more than one year after minimally invasive mitral valve repair and replacement surgery with sutures secured using automated titanium fasteners. ISMICS 2013 Abstract.
5. Grapow M, Mytsyk M, Fassl J, et al. Automated fastener versus manually tied knots in minimally invasive mitral valve repair: impact on operation time and short-term results. *J Cardiothorac Surg.* 2015;10:146.
6. Nichols HT, Blanco G, Uricchio JF, et al. Open-heart surgery for mitral regurgitation and stenosis. *Arch Surg.* 1960;82:128–137.
7. Clowes GH, Neville WE, Sancetta SM, et al. Results of open surgical correction of mitral valvular insufficiency and description of technique for approach from the left side. *Surgery.* 1962;51:138–154.
8. Bastidas JG, Razzouk AJ, Hasaniya NW, et al. Left thoracotomy: an ideal approach for mitral valve replacement in patient with severe chest wall deformity. *Ann Thorac Surg.* 2013;96:e63–e64.
9. Pezzella AT, Utley JR, Vander Salm TJ. Operative approaches to the left atrium and mitral valve: an update. *Op Tech Thorac Cardiovasc Surg.* 1998;3(2):74–94.

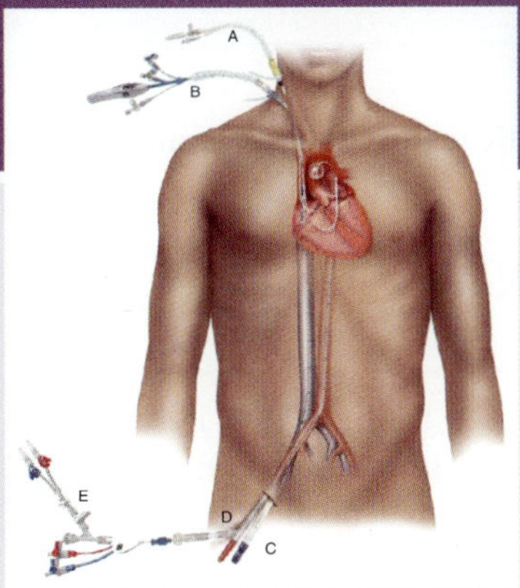

14

Myocardial Protection and Perfusion Techniques in Mitral Valve Surgery

Basel Ramlawi, Michel Pompeu Sá, Vishal N. Shah, Serge Sicouri

CHAPTER OUTLINE

LEARNING OBJECTIVES

1. The mitral valve surgeon should become familiarized with all types of myocardial protection, including routes of administration and cardioplegic solutions.
2. The mitral valve surgeon should know how to select patients for beating heart procedures (being fully aware of its advantages and disadvantages).
3. When choosing the route of cannulation for cardiopulmonary bypass, the surgeon should consider both central and peripheral cannulation as options, securing both adequate arterial flow and venous drainage.
4. Minimally invasive procedures should become the standard for mitral valve repair or replacement.

INTRODUCTION

Despite major advances in technologies and strategies aimed at reducing the proinflammatory effects of cardiopulmonary bypass (CPB) on the myocardium, myocardial ischemia and postischemic myocardial dysfunction can still occur. Myocardial damage is an independent predictor of adverse outcomes and reduced long-term survival following heart valve surgery.[1] Myocardial protection and perfusion techniques are key factors to achieve successful outcomes, primarily related to their ability to attenuate ischemia-reperfusion injury on CPB and subsequent tissue damage and organ dysfunction. This chapter is a brief review of myocardial protection and perfusion techniques as currently applied in mitral valve surgery.

MYOCARDIAL PROTECTION AND CARDIOPLEGIA

The two cornerstones of myocardial protection[2] during CPB are hypothermia and electromechanical cardiac arrest. Cardioplegia literally means "heart paralysis"; it relates to the intentional and temporary cessation of cardiac activity during surgery. The main objectives of cardioplegic solutions are the arrest of the heart in diastole and preservation of myocardial function (Table 14.1). Additional protection is provided by the addition of acid–base buffers, energy substrates, additives, or oxygenated blood to the cardioplegia infusion. Electromechanical arrest reduces myocardial metabolism, thereby allowing the patient to tolerate intermittent periods of ischemia. Electromechanical

TABLE 14.1 Main Aims of Cardioplegia
• Induction and maintenance of electromechanical diastolic cardiac arrest
• Myocardial hypothermia
• Limit development of myocardial edema
• Provide effective buffer capacity
• Minimize ischemia-reperfusion injury

arrest is usually achieved with potassium infusion, which leads to diastolic cardiac arrest. The cardioplegic solutions are dissolved in crystalloid fluids or in the blood of the patient, being delivered intermittently or continuously, using antegrade (aortic root or coronary ostia), retrograde (coronary sinus), or both routes of administration. There are two types of crystalloid cardioplegic solutions: the intracellular type and the extracellular type.[2] The intracellular types are characterized by absent or low concentrations of sodium and calcium. The extracellular types contain relatively higher concentrations of sodium, calcium, and magnesium. Both types avoid concentrations of potassium greater than 40 mmol/L (typical range is 10 to 40 mmol/L), contain bicarbonate for buffering, and are osmotically balanced.

Cardiopulmonary Bypass

CPB is usually instituted by placing two right-angled cannulas into the superior and inferior vena cava or one cannula into the right atrial appendage. A small (22 Fr) plastic or metal cannula is placed directly into the superior vena cava (SVC), above the sinoatrial node. The inferior caval cannula is placed at the entrance of the inferior vena cava, low in the right atrium. Bypass flows above 1.5 L/m^2/min and mild hypothermia is used with vacuum-assisted suction. In the setting of a minimally invasive procedure, the selection of cannulas and cannulation sites is of paramount importance for a stable CPB and bloodless exposure of the mitral valve. Particularly in this scenario, we use a 22 to 26 Fr percutaneous multi-stage venous cannula placed into the right atrium, at the SVC junction, via the right common femoral vein under transesophageal echocardiographic (TEE) guidance. Because the cannula has multiple holes (multi-stage) and flexibility, reaching the inferior vena cava, the drainage of both vena cava can be easily secured. If a concomitant coronary artery bypass procedure requiring a full sternotomy is to be performed, then venous cannulation should be bicaval via the atria. One curved venous cannula should be placed in the SVC above the cavoatrial junction and the other through the lowest part of the right atrium into the mouth of the inferior vena cava. The arterial cannula should be placed directly into the distal ascending aorta. Myocardial protection includes antegrade and retrograde blood cardioplegia and profound myocardial hypothermia. Retrograde cardioplegia is useful for all valvular surgery to protect the ischemic left ventricle and help remove air from the ascending aorta. Antegrade cardioplegia, used as an initial loading dose, is augmented by intermittent retrograde cardioplegia every 20 minutes. This provides safer delivery of cardioplegia because when the atrium is retracted during valve replacement, the aortic valve is distorted, and antegrade cardioplegia tends to fill the ventricle due to aortic regurgitation causing left ventricular distension.

MYOCARDIAL PROTECTION AND HYPOTHERMIA

Hypothermic cardioplegia, introduced in the 1960s, is effective in decreasing myocardial metabolism and reducing myocardial oxygen consumption. Electromechanical arrest leads to a 90% reduction in oxygen consumption. By decreasing the metabolic rate, hypothermia reduces oxygen demand and increases the tolerance to ischemia. Also, hypothermia reduces the amount of potassium required for the induction of cardiac arrest and inhibits the intracellular accumulation of calcium. However, hypothermia has a potential harmful influence on tissues due to oxidative stress (production of free-radicals) as well as inflammation (production of cytokines). Although both solutions can induce electromechanical cardiac arrest, hypothermic blood cardioplegia has been shown to be superior to crystalloid-based solutions in terms of myocardial protection in experimental studies when comparing the release of cardiac enzymes and metabolic response,[3] in part because of the characteristics of its blood-based composition. Noteworthy, the two largest clinical trials comparing blood and crystalloid cardioplegia[4,5] showed no statistical differences in terms of postoperative clinical outcomes. Furthermore, the largest meta-analysis (including 36 randomized controlled trials [RCTs]) showed similar results in terms of in-hospital death, perioperative myocardial infarction, and low cardiac output.[6]

Topical Hypothermia

Topical hypothermia with iced slush has been previously used as an adjunct to myocardial protection. Although some studies have demonstrated some efficacy in topical cooling, other studies have shown no additional cardioprotective benefit above systemic hypothermia and cold blood cardioplegia alone.[7] Moreover, several studies have demonstrated that the use of topical hypothermia is associated with increased diaphragmatic paralysis due to phrenic nerve palsy and pulmonary complications.[8] Topical hypothermia became less important in recent years to the point that it was not even a matter of discussion in the section for cardioplegia of the last European Association for Cardio-Thoracic Surgery (EACTS) European Association of Cardiothoracic (EACTA) European Board of Cardiovascular Perfusion (EBCP) guidelines on CPB in adult cardiac surgery.[3]

Normothermia Versus Hypothermia

Normothermic myocardial protection is usually performed by the continuous delivery of hyperkalemic normothermic blood during aortic cross-clamping. Warm blood cardioplegia offers adequate myocardial protection during CPB. The benefits obtained by normothermia include a constant oxygen supply and the preservation of aerobic metabolism, low adrenergic response with a subsequent better cardiac index. Lower incidence of ventricular arrhythmias after cross-clamp release with the use of warm heart protection has been reported.[9] Furthermore, the technique of using normothermic CPB and utilization of warm blood cardioplegia may be particularly helpful to mitigate the potential risk of cold agglutination such as in patients with cryoglobulinemia. Although normothermia protects the heart, it has been associated with increased neurological complications.[10] The safe duration of a cardioplegia administration during normothermia is still under debate, and mild (32°C to 35°C) to moderate (28°C to 32°C) hypothermia cardioplegia constitutes an alternative method. Moderate hypothermia has been shown to be associated with similar myocardial oxygen consumption, but less anaerobic lactate washout than normothermic cardioplegia.[11] A systemic temperature of 32°C to 35°C maintained via CPB, combined with mild hypothermic blood cardioplegia appears to best reduce the risks of neurologic complications, limit myocardial injury, and induce better functional myocardial recovery.

CARDIOPLEGIC SOLUTIONS: ROUTES OF ADMINISTRATION

Cardioplegia is effective only if it is well distributed. Adding retrograde perfusion via transatrial cannulation of the coronary sinus improves subendocardial perfusion, limits the removal of retractors during mitral procedures, avoids ostial cannulation during concomitant aortic valve procedures, and permits flushing of air and atheromas during concomitant coronary reoperations. Experimentally, right ventricular nutritive flow is limited by retrograde perfusion. Antegrade or retrograde cardioplegia alone are each inhomogeneous in their distribution in animals with normal coronary arteries as demonstrated in microsphere studies. Therefore, both are needed to ensure a uniform distribution in the myocardium. Noncoronary collateral flow from mediastinal collaterals displaces cardioplegia with warmer systemic blood. As mentioned previously, topical hypothermia slows rewarming but may cause pulmonary complications (phrenic palsy) without adding cardioprotective effects. Hence, continuous or intermittent cardioplegia is required. Continuous cardioplegic perfusion has been advocated to avoid ischemia, but adequate protection may not be achieved at usual flow rates, and the surgeon's vision becomes obscured during infusion. Intermittent cardioplegia, delivered at 10- to 20-minute intervals, maintains arrest, slows rewarming, and restores substrates depleted during ischemia. In addition, it flushes accumulated metabolites and counteracts acidosis and edema. A dedicated pump on the CPB machine for cardioplegic perfusion is required for specific cannulas for antegrade and retrograde cardioplegia administration and a monitoring-infusion system (Fig. 14.1).

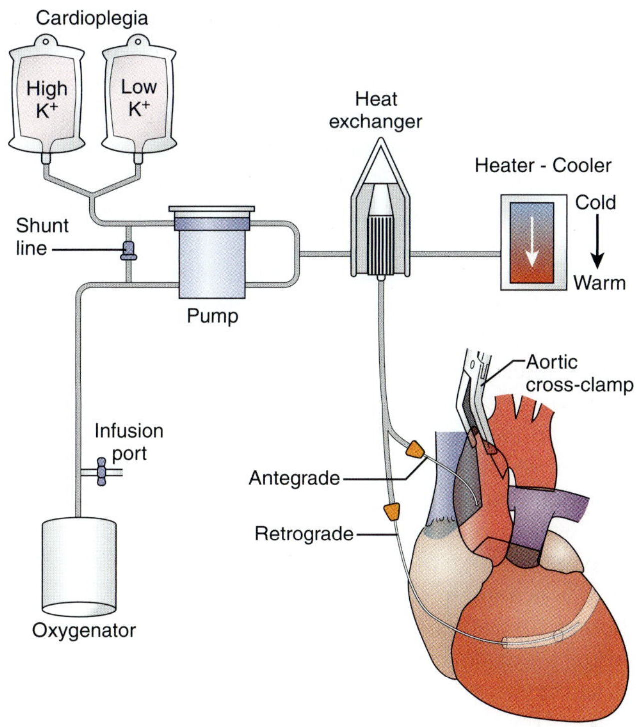

Fig. 14.1 Routes of Cardioplegia Administration. Antegrade versus retrograde.

Antegrade Cardioplegia

An antegrade cardioplegia cannula is placed in the ascending aorta below the site chosen for the aortic cross-clamp. An antegrade cannula is placed high on the ascending aorta and slightly to the right side. This cannula contains a pressure line and a vent port to suction air and blood between infusions. A 4-0 purse-string polypropylene suture is used to secure the cannula. When the CPB is running and the heart is empty, thanks to effective systemic venous drainage, the aorta is clamped, and blood antegrade cardioplegia is delivered for 2 minutes at a rate of 200 mL/min. According to the 2019 EACTS/EACTA/EBCP guidelines,[3] during antegrade infusion, aortic root pressure must be maintained between 60 and 100 mm Hg at a flow rate of 200 mL/min or, in hypertrophied hearts, 250 mL/min. Blood cardioplegia is given over time to ensure maximal oxygen delivery. Failure to arrest means inadequate systemic venous drainage (full heart), incomplete aortic clamping, or aortic insufficiency. Aortic pressure below 30 mm Hg means that antegrade flow is insufficient and only retrograde infusion should be used.

Retrograde Cardioplegia

Retrograde cardioplegia delivery is performed through the coronary sinus via the right atrium or direct ostial cannulation. The retrograde cannula has a self-inflating or manually inflated balloon at its tip; it also contains a line for monitoring-infusion pressure. It is placed low in the right atrium, anterior to the venous cannula, and just above the caval junction. It is directed into the coronary sinus by aiming at the patient's left shoulder. The cannula is advanced until it meets resistance within the coronary sinus, usually adjacent to the left atrial appendage. Coronary sinus cannulation can be performed before venous cannulation to prevent the venous cannula from being an obstacle to the insertion of the retrograde cannula. Otherwise, coronary sinus cannulation can be done on partial bypass with the right atrium slightly distended, with the aim of keeping the sinus ostium open. TEE-guided techniques or surgeon palpation are effective methods to guide the retrograde cannula into its correct position. Commercially available retrograde cannulas usually have a malleable stylet and inflatable balloon cannula. The site of introduction on the atrial wall is secured with a 4-0 purse-string polypropylene suture around the cannula. The coronary sinus can be injured by forceful cannulation or continued administration of cardioplegia when coronary sinus pressure exceeds 50 mm Hg. The perfusionist notes high pressure, then low pressure as a consequence of acute perforation, or the surgeon sees red blood accumulate in the pericardial well. Perforation can be repaired directly with 5-0 polypropylene sutures or pericardial pledgets if the tear site is not distinct. Hematomas are often self-contained after heparin reversal. During retrograde infusion, coronary sinus pressure is maintained between 30 and 50 mm Hg at a flow of 200 to 400 mL/min.[12] A coronary sinus pressure greater than 50 mm Hg means improper positioning or cardiac retraction. This is corrected by reducing the flow rate immediately, repositioning the catheter, and then resuming the flow. If severe aortic valve insufficiency is present, direct coronary ostial administration or retrograde cardioplegia can be delivered. If there is concomitant coronary artery disease, myocardial protection in this circumstance should be antegrade and retrograde to ensure adequate distribution of the cardioplegia,[13,14] considering that the coronary artery bypass graft/mitral operation presents one of the highest-risk operative settings in cardiac surgery.

BASIC CONCEPTS IN CARDIOPLEGIA-STANDARD VS MICROPLEGIA

Cardioplegic solutions are classified as crystalloid or blood-based solutions delivered either warm or cold. Cold blood cardioplegia is the most commonly used cardioplegic technique. The rationale for using blood for hypothermic potassium-induced cardiac arrest is that (a) it provides an oxygenated environment and a method for intermittent reoxygenation of the heart during arrest; (b) limits hemodilution when large volumes of cardioplegic solution are used; (c) affords an excellent buffering capacity and osmotic properties; (d) allows for electrolyte composition and pH that are physiologic; (e) offers a number of endogenous antioxidants and free-radical scavengers; and (f) is less complex to prepare than other solutions. The early development of cardioplegia used crystalloid-containing solutions only, which permits rapid cardiac arrest via the effects of high potassium, cold temperature, and hypoxia induced by the absence of oxygen. Generally, crystalloid solutions cause myocardial arrest induced by depolarization. Solutions that depolarize contain high extracellular potassium, which may lead to myocardial dysfunction during the post-CPB period due to accumulation of intracellular calcium and sodium during the arrest period. Recently, several crystalloid solutions have been reintroduced. The two most common solutions used are the del Nido solution[15] and Custodiol-HTK solution.[16] Both arrest the heart in diastole although by different mechanisms. In the del Nido solution, the high potassium concentration prevents repolarization, so the cell stays depolarized. When the resting potential approaches −50 mV, sodium channels are inactivated resulting in a diastolic arrest of cardiac activity. In Custodiol-HTK solution, the low extracellular sodium reduces the transmembrane sodium gradient so that not enough sodium can enter the myocyte during phase 0 of the cardiac action potential to cause depolarization, the myocyte membrane remains hyperpolarized, and is arrested in diastole. These solutions are thought to provide superior myocardial protection and increase the duration of time before repeat cardioplegia is required, allowing prolonged uninterrupted surgery.[17,18] This may reduce the aortic cross-clamp and CPB times and potentially the need for a retrograde catheter, as suggested by LeBon et al.[19] Limitations of a purely crystalloid approach are that high volumes are administered and lack of oxygen is delivered to the myocardium. Blood cardioplegia adds blood to the crystalloid solution. These typically consist of 4:1 ratios of blood to cardioplegia, but this may be greatly reduced in the microplegia systems available today. The dose of additional crystalloid used in microplegia is small, thus allowing large volumes of cardioplegia to be delivered without causing hemodilution or myocardial edema.

Composition of Cardioplegic Solutions

The rationale for the distinct ingredients of cardioplegic solutions has been based on the need to: (a) induce a rapid cardiac arrest using potassium or magnesium; (b) reduce energy demand and conserve adenosine triphosphate (ATP) reserves using hypothermia; (c) maintain intracellular ionic and metabolic homeostasis; (d) lower myocardial oxygen consumption; (e) enhance anaerobic and aerobic energy production utilizing glucose and amino acids; (f) stabilize the pH using bicarbonate, phosphate, or histidine buffers; (g) stabilize cellular membranes by using steroids, oxygen free-radical scavengers such as glutathione, calcium antagonists, and/or procaine; (h) avoid intracellular calcium overload by providing a hypocalcemic environment and adding magnesium; and (i) prevent cellular edema by the addition of colloids such as mannitol to maintain normal oncotic pressures. Although there is a concern that crystalloid cardioplegia lacks blood components and therefore has a limited oxygen-carrying capacity, this has not been shown to be clinically relevant. In fact, numerous clinical studies demonstrate that crystalloid cardioplegia is as effective as blood cardioplegia,[6] particularly in centers where it is the primary form of protection. The compositions of the different cardioplegic solutions in use are described below:

- **St. Thomas' Hospital solution #1** (STH-1) is a pure crystalloid cardioplegic solution with moderately elevated potassium (20 mM) and magnesium (16 mM) and a small additive of procaine (1 mM) in an extracellular ionic matrix. Further preclinical studies confirmed the importance of maintaining near to normal extracellular concentrations of calcium and sodium avoiding major fluctuations in these key ions during and following coronary infusion of cardioplegic solutions.
- **St. Thomas' Hospital solution #2** (STH-2) is a crystalloid solution with moderate elevations of potassium (16 mM) and magnesium (16 mM) together with near normal sodium (120 mM) and calcium (1.2 mM) and a minor content of bicarbonate (10 mM) for initial pH control. This solution can be applied for single-dose or multi-dose cardioplegia depending on the duration of aortic occlusion and on washout by noncoronary collateral blood flow. Commercially

TABLE 14.2 Composition of St. Thomas' Hospital Cardioplegic Solutions

Component (mM)	STH-1	STH-2
Sodium chloride	144	120
Sodium bicarbonate	—	10
Potassium chloride	20	16
Magnesium chloride	16	16
Calcium chloride	2.2	1.2
Procaine hydrochloride	1	—
pH	5.5–7.0	7.8
Osmolality (mOsm/Kg H_2O)	300–320	285–300

available STH-2 (Plegisol, Hospira Inc., Lake Forest, IL, USA) and STH-1 are still in clinical use (Table 14.2).

- **Cold blood cardioplegia** combines advantages of hypothermia and blood solutions and appears to allow myocardial recovery after long periods of ischemia in normal hearts. Blood cardioplegia consists of 4 parts of blood to 1 part of crystalloid solution. This limits the hemodilution occurring with crystalloid cardioplegia during repeated infusions. High-dose potassium (20 to 30 mEq/L) allows cardiac arrest during both warm and cold induction.
- **The del Nido cardioplegia solution,** initially used in pediatric cardiac surgery,[20] has been proven to be effective in inducing 90 minutes of cardioplegic arrest in a single-dose administration.[15] It has gained popularity in adult valvular surgery and is the standard preservation solution at our institution. The del Nido solution is a nonglucose-based solution containing low calcium and high lidocaine concentrations, indirectly preventing intracellular Ca^{2+} accumulation during ischemia and preventing reperfusion arrhythmias. Compared with the standard 4:1 blood cardioplegia, the del Nido cardioplegia is more dilute (1:4 blood:crystalloid), has 75% less calcium, and adds magnesium and lidocaine to the crystalloid component. The high potassium concentration of the del Nido solution prevents electrical repolarization, sodium channels are inactivated at depolarized potentials resulting in diastolic arrest. The del Nido solution is administered as a single bolus and can provide protection for a period of over 2 hours. Crystalloid components of the del Nido solution are listed in Table 14.3.
- **Custodiol, Histidine-tryptophan-ketoglutarate (HTK), or Bretschneider solution,** first proposed by Bretschneider in the 1970s, is an intracellular, crystalloid cardioplegia characterized by low sodium and calcium content. The mechanism of action is based on sodium depletion of the extracellular space, which causes hyperpolarization, inducing cardiac arrest in diastole. It contains histidine for buffering capacity, tryptophan to protect cell membrane, ketoglutarate which stabilizes the cell membrane and provides ATP during reperfusion, and mannitol which reduces edema. This intracellular-based crystalloid cardioplegic solution is mainly used for organ preservation in transplant surgery. Like the del Nido solution, it is administered as a single dose and can lead to up to 3 hours of myocardial protection without requiring frequent reinfusions. The components of Custodiol-HTK solution are listed in Table 14.4. A single, large bolus infusion (20 to 25 mL/kg) at 4°C to 6°C is given, and a half-dose is added after 1 hour.

TABLE 14.3 Crystalloid Components of the del Nido Cardioplegia Solution

Component	Volume (mL)
Plasma-Lyte A base solution	1000
Mannitol 20%	16.3
Magnesium sulfate 50%	4
Sodium bicarbonate 8.4%	13
Potassium chloride (2 mEq/mL)	13
Lidocaine 1%	13

TABLE 14.4 Composition of Custodiol-Histidine-Tryptophan-Ketoglutarate Solution

Ingredient	Value
Sodium	15 mmol/L
Potassium	9 mmol/L
Magnesium	4 mmol/L
Calcium	0.015 mmol/L
Histidine	198 mmol/L
Tryptophan	2 mmol/L
Ketoglutarate	1 mmol/L
Mannitol	30 mmol/L
pH	7.02–7.20

Additives in Cardioplegia Solutions

Adjuncts to cardioplegia include calcium-blockers, magnesium, beta-blockers, local anesthetics, nitric oxide, and ischemic preconditioning. Their possible advantages in myocardial preservation are described in Table 14.5.

TABLE 14.5 Additives in Cardioplegia Solutions

Adjunct	Possible Advantages
Calcium-blockers	• Improved myocardial metabolism • Reduced ischemic injury
Magnesium	• Reduction in incidence of new-onset postoperative afib
Beta-blockers (esmolol)	• Prevent or treat arrhythmias and myocardial ischemia
Local anesthetics (lidocaine, procaine)	• Membrane stabilization • Spontaneous return to sinus rhythm after surgery
Nitric oxide (NO) donors (L-arginine)	• Reduce myocardial injury and inflammatory response
Ischemic preconditioning	• Postoperative improvement of cardiac function • Reduced need for inotropic support • Antiarrhythmic effects

EXPEDITIOUS PROCEDURE (LIMITED ISCHEMIA)

Expeditious procedures with limited ischemia are performed in patients presenting with emergent indications for operative intervention such as papillary muscle rupture, a complication of ischemic heart disease. Expeditious surgical treatment offers optimal chances of survival in these patients because acute mitral regurgitation in this setting is poorly tolerated and may lead to hemodynamic collapse. In these patients, coronary artery bypass graft surgery (CABG) is most frequently performed concurrently with mitral valve repair or replacement (in the setting of severe ischemic mitral regurgitation). Patients in cardiogenic shock or profound organ dysfunction benefit from preoperative inotropes or preoperative or intraoperative placement of mechanical support devices such as intraaortic balloon pump, Impella, or extracorporeal membrane oxygenation (ECMO), which may stabilize hemodynamics and expedite operative intervention.[21]

BEATING HEART (CARDIOPULMONARY BYPASS ASSIST) MITRAL VALVE SURGERY

Beating heart mitral valve surgery is used in high-risk patients for conventional operations. Patients with low cardiac function due to ischemic cardiomyopathy or dilated cardiomyopathy, in cardiogenic shock, severe endocarditis, previous sternotomy, or prior patent coronary bypass grafts are good candidates for beating heart mitral valve surgery using either a median sternotomy or right thoracotomy approach with CPB but without cardioplegic arrest and aortic cross-clamping. Some centers have reported equivalent results with beating heart compared to conventional mitral valve surgery with cardiac arrest. A recent retrospective study of 120 consecutive high-risk patients undergoing mitral valve surgery reported positive postoperative outcomes after the beating heart approach as compared with cardioplegic arrest.[22] A meta-analysis of beating heart procedures also demonstrated good safety outcomes.[23] Beating heart surgery with aortic cross-clamp and coronary perfusion and that without aortic cross-clamp are also available. Of great importance during beating heart surgery without aortic cross-clamp is to vent the left ventricle and maintain aortic root pressure, resulting in constant closure of the aortic valve. If beating or ventricular fibrillation (VF) heart surgery is used instead of aortic cross-clamping, the patient is placed in the Trendelenburg position slightly rotated to the left (to elevate the left atrium relative to the left ventricle) and the aorta is vented whenever possible. Fibrillation is induced by either cooling the patient to 28°C to 30°C or by electrical stimulation. A balloon catheter (e.g., 8 Fr Foley catheter) may be used to vent the left ventricle, especially in patients with mild aortic regurgitation or previous mechanical aortic valve replacement. At the end of the procedure, ventilation is resumed once the left atrium has been completely de-aired, as assessed by TEE. Although many of these high-risk patients are now being treated with MitraClip (Abbott Laboratories - Structural Heart- Westfield, IN), beating heart mitral valve surgery should also be considered in patients unsuitable for MitraClip or after failed MitraClip implantation.

- **Advantages of the beating heart technique:** In addition to permitting to operate on high-risk patients by avoiding aortic cross-clamping and cardioplegia, this strategy eliminates additional ischemic insult to the heart. Cardioplegic arrest is a major cause of postoperative morbidity in patients with severely reduced left ventricular function. Compared to patients with cardioplegic arrest, those undergoing beating heart surgery have demonstrated lower levels of postoperative creatine kinase-MB levels and shorter period of postoperative inotropic and ventilatory support, therefore improving early postoperative outcomes.[24] Another advantage is that it facilitates reoperation in patients with multiple previous cardiac operations.[25] Patients with diffuse severe calcification of the ascending aorta or "porcelain" aorta would also benefit from this approach.
- **Disadvantages of the beating heart technique:** They relate to the difficulty for the surgeon to operate on a beating heart. In addition, air embolization can occur with this technique.

MINIMALLY INVASIVE CONSIDERATIONS

Minimally invasive approaches to both minimally invasive mitral valve replacement (MIMVR) include upper or lower hemisternotomy, direct-vision right minithoracotomy, endoscopic right minithoracotomy, and robotic-assisted right minithoracotomy. In select patients, MIMVR is now the preferred approach due to improved postoperative outcomes including less bleeding and atrial fibrillation, reduced incidence of wound infection, shorter hospital stay, faster recovery, and improved cosmesis compared to full sternotomy conventional approaches. A recent consensus document by Ailawadi et al.[26] provides current best practice guidelines for undertaking minimally invasive mitral procedures particularly in the maintenance of adequate cannulation and perfusion, appropriate myocardial protection, optimal exposure, and procedures appropriate to the patient's specific pathology (Fig. 14.2).

Myocardial Protection and Aortic Occlusion in Minimally Invasive Approaches to Both Mitral Valve Repair and Replacement

Since most MIMVR procedures are performed with peripheral cannulation, the strategies for myocardial protection and aortic occlusion are different from those of conventional full sternotomy. Myocardial protection avoiding aortic occlusion and cardioplegic arrest can be performed by using either VF or a beating heart strategy (previously described). The VF technique for mitral valve surgery has been shown to induce a higher perioperative stroke rate compared to aortic occlusion and cardioplegic arrest possibly due to air entrainment in the left ventricular without the ability to capture air that is pushed into the ascending aorta. Suboptimal de-airing may explain worse outcomes with this approach. Moreover, VF cannot be used in the presence of aortic regurgitation, which obscures the surgical field. VF technique may be preferred in reoperations involving prior patent coronary bypass grafts or aortic valve replacement.

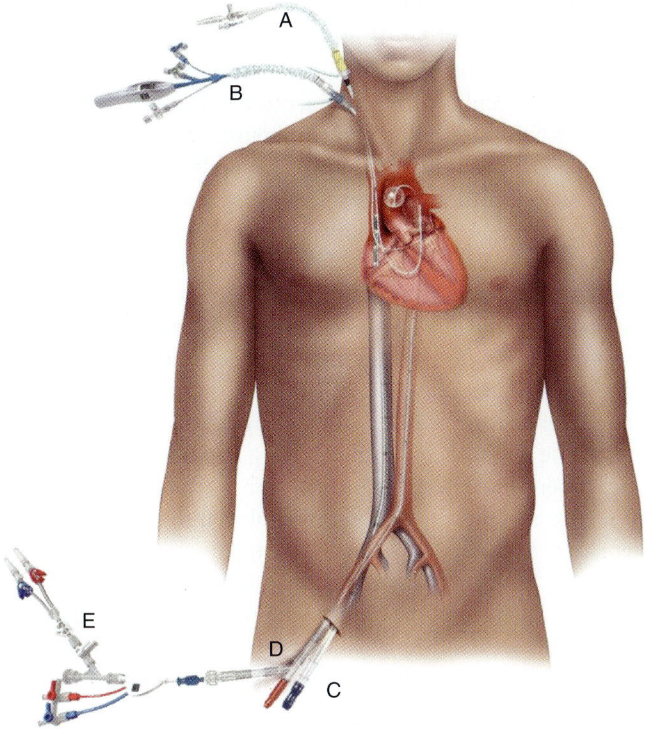

Fig. 14.2 Placement of Perfusion Catheters and Cannulas in Minimally Invasive Mitral Valve Repair and Replacement. (A) Pulmonary artery vent catheter. (B) Coronary sinus catheter. (C) Femoral venous cannula. (D) Femoral arterial cannula. (E) Endoaortic balloon occlusion catheter. (From Ailawadi G, Agnihotri AK, Mehall JR, et al. Minimally invasive mitral valve Surgery I: patient selection, evaluation, and planning. *Innovations (Phila)*. 2016;11[4]:243–250.)

Cardioplegia-based Strategies in Minimally Invasive Approaches to Both Mitral Valve Repair and Replacement

When using cardioplegia, an antegrade approach alone or a combined antegrade and retrograde approach can be used. The del Nido cardioplegia or Custodiol-HTK crystalloid cardioplegia solutions can be used in a single dose and may reduce the need for the placement of a retrograde cardioplegia catheter.[27] Any degree greater than mild aortic valve regurgitation should lead to the use of retrograde cardioplegia. Antegrade cardioplegia can be delivered by two approaches. The first is by way of the aortic root through an externally inserted cardioplegia needle. This is typically brought out through the working port but can be placed through a separate small incision in the right chest. In this scenario, a transthoracic cross-clamp is required. The alternative is to use an endoaortic balloon to occlude the aorta internally via the femoral vessels. With this technique, antegrade cardioplegia is delivered through the endoaortic balloon to the aortic root. If retrograde cardioplegia is planned, there are two main options for insertion. One is through the right atrium into the coronary sinus; the other uses percutaneous coronary sinus cannulation through the right internal jugular vein.

Aortic Occlusion in Minimally Invasive Approaches to Both Mitral Valve Repair and Replacement

Aortic occlusion in MIMVR can be with a transthoracic cross-clamp or through endoaortic balloon occlusion. Transthoracic cross-clamping allows direct clamping of the aorta as typically done through a sternotomy. The transthoracic cross-clamp is placed through an entry site in the chest wall, anterior to the SVC. Alternate to the transthoracic cross-clamp is endoaortic balloon occlusion. With an endoaortic balloon, there is no need for a separate antegrade cardioplegia catheter because cardioplegia delivery and root venting are performed through the endoaortic balloon catheter itself. This eliminates any issues with suturing the aorta or bleeding from the puncture site and minimizes clutter in the reduced surgical field. Other advantages are that it is inserted into the ascending aorta before initiating CPB and can shorten CBP and aortic cross-clamp times. It is also ideal for use in reoperations. Disadvantages of endoaortic balloon occlusion include the need to place the catheter through the arterial cannula, hence reducing the effective size of the arterial cannula. If this results in excessively high line pressures or inadequate flow, then the option exists to place the balloon through a separate arterial cannulation site. Retrospective data comparing transthoracic cross-clamping and endoaortic balloon occlusion showed no significant difference in outcomes safety profiles between the two techniques.[28]

PERFUSION TECHNIQUES

Key Concepts of Perfusion in Mitral Valve Surgery: Left and Right Ventricle Decompression, Drainage, and Venting

De-Airing

The main goals of perfusion in mitral valve surgery are to provide complete drainage of the heart, establish adequate systemic perfusion, and minimize risks of malperfusion or vascular injury. Adequate venous drainage and decompression of the heart are absolutely necessary. Two key components for accomplishing adequate drainage are cannula size and vacuum assistance. During conventional full sternotomy procedures, venous drainage is often accomplished via gravity and without vacuum assistance. Cannula size may vary depending on the type of cannula and patient body surface area. With all modes of venous cannulation for MIMVR, vacuum assist is necessary for effective drainage and prevention of air entrapment. Vacuum pressures are started at −30 mm Hg and can go as high as −60 mm Hg; higher vacuum pressures have been associated with gaseous microemboli. A disadvantage of new minimally invasive CPB circuits is their inability to use vacuum assist, potentially impeding venous drainage.

Central Cannulation

Direct distal ascending aorta cannulation (Fig. 14.3) is used for conventional full sternotomy as well as in some cases of

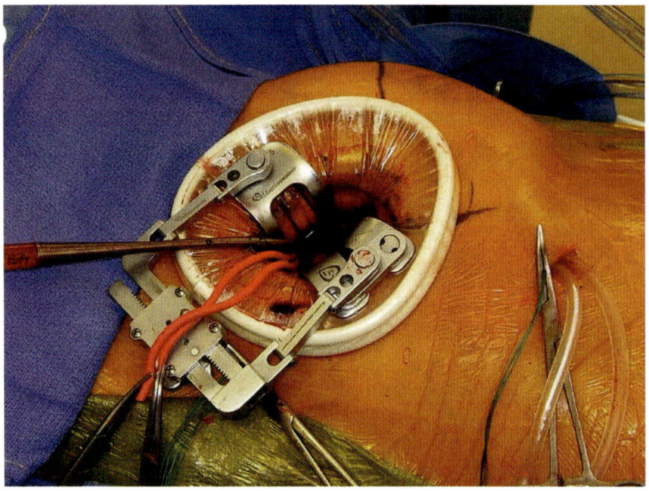

Fig. 14.3 Central Aortic Cannulation: The aorta is directly cannulated for a mitral valve surgery. (From Lamelas J, Aberle C, Macias AE, et al. Cannulation strategies for minimally invasive cardiac surgery. *Innovations (Phila)*. 2020;15[3]:261–269.)

MIMVR generally when the axillary artery is too diseased for safe cannulation. The aorta is identified and mobilized toward the operative field with the use of pericardial sutures. Concentric purse-string sutures are placed and secured with tourniquets. Aortic cannulation is accomplished through the purse-strings using the Seldinger technique. The cannula is secured with the tourniquets and additionally to the skin. Although central cannulation is possible via any MIMVR approach, it may limit exposure in an already reduced surgical field. As such, if the need for central access is necessary, upper hemisternotomy may provide better exposure and a more convenient approach.[29] Furthermore, if the aorta is extremely shifted to the left, a minithoracotomy approach may prove challenging for central cannulation and an inverted T-shaped ministernotomy may optimize exposure in this case. A CT angiogram of the chest may help guide the choice of which approach is more suitable.

Peripheral Cannulation

Femoral Cannulation. Femoral cannulation (Fig. 14.4) is the most commonly utilized cannulation strategy for MIMVR approaches, particularly minithoracotomy. Femoral cannulation can be accomplished either percutaneously or directly via femoral cutdown. The cannula size is based on body surface area (Table 14.6). During MIMVR cases, smaller cannula sizes may be occasionally utilized. A small femoral artery or presence of significant atherosclerotic disease should prompt the use of an alternative cannulation site such as the axillary artery. Percutaneous femoral cannulation is done by using ultrasound in order to ensure that the cannulation site is in the proximal common femoral artery and identify anatomical variations. The puncture site is positioned over the femoral head obtaining access by puncturing at a point one-third of the distance along an oblique line from the pubic tubercle to the anterior superior iliac spine. After needle access, the Seldinger technique is employed to pass a guidewire. Thereafter, a ProGlide System (Abbott Vascular Devices, Santa Clara, CA, USA) is passed over the guidewire for percutaneous suture-mediated closure. This device places suture through the anterior wall of the artery which is subsequently tightened following sheath or cannula removal. The Perclose ProGlide device is approved for closure of 5 to 21 Fr arterial sheaths or cannulas and should only be used on 5-mm or larger vessels. Other percutaneous closure device options are available, including AngioSeal (Terumo Europe NV -Leuven (Belgium)) and Manta (Teleflex-Morrisville, NC) devices. This is followed by progressive dilatation and ultimately passage of the arterial cannula. Direct (open) cannulation of the femoral artery following cutdown is a safe alternative to percutaneous access. Preferentially, the left femoral artery is utilized for this approach as the right femoral artery is often used for access during cardiac catheterization, and may result in scarring, hematoma, and more difficult right-sided access. A 1 to 2 cm vertical skin incision is made overlying the femoral vessels, above the groin crease. The inguinal ligament is retracted, and the vessel is exposed proximally on the common femoral artery. A 5–0 Prolene U-stitch is placed, and the artery is cannulated through the purse-string suture using the Seldinger technique.

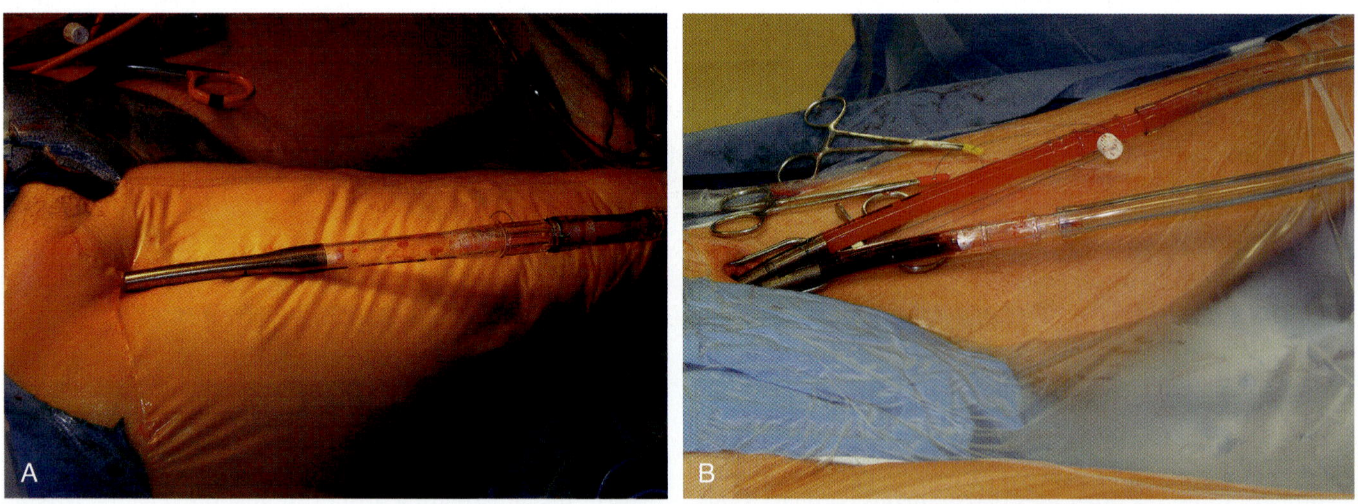

Fig. 14.4 Peripheral Femoral Cannulation. (A) Percutaneous cannulations. (B) Direct canulation (Seldinger technique). (From Lamelas J, Aberle C, Macias AE, et al. Cannulation strategies for minimally invasive cardiac surgery. *Innovations (Phila)*. 2020;15[3]:261–269.)

Axillary/Subclavian Cannulation. In case of significant peripheral vascular disease in the femoral artery, alternate axillary or subclavian arterial access should be used (Fig. 14.5). A 2-cm skin incision is made 1 cm beneath the clavicle, medial to the deltopectoral groove. The pectoralis muscles are separated or divided, and finger guidance of the axillary arterial pulse facilitates localization. Proximal and distal control of the vessel is obtained using silastic vessel loops. The distal loop is retracted, and the proximal aspect of the artery is clamped with a vascular clamp. A direct arteriotomy on the vessel is recommended to avoid injury, which may occur with blunt dilation of the fragile vessel with the Seldinger technique. After cutdown, a 6 Fr sheath is introduced followed by a guidewire. Visualization of the guidewire with TEE in the ascending aorta or descending aorta is required prior to cannula advancement through the artery. Alternatively, fluoroscopy may be used to direct guidewire and cannula advancement (Fig. 14.5D). Location of the cannula can also be confirmed with angiography. With axillary/subclavian cannulation, a cannula one size smaller than that required for femoral cannulation can be utilized (see Table 14.6).

TABLE 14.6 Cannula Sizes Recommended for Femoral Cannulation

Cannulation Site	BSA	Cannula Size
Femoral artery	<1.6	15 Fr
	1.7–2.1	17 Fr
	>2.1	19 Fr
Femoral vein	All patients	>25 Fr

BSA, Body surface area; *Fr,* French sizing scale.

Minimally Invasive Options

The surgical approach will dictate the appropriate cannulation strategy needed to facilitate optimal exposure and ease of operation. Conventional full sternotomy procedures typically utilize central ascending aortic cannulation with right atrial or

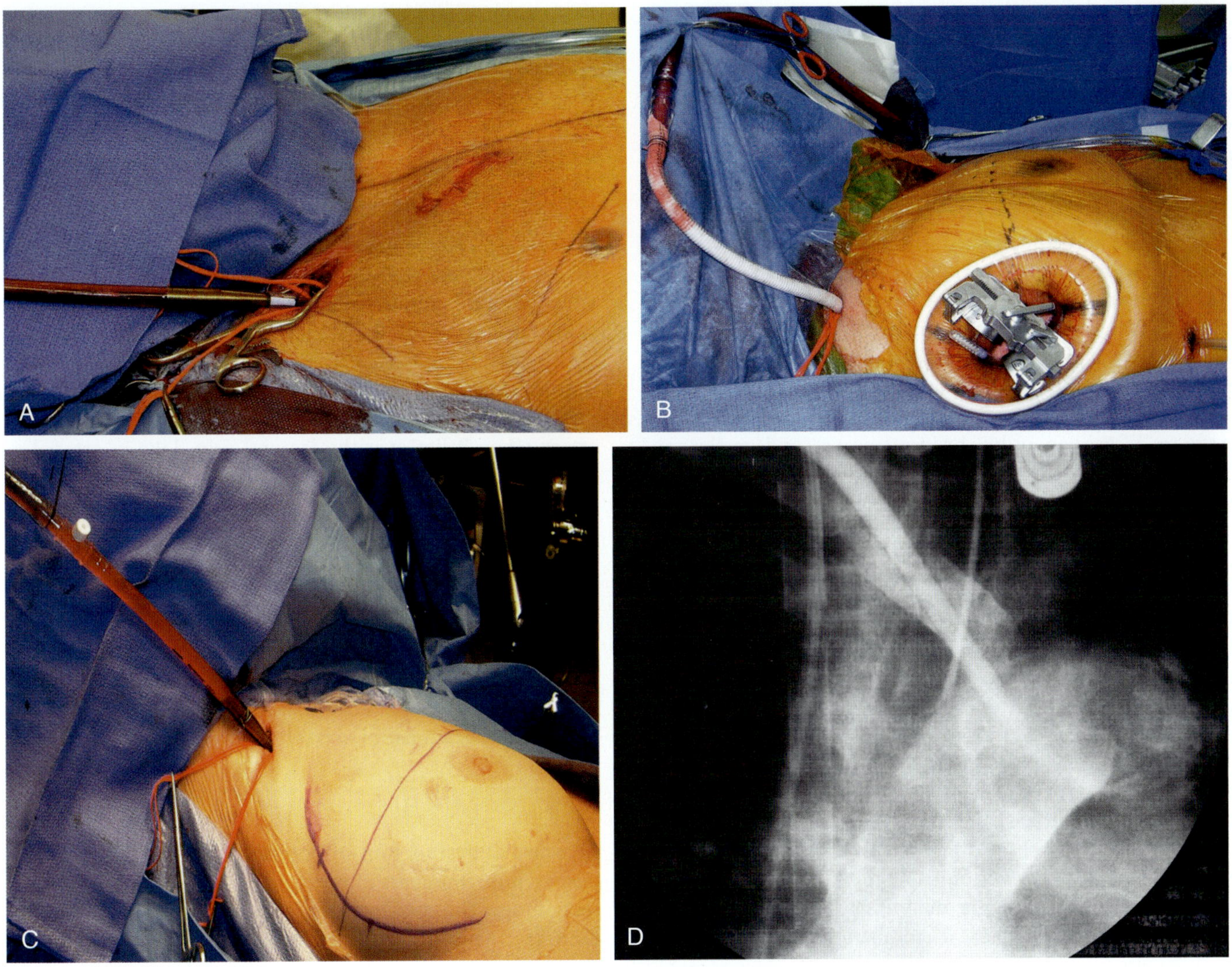

Fig. 14.5 Peripheral Axillary Cannulation. Subclavian artery cannulation: (A) via direct arteriotomy; (B) axillary artery cannulation in axilla with a graft; (C) axillo-axillary artery cannulation; (D) a fluoroscopy-guided axillary artery cannulation. (From Lamelas J, Aberle C, Macias AE, et al. Cannulation strategies for minimally invasive cardiac surgery. *Innovations (Phila).* 2020;15[3]:261–269.)

bicaval cannulation. In MIMVR approaches, several cannulation options are available. Hemisternotomy approaches often use central arterial and venous cannulation, although alternative peripheral options including percutaneous femoral venous cannulation, in combination with central arterial cannulation or a completely femoral approach may be utilized. In comparison to sternotomy and hemisternotomy, the minithoracotomy approach generally relies on peripheral cannulation strategies including femoral and/or axillary cannulation.

Arterial Cannulation and Perfusion in Minimally Invasive Approaches to Both Mitral Valve Repair and Replacement. In MIMVR, pericardial space is limited and offers limited visualization of the heart. Thus, arterial cannulation is typically done via the larger and less diseased common femoral artery. A 23 Fr side-arm arterial cannula should be used if femoral artery size will allow; if a 21 Fr side-arm cannula is used, a higher arterial line pressure should be anticipated. If the femoral arteries are too small to accommodate a 21 Fr cannula and if an endoaortic balloon is to be used, then a 19 Fr cannula can be placed in each femoral artery for perfusion and for the endoaortic balloon. Alternatively, to avoid bilateral femoral artery cannulation, the transthoracic aortic cross-clamp can be used. Importantly, CPB should be initiated slowly to prevent arterial spasm in these situations.

Venous Cannulation in Minimally Invasive Approaches to Both Mitral Valve Repair and Replacement. Venous drainage routinely uses a multistage femoral venous catheter, typically placed in the right femoral vein with advancement and final positioning in the SVC under TEE guidance. A second venous line (15 to 18 Fr) can be positioned into the SVC to aid in venous drainage from a right internal jugular approach. In this case, the femoral venous cannula would be advanced to IVC-right atrial junction. Two venous cannulas may alleviate concern about suboptimal drainage caused by left atrial retraction, but a single venous cannula with correct placement and vacuum assistance is often sufficient. In cases of inadequate venous drainage, it is helpful to "Y" the venous line by inserting a second smaller cannula directly into the right atrium. Another useful adjunct that can help with drainage is the use of a percutaneous pulmonary arterial vent that can be placed through the right jugular vein.

Cannulation in Robotic Procedures. The femoral artery is the most common site for perfusion in robotic-assisted cardiac surgery. The right side is more convenient, being more accessible when the robot is docked. Direct aortic cannulation is also possible in robotic mitral valve procedures when peripheral vascular disease prevents a femoral approach; however, limitations for robotic-assisted procedures include the need for an additional thoracotomy placed under the robotic arms, so access is limited. Alternatively, the cannula could be placed through a 12-mm port with purse-string sutures placed either robotically in a port-only approach or directly with a small-access thoracotomy. Optimal venous cannulation approach is still debated. Some surgeons prefer a single, dual-stage femoral venous cannula, whereas others use bicaval cannulation in an effort to ensure adequate venous drainage, gaining percutaneous access to the SVC by cannulating the right internal jugular vein. Vacuum or kinetic-assisted venous drainage provides better drainage when using femoral cannulation, thereby avoiding distention of the right side of the heart, improving exposure and maintaining myocardial hypothermia.

Importance of Preoperative Assessment for Cannulation in Minimally Invasive Approaches to Both Mitral Valve Repair and Replacement. Computed tomography angiography is used in the evaluation of several factors prior to MIMVR.[30] In this scenario, since CPB may be established by retrograde perfusion through femoral vessels, the femoral and iliac vessels should be of sufficient caliber to allow cannulation. Furthermore, the absence of significant atherosclerotic disease is essential for reducing risk of cerebral embolism or retrograde dissection.[31]

Complications of Cannulation

Arterial Complications. Although rare, severe complications including retrograde dissection, embolization, limb ischemia, and stroke have been correlated with arterial cannulation, including when the most commonly used femoral cannulation technique is employed. For procedures performed without aortic cross-clamp, techniques for removal of air should mimic the technique used during standard median sternotomy to help reduce the incidence of stroke. In 1501 consecutive patients undergoing a minithoracotomy valve procedure, LaPietra et al.[32] observed an incidence of stroke from femoral artery and axillary artery cannulation of 1.4% and 2.9%, respectively ($P = .15$). Lamelas et al.[33] evaluated 2645 patients who underwent femoral cannulation, including patients with a prior history of stroke or peripheral vascular disease and observed a lower incidence of stroke in the femoral cannulation group (1.17%) compared to axillary or central cannulation (2.6%). Conversely, risk-adjusted outcomes in MIMVR published by Bedeir et al.[34] showed a higher incidence of permanent stroke with femoral cannulation group when compared with aortic cannulation ($P = .032$).

Venous Complications. Vascular complications from venous cannulation performed via a direct cutdown approach are rare. Percutaneous venous cannulation may injure the femoral artery when it lies over the femoral vein. Like in arterial percutaneous access, we recommend the use of ultrasound-guided vessel puncture using a micro-puncture needle. In some cases, it may be advisable to expose the right common femoral vein via a small groin incision in order to avoid inadvertent injury to the common femoral artery particularly in cases of anatomical variations. Bleeding with localized hematoma formation may occur with or without femoral artery injury. Additionally, even with the use of TEE and/or fluoroscopic guidance, perforation of the SVC, IVC, right atrium, and right ventricle remains potential complications.

SUMMARY

Myocardial dysfunction still occurs following cardiac surgery despite improvements in myocardial protection and perfusion techniques. The cornerstones of myocardial protection during CPB are hypothermia and electromechanical cardiac arrest. Cardioplegic solutions arrest the heart in diastole and help preserve myocardial function. Cardioplegic solutions are classified as crystalloid or blood-based solutions. Cold blood cardioplegia, and crystalloid-based del Nido and Custodiol-HTK solutions are the most frequently used cardioplegic solutions in mitral valve surgery. Antegrade and retrograde cardioplegia are administered via the ascending aorta and coronary sinus, respectively, and should be used simultaneously when concerns for adequate myocardial protection exist. Beating heart mitral valve surgery is used in high-risk patients (e.g., low cardiac function due to ischemic cardiomyopathy or dilated cardiomyopathy, previous sternotomy, or prior patent coronary bypass grafts) for conventional operations. In select patients, minimally invasive approaches to mitral valve surgery are preferred due to improved postoperative outcomes. Goals of perfusion are to provide complete drainage of the heart, establish adequate systemic perfusion, and minimize risks of malperfusion or vascular injury. Adequate venous drainage and decompression of the heart are necessary. Canulations strategies include peripheral cannulation performed via femoral, axillary, or subclavian artery cannulations, and central cannulation performed via direct distal ascending aorta cannulation. Femoral cannulation is commonly used in minimally invasive approaches while central cannulation is used mainly for conventional full sternotomy or when peripheral vessels are too diseased for cannulation.

CASE-BASED ASSESSMENT

1. A 73-year-old woman is referred for mitral valve repair. During the surgical workup, a critical calcified lesion is found in the left main coronary artery and the patient also needs coronary artery bypass graft. You connect the patient to the cardiopulmonary bypass (with an arterial cannula in the aorta and one venous cannula in the right atrium) and start with an antegrade cardioplegia, however, you realize that the heart does not stop beating. What do you do?
   A. You ask the perfusionist to increase the pressure of infusion of the cardioplegic solution.
   B. You proceed with the surgical procedure (since you think that a beating heart procedure is advantageous).
   C. You change the cardioplegic solution (since you start to think that the one you are using now is not working well).
   D. You place a catheter with balloon in the right atrium and guide it into the coronary sinus to start retrograde cardioplegia.
2. About the del Nido cardioplegia for adults, it is composed of:
   A. Crystalloid component only
   B. Blood component only
   C. Mixture of blood and crystalloid solution (4 parts of blood and 1 part of crystalloid)
   D. Mixture of blood and crystalloid solution (4 parts of crystalloid and 1 part of blood)

See page 317 for the answers.

REFERENCES

1. Paparella D, Guida P, Caparrotti S, et al. Myocardial damage influences short- and mid-term survival after valve surgery: a prospective multicenter study. *J Thorac Cardiovasc Surg*. 2014;148(5):2373–2379. doi:10.1016/j.jtcvs.2013.10.061.
2. Russell S, Butt S, Vohra HA. In search of optimal cardioplegia for minimally invasive valve surgery. *Perfusion*. Jun 3, 2021. doi:10.1177/02676591211012554. Online ahead of print.
3. Wahba A, Milojevic M, Boer C, et al. EACTS/EACTA/EBCP Committee Reviewers. 2019 EACTS/EACTA/EBCP guidelines on cardiopulmonary bypass in adult cardiac surgery. *Eur J Cardiothorac Surg*. 2020;57(2):210–251. doi:10.1093/ejcts/ezz267.
4. Ovrum E, Tangen G, Tollofsrud S, et al. Cold blood cardioplegia versus cold crystalloid cardioplegia: a prospective randomized study of 1440 patients undergoing coronary artery bypass grafting. *J Thorac Cardiovasc Surg*. 2004;128:860–865. doi:10.1016/j.jtcvs.2004.03.032.
5. Ovrum E, Tangen G, Tollofsrud S, et al. Cold blood versus cold crystalloid cardioplegia: a prospective randomised study of 345 aortic valve patients. *Eur J Cardiothorac Surg*. 2010;38:745–749. doi:10.1016/j.ejcts.2010.03.052.
6. Sá MP, Rueda FG, Ferraz PE, et al. Is there any difference between blood and crystalloid cardioplegia for myocardial protection during cardiac surgery? A meta-analysis of 5576 patients from 36 randomized trials. *Perfusion*. 2012;27:535–546. doi:10.1177/0267659112453754.
7. Alassar A, Bazerbashi S, Moawad N, et al. What is the value of topical cooling as an adjunct to myocardial protection? *Interact Cardiovasc Thorac Surg*. 2014;19(5):856–860. doi:10.1093/icvts/ivu259.
8. Cassese M, Martinelli G, Nasso G, et al. Topical cooling for myocardial protection: the results of a prospective randomized study of the "shallow technique". *J Card Surg*. 2006;21(4):357–362. doi:10.1111/j.1540-8191.2006.00245.x.
9. James TM, Nores M, Rousou JA, et al. Warm Blood Cardioplegia for Myocardial Protection: Concepts and Controversies. *Tex Heart Inst J*. 2020;47(2):108–116. doi:10.14503/THIJ-18-6909.
10. Martin TD, Craver JM, Gott JP, et al. Prospective, randomized trial of retrograde warm blood cardioplegia: myocardial benefit and neurologic threat. *Ann Thorac Surg*. 1994;57(2):298–302. doi:10.1016/0003-4975(94)90987-3.
11. Baikoussis NG, Papakonstantinou NA, Verra C, et al. Mechanisms of oxidative stress and myocardial protection during open-heart surgery. *Ann Card Anaesth*. 2015;18(4):555–564. doi:10.4103/0971-9784.166465.
12. Dagenais F, Pelletier LC, Carrier M. Antegrade/retrograde cardioplegia for valve replacement: a prospective study. *Ann Thorac Surg*. 1999;68:1681–1685. doi:10.1016/s0003-4975(99)00837-1.
13. Radmehr H, Soleimani A, Tatari H, Salehi M. Does combined antegrade-retrograde cardioplegia have any superiority over antegrade cardioplegia? *Heart Lung Circ*. 2008;17:475–477. doi:10.1016/j.hlc.2008.04.009.
14. Onorati F, Renzulli A, De Feo M, et al. Does antegrade blood cardioplegia alone provide adequate myocardial protection in patients with left main stem disease? *J Thorac Cardiovasc Surg*. 2003;126:1345–1351. doi:10.1016/s0022-5223(03)00736-0.
15. Luo H, Qi X, Shi H, et al. Single-dose del Nido cardioplegia used in adult minimally invasive valve surgery. *J Thorac Dis*. 2019;11(6):2373–2382. doi:10.21037/jtd.2019.05.78.
16. Preusse CJ. Custodiol Cardioplegia: A Single-Dose Hyperpolarizing Solution. *J Extra Corpor Technol*. 2016;48(2):15–20. https://

www.ncbi.nlm.nih.gov/pmc/articles/PMC5001528/. Accessed July 12, 2021.

17. Hummel BW, Buss RW, DiGiorgi PL, et al. Myocardial Protection and Financial Considerations of Custodiol Cardioplegia in Minimally Invasive and Open Valve Surgery. *Innovations (Phila).* 2016;11(6):420–424. doi:10.1097/IMI.0000000000000314.
18. Misra S, Srinivasan A, Jena SS, et al. Myocardial Protection in Adult Cardiac Surgery With del Nido Versus Blood Cardioplegia: A Systematic Review and Meta-Analysis. *Heart Lung Circ.* 2021;30(5):642–655. doi:10.1016/j.hlc.2020.10.016.
19. Lebon JS, Couture P, Colizza M, et al. Myocardial Protection in Minimally Invasive Mitral Valve Surgery: Retrograde Cardioplegia Alone Using Endovascular Coronary Sinus Catheter Compared With Combined Antegrade and Retrograde Cardioplegia. *J Cardiothorac Vasc Anesth.* 2019;33(5):1197–1204. doi:10.1053/j.jvca.2018.11.042.
20. Matte GS, del Nido PJ. History and use of del Nido cardioplegia solution at Boston Children's Hospital. *J Extra Corpor Technol.* 2012;44(3):98–103. https://www.ncbi.nlm.nih.gov/pmc/articles/PMC4557532/. Accessed July 12, 2021.
21. Marbach JA, Chweich H, Miyashita S, et al. Temporary mechanical circulatory support devices: updates from recent studies. *Curr Opin Cardiol.* 2021;36(4):375–383. doi:10.1097/HCO.0000000000000880.
22. Pasic M, Sündermann S, Unbehaun A, et al. Beating heart mitral valve surgery: results in 120 consecutive patients considered unsuitable for conventional mitral valve surgery. *Interact Cardiovasc Thorac Surg.* 2017;25(4):541–547. doi:10.1093/icvts/ivx139.
23. Salhiyyah K, Taggart D. Beating-heart valve surgery: a systematic review. *Asian Cardiovasc Thorac Ann.* 2009;17:650–658. doi:10.1177/0218492309348942.
24. Babaroglu S, Yay K, Parlar AI, et al. Beating heart versus conventional mitral valve surgery. *Interact Cardiovasc Thorac Surg.* 2011;12(3):441–447. doi:10.1510/icvts.2010.255240.
25. Zhang H, Xu HS, Wen B, et al. Minimally invasive beating heart technique for mitral valve surgery in patients with previous sternotomy and giant left ventricle. *J Cardiothorac Surg.* 2020;15(1):122. doi:10.1186/s13019-020-01171-6.
26. Ailawadi G, Agnihotri AK, Mehall JR, et al. Minimally Invasive Mitral Valve Surgery I: Patient Selection, Evaluation, and Planning. *Innovations (Phila).* 2016;11(4):243–250. doi:10.1097/IMI.0000000000000301.
27. Braathen B, Jeppsson A, Scherstén H, et al. One single dose of histidine-tryptophan-ketoglutarate solution gives equally good myocardial protection in elective mitral valve surgery as repetitive cold blood cardioplegia: a prospective randomized study. *J Thorac Cardiovasc Surg.* 2011;141(4):995–1001. doi:10.1016/j.jtcvs.2010.07.011.
28. Rival PM, Moore THM, McAleenan A, et al. Transthoracic clamp versus endoaortic balloon occlusion in minimally invasive mitral valve surgery: a systematic review and meta-analysis. *Eur J Cardiothorac Surg.* 2019;56(4):643–653. doi:10.1093/ejcts/ezy489.
29. Lamelas J, Aberle C, Macias AE, et al. Cannulation Strategies for Minimally Invasive Cardiac Surgery. *Innovations (Phila).* 2020;15(3):261–269.
30. Rajiah P, Schoenhagen P. The role of computed tomography in pre-procedural planning of cardiovascular surgery and intervention. *Insights Imaging.* 2013;4(5):671–689. doi:10.1007/s13244-013-0270-8.
31. Schoenhagen P, Numburi U, Halliburton SS, et al. Three-dimensional imaging in the context of minimally invasive and transcatheter cardiovascular interventions using multi-detector computed tomography: from pre-operative planning to intra-operative guidance. *Eur Heart J.* 2010;31(22):2727–2740. doi:10.1093/eurheartj/ehq302.
32. LaPietra A, Santana O, Mihos CG, et al. Incidence of cerebrovascular accidents in patients undergoing minimally invasive valve surgery. *J Thorac Cardiovasc Surg.* 2014;148(1):156–160. doi:10.1016/j.jtcvs.2013.08.016.
33. Lamelas J, Williams RF, Mawad M, et al. Complications Associated With Femoral Cannulation During Minimally Invasive Cardiac Surgery. *Ann Thorac Surg.* 2017;103(6):1927–1932. doi:10.1016/j.athoracsur.2016.09.098.
34. Bedeir K, Reardon M, Ramchandani M, et al. Elevated Stroke Risk Associated With Femoral Artery Cannulation During Mitral Valve Surgery. *Semin Thorac Cardiovasc Surg.* 2015;27(2):97–103. doi:10.1053/j.semtcvs.2015.06.008 Summer.

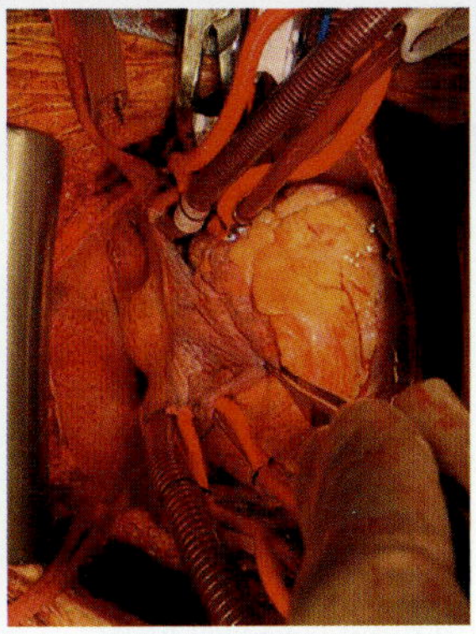

15

Mitral Operation: Sternotomy Approach

Michael Ibrahim, Michael A. Acker

CHAPTER OUTLINE

LEARNING OBJECTIVES

- Understand the indications for sternotomy approach to mitral valve surgery.
- Understand the standard setup and cannulation strategy for mitral valve surgery through sternotomy.
- Understand tips and tricks for optimizing exposure through sternotomy.
https://www.kollaborate.tv/link?id=6144de4daefe9

INTRODUCTION

Mitral repair or replacement via median sternotomy is the gold standard for surgical interventions upon the mitral valve and remains the most common approach.[1] Median sternotomy is universally available, safe, and provides. Cvalvular apparatus. In certain patients, for example, those with severe peripheral vascular disease or unsuitable anatomy for limited access approaches, it is the only option. In other patients, a limited approach to the mitral valve is converted to a sternotomy approach for a number of reasons. The sternotomy approach also provides considerable versatility in managing complex cases, extending exposure in challenging scenarios, and should be the foundational technique in a surgical mitral valve program, even one which includes or is starting a minimal access program.[2] Here we describe our practice of median sternotomy mitral valve surgery.

MEDIAN STERNOTOMY AND CANNULATION

We perform a limited skin incision and a full sternotomy to provide complete access to the heart and great vessels. Pericardial stay sutures are placed on the right side to allow the left atrium to be rotated and pulled into view. Following systemic heparinization, central cannulation is achieved with a dispersion tip aortic cannula in the lesser curve of the distal ascending aorta, allowing space for placement of an aortic root vent and any other concomitant procedures such as aortic valve replacement or coronary bypass grafts. The superior vena cava (SVC) is directly cannulated with a 20 to 22 Fr metal tip right angle drainage cannula, and the inferior vena cava (IVC) is cannulated with a single-stage 32 to 36 Fr venous drainage cannula. A coronary sinus cannula is placed through the body of the right atrium for retrograde cardioplegia. The oblique sinus is opened, and the SVC is dissected free from its pericardial connections to promote mobility of the heart which may be rotated around the great vessels. Cardiopulmonary bypass is commenced, the root vent is placed and the aorta is cross-clamped, and cold blood high-K^+ cardioplegia is administered for diastolic cardiac arrest. During this time, the sidebar of a standard Carpentier mitral retractor is attached. Once cardioplegia is complete, surgical access to the mitral valve begins. Fig. 15.1 demonstrates this standard setup.

LEFT ATRIOTOMY AND MITRAL EXPOSURE

We begin with deep dissection of the interatrial groove first described by Søndergaard in 1955, who used this dissection to facilitate extracardiac closure of atrial septal defects.[3] This is essential in order to provide adequate access to the left ventricle. A very safe way of conducting this dissection is using electrocautery or scissors beginning under the proximal SVC and working toward the oblique sinus which was previously dissected (Video 15.1). This dissection can be carried at least 1 to 2 cm into the interatrial groove, liberating the atria from

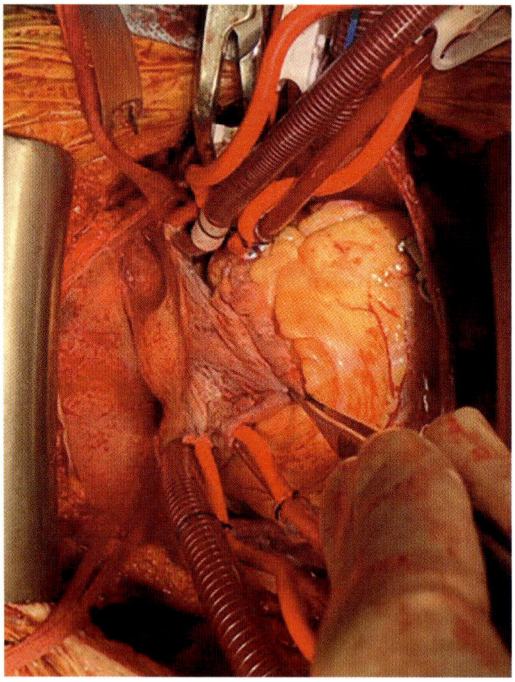

Fig. 15.1 Standard Cannulation Setup. Bicaval cannulation, with circumferential dissection of the SVC and IVC, and caval tapes are shown. *SVC*, superior vena cava; *IVC*, inferior vena cava.

one another. Then, using a number 15 blade, the left atrium is opened and cleared of blood with cardiotomy suction. The incision is extended in both lateral directions, along the previously dissected groove and 1.5 cm away from the os of the right pulmonary veins. Video 15.1 shows this dissection being performed with a long scalpel along the interatrial groove, concluding by entering the left atrium itself. Video 15.2 shows the extension of this incision with long scissors. We then place the first atrial retractor in the roof of the left atrium, which is carefully retracted and tightened by the assistant. A second atrial retractor is placed at the IVC margin of the roof of the left atrium, and in most cases, a third retractor is placed at right angles to the first two and secured on a side-arm. These retractors are serially tightened several times to provide optimal exposure according to the principles outlined by Cosgrove.[4] This step is critical to optimizing valve exposure. Together, this provides approximately 270-degree retraction on the atrium and has the effect of pulling the mitral valve into view and toward the surgeon. Figs. 15.2 and 15.3 show the excellent exposure of the mitral valve which can be achieved with this simple and safe technique. Placement of a retrograde cannula allows convenient administration of cardioplegia when it will not hinder operation, such as during suture placement through the annuloplasty ring.

VALVE INSPECTION AND REPAIR

From a sternotomy approach, surgical valve inspection commences with a hook to identify areas of valve dysfunction and determine a repair strategy according to the principles defined by Carpentier.[5] Fig. 15.3 shows that this approach provides excellent exposure of the mitral valve for complete valve analysis. Annuloplasty sutures are placed to pull the valve into view and facilitate leaflet repair. On occasion, an atrial retraction suture is placed to pull the mitral valve further into view. Our approach typically involves complete ring annuloplasty and limited resection or placement of neochordae.

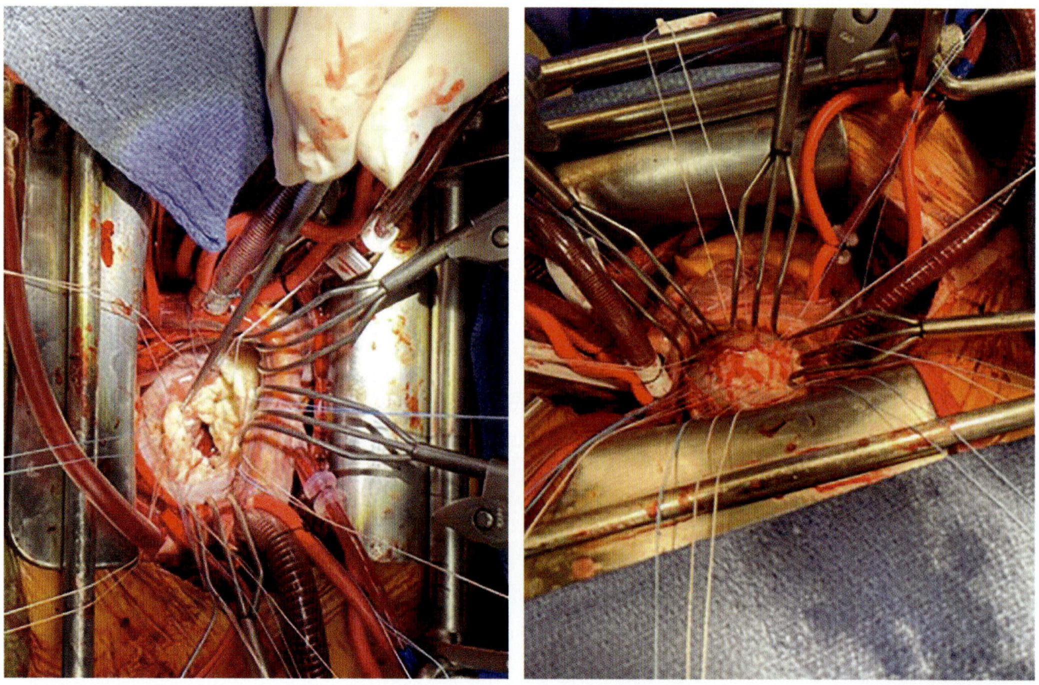

Fig. 15.2 Surgeon's View of Exposed Mitral Valve. Three atrial retractors as shown provide excellent exposure of the mitral valve. The effect of annular suture retraction can also be seen.

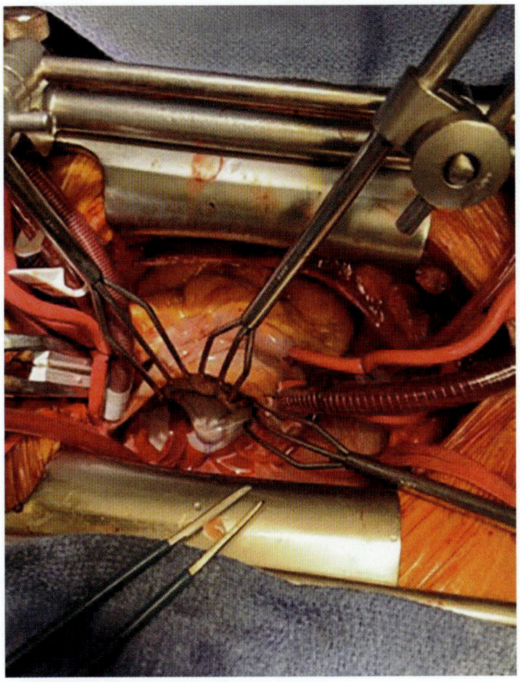

Fig. 15.3 Surgeon's View of Exposed Mitral Valve—Atrial Retraction. A pledgeted Prolene suture in the floor of the left atrium enables the mitral valve to be pulled into view.

PLACEMENT OF ANNULOPLASTY SUTURES

Mitral repair through sternotomy at the University of Pennsylvania is performed by a senior cardiac surgery resident on the surgeon's side and a faculty mitral surgeon on the assistant side. We have found this "two-surgeon" approach to be an excellent platform that facilitates not only education but also efficient conduct of the operation. Annuloplasty is an excellent example of this. Following left atriotomy as described, we begin with annuloplasty suture placement at the P2 segment using a 2-0 Ti-Cron suture using a simple forehand technique. This suture is normally placed by the surgeon on the left-hand side of the table who has a better view of P2. Using suture retraction, each suture facilitates placement of the next. Annuloplasty suture placement continues toward P3 using a combination of forehand and backhand sutures by turning one's body appropriately. Once the right fibrous trigone is reached, we then return to P2 and place sutures toward the left fibrous trigone. The surgeon at the left-hand side of the table places most of the anterior sutures that are forehand for a right-handed surgeon.

CHALLENGING EXPOSURE

A number of situations represent challenges for exposure and can be tackled with modification of the standard sternotomy approach we describe. We must emphasize that formal dissection of Søndergaard's groove is critical and enhances exposure significantly. The left atriotomy can be extended under the IVC which in challenging cases will sometimes be enough to provide adequate exposure. In some situations, for example in an especially deep chest, we place a pledgeted atrial retraction suture to move the valve closer to the surgeon, as shown in Fig. 15.3. We have rarely required the transseptal approach, except in some re-operations with limited cardiac mobility.

The transseptal approach begins with a standard extended right atriotomy after both SVC and IVC have been snared.[6] This incision should be parallel to the atrioventricular groove and at least 2 cm away from it. Then, the interatrial septum is sharply incised beginning at the location of the fossa ovalis and extended superiorly to join the right atrial incision. Lastly, the incision is carried onto the dome of the left atrium, being sure to give wide clearance to the aortic root. This approach can be useful in situations where it is unsafe or impractical to perform a wide dissection of the heart in the re-operative setting. The pitfalls of this technique are injury to the atrioventricular groove, injury to the aortic root, and residual septal defect. There is concern about an increase in non-sinus rhythms due to injury to the SAN artery, but this is likely avoidable with careful attention to detail.[7] In general, we prefer deep dissection of Søndergaard's groove to the transseptal approach. Situations in a first-time operation where this approach can be useful are when the left atrium is diminutive or when a large mass such as a left atrial or mitral-based tumor is being resected.

In situations where exposure is inadequate with standard left atriotomy, we snare the cavae and transect the SVC to facilitate retraction of the interatrial septum as described by Selle.[8] Fig. 15.4 shows this provides excellent exposure to the valve, especially in complex re-operations where the maneuvers described hitherto have been ineffective. The SVC is first dissected free from its pericardial connections. It is encircled, snared, and transected away from the sinoatrial node. After completion of the mitral valve and closure of the left atrium, the SVC is re-anastomosed with a running 5-0 Prolene suture.

MITRAL ANNULAR CALCIFICATION

Mitral annular calcification (MAC) represents one of the most challenging subsets of mitral pathologies and often coincides with an increased comorbidity burden.[9] In situations of severe MAC, we typically avoid minimal access strategies and opt for sternotomy. This allows more flexibility and control of MAC including the use of ultrasonic devices to penetrate dense areas where sutures are required. We also feel that sternotomy provides an additional layer of safety in the setting of a higher risk case and allows us to rapidly detect and respond to complications such as groove disruptions that occur with higher frequency in the setting of MAC. The sternotomy approach also allows direct visual inspection of the annulus and immediate tactile feedback using regular instruments.

RE-OPERATION

Re-operation may follow any previous cardiac operation through either conventional sternotomy or minimal access. The first and most important step is preoperative assessment with a CT scan. We review the proximity of critical structures including the innominate vein, the ascending aorta, the right ventricle, and any patent coronary bypass grafts. We routinely place femoral arterial

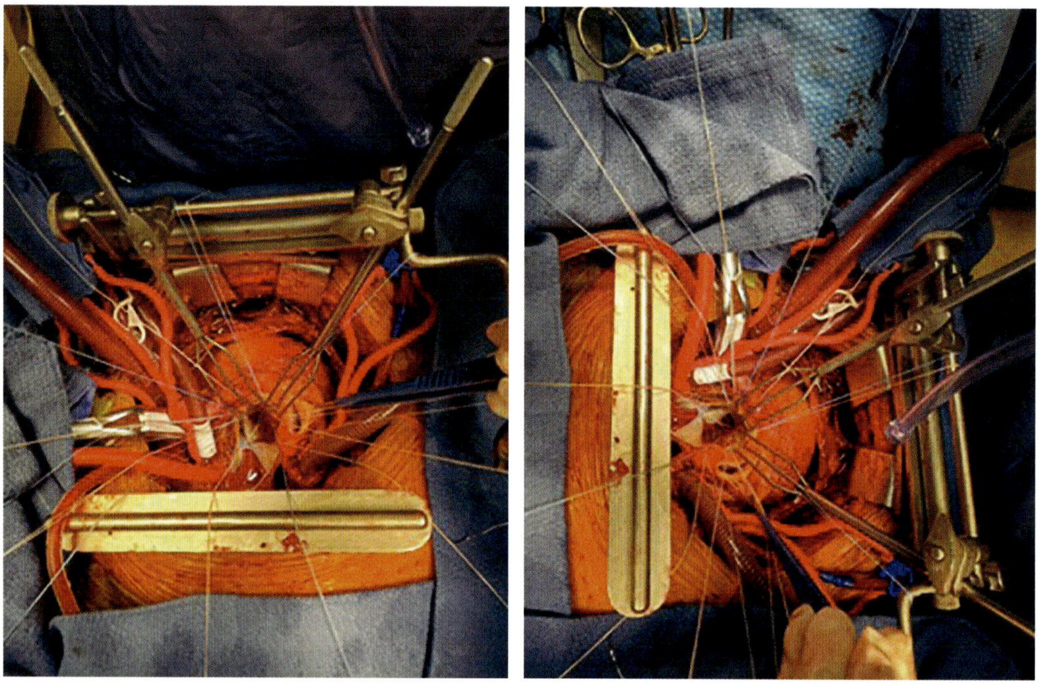

Fig. 15.4 Division of the SVC for Mitral Valve Exposure. The divided SVC can be seen at the tip of the forceps. In this case, extremely challenging exposure of the mitral valve was handled by mobilization, division, and retraction of the SVC. *SVC*, Superior vena cava.

and venous access sheaths in the groin vessels prior to incision and ensure that six units of cross-matched blood are available and checked. In the case of previous minimal access approaches, sternotomy is achieved with a regular saw assuming the CT scan is reassuring. In the case of previous sternotomy, we re-open the previous incision and divide sternal wires. Then, an oscillating saw is used to divide the anterior table. Only then are the wires removed and division of the posterior table is completed. The heart is dissected out so that cannulation may be achieved. Following the commencement of cardiopulmonary bypass, the lateral heart is dissected free which is important in allowing sufficient mobility and exposure. We favor deep dissection of Søndergaard's groove and left atrial incision as a primary approach in re-operations. We have generally found that this allows excellent exposure of the valve. It is critical that the apex is released to facilitate cardiac rotation. In certain circumstances, we perform a transseptal approach or divide the SVC as described if exposure is inadequate.

CONCOMITANT OPERATIONS

One of the most important indications for and advantages of the sternotomy approach is the ability to perform concomitant operations (Fig. 15.5). Most commonly, these are coronary artery bypass grafting, right-sided valve operations, and surgery for atrial fibrillation. The order of operation is dictated by the imperative to avoid cardiac distraction following implantation of a rigid mitral prosthesis or annuloplasty device. For arrhythmia surgery, sternotomy provides access to both left- and right-sided veins and allows external resection and primary closure of the left atrial appendage. Distal coronary bypass grafts are typically constructed prior to mitral operation. In the case of combined aortic and mitral operation, our standard approach is to complete the mitral operation first and then address the aortic valve. Some authors prefer to excise the aortic valve prior to mitral operation, but we have not found this necessary in most cases. It is critical

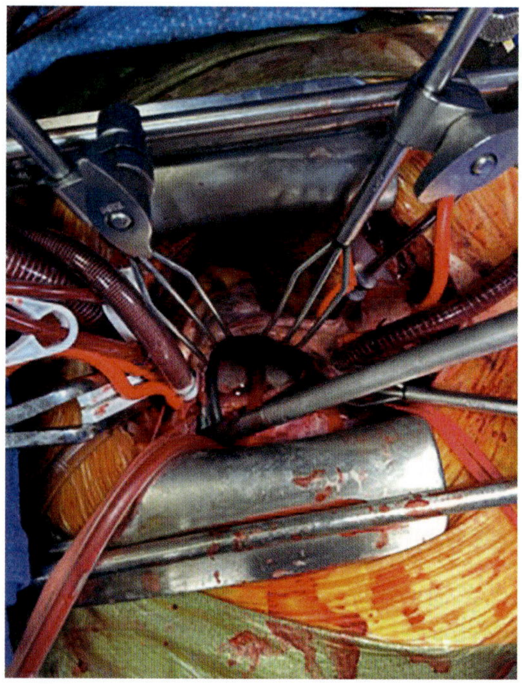

Fig. 15.5 Sternotomy Provides Complete Access for Concomitant Operations. Radiofrequency ablation device can be seen traversing the posterior left atrium. Sternotomy is an ideal approach for patients who require concomitant operation, including coronary and multi-valve surgery.

to avoid aortic valve replacement prior to mitral operation and to consider both valves when making sizing decisions. Operations on the tricuspid valve are typically performed after the left atriotomy is closed, with or without the aortic cross-clamp.

SUMMARY

The sternotomy approach is the gold standard approach to mitral operation against which new, minimal access approaches will be judged. It is important that all mitral surgeons be familiar with the sternotomy approach which will facilitate appropriate selection of candidates for sternotomy and minimal access approaches and allow safe conversion when necessary. This strategy will produce equivalent results for either strategy.[10] There are a multitude of ways of enhancing exposure through a sternotomy which we have outlined. One of the advantages of sternotomy is the ability to combine mitral operation with any other cardiac or aortic procedure.

CASE-BASED ASSESSMENT

A 51-year-old female is worked up for shortness of breath. Her echocardiogram reveals severe mitral valve insufficiency with an ejection fraction of 0.2. She undergoes preoperative cardiac catheterization which reveals a right dominant coronary circulation with a 95% diffuse mid-stenosis of the right coronary artery and what appears to be heavy posterior mitral annular calcification (MAC).

1. What is her indication for a sternotomy approach?
   a. MAC
   b. Right coronary lesion
   c. Impaired LV function
2. You use ultrasonic debridement to manage severe MAC and are able to repair the valve. Upon closure, you lift the heart to place a pacing wire. A short while after this, the patient becomes hemodynamically unstable and blood accumulates from behind the heart. You must rule out which feared complication?
   a. AV groove disruption
   b. Left atrial dissection
   c. Aortic dissection
3. This complication is best treated by which of the following?
   a. Administration of blood products
   b. Patch exclusion from the exterior LV surface
   c. Re-atriotomy, removal of prosthesis, patch closure of defect, and redo MV replacement
   d. Intra-aortic balloon pump placement

See page 317 for the answers

REFERENCES

1. Vemulapalli, S, Grau-Sepulveda, M, Habib, R, et al. (2019). Patient and hospital characteristics of mitral valve surgery in the United States. *JAMA Cardiol, 4*(11), 1149–1155.
2. Kastengren, M, Svenarud, P, K ä llner, G, et al. (2020). Minimally invasive versus sternotomy mitral valve surgery when initiating a minimally invasive programme. *Eur J Cardiothorac Surg, 58*(6), 1168–1174.
3. Sondergaard, T, Gotzsche, H, Ottosen, P, et al. (1955). Surgical closure of interatrial septal defects by circumclusion. *Acta Chir Scand, 109*(3–4), 188–196.
4. McCarthy, JF, & Cosgrove, DM, 3rd (1998). Optimizing mitral valve exposure with conventional left atriotomy. *Ann Thorac Surg, 65*(4), 1161–1162.
5. Carpentier, A, Deloche, A, Dauptain, J, et al. (1971). A new reconstructive operation for correction of mitral and tricuspid insufficiency. *J Thorac Cardiovasc Surg, 61*(1), 1–13.
6. Bowman, FO Jr, & Malm, JR. (1965). The transseptal approach to mitral valve repair. *Arch Surg, 90*, 329–331.
7. Nienaber, JJ, & Glower, DD. (2006). Minitransseptal versus left atrial approach to the mitral valve: a comparison of outcomes. *Ann Thorac Surg, 82*(3), 834–839; discussion 839.
8. Selle, JG. (1984). Temporary division of the superior vena cava for exceptional mitral valve exposure. *J Thorac Cardiovasc Surg, 88*(2), 302–304.
9. Edelman, JJ, Badhwar, V, Larbalestier, R, et al. (2021). Contemporary surgical and transcatheter management of mitral annular calcification. *Ann Thorac Surg*. Feb.;111(2):390–397. doi: 10.1016/j.athoracsur.2020.04.148.Epub 2020 Aug 14.
10. Moscarelli, M, Fattouch, K, Gaudino, M, et al. (2020). Minimal access versus sternotomy for complex mitral valve repair: a meta-analysis. *Ann Thorac Surg, 109*(3), 737–744.

16

Mitral Valve Surgery: Right Thoracotomy Approach

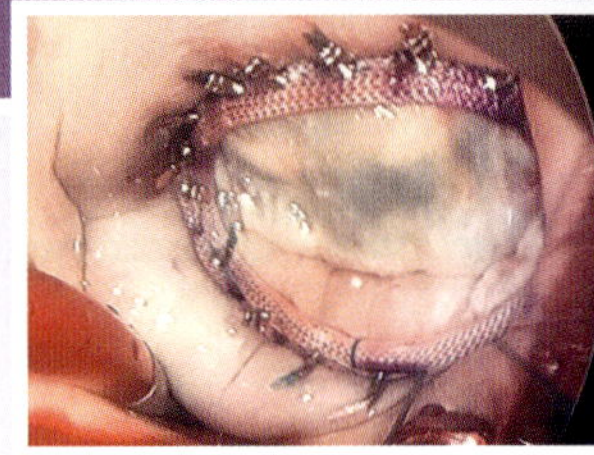

Nicolas H. Pope, Gorav Ailawadi

CHAPTER OUTLINE

LEARNING OBJECTIVES

1. To describe basic patient positioning, special equipment, and cannulation strategies for right-thoracotomy/port-access mitral valve surgery
2. To describe the advantages of right-thoracotomy port-access mitral intervention over traditional sternotomy approach
3. To describe the utility of the right-thoracotomy port-access approach in patients with prior sternotomy
4. To discuss strategies to maximize cardioprotection during right-thoracotomy port-access mitral valve intervention

INTRODUCTION

One of the more time-tested alternative, nonsternotomy approaches to the mitral valve is through a right thoracotomy. Over time, this approach has evolved into a minimally invasive technique through a "port access" right anterior minithoracotomy. While various strategies exist for cannulation, cardioprotection, aortic cross-clamping, and exposure of the mitral valve, the basic tenants of peripheral cannulation and a more anatomic approach to the mitral valve offer several advantages. First, such less-invasive approaches have been shown to decrease postoperative pain, decrease need for blood transfusion, and decreased length of stay.[1,25] Additionally, this approach allows for evaluation and testing of the mitral valve in the natural, anatomic orientation of the mitral annulus, which theoretically can increase the likelihood of repair. The right thoracotomy approach also offers a distinct advantage in patients who have had a previous sternotomy as it typically requires less adhesiolysis and less need for blood products. Several challenges are also conferred by this approach, including cannulation, cardioprotection, aortic cross-clamping, and visualization. Herein, we present our preferred right anterior minithoracotomy port-access technique with thoracoscopic assistance and highlight the challenges and solutions to common problems this technique affords.

COMPARISON OF RIGHT THORACOTOMY TO STERNOTOMY

The mini-right thoracotomy approach to the mitral valve first gained popularity in the late 1990s.[2,3] Despite several decades of experience, only 25% of isolated mitral operations were undertaken through minimally invasive approaches as of 2009.[4] Compared to sternotomy, patients undergoing minimally invasive operations had comparable rates of stroke and mortality while requiring fewer reoperations for postoperative hemorrhage and had shorter length of stay.[5,6] While patients in the minimally invasive cohort in this study had longer cardiopulmonary bypass and aortic cross-clamp times, these importantly did not result in an increase in morbidity or mortality.[1]

Additionally, the lateral approach to the mitral valve allows for evaluation of the mitral valve in a more anatomic position than when approached via sternotomy. This allows for testing of the repaired valve with minimal distortion of the geometry of the mitral apparatus and has, in our experience, facilitated repairs with no residual regurgitation. While there was no reported increase in reoperation, patients with mild residual mitral regurgitation (MR) after repair were shown to have more frequent progression to moderate (17% vs. 7%, $P = .03$) or severe (6% vs. 1%, $P = .016$) regurgitation as compared to patients with no residual MR, suggesting that these small differences in residual MR improve long-term outcomes.[7]

Furthermore, avoidance of sternotomy also avoids potential sternal wound complications and may decrease postoperative pain.[1,8,9] While pain following thoracotomy certainly can prove significant, adjuncts such as indwelling local anesthetic catheters, intercostal nerve cryoablation, and intercostal nerve block with long-acting local anesthetics have been shown to significantly decrease postoperative pain after thoracotomy.[10–12] As part of a multimodal, multidisciplinary approach, institution of "enhanced recovery" pathways, which include the intraoperative use of such adjuncts, have been shown to decrease postoperative morphine equivalents, length of stay and hospital cost in patients undergoing general thoracic surgery by thoracotomy.[13] The study of such pathways in minimally invasive cardiac surgery remains ongoing.

While not rising to the level of importance of the quality of the operation performed, it should also be mentioned that overall cosmesis from port-access mitral surgery is generally excellent, consisting of a single 3 to 6 cm incision of the right anterolateral chest that can often be placed in the inframammary fold in women, and a 1 to 2 cm femoral incision to allow for cannulation for cardiopulmonary bypass. Avoidance of a sternotomy may be particularly advantageous in frail patients. Additionally, patient perception of minimally invasive techniques remains positive, and demand for such operations remains high with both referring cardiologists and patients alike.

Finally, our described strategy for direct visualization of the operation through a well-placed right thoracotomy aided by placement of a thoracoscopic port allows for the surgeon, the trainee, and the assistant to have excellent, simultaneous visualization of the operative field. This allows for ease of demonstration of technique ("watch the way I do this") and supervised practice ("let me watch you do this"), which can be difficult without the use of a thoracoscope or with open mitral surgery.

SET UP

Preoperative Considerations

The preoperative workup for patients being considered for port-access mitral valve surgery must be thorough and thoughtful, in addition to the standard workup for those undergoing mitral valve surgery (echocardiography to determine mechanism of valvular pathology and assess for other valvular lesions, coronary artery assessment, carotid duplex, and pulmonary function testing where appropriate).

First, we routinely obtain a computed tomography (CT) scan of the chest, abdomen, and pelvis. It is critical to assess the presence of significant ascending or aortic arch calcification that may preclude a minimally invasive approach, particularly when cross-clamping at the level of the transverse sinus. Historically, minimally invasive (MIS) mitral surgery was associated with higher stroke risk related to peripheral cannulation.[14] To minimize this risk, preoperative assessment of the femoral vessels encourages safe peripheral cannulation for cardiopulmonary bypass. Alternative arterial cannulation through a right axillary graft can be used in cases where the femoral arteries are of inadequate size or are heavily calcified. Likely due to more careful cannulation strategies, contemporary data from the STS National Database suggests stroke risk is now equivalent with MIS and sternotomy.[4]

Left heart catheterization or coronary artery CT is required to rule out concomitant coronary artery disease that warrants intervention, as well as document coronary dominance and risk of injury during annular suture placement. Presence of significant obstructive coronary disease is typically an indication for an open approach with concomitant coronary artery bypass grafting, although a hybrid port-access approach with percutaneous coronary intervention can be considered for select patients (e.g., those with low SYNTAX score and non-LAD [left anterior descending artery disease]). When left heart catheterization is required, our preference is via a radial approach in order to preserve a virgin plane for femoral cutdown for cannulation. Femoral artery access for coronary catheterization can result in focal femoral arterial dissection and lead to retrograde aortic dissection during peripheral cannulation.[15]

Pulmonary function testing is also routinely performed prior to consideration of a mini-right thoracotomy approach in those patients with history of smoking, asthma or other lung disease, as brief periods of single lung ventilation are required prior to and following institution of cardiopulmonary bypass. Because these periods are relatively short and intermittent dual lung ventilation is possible, even patients with moderately severe lung disease may be considered for port-access approach, with the understanding that sternotomy remains the backup plan should single lung isolation not be tolerated.

Positioning

While important with any cardiac operation, subtle changes in positioning and preparation of the patient can be the difference between success and challenging exposure when attempting minimally invasive techniques. The patient is positioned supine on the operative table, at a point in the bed which allows operators to comfortably stand on the right of the bed near the level of the right shoulder. This typically is at a point further towards the foot of the bed than in positioning for sternotomy to allow two operators (surgeon and trainee).

An inflatable bump is placed length-wise under the patient's right shoulder and inflated to allow for sterile access to the right hemithorax. We prefer the use of an inflatable device to a fixed "bump," as this allows for quick deflation should a sternotomy be required. When using a conventional cross-clamp, invasive and noninvasive blood pressure monitoring should be performed in the left arm to minimize disruption of the operation with inflation of the cuff on the right arm or need to access the right radial artery if nonfunctional.

After inflation of the bump, the hips are reoriented in a flat, supine position in order to allow for easy access to the bilateral femoral vessels. The right arm is tucked away from the body and below the level of the bed to allow access to the lateral chest. An ether screen is used to allow for separation of the operative field while maintaining easy access to both the endotracheal tube and the transesophageal echocardiography (TEE) probe, both

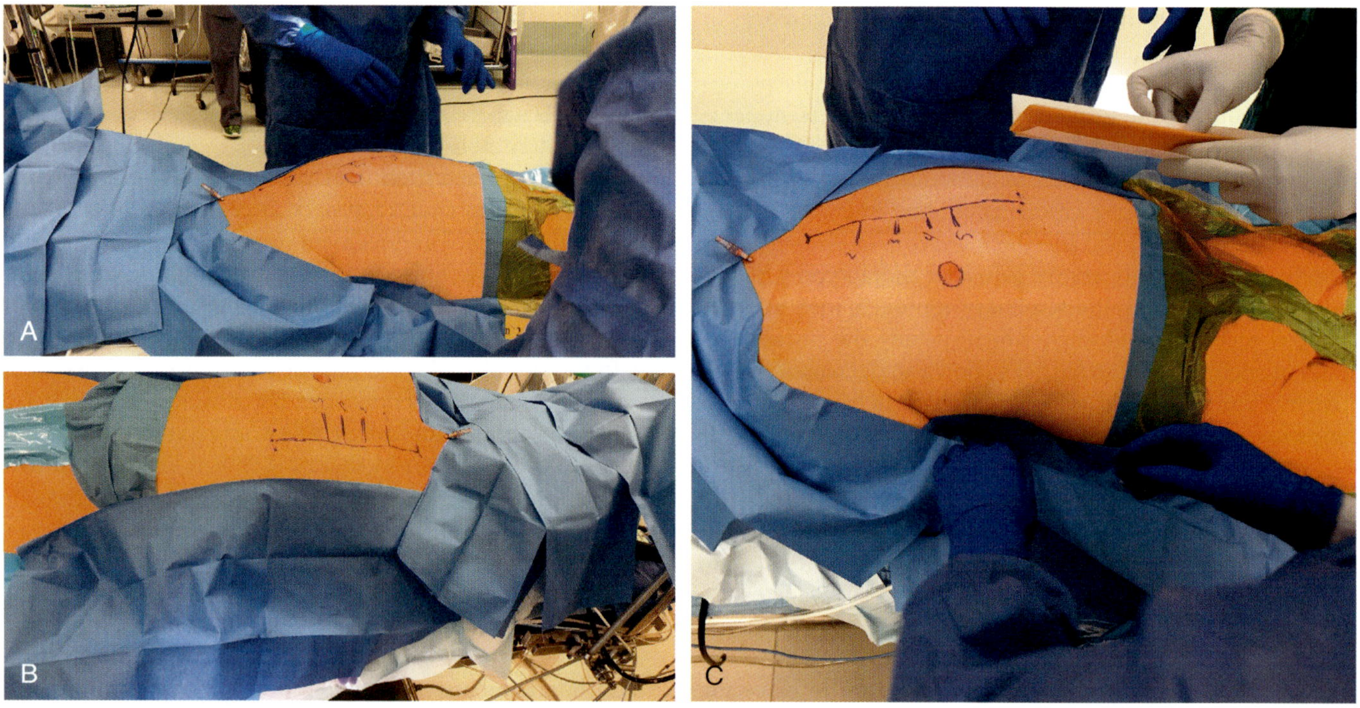

Fig. 16.1 Patient Positioning for Port-access Mitral Valve Access via Right Mini-thoracotomy. After prepping, the areola (A) and sternal landmarks (B) are marked prior to placement of sterile adhesive skin barriers (C), as these get distorted with positioning.

of which require more frequent access for a minimally invasive operation. After prepping, the areola and sternal landmarks are marked prior to placement of sterile adhesive skin barriers, as these get distorted with positioning (Fig. 16.1). Moreover, rapid midline sternal incision can be performed when premarked. We utilize a table-mounted sterile camera holder for the thoracoscope. The attachment for the camera holder is placed on the operating room table at the level of the right hip.

Anesthetic Concerns

As periods of single lung ventilation are required prior to and following cardiopulmonary bypass, single lung ventilation of the left lung is required. This can be accomplished either by intubation with a double lumen endotracheal tube or with bronchoscopic guided placement of an endobronchial blocker. While either typically provides excellent exposure, it has been our preference to use a bronchial blocker, as intubation with a double lumen endotracheal tube can be technically challenging and can require reintubation with a single lumen endotracheal tube at the end of the case should the patient not meet criteria for extubation in the operating room.

In order to provide access for future superior vena cava (SVC) cannulation, ultrasound-guided placement of a large bore (typically 16G) peripheral venous catheter is placed by the anesthesia team proximal to the introducer sheath at the time of central line placement. This catheter is prepped into the sterile field and allows access for dilation of the tract and percutaneous SVC cannulation after systemic heparinization.

Because internal defibrillation is difficult through a right mini-thoracotomy, careful placement of external defibrillator pads is of utmost importance. The right-sided pad is placed along the right scapula, while the left pad is placed more anteriorly, just below the left inframammary fold in order to create a vector across the heart. Because of their proximity to the field, these are excluded with adhesive drapes prior to prepping in order to keep dry, avoid difficulty with conduction, and decrease fire risk.

Intraoperative TEE is necessary for port-access mitral surgery. In addition to the information typically gained at the time of all mitral operations, including more precise evaluation of the mechanism of mitral pathology, risk of systolic anterior motion such as the C-sept (coaptation to septal distance) and aorto-mitral angle, and intraoperative assessment postsurgical repair, TEE is crucial for several key portions of the port-access technique. First, evaluation of aortic insufficiency is vital, as a retrograde cardioplegia catheter is not routinely placed. While percutaneous coronary sinus catheters are routinely used by some centers, we generally see severe aortic insufficiency as an indication for an open procedure and lesser degrees can be managed with our standard minimally invasive approach. Second, TEE is used to guide peripheral cannulation for cardiopulmonary bypass, ensuring safe passage of wires and cannula to their desired locations under direct visualization. Lastly, evaluation for left ventricular distention, particularly during administration of cardioplegia, is only accomplished by echocardiography, as visualization of the left ventricle is limited, and direct visualization or palpation is not possible.

Equipment

The advent of specialty equipment designed specifically for port-access mitral valve surgery has greatly aided in the ease of exposure and the development of novel techniques. We provide a list of commercially available equipment we routinely use as a point of reference.

In order to achieve adequate exposure through a relatively small thoracotomy, we utilize a small Alexis Soft Tissue Retractor (Applied Medical, Rancho Santa Margarita, CA, USA). Next, a low-profile adjustable Finochietto-type retractor is used. We utilize the Estech Window Access SI Retractor Body (AtriCure, Mason, OH, USA) with standard blades, the depth for which is chosen according to the amount of soft tissue above the chest wall.

Various methods of aortic cross-clamping have been described, including endoaortic balloon occluders (IntraClude device, Edwards Lifesciences, Irvine, CA, USA) and direct aortic cross-clamping with intrathoracic cross-clamps placed through stab incisions and specifically designed for minimally invasive applications (Chitwood or Mohr clamps).[3] While there were initial concerns with reports of clamp movement or aortic injury with early generations of the endoaortic clamp, later generations appear to have remedied these safety concerns in experienced hands, and this is a safe alternative to direct aortic cross-clamping.[16–18] We prefer the use of a Glauber Aortic Cross Clamp (Sorin, Arvada, CO, USA). This direct aortic clamp is deployable completely within the chest, allowing for more working room. As it does not protrude through the chest wall, there are benefits with less theoretic risk of accidental manipulation or injury to the aorta.

Retraction of the left atrium and exposure of the mitral valve is achieved with an atrial lift retractor, and we use the Atrial Lift (AtriCure, Mason, OH, USA). Extended, single shaft instruments are used throughout the case directly through the thoracotomy. A knot pusher is used for intracorporeal tying; however, the annular sutures and the aortic root vent sites are secured with a long Cor-Knot (LSI Solutions, Victor, NY, USA) device, which allows for easier adjustment of tension on each knot with minimal manipulation.

Cannulation Strategies

Many of the potential life-threatening complications from less-invasive cardiac surgery are generated by difficulty with nontraditional cannulation for cardiopulmonary bypass. Routine cannulation for peripheral bypass is accomplished through a 2 to 3 cm vertical incision overlying the common femoral artery. We found that vertical incisions are less disruptive to the lymphatic system and anecdotally result in fewer groin seromas. Preoperative CT with or without contrast through the femoral vessels provides important information for choosing an appropriate cannulation site. As mentioned above, avoidance of cutdown and cannulation at a site of recent femoral access avoids interaction with any scar or focal dissections as a result of the left heart catheterization. Care is taken to avoid lymphatics when possible and clip any which must be divided.

Once the femoral vessels have been minimally exposed, a proximal and distal purse-string are placed in the common femoral artery, the proximal for the arterial cannula (OptiSite, Edwards Lifesciences, Irvine, CA, USA) and the distal for a 5 Fr rapid infusion catheter (Teleflex Inc., Morrisville, NC, USA), which is used for distal limb perfusion. While some centers choose not to utilize distal limb perfusion routinely, we have found that this relatively simple step avoids potentially tragic limb complications postoperatively. An additional purse-string is placed in the common femoral vein. A 23 to 25 Fr Estech femoral venous cannula (Livanova, London, UK) is typically selected, and the arterial cannula is based on patient body surface area and the size of the femoral artery.

After administration of heparin for cardiopulmonary bypass and using the Seldinger technique, these vessels are accessed, and wire placement confirmed in the appropriate proximal structure by TEE. The cannulas are deaired and secured and a doxycycline-soaked sponge is placed in the inguinal incision to dwell for the remainder of the case, in an attempt to promote lymphatic sclerosis and avoid seroma formation postoperatively.

SVC cannulation is accomplished by obtaining wire access into the IVC through the previously placed second internal jugular access obtained at the time of central line placement. Serial dilation to a 15 Fr arterial cannula (Bio-Medicus, Medtronic, Minneapolis, MN, USA) provides excellent bicaval drainage for mitral operations. In the case when concomitant tricuspid intervention is planned, this SVC catheter is upsized to a 17 Fr cannula to allow for better drainage to facilitate opening of the right atrium. Encircling and snaring of the cava is not routinely needed; however, large bulldog clamps can be used to occlude the cava distal to the cannula if needed. Occasionally, if placing the SVC cannula is difficult (i.e., chronic hemodialysis patient with occluded SVC), a 20 Fr venous cannula may be placed through a purse-string in the SVC directly through the thoracotomy; however, this is only performed as a secondary alternative as this occupies working room within the incision.

In the event that femoral arterial access is not possible, a right axillary cutdown with placement of an 8 mm Dacron graft in an end-to-side fashion can be used for arterial access for cardiopulmonary bypass. In this scenario, IVC access is typically accomplished percutaneously through the femoral vein and controlled with manual pressure after removal of the cannula at the termination of the bypass run.

OPERATIVE PROCEDURE

Patient positioning and anesthetic concerns are addressed above. The site for the right anterolateral mini-thoracotomy is chosen based on a combination of physical exam and preoperative imaging. For the majority of patients, the right third interspace provides excellent exposure to the Waterston groove. Occasionally, the fourth interspace is chosen based on the location of the pulmonary vein orifices. A 3 to 6 cm incision is made above the chosen interspace 1 to 2 cm inferior and posterior to the right areola in men or the right inframammary fold in women. The creation of subcutaneous flaps allows for a larger thoracotomy to be performed through a relatively smaller incision. Lung isolation allows for safe entry into the right pleural space without injury to the underlying lung. The thoracotomy at the level of the chest wall is made large enough to ensure good positioning relative to the right pulmonary veins and the thoracotomy is then extended medially and laterally. If needed, a diaphragmatic retraction stitch using a 0-silk suture can be placed in the central tendon of the diaphragm and brought out through an inferior stab incision to aid in exposure. Meticulous attention to hemostasis is necessary as small areas of bleeding may obscure the field of view. Simultaneous to this, the assistant begins the femoral cutdown for cannulation for cardiopulmonary bypass.

Prior to administration of heparin for cardiopulmonary bypass, a long spinal needle is used to perform a posterior right intercostal nerve block under direct visualization using exparel: nontrade name: liposomal bupivicaine Pacira (Parsippany, NJ). Alternatively, cryoablation (AtriCure, Mason, OH, USA) of the intercostal nerves can be performed with 2″ to 3″ lesions in each intercostal space. The mediastinal fat pad is carefully removed using care to identify and protect the right phrenic nerve with the Bovie coagulation turned low. Heparin is then administered, and cannulation proceeds as described above. Following institution of cardiopulmonary bypass, the pericardium is opened longitudinally well anterior to the right phrenic nerve. Silk stay sutures are placed to retract the pericardium and are brought out through the chest wall through sperate stab incisions using an Endo Close device (Medtronic, Minneapolis, MN, USA).

A location on the proximal ascending aorta is chosen for placement of aortic root cannula (Fig. 16.2A). A double-pledgeted 3-0 braided, permanent suture (Ethibond, Ethicon, Cornelia, GA, USA) is used to make a purse-string approximately at the level of the aortic fat pad (Fig. 16.2B). Exquisite care must be taken to ensure proper placement of these sutures with minimal torque on the needle. The aortic root cannula is then guided along the sutures into the ascending aorta, secured, and deaired.

The Waterston groove is then dissected with the electrocautery (Fig. 16.2C). Care must be taken to adequately carry this dissection medially in order to allow for eventual closure of the left atrial suture line without impingement on the right pulmonary vein orifices.

Next, the site for the Atrial Lift retractor is chosen lateral to the right internal mammary artery in the interspace over the pulmonary vein bifurcation. Bovie electrocautery is used to enter the chest wall and the track is dilated with a 5 mm laparoscopic port dilator. The atrial lift shaft is inserted through the chest wall and secured in place to the chest wall with an atrial lift holder (Delacroix-Chevalier, Paris, France).

Now ready for cross-clamping, arterial flows are then decreased and the Glauber aortic cross-clamp is carefully guided into position with the posterior tong through the transverse sinus. Careful attention must be paid to ensure the clamp is across the entirety of the ascending aorta, but free of the left atrial appendage or left main artery, which can be in close proximity (Fig. 16.2D). Arterial flows are increased and adequate decompression of the aortic root through the previously placed aortic root cannula ensured prior to institution of antegrade cardioplegia.

We utilize a standard of 1500 mL of del Nido cardioplegia antegrade. TEE is used to confirm distension of the aortic root, flow in the coronary arteries, and that the left ventricle remains decompressed. The left atrium is opened in the Waterston groove and vented with a pump sucker. Cardioplegia is redosed at 45-minute intervals. Cardioprotection is of utmost importance during minimally invasive mitral surgery. In order to ensure excellent delivery of cardioplegia at every dose, the atrial retractor is lowered prior to subsequent dosing to ensure

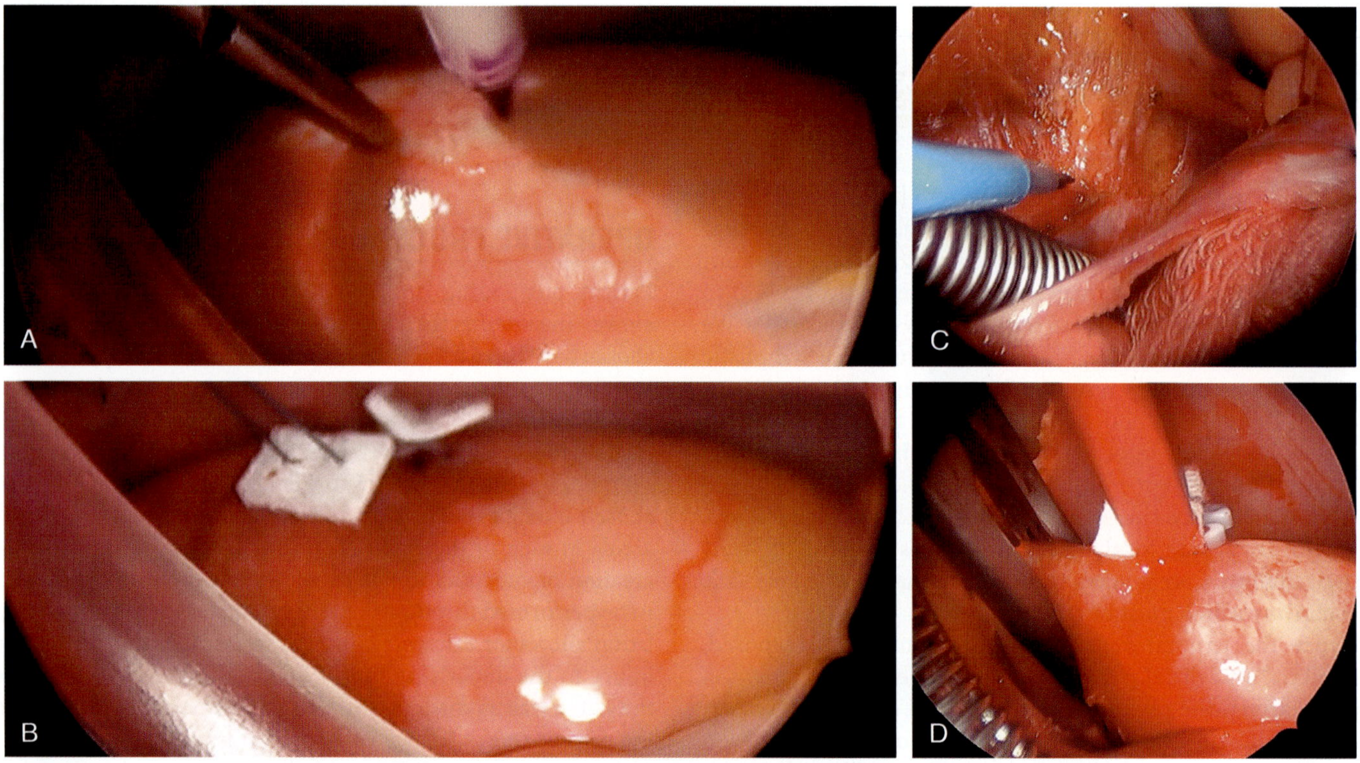

Fig. 16.2 Following institution of peripheral cardiopulmonary bypass, the proximal ascending aorta is marked (A) and pledgeted permanent suture is used to form a purse-string for the aortic root vent (B). Waterston groove is then dissected (C) prior to aortic cross-clamp placement (D).

competence of the aortic valve. Additionally, testing of the valve is accomplished with cold del Nido irrigation rather than saline, as large doses of saline used for testing may tend to wash out the infrequently dosed del Nido cardioplegia. Of note, we re-dose cardioplegia every 45′ with 500 mL del Nido. We ensure there is no air in the aorta by filling the ventricle and aorta with del Nido as described above.

After adequate cardioplegic arrest, the left atriotomy is opened in the Waterston groove. The Atrial lift retractor blade is placed within the left atrium and mounted. The flexible pump sucker is placed in the left pulmonary vein orifice and secured in place with a silk suture, retracting this out of the visual field. This typically provides excellent exposure to the mitral valve (Fig. 16.3A). From here, standard repair and replacement techniques can be utilized to address a wide variety of mitral pathologies. Our typical repair begins with the placement of 2-0 Ethibond annular sutures which at the fibrous trigones, followed by at the base of P2 (Fig. 16.3B). The remaining annular sutures are places to aid in valve exposure. Valve testing using a laparoscopic suction irrigator (Stryker, Kalamazoo, MI, USA) filled with del Nido cardioplegia is used to rapidly distend the left ventricle. A subtle but important technique is to maintain the root vent on high suction. When testing the mitral valve, only when all the air has exited through the root vent is it clamped, minimizing air entering the coronary arteries. Areas of prolapse are identified and marked.

We primarily use a respect approach with artificial cords in the majority of patients. A replacement valve sizer (Jude Epic, Abbott Laboratories, Santa Clara, CA) with a long shaft may aid in exposure of the subvalvular apparatus to aid in chordal replacement (Fig. 16.3C). We utilize pledgeted CV4 PTFE (Gore Medical, Flagstaff, AZ, USA) and gently tie this suture at the level of the papillary muscle (Fig. 16.3D). The PTFE is then passed through the segments of prolapse approximately 5 to 7 mm from the free edge. After the annular ring is chosen and secured in place, the final check of the chordal length is performed (Fig. 16.3E). A 5mm laparoscopic clip (Ethicon Inc., Raritan, NJ, USA) is used to mark the appropriate chordal length while tying and the clip is removed. A final image of the repaired valve is routinely stored (Fig. 16.4). Anterior leaflet prolapse may also be successfully repaired with this approach (Fig. 16.5).

The left atrium is closed, and an LV vent is left across the atrial suture line. The cardioplegia in the heart is flushed out with 500 mL of warm blood through the aortic root. The aortic cross-clamp is carefully removed with the patient in Trendelenburg and positioned with the left side down. Defibrillation is rarely required with del Nido cardioplegia, but when needed, the lungs must be inflated prior to external defibrillation to allow for electrical conduction. Ventricular pacing wires are placed on the inferior surface of the right ventricle and are guided out through the thoracotomy by passing through a chest tube to assist in tunneling. Pacing wire site bleeding should be addressed before coming off pump as visualization becomes difficult.

Following deairing and confirmation of valve function, cardiopulmonary bypass is fully reinstated to allow for safe removal of the aortic root vent. Use of 3-0 Ethibond suture allows for

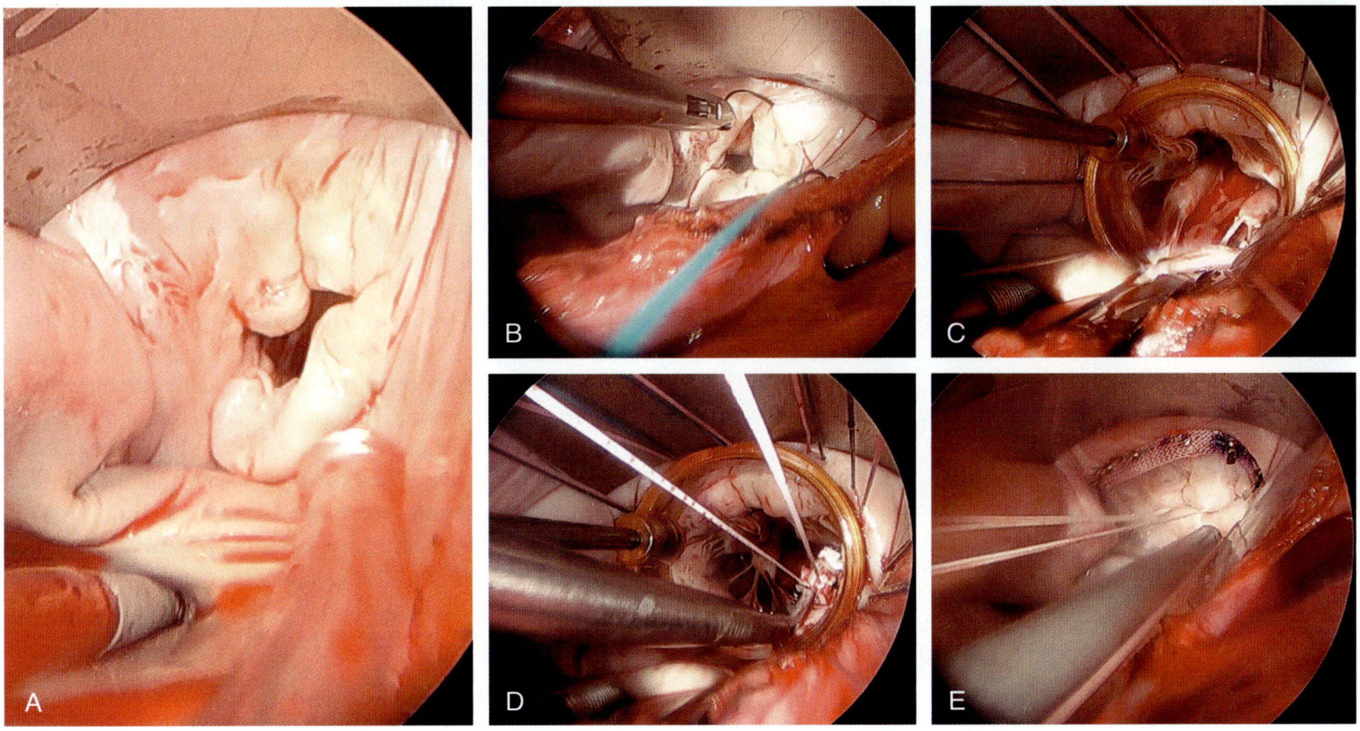

Fig. 16.3 (A) Placement of the atrial retractor reveals excellent visualization of the mitral valve. (B) Annular sutures are placed, beginning at the fibrous trigones. (C) A replacement valve sizer allows for excellent exposure of the subvalvular apparatus and (D) allows for NeoChord attachment to the papillary muscles. (E) After placement of the annuloplasty ring, the final chordal length is determined by filling the ventricle with cardioplegia.

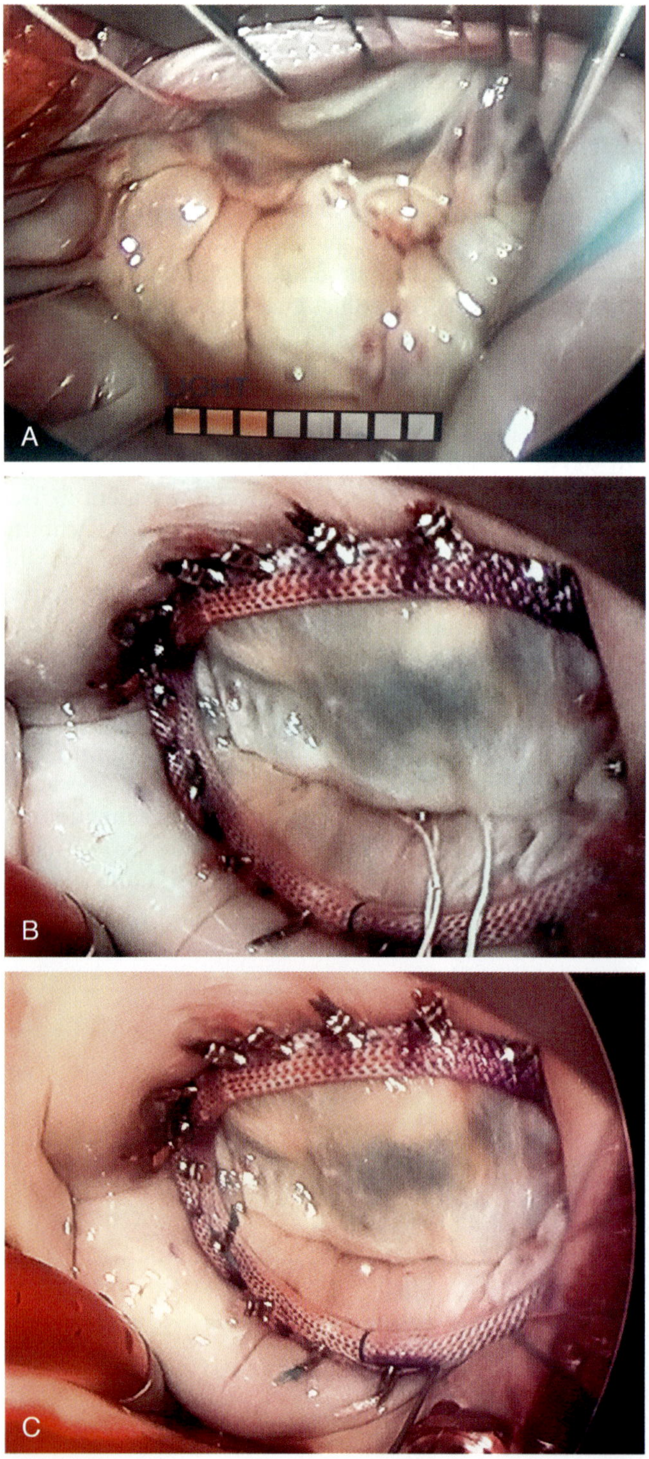

Fig. 16.4 Posterior Leaflet Prolapse Repair With Annuloplasty Ring and NeoChords Via Right Mini-Thoracotomy. (A) Annular sutures are placed first, which aids in visualization and will allow for future ring annuloplasty. (B) Semi-rigid annuloplasty ring is secured with a Cor-Knot device prior to adjustment of final NeoChord length. (C) Completed repair.

safe and reliable fixation with a Cor-Knot device, rather than relying on intracorporeal knot tying, while maintaining adequate tension to maintain hemostasis. Importantly, the metal tab remaining on the back of the Cor-Knot is both rigid and relatively fixed in position. This can injure nearby structures, such as the right atrial appendage. We routinely cover the Cor-Knot device with a single layer of hemostatic matrix to both aid in adventitial hemostasis and protect the right atrium from injury by the Cor-Knot. Once weaned from cardiopulmonary bypass, the cannulas are removed, and the circulating heparin is reversed with protamine. Femoral purse strings are tied and reenforced with additional Prolene suture. Two Blake chest tubes (Blake chest tubes: Ethicon, Sommerville, NJ) are left, one in the right pleural space and one within the mediastinum in the oblique sinus. The thoracotomy is reapproximated with #2 Vicryl suture on a blunt needle and the right lung is inflated under direct visualization prior to closure of the chest. The fascia and subcutaneous tissue are then closed in layers. Extubation in the operating room is not uncommon in hemodynamically stable patients with adequate pulmonary reserve.

SPECIAL CONSIDERATIONS

Previous Median Sternotomy

Multicenter studies have reported a high operative risk of repeat mitral surgery via repeat median sternotomy compared to port access.[19] First, structures near or adherent to the posterior table of the sternum are at risk for injury at the time of resternotomy. In addition, presence of live bypass grafts traveling from the aorta to their distal targets may cross the midline, thus putting their safety on resternotomy at risk. Additionally, redo sternotomy increases the risk of sternal complications postoperatively.[20] Finally, the extent of dissection and bleeding are substantially greater with resternotomy. Approaches, such as the described port-access right thoracotomy approach, have been shown to be safe and effective in patients with previous sternotomy and avoid many of the potential complications of redo sternotomy.[21]

When approaching a patient with previous sternotomy for port-access mitral surgery, it is important to note the presence and locations of "live" right-sided bypass grafts. Additionally, previous operative reports may be helpful in identifying patients in whom the right pleural space was entered, as this may be predictive of intrapleural adhesions. Dissection of the ascending aorta remains challenging from a right-sided approach when utilizing a conventional cross-clamp; however, the native issue planes are typically maintained if surgery on the proximal ascending aorta has not been performed. Previous left anterior descending arterial grafts are not able to be accessed from a right-sided approach, and further cooling may be necessary to achieve adequate cardioprotection. Even in rare settings where cross-clamping is not feasible and fibrillatory arrest is required, we prefer to place an aortic root vent to aid in deairing. In the setting of previous CABG, there is often a virgin plane along the left atrium in which to make a left atriotomy if further dissection of Waterston groove is undertaken.

Mitral Annular Calcification

Severe mitral annular calcification presents a challenging clinical situation. While a variety of invasive treatment options are available, port-access intervention offers several distinct advantages over a midline approach. First, a right thoracotomy approach allows for visualization of the mitral valve

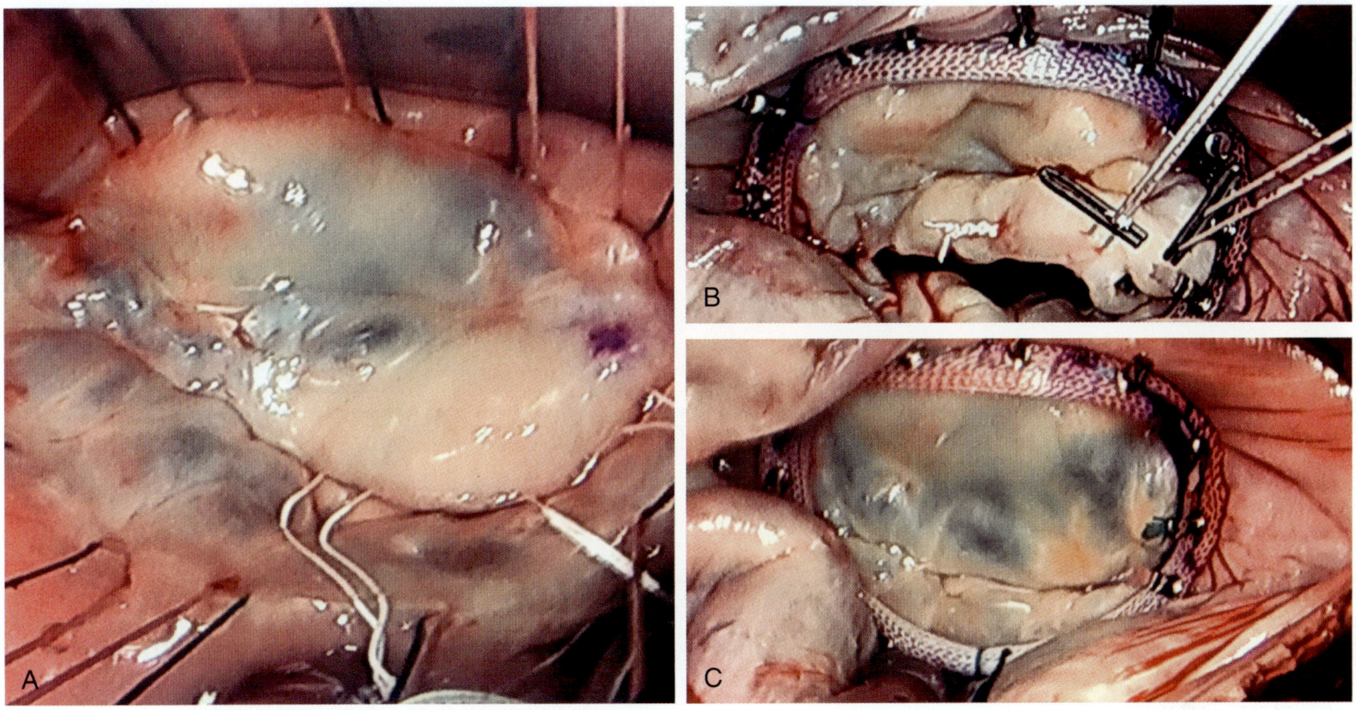

Fig. 16.5 Anterior Leaflet Prolapse Repair. (A) Annular sutures and Gor-Tex NeoChords are placed. (B) After securing the annuloplasty ring, NeoChord height is adjusted to eliminate anterior leaflet prolapse. (C) Repaired valve without residual regurgitation.

without the need for excess tension or disruption of the natural anatomic position of the heart. Atrioventricular groove disruption is the most feared complication in operation on a heavily calcified mitral annulus, with reported mortality of up to 75%.[22] While AV disruption is still possible with a lateral approach, the smaller amount of force transmitted to the annulus required to gain adequate exposure makes this approach more attractive in these difficult patients. The port-access approach still allows for several of the adjuncts utilized in a midline approach, including ultrasonic debridement (Sonopet, Stryker, Kalamazoo, MI, USA) of the annulus or placement of a balloon-expandable percutaneous aortic valve (S3, Edwards Lifesciences) within a severely calcified mitral annulus (Fig. 16.6). In these surgical implantation

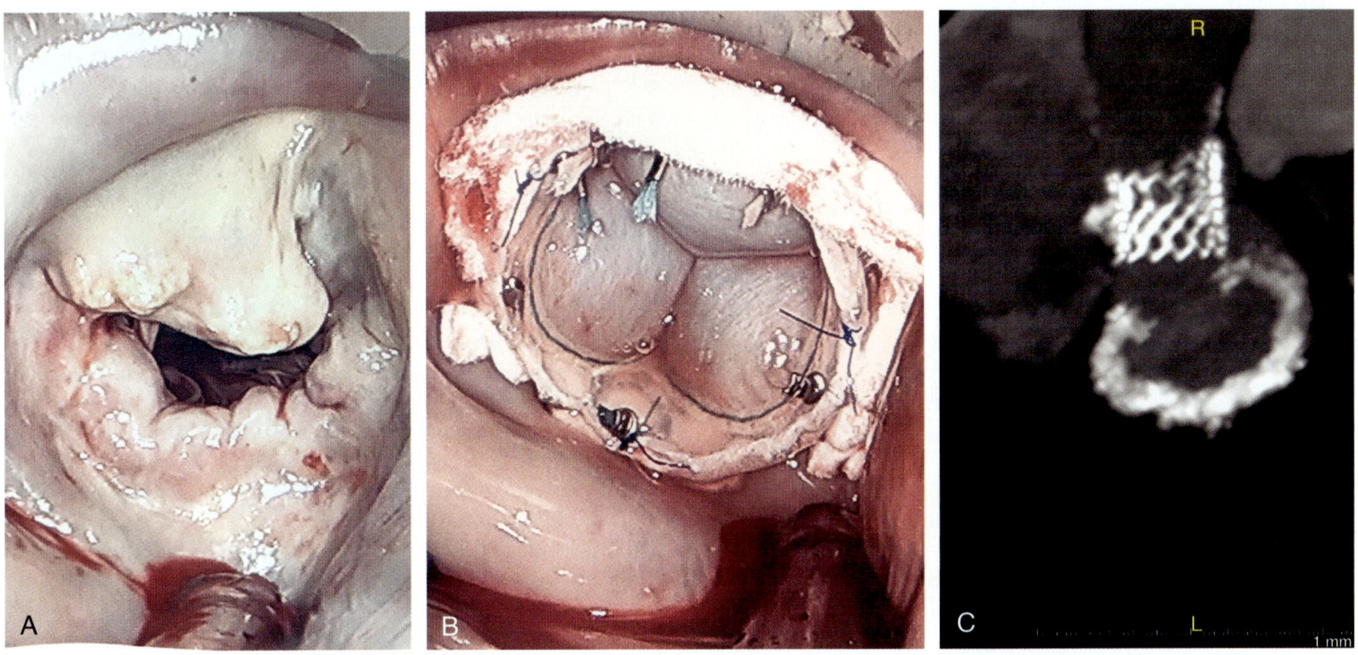

Fig. 16.6 (A) Severely calcified mitral annulus. (B, SITRAL) Placement of Sapien 3 aortic bioprosthesis in the mitral position. (C) Computed tomography prior to SITRAL mitral valve replacement.

of transcatheter valve in native mitral annular calcification (SITRAL, Clinical Trial NCT02830204) cases, a septal resection through the left atriotomy is possible to avoid left ventricular outflow obstruction.[23,24]

SUMMARY

Port-access mitral valve intervention offers a less invasive, but highly effective and versatile, approach to the mitral valve. While technical considerations including exposure, peripheral cannulation, and cardioprotection require special attention, various established open techniques for valve repair or replacement are possible through this approach with only modest modification. This technique offers excellent visualization of the mitral apparatus and may be preferential for teaching or those patients with small left atria, as open visualization in such cases is often difficult. Finally, the port-access approach offers distinct advantages in patients who have undergone a previous sternotomy or in those whom there is severe mitral annular calcification.

CASE-BASED ASSESSMENT

A 63-year-old woman is referred to your clinic with increasing shortness of breath and severe mitral regurgitation. A recent TTE demonstrates severe mitral regurgitation with suspected P2 prolapse and normal biventricular function. There are no other valvular pathologies. She has a 20-pack-year history of smoking. She does not use home oxygen. She is otherwise healthy. She is interested in less-invasive surgical intervention.

1. All of the following are part of a standard workup for right-thoracotomy mitral valve repair *EXCEPT:*
   A. Left heart catheterization
   B. Intraoperative TEE
   C. Cardiac MRI
   D. CT chest/abdomen/pelvis
2. The patient has PFTs which demonstrate moderate obstructive lung disease with an FEV1 58% predicted. The patient should be counseled that:
   A. She is not a candidate for right-thoracotomy mitral valve surgery based on her PFTs
   B. Single lumen ETT is required as she should not tolerate double lumen ETT
   C. She will require several hours of single lung ventilation during her surgery
   D. Her PFTs should be repeated with the bronchodilators
3. A CTA demonstrates moderate mitral annular calcification along the posterior mitral annulus. Which of the following is true of right-thoracotomy mitral valve surgery.
   A. Right-thoracotomy mitral valve surgery is not advised in the setting for mild or moderate mitral annular calcification.
   B. Surgical implantation of a Sapien 3 valve in the mitral position for severe mitral annular calcification is not possible through a right thoracotomy approach.
   C. Right-thoracotomy mitral valve surgery increases the risk of atrial-ventricular dissociation in the setting of severe mitral annular calcification compared to a sternotomy approach as this requires greater manipulation to provide adequate exposure.
   D. Careful debridement of a calcified mitral annulus is possible through a right thoracotomy approach.
4. CTA also demonstrates bilateral 6 mm common femoral arteries with significant anterior calcification along the entire length of the artery. The best cannulation strategy for right-thoracotomy mitral surgery for this patient includes:
   A. Left femoral cutdown and arterial and venous cannulation with percutaneous superior vena cava cannulation.
   B. Right axillary cutdown with placement of an 8 mm end-to-side graft to the right axillary artery and right femoral cutdown for IVC cannulation with placement of a percutaneous SVC cannula.
   C. Right axillary cutdown with placement of an 8 mm end-to-side graft to the right axillary artery and right femoral percutaneous ICV cannulation with placement of a percutaneous SVC cannula.
   D. Minimally invasive mitral valve surgery through right thoracotomy is not possible for patients with peripheral arterial disease.
5. To ensure adequate cardioprotection during port-access mitral valve repair, one should do all of the following *EXCEPT:*
   A. Close the root vent prior to beginning to deliver antegrade cardioplegia to ensure adequate coronary perfusion pressure throughout administration of cardioplegia.
   B. Release tension on the atrial retractor to ensure a competent aortic valve.
   C. Use del Nido cardioplegia to fill the left ventricle in order to test the repair to avoid saline washout of cardioplegia and prevents air embolism.
   D. Ensure the left ventricle is not distending by TEE during initial administration of antegrade cardioplegia.

See page 317 for the answers

REFERENCES

1. Modi P, Hassan A, Chitwood Jr WR. Minimally invasive mitral valve surgery: a systematic review and meta-analysis. *Eur J Cardiothorac Surg.* 2008;34(5):943–952.
2. Chitwood Jr WR, Elbeery JR, Moran JF. Minimally invasive mitral valve repair using transthoracic aortic occlusion. *Ann Thorac Surg.* 1997;63(5):1477–1479.
3. Chitwood Jr WR, Wixon CL, Elbeery JR, et al. Video-assisted minimally invasive mitral valve surgery. *J Thorac Cardiovasc Surg.* 1997;114(5):773–780; discussion 780–782.
4. Nissen AP, Miller CC 3rd, Thourani VH, et al. Less invasive mitral surgery versus conventional sternotomy stratified by mitral pathology. *Ann Thorac Surg.* 2020;111(3):819–827.
5. Downs EA, Johnston LE, LaPar DJ, et al. Minimally invasive mitral valve surgery provides excellent outcomes without increased cost: a multi-institutional analysis. *Ann Thorac Surg.* 2016;102(1):14–21.
6. Hawkins RB, Mehaffey JH, Kessel SM, et al. Minimally invasive mitral valve surgery is associated with excellent resource utilization, cost, and outcomes. *J Thorac Cardiovasc Surg.* 2018;156(2):611–616.e3.
7. Imielski B, Malaisrie SC, Pham DT, et al. The impact of intraoperative residual mild regurgitation after repair of degenerative mitral regurgitation. *J Thorac Cardiovasc Surg.* 2019;161(4):1215–1224.
8. Cohn LH, Adams DH, Couper GS, et al. Minimally invasive cardiac valve surgery improves patient satisfaction while reducing costs of cardiac valve replacement and repair. *Ann Surg.* 1997;226(4):421–426; discussion 427–428.

9. Glower DD, Landolfo KP, Clements F, et al. Mitral valve operation via port access versus median sternotomy. *Eur J Cardiothorac Surg*. 1998;14(Suppl 1):S143–S147.
10. Keller BA, Kabagambe SK, Becker JC, et al. Intercostal nerve cryoablation versus thoracic epidural catheters for postoperative analgesia following pectus excavatum repair: preliminary outcomes in twenty-six cryoablation patients. *J Pediatr Surg*. 2016;51(12):2033–2038.
11. Kolettas A, Lazaridis G, Baka S, et al. Postoperative pain management. *J Thorac Dis*. 2015;7(Suppl 1):S62–S72.
12. Mehra MR, Uriel N, Naka Y, et al. A fully magnetically levitated left ventricular assist device - final report. *N Engl J Med*. 2019;380(17):1618–1627.
13. Martin LW, Sarosiek BM, Harrison MA, et al. Implementing a thoracic enhanced recovery program: lessons learned in the first year. *Ann Thorac Surg*. 2018;105(6):1597–1604.
14. Gammie JS, Zhao Y, Peterson ED, et al. J. Maxwell chamberlain memorial paper for adult cardiac surgery. Less-invasive mitral valve operations: trends and outcomes from the society of thoracic surgeons adult cardiac surgery database. *Ann Thorac Surg*. 2010;90(5):1401–1408 1410.e1; discussion 1408–1410.
15. Prasad A, Compton PA, Prasad A, et al. Incidence and treatment of arterial access dissections occurring during cardiac catheterization. *J Interv Cardiol*. 2008;21(1):61–66.
16. Hesselvik JF, Ortega RA, Treanor P, et al. Intraoperative rupture of the endoaortic clamp balloon in a patient undergoing port-access mitral valve repair. *J Cardiothorac Vasc Anesth*. 1999;13(4):462–465.
17. Ius F, Mazzaro E, Tursi V, et al. Clinical results of minimally invasive mitral valve surgery: endoaortic clamp versus external aortic clamp techniques. *Innovations (Phila)*. 2009;4(6):311–318.
18. Schneider F, Falk V, Walther T, et al. Control of endoaortic clamp position during port-access mitral valve operations using transcranial doppler echography. *Ann Thorac Surg*. 1998;65(5):1481–1482.
19. Launcelott S, Ouzounian M, Buth KJ, et al. Predicting in-hospital mortality after redo cardiac operations: development of a preoperative scorecard. *Ann Thorac Surg*. 2012;94(3):778–784.
20. Balachandran S, Lee A, Denehy L, et al. Risk factors for sternal complications after cardiac operations: a systematic review. *Ann Thorac Surg*. 2016;102(6):2109–2117.
21. Mehaffey HJ, Hawkins RB, Schubert S, et al. Contemporary outcomes in reoperative mitral valve surgery. *Heart*. 2018;104(8):652–656.
22. Kwon JT, Jung TE, Lee DH. The rupture of atrioventricular groove after mitral valve replacement in an elderly patient. *J Cardiothorac Surg*. 2014;9:28.
23. Albacker TB, Bakir B, Eldemerdash A, et al. Surgical mitral valve replacement using direct implantation of sapien 3 valve in a patients with severe mitral annular calcification without adjunctive techniques, a case report. *J Cardiothorac Surg*. 2020;15(1):42.
24. El-Eshmawi A, Alexis SL, Sengupta A, et al. Surgical management of mitral annular calcification. *Curr Opin Cardiol*. 2020;35(2):107–115.
25. Pavan Atluri, Stetson Robert, Hargrove W Clark. Minimally invasive mitral valve surgery is associated with equivalent cost and shorter hospital stay when comparted with traditional sternotomy. *Journal of Thoracic and Cardiovascular Surgery*. 2016;151(2):385–388.

17

Mitral Operation: Endoscopic Approach

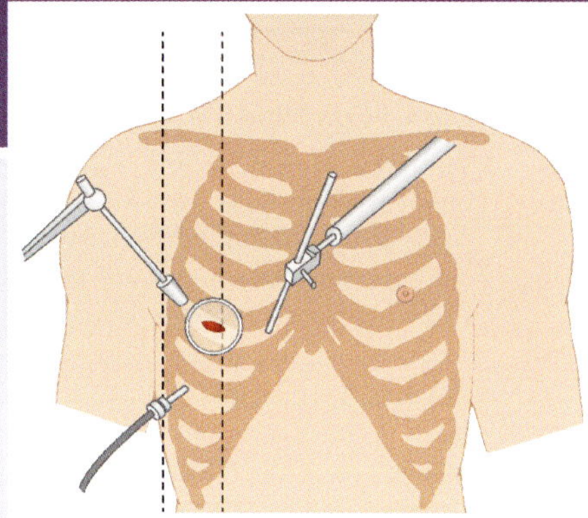

Michael Ibrahim, Pavan Atluri, W. Clark Hargrove III

CHAPTER OUTLINE

LEARNING OBJECTIVES

- Understand the indications and contraindications for endoscopic approach to mitral valve surgery.
- Understand the standard setup and cannulation strategy for mitral valve surgery through an endoscopic approach.
- Understand tips and tricks for optimizing exposure and dealing with challenges in endoscopic mitral valve surgery.

INTRODUCTION

Mitral repair or replacement via median sternotomy is the gold standard for surgical interventions upon the mitral valve and remains the most common approach.[1] However, mitral operation began with non-sternotomy approaches. In certain patients, such as those with severe peripheral vascular disease or unsuitable anatomy for limited access approaches, sternotomy is the only option. Here we describe our practice of endoscopic mitral valve surgery. This procedure may also be known as HeartPort or port access mitral surgery.

HISTORICAL PERSPECTIVE

While today median sternotomy is the most common approach to mitral valve surgery, mitral operations began with non-sternotomy approaches. Indeed, the first mitral operation in 1923 was through a transapical approach via thoracotomy.[2] Thoracotomy approaches continued to dominate surgical approach to the mitral valve, particularly operations for mitral stenosis. This lasted until the routine establishment of sternotomy in the 1960s. In 2003, Casselman et al.[3] described their approach to endoscopic mitral valve repair, declaring that "mitral valve surgery can now routinely be performed endoscopically."[3] Over the last several decades, endoscopic approach mitral surgery has expanded in its use substantially but has not yet supplanted median sternotomy, despite data showing comparative outcomes for mitral valve repair. There has also been a suggestion of improved outcomes such as shorter length of stay, reduced bleeding, better cosmesis, and possibly less postoperative pain.[4] The hesitancy to use a thoracotomy approach is likely due to the learning curve of this procedure and, until recently, the anxiety surrounding the mitral valve repair. In this chapter, we will discuss many of these aspects with respect to our own substantial experience.[5–8]

PATIENT SELECTION

One of the most important elements in minimal access mitral valve surgery is proper patient selection. This relates to two specific elements: clinical factors and vascular assessment. Body habitus is one of the most important elements in determining how challenging endoscopic access surgery will be. Patients who have a body mass index (BMI) above 40 or who have chest wall deformities may be challenging operative candidates from an endoscopic approach. These patients are best avoided in the early experience of new surgeons. For patients needing reoperative mitral surgery, including those with previous coronary artery bypass grafting (CABG), aortic valve replacement (AVR), or mitral valve replacement (MVR), thoracotomy is our preferred approach. This necessitates the use of the endoballoon, so again we would recommend against this technique early in one's experience. In patients with a diminutive left atrium, thoracotomy provides excellent exposure as opposed to sternotomy. Standard elements of the preoperative assessment are shared with the approach to a patient undergoing sternotomy. These include left and right cardiac catheterizations to define any pulmonary hypertension, visualize the coronaries (including dominance and proximity of the circumflex artery), and the extent of mitral annular calcification. In some younger patients we will accept computerized tomographic angiogram (CTA) as a screening tool and not require catheterization. Elements which make a patient a higher-risk sternotomy candidate also make them a higher-risk endoscopic candidate. This includes poor left ventricular function, severe pulmonary hypertension, and severe lung disease. Early in one's experience, it is advisable to select mitral cases requiring straightforward repair in patients with normal BMI and without chest wall deformity. For example, a repair requiring a P2 management (resection or chords) and annuloplasty band would be more appropriate than a complex bileaflet repair approach in a sick patient.[9]

The second category of factors relates to the suitability of the patient for peripheral cannulation for cardiopulmonary bypass. First, the common femoral artery must be relatively free of calcification. We have not found vessel caliber to be an important factor and have not routinely placed an antegrade perfusion limb for the lower extremity. The abdominal and thoracic aorta should be of a reasonable quality without heavy calcification or severe tortuosity. In particular, "shaggy" calcium in the lumen of the aorta may be dislodged and result in ischemic stroke, while mural calcification is less problematic. Although in the first 1000 cases we did not routinely do computed tomography (CT) scans (non-con) of the chest, abdomen, and pelvis, that is currently part of our preoperative assessment. Much can be learned about the burden of atherosclerosis on the basis of the views of the descending thoracic aorta and arch on transesophageal echocardiogram (TEE).[9]

SETUP

Here we briefly describe our setup. It is important to stress the impact the entire operative team has on the success of minimal access mitral surgery, including endoscopic approaches. Skilled and experienced physician assistants should train with the surgical proctors, as should the scrub team to learn how to conduct the operation together.

The anesthesiologists routinely provide double-lumen tracheal intubation, a 16 to 18 Fr superior vena cava (SVC) venous drainage cannula via the internal jugular vein. We do not use an endopulmonary vent. We routinely use this bi-caval cannulation method. There are groups, however, that use a single venous cannula from the groin. If this single venous cannula does not provide adequate venous drainage, then the surgeon will experience a couple of miserable hours with difficult exposure. The patient is prepared in the usual fashion, with a bump used to elevate the right hemithorax. The patient's pertinent surface anatomy is marked, including the nipple and the site of the mid-sternum. The right costal margin and clavicle are marked to define the midpoint of the thorax. A pulmonary artery catheter is inserted. A complete echocardiographic assessment of the valve is performed including three-dimensional reconstruction.

Operation is begun in the groin crease, with exposure of the femoral vessels via a limited oblique incision. Only the anterior surface of these structures is exposed. This is to minimize dissection in order to limit nerve and lymphatic injury. Once we have secured sites for arterial and venous cannulation, we open the right hemithorax with an incision approximately 2 to 3 inches long, immediately below the right nipple (typically the fourth interspace). In women, we take care to place this just above the inframammary crease to prevent bra friction. The patient is now ventilated selectively through the left lung on single-lung anesthesia. We initially open the chest through a small wound and palpate the diaphragm to determine how close it is. If it is very close, the thoracotomy is placed one space higher up. If diaphragmatic retraction is necessary, a heavy braided retraction suture is placed in the central tendon and brought out to the chest wall under tension (it is important to tie this suture to prevent diaphragmatic bleeding). Care also must be taken not to place too much tension on the phrenic nerve by pulling the diaphragm down. The "working" port is then enlarged to approximately 2.5 inches. Reaching in the wound, the intercostal space two below the working port is identified. A trocar is inserted, and CO_2 infusion begun. The left ventricular vent is subsequently placed through this trocar. A soft tissue wound protector is then placed through the working port, and the deflated lung is retracted. A good landmark to confirm that the incision will provide adequate exposure to the mitral valve is that the right-sided pulmonary veins should be evident in the center of the incision. A 5-mm camera port is placed in the same rib space as the thoracotomy, a bit more laterally. This initially contains a 0-degree thoracoscope which is later exchanged to a 30-degree thoracoscope. An angiocath is placed superomedially to the thoracotomy. Through this a 24-gauge steel wire is placed that will be used to retract annular sutures and enhance the surgeon's view later (Vanermen maneuver). Finally, it may be necessary to place a retractor into the incision to facilitate exposure, although frequently the soft tissue retractor suffices (Fig. 17.1).[10]

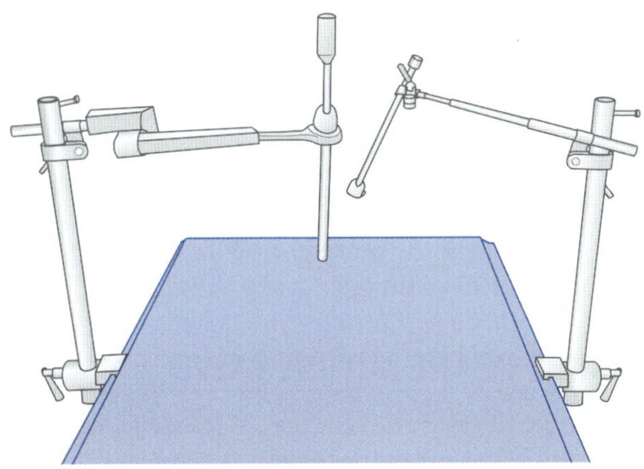

Fig. 17.1 Standard Endoscopic Setup of Retractors.

BYPASS MANAGEMENT

The patient is cannulated for bypass through the groin. Using the Seldinger technique, a wire is passed into the right atrium and a 25 Fr venous cannula is passed to the SVC-atrial junction. The SVC drain placed by anesthesia is brought through the drapes, and the two venous cannulae are Y-ed together and connected to the CP bypass machine. Again, using Seldinger technique, a wire is introduced into the femoral artery and advanced into the thoracic aorta under echo guidance. Once wire position is confirmed, serial dilation is performed to an arterial cannula size of 18 to 21 Fr. We routinely use arterial cannulas compatible with the endoclamping technique (21 Fr). If the femoral artery appears too small to accommodate this cannula, then we would opt for the Chitwood clamp. The side port of the endoballoon cannula is deaired. Following this, the endoballoon is advanced to the 15-cm mark. The wire is then passed to the level of the sinotubular junction (STJ), over which the endoballoon is advanced to the level of the STJ, and the screw on the side-port is tightened to keep it in place. TEE guidance is used to pass and confirm all cannula placements. (Note: Never, ever force a guidewire!)

It is imperative to prevent inadvertent wire perforation of the aortic valve leaflets during these maneuverers. Cardiopulmonary bypass is then instituted, and ventilation is ceased. The pericardium is opened parallel and approximately 2 cm above the phrenic nerve. Pericardial stay sutures are placed along the superior and inferior margins of this pericardial cradle. The inferior pericardial stays are brought out through punctures in the chest wall using an endo-catch. The interatrial groove is minimally dissected and, using blunt dissection, the oblique sinus is opened under the inferior vena cava (IVC). At this point, we confirm the endoballoon position. The endoballoon is then inflated under TEE guidance using 30 cc of heparinized saline through the blue port to achieve a pressure of 300 to 400 mm Hg, while adenosine is infused through the red port to rapidly arrest the heart. Fine manipulation and close attention to monitored balloon pressures are needed to ensure stable balloon placement. Del Nido cardioplegia is infused into the aortic root, while the left ventricle (LV) is monitored by echocardiography to ensure it is not distended. After most of the cardioplegia has been infused, the left atrium is opened and vented.

If a Chitwood clamp is being used, a purse string is placed in the proximal ascending aorta. The cardioplegia needle is normally placed through the working port and secured in place. The aorta is cross-clamped, taking care to avoid injury to the right pulmonary artery and left atrial appendage (LAA). Cardioplegia is then infused as when using the endoballoon. We also selectively use the Chitwood cross-clamp in patients with enlarged proximal aortas (>4.2 cm) as well as small femoral arteries. When the Chitwood clamp is used, the cardioplegia site is closed at the end of the procedure with a Cor-Knot after the cardioplegia needle is removed.

EXPOSURE OF THE MITRAL VALVE

The left atriotomy made to vent the LV is extended superiorly and inferiorly in the intra-atrial groove. A suture is placed in the superior margin of the atrial wall, and this is retracted through the working port. A small stab incision is made on the right (medial) side of right internal mammary artery. The axle of an atrial retractor is brought through. This is secured to a metal arm which is framed onto the operating table (see Fig. 17.1).[10] We place a single-superior atrial retractor blade which can be angulated to enhance mitral exposure. To this atrial retractor, a flexible arm is attached which posteriorly displaces the floor of the left atrium, bringing into view the mitral valve (Obadia II 3D Atrial Tripod Lift System, Delacroix-Chevalier, Paris, France). A floppy cardiotomy suction is advanced into the right pulmonary veins through the CO_2 port. The camera is then switched to a 5 mm 30-degree endoscope which directs the view onto the valve (Fig. 17.2).[10] To facilitate visualization of the subvalvular apparatus, we frequently place a Fehling retractor in the mitral orifice. This is a coiled spring retractor which laterally displaces the leaflets allowing excellent exposure of the subvalvular apparatus.

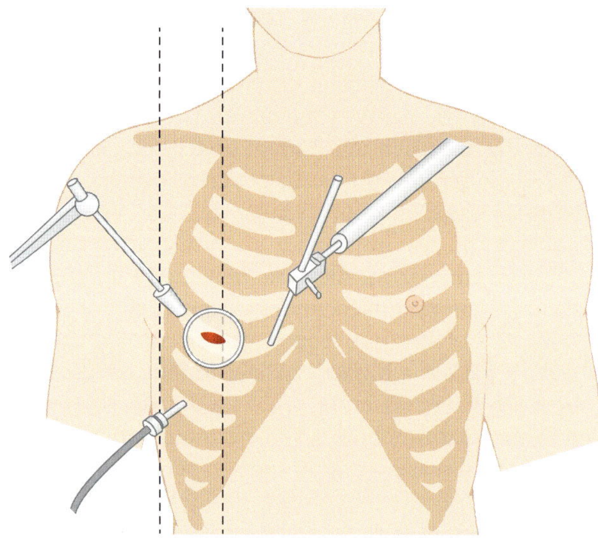

Fig. 17.2 Standard Atrial Retractors and Suture Guides.

We begin with valve inspection and analysis using an endoscopic hook and long-shafted forceps. All instruments are long-shafted and designed for endoscopic cardiac surgery.

ENDOSCOPIC APPROACH TO MITRAL REPAIR

At this point, we have good visualization of the valve (Fig. 17.3).[10] The leaflet work can be done at this time or, if the exposure is not optimal, there is the option of first placing the annular sutures to enhance this exposure. Annular suture placement is begun at the left fibrous trigone and worked counterclockwise radially towards the right fibrous trigone. After three to four have been placed along the P1 region then we use the previously placed 24-gauge wire to distract the sutures laterally allowing clear visualization of the valve (Vanermen maneuver). The remainder of the annular sutures are then placed. Each suture is placed with the aid of suture retraction on existing sutures. These sutures are put on suture guides, which have the effect of pulling the entire mitral valve toward the surgeon. If not done before placement of the annular sutures, then at this point we perform

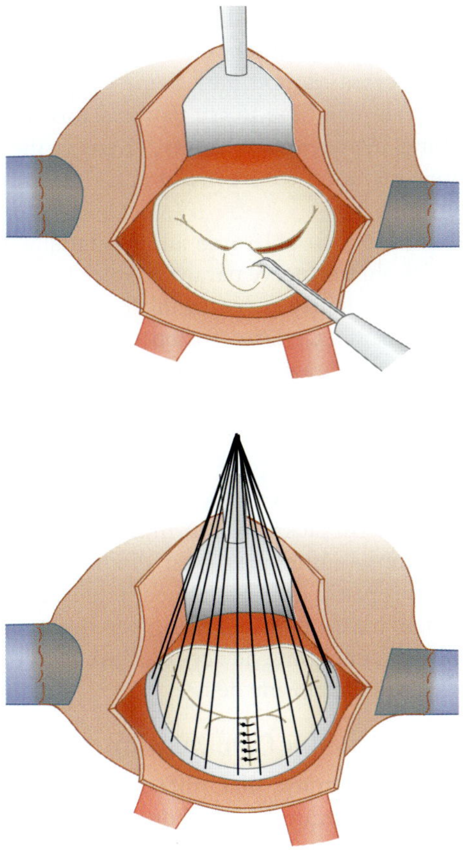

Fig. 17.3 Surgeon's View of Exposed Mitral Valve—Atrial Retraction.

leaflet reconstruction or placement of artificial neochordae as needed. We generally prefer the use of flexible mitral annuloplasty bands with the size based on the intertrigonal distance and size of the anterior mitral leaflet. Sizers are marked with a long silk to facilitate removal. Complete annuloplasty rings can be used depending on pathology and surgeon preference. Annuloplasty sutures are secured with the Cor-Knot device and monofilament sutures are secured with a long-shafted knot tying device.

Following valve testing, the LV vent is placed through the valve. The atrium is closed in standard fashion beginning at the margins. These sutures are snared down around the LV vent exiting the atrial incision. Before snaring, the left heart is de-aired by filling and ventilation. Before deflating the endo-clamp, we place a bipolar ventricular pacing wire. The remainder of the operation proceeds as for sternotomy, with care taken to ensure the heart is de-aired and the repair has been successful, monitored by TEE control. Because of constant CO_2 infusion, there is usually very little air in the heart, barring excessive valve testing.

OPERATIONS IN SPECIAL POPULATIONS

Some patients represent unique challenges. These include the obese, those with a high burden of comorbidities, and those with poor ventricular function. One particular challenge is the patient with significant pulmonary disease. These patients will struggle with single-lung isolation and great care should be expended to undertake a rigorous assessment of their pulmonary status, including blood gas analysis, pulmonary function testing, and possible screening by a pulmonologist. Patients with significant pulmonary hypertension are also considered higher risk, but recent data suggests they can be operated on without compromising outcomes.[8] Such patients are better avoided in the early experience of an endoscopic mitral surgeon. The same is true for those with significant chest wall deformities, such as pectus excavatum.

RE-OPERATIONS

In patients with prior sternotomy, endoscopic approach is our preferred method for re-operation. If the pericardium covers the rightward aspect of the left atrium, there is often a helpful tissue plane here. If dense adhesions between the lung and chest wall are encountered, then the endoscopic approach may have to abandoned. Likewise, we do not consider repeat re-operation through the right thoracotomy to be unreasonable. On primary operations we routinely re-approximate the right-sided pericardium to prevent lung adhesions to the heart and allow for an easier re-operation. We always expose the femoral vessels routinely prior to moving to the chest, whether in re-operations or primary operations.

MITRAL REPLACEMENT AND CONCOMITANT OPERATIONS

Mitral replacement makes for an ideal first operation for the early-stage endoscopic mitral surgeon, so long as the patient is a reasonable surgical candidate. The anterior leaflet is retracted posteriorly by a nerve hook and is incised. We prefer to spare the subvalvular apparatus by suspending the divided and trimmed segments of the anterior leaflet from the anterior and posterior commissures. For mechanical valves, the sutures are placed in a supra-annular fashion. For tissue valves, the sutures are placed intra-annular. Suture retraction aids in placing the sutures, and Cor-Knot allows secure tying down of the prosthesis with almost no incidence of paravalvular leak.

A range of concomitant operations can be added on to mitral repair or replacement. These include tricuspid valve repair, operation on the atrial septum, limited septal myectomy, and atrial ablation, including placing a clip on the LAA. This clip (AtriClip, AtriCure, Mason, OH) is placed through the transverse sinus under direct camera visualization. This is facilitated by lifting the aorta, grasping the appendage, and placing an appropriately sized clip along its base. An alternative is to close the appendage from the endocardial surface at the time of mitral operation, using a running monofilament suture, although this has a high incidence of recannulization.[11] For operations involving exploration of the right heart, the cavae are snared. To do this, we bluntly dissect then encircle the cavae with tapes and snare them. Operations on the mitral and tricuspid in the same patient require separate atrial incisions and cannot be done transseptally as with the sternotomy approach.

POSTOPERATIVE CARE AND OUTCOMES

Typical postoperative care is not substantially different to that following sternotomy. Patients undergoing minimal access mitral surgery are more likely to be candidates for early extubation. This is facilitated by assiduous pain control, including intraoperative nerve blocks with long-lasting liposomal bupivacaine infiltrated into the surrounding intercostal nerve bundles. Chest drains and pacing wires are removed as normal in the first several postoperative days.[12]

Outcomes for endoscopic mitral surgery are excellent and compare favorably with the gold standard sternotomy approach, even in complex mitral disease.[3] In a recent meta-analysis focusing on long-term relief from mitral insufficiency, matched minimally invasive and sternotomy approach patients had similar long-term outcomes including valve function, requirement for re-operation, and survival. This came at a cost of increased operative times.[7]

Complications and Caveats

As with any operation there are potential complications. We classify these into catastrophic, troublesome, and nuisance. The three catastrophic and potentially fatal complications of endoscopic mitral operations are: (1) aortic dissection, (2) ligation of the circumflex coronary artery, and (3) unilateral pulmonary edema. All are rare, and only unilateral pulmonary edema is unique to the endoscopic approach. Aortic dissection is best avoided by preoperative screening with computed tomography (CT) scanning of the aorta and peripheral vessels and meticulous adherence to catheter placement techniques. If this occurs, conversion to sternotomy is required and standard treatment of Type A dissection is undertaken. If Type B dissection occurs, then depending on the stage of the procedure, it can be abandoned to restore antegrade flow. Ligation of the circumflex is more likely to occur in a patient with left-dominate coronary circulation. Care should be taken in all mitral repairs when placing the annuloplasty sutures from the left fibrous trigone to the junction of P1 and P2 (the area where the circumflex comes closest to the mitral annulus). Although this may also occur during sternotomy, the angle of the needle in the endoscopic approach is different than in the sternotomy approach. Unilateral pulmonary edema is more likely to occur with prolonged cross-clamp times. Some surgeons choose not to use a double-lumen tube to try to avoid this complication. If the resulting hypoxemia is severe, there is the option of extracorporeal membrane oxygenator (ECMO) in the current armamentarium.

A less serious, but troublesome and potentially debilitating complication, is phrenic nerve paralysis. Since it is always in the field of view, direct injury is very unlikely. The most common cause, we believe, is excessive tension on the traction suture when pulling the diaphragm out of the surgical field.

Finally, a nuisance complication is a lymphocele or draining lymph fistula in the groin where the femoral arteries have been cannulated. When dissecting the femoral vessels, care must be taken to avoid lymph nodes and lymphatics. Our current practice is to leave a small Jackson-Pratt in the groin incision until the drainage stops—sometimes even discharging the patient with the drain in place. This has almost totally eliminated the problem. Others have advocated using percutaneous cannulation with subsequent closing device. We have not done this because of the cost of the closing device.

Caveat-Mitral Annular Calcification

All mitral surgeons know that mitral annular calcification (MAC) can pose a technical hazard during mitral operations. For this reason, we have generally been conservative and have used the endoscopic approach in these patients on a selected basis. However, if the patient has severe circumferential MAC, then we have used a transcatheter aortic valve replacement (TAVR) valve to replace the mitral valve via the endoscopic approach. One must carefully measure the mitral annulus on CT scan to assure that the prosthesis will fit.

SUMMARY

Endoscopic approach mitral valve surgery represents the most accessible form of minimal access mitral surgery since it preserves the surgeon's tactile interaction with the tissues and does not involve prohibitively expensive new technology. A large body of data suggests outcomes are excellent. While there is certainly a learning curve, any dedicated mitral surgeon can invest in the time and resources (and mentorship) required to develop an endoscopic mitral valve practice which is safe and effective.[13]

CASE-BASED ASSESSMENT

1. What is the major risk associated with endoscopic mitral regurgitation?
   A. Stroke
   B. Groove disruption
   C. Bleeding
2. Which feature is a prohibitive risk for endoscopic mitral surgery?
   A. High risk of needing replacement
   B. Severe calcific aortic disease
   C. Aortic stenosis (moderate)
3. Concomitant procedures possible endoscope approaches are:
   A. ASD closure
   B. Tricuspid repair
   C. Aortic replacement
   D. Coronary bypass

See page 317 for the answers.

REFERENCES

1. Vemulapalli S, Grau-Sepulveda M, Habib R, et al. Patient and hospital characteristics of mitral valve surgery in the united states. *JAMA Cardiol*. 2019;4(11):1149–1155.
2. Cutler EC, Levine SA. Cardiotomy and valvulotomy for mitral stenosis: experimental observations and clinical notes concerning an operated case with recovery. *Boston Med Surg J*. 1923;188:1023–1027.
3. Casselman FP, Van Slycke S, Wellens F, et al. Mitral valve surgery can now routinely be performed endoscopically. *Circulation*. 2003;108(suppl 1):II48–II54.
4. Falk V, Cheng DC, Martin J, et al. Minimally invasive versus open mitral valve surgery: a consensus statement of the international society of minimally invasive coronary surgery (ISMICS) 2010. *Innovations*. 2011;6:66–76.
5. Goldstone AB, Atluri P, Szeto WY, et al. Minimally invasive approach provides at least equivalent results fo surgical correction of mitral regurgitation: A propensity-matched comparison. *J Thorac Cardiovasc Surg*. 2013;145:748–756.
6. Atluri P, Goldstone AB, Fox J, et al. Port access cardiac operations can be safely performed with either endoaortic balloon or chitwood clamp. *Ann Thorac Surg*. 2014;98:1579–1584.
7. Moscarelli M, Fattouch K, Gaudino M, et al. Minimal access versus sternotomy for complex mitral valve repair: a meta-analysis. *Ann Thorac Surg*. 2020;109(3):737–744.
8. Helmers MR, Kim ST, Altshuler P, et al. Mitral valve surgery in pulmonary hypertension patients: is minimally invasive surgery safe?. *Ann Thorac Surg*. 2021;111(6):2012–2019.
9. Ailawadi G, Agnihotri AK, Mehall JR, et al. Minimally invasive mitral valve surgery I patient selection, evaluation, and planning. *Innovations*. 2016;11:243–250.
10. Grau J, Eckhauser AW, Hargrove WC. Endoscopic mitral repair: evolution to robotics-endo-balloon aortic occlusion technique. In: Chitwood WR Jr, ed. *Atlas of Robotic Cardiac Surgery*. London: Springer Verlag; 2014.
11. Kanderian AS, Gillinov AM, Pettersson GB, et al. Success of surgical left atrial appendage closure: assessment by transesophageal echocardiography. *J Am Coll Cardiol*. 2008; 52:924–929.
12. Wolfe JA, Malaisrie SC, Farivar RS, et al. Minimally invasive mitral valve surgery II surgical technique and postoperative management. *Innovations*. 2016;11:251–259.
13. Lehr EJ, Guy TS, Smith RL, et al. Minimally invasive mitral valve surgery III training and robotic-assisted approaches. *Innovations*. 2016;11:260–267.

18

Mitral Operation: Robotic Approach

Amber M. Edwards, Evelio Rodriguez

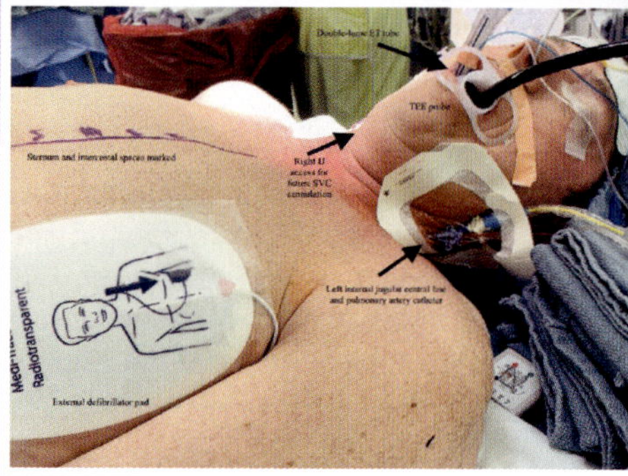

CHAPTER OUTLINE

LEARNING OBJECTIVES

- Gain an understanding of the history of robotics.
- Identify and understand contraindications for mitral valve repair and/or replacement.
- Learn how to assess patients to determine suitability for robotic surgery.
- Gain an understanding of techniques, complications, and patient outcomes.

HISTORICAL PERSPECTIVE

The history of robotic mitral valve surgery is relatively short, with the first robotic mitral valve operation performed in 1998 by Dr. Carpentier.[1] This operation was prefaced by a movement in mitral valve surgery to become less invasive, starting with minimal access incisions in the right chest by Cohn and Cosgrove in the 1990s.[2] Their operation, performed under direct visualization via a right posterolateral thoracotomy, allowed for arguably better visualization of the mitral valve due to the sagittal nature of the plane of the valve in the human body. Minimal access incisions were shortly followed by video-assisted mitral valve surgery, which allowed for even better visualization of the mitral valve; and, again, the first was reported by Dr. Carpentier, this time in 1998.[3] These initial pioneering case series and reports showed that minimally invasive mitral valve surgery could be performed with acceptable short-term mortality rates.

Shortly following Dr. Carpentier's work, the first robotic cardiac surgery was reported in the United States in 2000 by Dr. Chitwood. Again, this operation was a mitral valve repair for P2 prolapse involving a P2 resection and annuloplasty.[4] Pivotal to the advancement of robotic mitral valve surgery were two trials in the early 2000s showing that the da Vinci surgical system (Intuitive Surgical, Inc., Mountain View, CA) was safe and effective for mitral valve repair. Furthermore, the system provided three-dimensional, magnified visualization and articulated wrist movements via seven degrees of freedom that enabled precise surgical manipulation in this complex surgery.[5,6] Over the past 20 years, the da Vinci surgical system has continued to evolve to optimize patient safety and surgeon experience.

INDICATIONS AND PREOPERATIVE ASSESSMENT

Indications for robotic mitral valve repair or replacement follow the American College of Cardiology (ACC) American Heart Association (AHA) guidelines for valvular heart disease, essentially the same as a sternotomy approach.[7] Large series of concomitant mitral valve surgery with the Cox-Maze procedure or the modified Cox-Maze procedure or with concomitant tricuspid valve surgery have also been reported with excellent outcomes.[8]

In the initial building of a robotic mitral valve surgery team, patient selection is key. More straight-forward repairs and replacement should be performed, and as experience increases so can the complexity of the operations.

Preoperative workup is fairly similar to patients undergoing cardiac surgery via sternotomy. All patients should have electrocardiography (ECG), chest x-ray, coronary angiogram if age appropriate, transthoracic echocardiogram, and pulmonary function tests. Transesophageal echocardiogram should be performed preoperatively if valve anatomy or pathology is unclear on transthoracic imaging. Specific to robotic mitral valve surgery, we recommended obtaining preoperative computed tomography (CT) angiogram of the chest, abdomen, and pelvis.[9] This is an

TABLE 18.1 Contraindications to Robotic Mitral Valve Surgery

Relative Contraindications	Absolute Contraindications
• Pulmonary disease	• Emergency Operation
• Peripheral vascular disease	• Major trauma
• Prior right chest surgery	• Atherosclerotic or aneurysmal ascending aorta
• Poor left ventricular ejection fraction	
• Multiple valve repair or replacement	
• Associated coronary artery bypass grafting	

assessment of several factors: chest wall and intercostal anatomy; cardiac anatomy including aortic calcifications and left atrial size and orientation; lung pathology; peripheral arterial atherosclerotic disease; and central and peripheral venous anatomy.

CONTRAINDICATIONS

Absolute and relative contraindications are shown in Table 18.1.

SURGICAL TECHNIQUE

Anesthetic Considerations

As with standard cardiac surgery, the patient should have hemodynamic monitoring and vascular access. This includes arterial line, central venous line(s), peripheral venous access, and a pulmonary artery catheter. During the lining process, we have our anesthesiologist colleagues place an additional low right internal jugular line which we later dilate and use for peripheral superior vena cava (SVC) cannulation.

A double-lumen endotracheal tube is needed to allow for left single-lung ventilation during the operation prior to cardiopulmonary bypass. A single-lumen endotracheal tube with bronchial can also be placed in lieu of a double-lumen tube.

A transesophageal echocardiogram is performed at the time of surgery. This confirms pathology, anatomy, and cardiac function; in addition, it aids in separation from cardiopulmonary bypass. Transesophageal echo is also used to confirm correct placement of cannulas for cardiopulmonary bypass.

Prepping and Draping

The operation is done with the patient in the supine position. A pillow, roll, or inflatable device is placed under the right scapula to elevate the right hemithorax. The right arm is tucked loosely and somewhat hanging with the elbow slightly flexed to facilitate access to the axillary anatomy. Padding or pillows should be placed under the ankles and knees to avoid compression points on the operating table. External defibrillator pads should be placed behind the right scapula and on the left anterolateral chest wall (Fig. 18.1).

The patient is prepped from the neck to the knees. Key areas that the surgeon needs access to include the previously placed right internal jugular central line, right chest including the anterior axillary and infraclavicular areas, sternum, and bilateral groins (Fig. 18.2).

Incisions

A 4-cm right submammary posterolateral incision is made and is the primary working incision. Dissection is carried down to the chest wall, and the thorax is entered in the fourth intercostal space. A small intercostal retractor is used to visualize the intrathoracic contents. Typically, this step is performed prior to peripheral cardiopulmonary bypass access to ensure that the right hemothorax has no anatomic considerations, such as dense adhesions, that would preclude proceeding with a minimally invasive, robotic operative approach.

Additional ports are triangulated around the working incision. These include the right hand, left hand, and camera ports. Location of the right-hand port is typically in the sixth intercostal space in the anterior axillary line. Location of the left-hand port is typically in the second intercostal space in the anterior axillary line. Location of the camera is typically anterior to the working incision and in the same intercostal space (Fig. 18.3).

The pericardium is then opened and put up on stay sutures that are brought through the chest wall. When opening the pericardium, the phrenic nerve is visualized and care is made to make the pericardiotomy a minimum of 1-cm anterior to the nerve. The pericardium is opened from the diaphragm to the pericardial reflection on the ascending aorta.

Cardiopulmonary Bypass

After appropriate anatomy is confirmed via preoperative imaging, the surgeon can proceed with setup for peripheral cardiopulmonary bypass. First, a small right femoral cutdown incision is made. Both the femoral artery and vein are exposed and peripherally cannulated in Seldinger fashion using transesophageal echocardiography (TEE) guidance. If the femoral artery has significant peripheral vascular disease that prevents safe cannulation, an axillary artery cutdown is performed, and the axillary artery is used for arterial access for cardiopulmonary bypass. If the axillary artery is used, then the femoral vein is accessed percutaneously, instead of via cutdown (Fig. 18.4).

Next, the superior vena cava cannula is placed in a previously placed introducer in the right internal jugular vein. A stiff wire is placed through the introducer, the vein is serially dilated using Seldinger technique, and then the cannula is placed with the tip in the superior vena cava.

Cardiopulmonary bypass is instituted using both venous cannulas and the single arterial cannula. An antegrade cardioplegia catheter is placed in the ascending aorta. The Chitwood clamp is introduced into the chest posterior to the working incision. The Chitwood aortic cross-clamp is applied, and 1.5 to 2.0 L of Custodial cardioplegia solution is given in the aortic root. During this time, the left atrium is partially opened and vented, and the surgeon moves away from the operating room table. The surgical assistant facilitates docking the robot at this time.

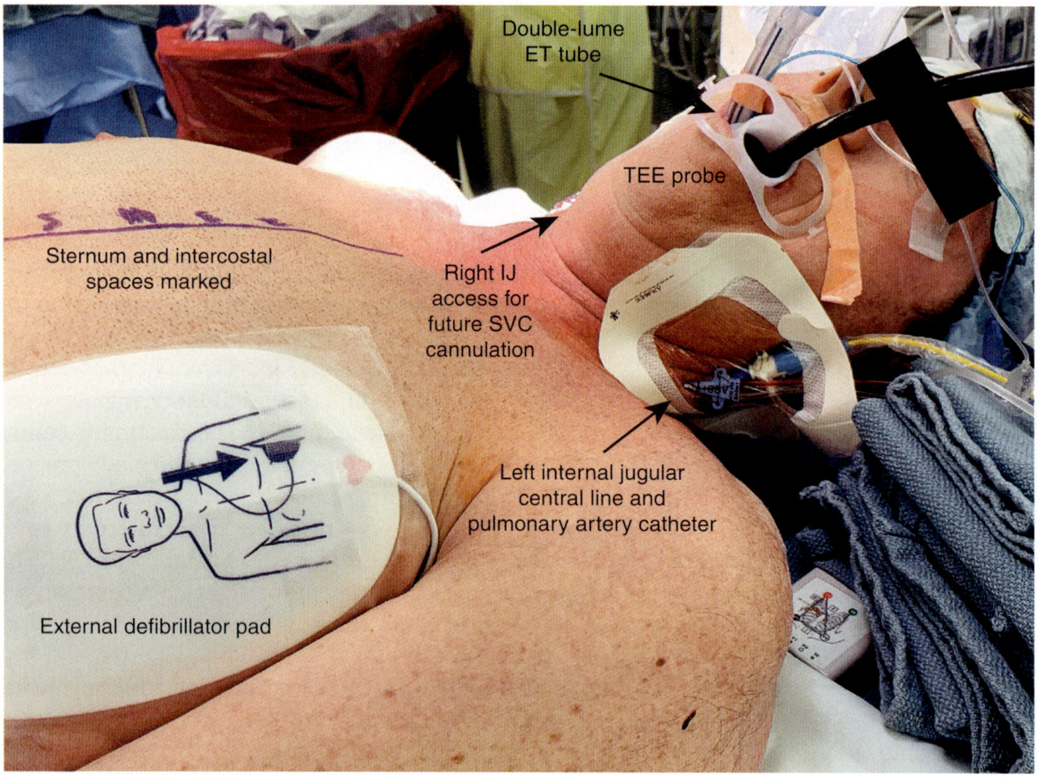

Fig. 18.1 Patient Access and Anesthetic Setup.
ET, Endotracheal; *IJ*, internal jugular; *SVC*, superior vena cava; *TEE*, transesophageal echocardiography.

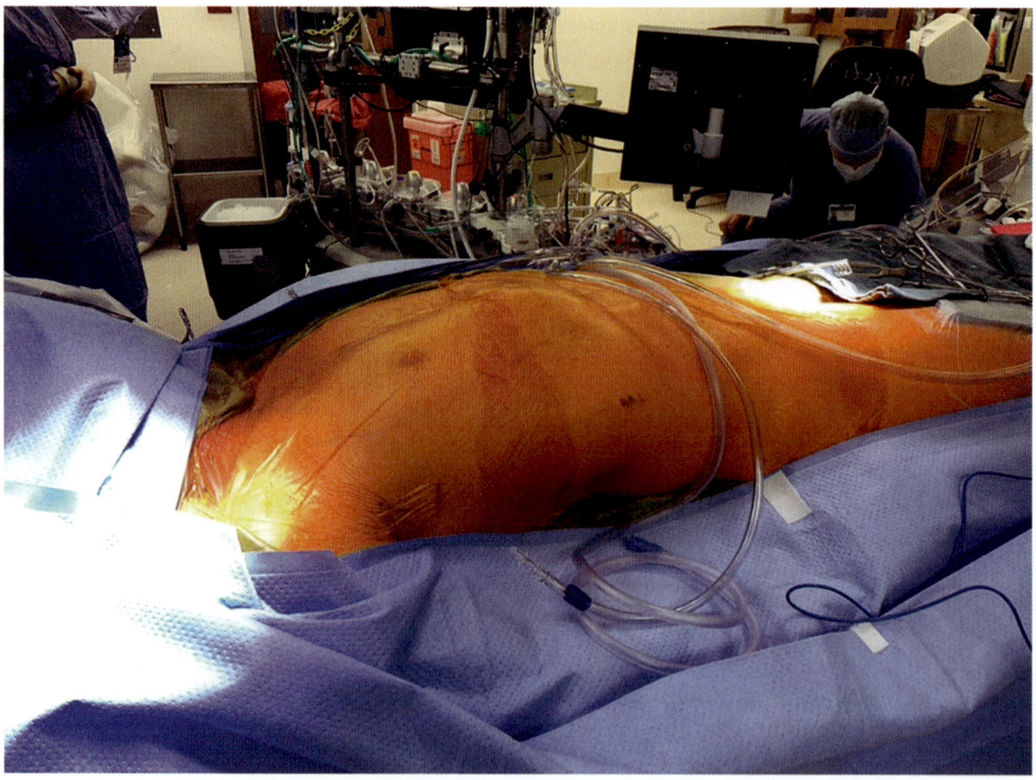

Fig. 18.2 The Patient Is Prepped From the Neck to the Knees. Key areas that the surgeon needs access to include the right internal jugular central line, right chest including the anterior axillary and infraclavicular areas, sternum, and bilateral groins.

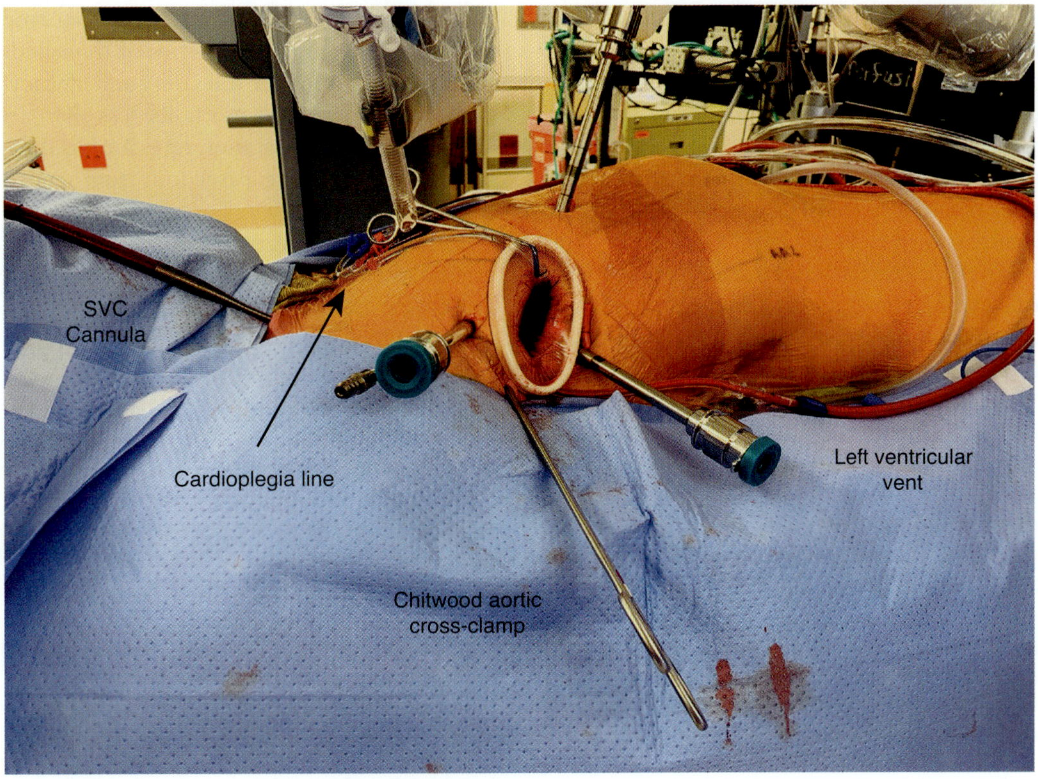

Fig. 18.3 Working and Port Incisions.

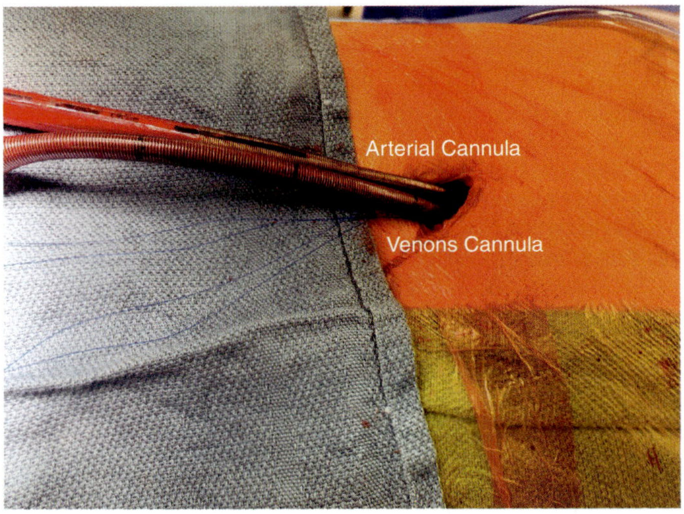

Fig. 19.4 Setup for Peripheral Cardiopulmonary Bypass.

Mitral Valve Repair and Replacement

The surgeon then moves to the robotic console. The mitral valve is exposed with the aid of a left atrial retractor. The diseased valve is evaluated and the pathology confirmed. The same options for mitral valve repair are used as in the classic sternotomy approach: either resection, chordal replacement, chordal transfer, etc. Following leaflet repair, an annuloplasty ring is placed and secured with commercially available titanium fasteners in lieu of traditional hand-thrown knots. The valve is then tested using saline injection into the left ventricle for competency. The left atrium is de-aired and closed with a running suture.

If the valve is unable to be repaired and instead has to be replaced, the technique is similar to traditional mitral valve replacement. The left atrium is opened, and the valve is exposed the same as for a repair. Chordal-sparing valve excision is then performed. Interrupted pledgeted valve sutures are placed around the annulus. The valve is then appropriately sized and seated on the previously placed sutures. The valve sutures are secured with a titanium fastener.

SURGICAL COMPLICATIONS

The postoperative complication profile of robotic mitral valve surgery has similarities and differences to that of classic mitral valve surgery via a sternotomy. Those that are unique to the robotic approach with associated incidence include:[10–17]

- conversion to midline sternotomy (<1%)
- hemothorax (1% to 4%)
- unilateral pulmonary edema (2%)
- phrenic nerve injury (0% to 3%)
- inadequate myocardial protection
- stroke from retrograde arterial perfusion (1.5% to 3.5%)
- vascular complications related to peripheral cannulation for cardiopulmonary bypass

OUTCOMES

Since the origination of robotic mitral valve surgery in the late 1990s, there has been a plethora of evidence published on outcomes after robotic valve surgery. From these data, the operative indications have broadened from simple to complex repairs, reoperative mitral surgery, and concomitant operations. Cross-clamp and operative times have shortened for all complexities of repair.[12] Compared with conventional sternotomy, robotic mitral valve surgery has also been shown to have decreased postoperative atrial fibrillation, blood transfusions, intensive care unit and hospital stay, and faster return to normal activity.[12–14] These superior results also translate over to older patient populations, as recently shown by Wang et al.[15]

The early studies in the 2000s looked at the immediate perioperative and short-term outcomes. Cross-clamp and operative times were longer than traditional sternotomy mitral valve surgery, but perioperative morbidity and mortality were no different.[15] Shortly thereafter, a larger series of more than 100 patients verified these acceptable short-term outcomes, reporting no conversion to median sternotomy, perioperative mortality of less than 1%, and a 5-year freedom from reoperation of 90%.[10] Contemporary large-scale series of thousands of patients have continued to reproduce the safety and efficacy of this operation, showing perioperative mortality less than 1% and stroke rate 0.6% to 2%, low reoperation rates for bleeding of 2% to 4%, and greater than 90% 5-year freedom from reoperation for valvular abnormalities.[11,17]

Midterm and longer-term data have also been favorable for robotic mitral valve repair. Suri and colleagues reported excellent 5-year data for this operation: they showed 5-year survival of 99.5%, freedom from mitral regurgitation 94.6%, and freedom from reoperation for mitral regurgitation of 97.7%.[18] Ten-year Chinese data were presented from Dr. Wang recently, showing survival rate of 91.6%, stroke rate 8.8%, and freedom from reoperation of 95%.[19]

CASE-BASED ASSESSMENT

1. A 65-year-old male presents with new-onset fatigue and dyspnea on exertion. Physical examination reveals a holosystolic murmur, which radiates from the apex to the base and is otherwise unremarkable. A transthoracic echocardiogram is performed. A dilated left ventricle with preserved systolic function and severe mitral regurgitation with posterior leaflet prolapse and possible ruptured chords are noted. An Electrocardiogram (EKG) shows T-wave inversion laterally. He is referred for possible robotic mitral valve surgery.
What two studies would be necessary to determine if this patient is a candidate for robotic mitral valve surgery?
   A. Transesophageal echocardiogram and stress test
   B. Right heart catheterization and pulmonary function test
   C. Coronary angiography and computed tomography (CT) angiogram of the chest, abdomen, and pelvis
   D. Cardiac magnetic resonance imaging (MRI) and extended cardiac monitor to rule out atrial fibrillation

See page 317 for the answers.

REFERENCES

1. Carpentier A, Loulmet D, Aupécle B, et al. Computer assisted open heart surgery. First case operated on with success. *C R Acad Sci III*. 1998;321:437–442.
2. Cohn LH, Adams DH, Couper GS, et al. Minimally invasive cardiac valve surgery improves patient satisfaction while reducing costs of cardiac valve replacement and repair. *Ann Surg*. 1997;226:421–426; discussion 427–428.
3. Navia JL, Cosgrove 3rd DM. Minimally invasive mitral valve operations. *Ann Thorac Surg*. 1996;62:1542–1544.
4. Chitwood Jr WR, Nifong LW, Elbeery JE, et al. Robotic mitral valve repair: trapezoidal resection and prosthetic annuloplasty with the da vinci surgical system. *J Thorac Cardiovasc Surg*. 2000;120:1171–1172.
5. Nifong LW, Chu VF, Bailey BM, et al. Robotic mitral valve repair: experience with the da Vinci system. *Ann Thorac Surg*. 2003;75:438–442; discussion 443.
6. Nifong LW, Chitwood WR, Pappas PS, et al. Robotic mitral valve surgery: a United States multicenter trial. *J Thorac Cardiovasc Surg*. 2005;129:1395–1404.
7. Nishimura RA, Otto CM, Bonow RO, et al. 2014 AHA/ACC Guideline for the Management of Patients With Valvular Heart Disease: A Report of the American College of Cardiology/American Heart Association Task Force on Practice Guidelines. *JACC*. 2014;63:22.
8. Nifong LW, Rodriguez E, Chitwood WR. 540 Consecutive robotic mitral valve repairs including concomitant atrial fibrillation cryoablation. *Ann Thorac Surg*. 2011;94(1):38–43.
9. Moodley S, Schoenhagen P, Gillinov AM, et al. Preoperative multidetector computed tomography angiography for planning of minimally invasive robotic mitral valve surgery: impact on decision making. *J Thorac Cardiovasc Surg*. 2013;146:262–268.
10. Nifong LW, Chu VF, Bailey BM, et al. Robotic mitral valve repair: experience with the da Vinci system. *Ann Thorac Surg*. 2003;75:438–443.
11. Nifong LW, Chitwood W, Pappas P, et al. Robotic mitral valve surgery: a United States multicenter trial. *J Thorac Cardiovasc Surg*. 2005;129:1395–1404.
12. Paul S, Isaacs AJ, Jalbert J, et al. A population-based analysis of robotic-assisted mitral valve repair. *Ann Thorac Surg*. 2015;99:1546–1553.
13. Wang A, Brennan JM, Zhang S, et al. Robotic mitral valve repair in older individuals: an analysis of the Society of Thoracic Surgeons Database. *Ann Thorac Surg*. 2018;106:1388–1393.
14. Mihaljevic T, Koprivanac M, Kelava M, et al. Value of robotically assisted surgery for mitral valve disease. *JAMA Surg*. 2014;149:679–686.
15. Wang A, Brennan JM, Zhang S, et al. Robotic mitral valve repair in older individuals: an analysis of the Society of Thoracic Surgeons database. *Ann Thorac Surg*. 2018;106:1388–1393.
16. Nifong LW, Chu VF, Bailey BM, et al. Robotic mitral valve repair: experience with the da Vinci system. *Ann Thorac Surg*. 2003;75:438–443.
17. Suri RM, Taggarse A, Burkhart HM, et al. Robotic mitral valve repair for simple and complex degenerative disease: mid-term clinical and echocardiographic quality outcomes. *Circulation*. 2015;132:1961–1968.
18. Murphy DA, Moss E, Binongo J, et al. The expanding role of endoscopic robotics in mitral valve surgery: 1257 consecutive procedures. *J Thorac Cardiovasc Surg*. 2015;100:1675–1682.
19. Wang R, Zhang H, Gao C. *Long-term Follow-up Results of Robotic Mitral Valve Surgery*. ISMICS 2019 poster presentation, New York, NY.

19

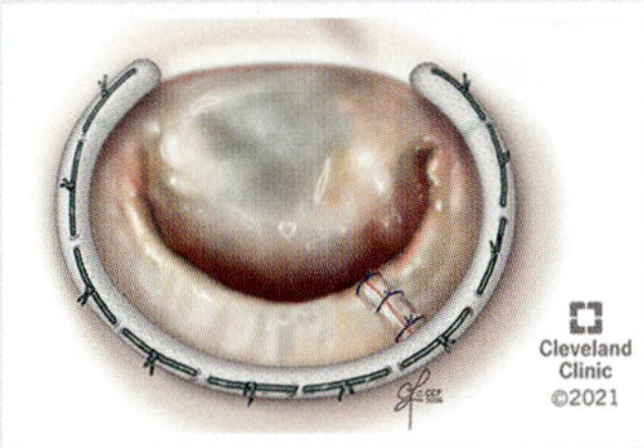

Surgical Repair of the Mitral Valve

Ryan A. Moore, Per Wierup, Daniel J.P. Burns, Gosta B. Pettersson, A. Marc. Gillinov

CHAPTER OUTLINE

LEARNING OBJECTIVES

1. Review the advantages that mitral valve repair confers over mitral valve replacement in degenerative disease.
2. Discuss the preoperative and intraoperative assessment of the mitral valve used in determining candidacy for valve repair.
3. Describe how disease etiology and mechanism of mitral regurgitation inform the decision to repair or replace the mitral valve.
4. Highlight key mitral valve repair techniques commonly employed in the treatment of mitral regurgitation.
5. Describe our general philosophy concerning the approach to mitral valve repair.

INTRODUCTION

When surgical intervention is indicated, mitral valve repair is the procedure of choice across most causes of mitral regurgitation (MR). This is owed to significant advantages over mitral valve replacement concerning long-term survival, freedom from reoperation, preservation of ventricular function, and avoidance of complications related to anticoagulation, particularly in those with degenerative mitral valve disease.[1–7] Over the last 50 years the techniques for mitral valve repair have been refined, with over 95% of patients with degenerative disease being candidates for valve repair.[8,9]

Beginning with Dr. Carpentier's famous description of the French Correction,[10,11] the utility and applicability of mitral valve repair has continued to evolve, with surgeons now employing a number of different repair techniques to achieve successful repair. Along with the emergence of the "respect versus resect" philosophy concerning the treatment of leaflet tissue at the time of repair, techniques such as artificial chord repair, pericardial patch reconstruction, and other nonresectional strategies have emerged and broadened the applicability of mitral valve repair in the modern era.

In this chapter we will explore the surgical considerations that go into determining the feasibility of mitral valve repair, as well as various techniques that surgeons have at their disposal to perform successful valve repair. We will conclude by describing our philosophy in the approach to mitral valve repair in modern surgical practice.

CANDIDACY FOR VALVE REPAIR

Preoperative Evaluation (Demographics and Echocardiography)

Routine preoperative assessment considering a patient's medical history, baseline cardiac function, and echocardiographic findings is fundamental in ascertaining the likelihood of successful valve repair. Depending on the course of surgery, this evaluation may influence whether valve repair or replacement should be undertaken. For example, sicker patients may benefit from a shorter operative duration, in which case a simple and quick mitral valve replacement might be preferable to a complex and time-consuming mitral valve repair.

The routine review of preoperative transthoracic echocardiography (TTE) coupled with intraoperative transesophageal echocardiography (TEE) is essential for surgical planning and avoiding unanticipated findings at the time of surgery. Morphological assessment of the mitral valve should include evaluation of both leaflets, the mitral annulus, as well as the subvalvular apparatus.[12] TTE can identify leaflet abnormalities, detect annular calcification and provide information on ventricular size and function, while the superior diagnostic accuracy of TEE is useful for real-time intraoperative management. Newer imaging modalities such as 3D echocardiography, cardiac magnetic resonance imaging (MRI), and intracardiac ultrasound are being evaluated to see if they offer advantages in the setting of mitral valve disease.[13]

Surgical Approach

For many cardiac surgeons, sternotomy is the default approach to mitral valve repair, owing to optimal exposure and greater control over operative conduct. This is particularly beneficial in cases where unanticipated findings are encountered and/or when concomitant procedures are required. Minimally invasive chest wall approaches, such as partial sternotomy or right thoracotomy, have been developed and can be employed at the discretion of the surgeon in select patients. Innovations in robotic surgery have facilitated the emergence of robotic-assisted mitral valve repair, where this minimally-invasive alternative to the conventional approach maintains the advantages that valve repair has over valve replacement.[14–16] In our practice, we employ a screening algorithm to identify patients who would benefit from robotic-assisted repair.[17] Illustration of the various chest wall approaches utilized in mitral valve surgery can be found in Fig. 19.1.

Technical Implications of Mitral Regurgitation Etiology

The majority of cases requiring surgery for MR are due to degenerative disease. Additional common causes of MR include

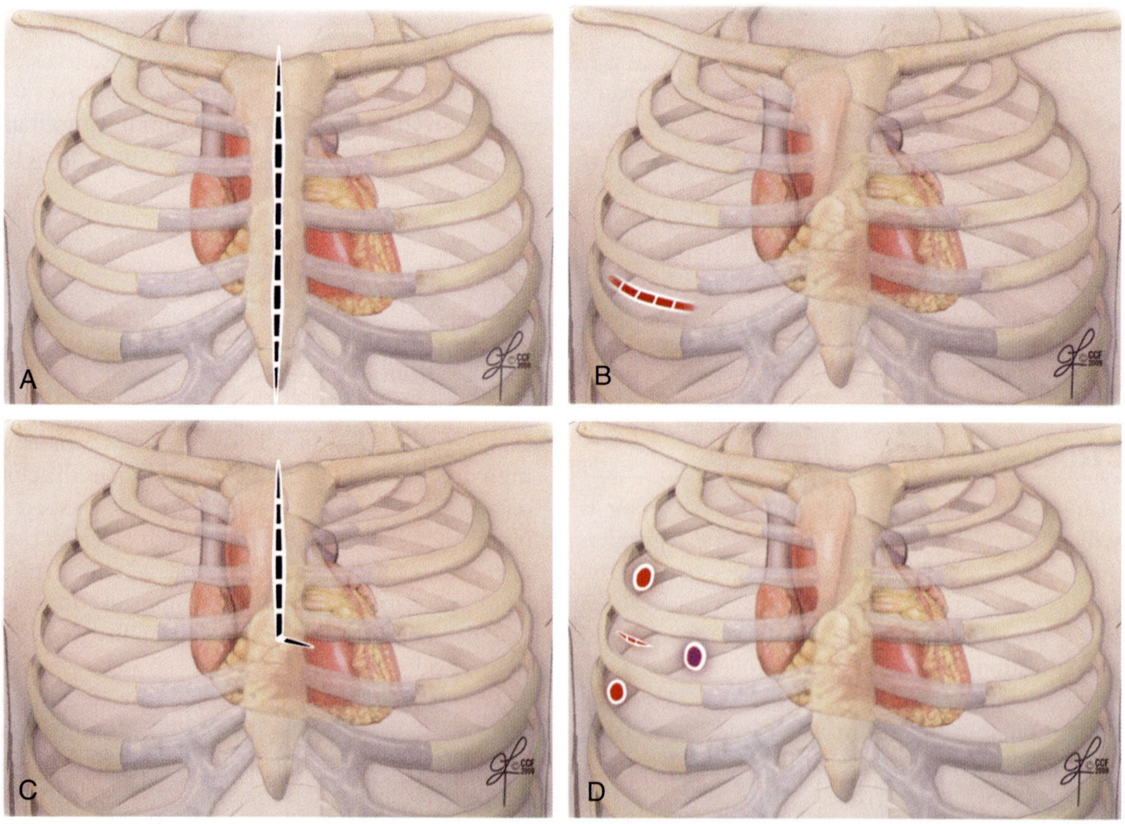

Fig. 19.1 Illustration of Chest Wall Approaches Utilized for Mitral Valve Surgery. (A) Full sternotomy. (B) Right thoracotomy. (C) Partial sternotomy. (D) Robotic-assisted approach. *Reprinted with permission,* Cleveland Clinic Center for Medical Art & Photography ©2021. All Rights Reserved.

endocarditis, rheumatic heart disease (RHD), ischemic cardiomyopathy (ICM), and others (i.e., congenital, hypertrophic obstructive cardiomyopathy [HOCM], drug-induced, etc.).[18] Here we'll discuss the surgical and technical implications of some of the more common causes of MR encountered by cardiac surgeons.

Degenerative Prolapse

Degenerative disease is the most common cause of MR in patients undergoing mitral valve surgery[19] and is also the most repairable. In many cases, the mitral valve exhibits a primary flail segment with myxomatous degeneration localized to one area with otherwise normal valve morphology.[18] Alternatively, the mitral valve may undergo diffuse myxomatous degeneration which results in large billowing leaflets as classically seen in Barlow disease.[20] Mitral valve repair is achievable in more than 95% of cases due to degenerative prolapse with very low rates of morbidity and mortality, with surgeons employing a number of different techniques in modern practice.[21–24]

Rheumatic Heart Disease and Mitral Stenosis

Patients with RHD may develop MR and/or mitral stenosis due to the autoimmune inflammatory process associated with the disease. Most often, patients with RHD exhibit extensive chordal and leaflet retraction associated with the mitral valve, and when compounded by annular dilatation, this leads to loss of leaflet coaptation.[18] Patients with mitral stenosis present unique surgical considerations, whether due to RHD, radiation changes, or other inflammatory processes. The feasibility of mitral valve repair in this setting often depends on the presence of calcification and the thickness/pliability of leaflet tissue. While valve repair should always be considered, annular and leaflet calcification and fibrosis limit the ability to achieve a successful repair, and the ongoing inflammatory process decreases the longevity of the repair.

Endocarditis

Historically, the application of mitral valve repair in the setting of endocarditis has been limited, with repair rates reported around 40%, largely owing to concerns over tissue destruction and repair durability. In practice, concerns persist despite studies demonstrating a survival benefit for patients who undergo valve repair in this setting.[25–28] The case for valve repair is further supported by newer studies, showing lower rates of recurrent infection and reoperation with valve repair, all while avoiding the risks of therapeutic anticoagulation.[29,30] We recommend valve repair in this setting whenever contextually feasible, and surgeons have a multitude of techniques at their disposal to perform valve repair or reconstruction based on the pathology encountered at the time of surgery. The employment of artificial chord repair and pericardial patch construction have increased the feasibility of valve repair in cases where otherwise prohibitive tissue destruction has occurred. Successful valve repair hinges upon radical debridement, the restoration of valve integrity, and annular continuity in cases of invasive disease.

Ischemic Cardiomyopathy

MR secondary to ICM rarely arises from an organic mechanism, such as papillary muscle rupture, and often represents a more chronic pathophysiology.[18] The valve leaflets usually display normal morphology, but the mechanism of MR in this setting is functional, owing to ischemic ventricular remodeling that leads to valvular dysfunction. Ischemic remodeling causes apical and lateral papillary muscle displacement that leads to valve tenting. When coupled with annular dilatation, leaflet tethering and decreased myocardial contractility, which represent the natural history of ICM, a loss of leaflet coaptation occurs.[31–33] Valve repair in this setting has traditionally relied upon placement of an undersized, rigid annuloplasty ring. This sort of valve repair has limited durability. While some have added subvalvular procedures to annuloplasty in patients with this sort of functional MR, durability of this approach is unknown. Valve replacement is often pursued in these patients due to concerns over repair durability.

Hypertrophic Obstructive Cardiomyopathy

Patients with HOCM often exhibit some degree of MR secondary to systolic anterior motion (SAM) of the mitral valve (Fig. 19.2). In patients undergoing surgery to relieve left ventricular outflow tract obstruction secondary to HOCM, the MR is often addressed by septal myectomy alone, with acceptable late survival and relief of elevated gradients.[34–38] In cases where additional intervention on the mitral valve is required to eliminate MR, mitral valve repair is preferable to valve replacement, due to better overall survival and lower rate of thromboembolic events.[39–42] The goal of surgery in the setting of HOCM is to relieve left ventricular outflow tract obstruction (LVOTO) with septal myectomy while eliminating/preventing SAM, which is done by reorienting the zone of leaflet coaptation well posteriorly.

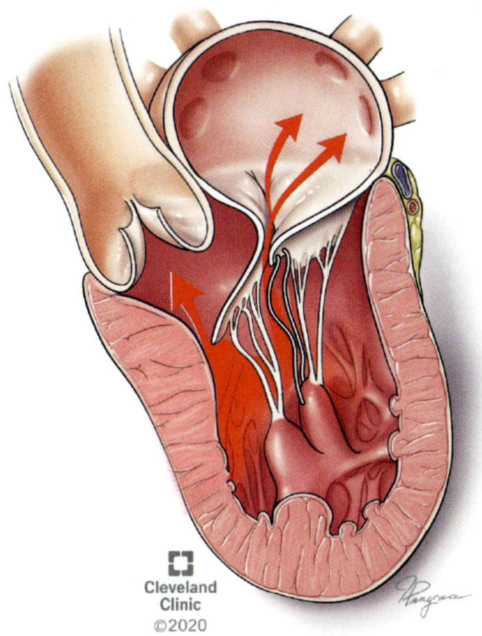

Fig. 19.2 Mechanism of Mitral Regurgitation in Hypertrophic Obstructive Cardiomyopathy. *Reprinted with permission,* Cleveland Clinic Center for Medical Art & Photography ©2021. All Rights Reserved.

COMMON TECHNIQUES FOR MITRAL VALVE REPAIR

The French Correction—Classic Resectional Techniques

Dr. Carpentier first described the techniques for mitral valve repair after publishing his classification of MR for degenerative prolapse.[10,11] His techniques have been the cornerstone of advances in mitral valve repair and are performed routinely to this day. Quadrangular resection, as classically described, is performed on the posterior leaflet and involves excision of the diseased segment from the free margin to the level of the annulus. Leaflet continuity is then directly restored with suture with the option for annular plication to reduce leaflet height or orifice size. Subsequently, Dr. Carpentier described the sliding plasty with quadrangular resection to reduce posterior leaflet height and reduce the risk of SAM after mitral valve repair. Once quadrangular resection has been performed, the remaining leaflet tissue is then mobilized along the posterior annulus, creating a sliding plasty prior to reapproximating the leaflet tissue with suture (Fig. 19.3). Modifications to these techniques, including the use of folding valvuloplasty, the Butterfly technique, and others, have emerged as alternatives for addressing discrepancies in leaflet height, eliminating the need for annular plication.

Triangular resection eliminates the need for annular plication/ sliding plasty and may be preferred in cases where limited tissue

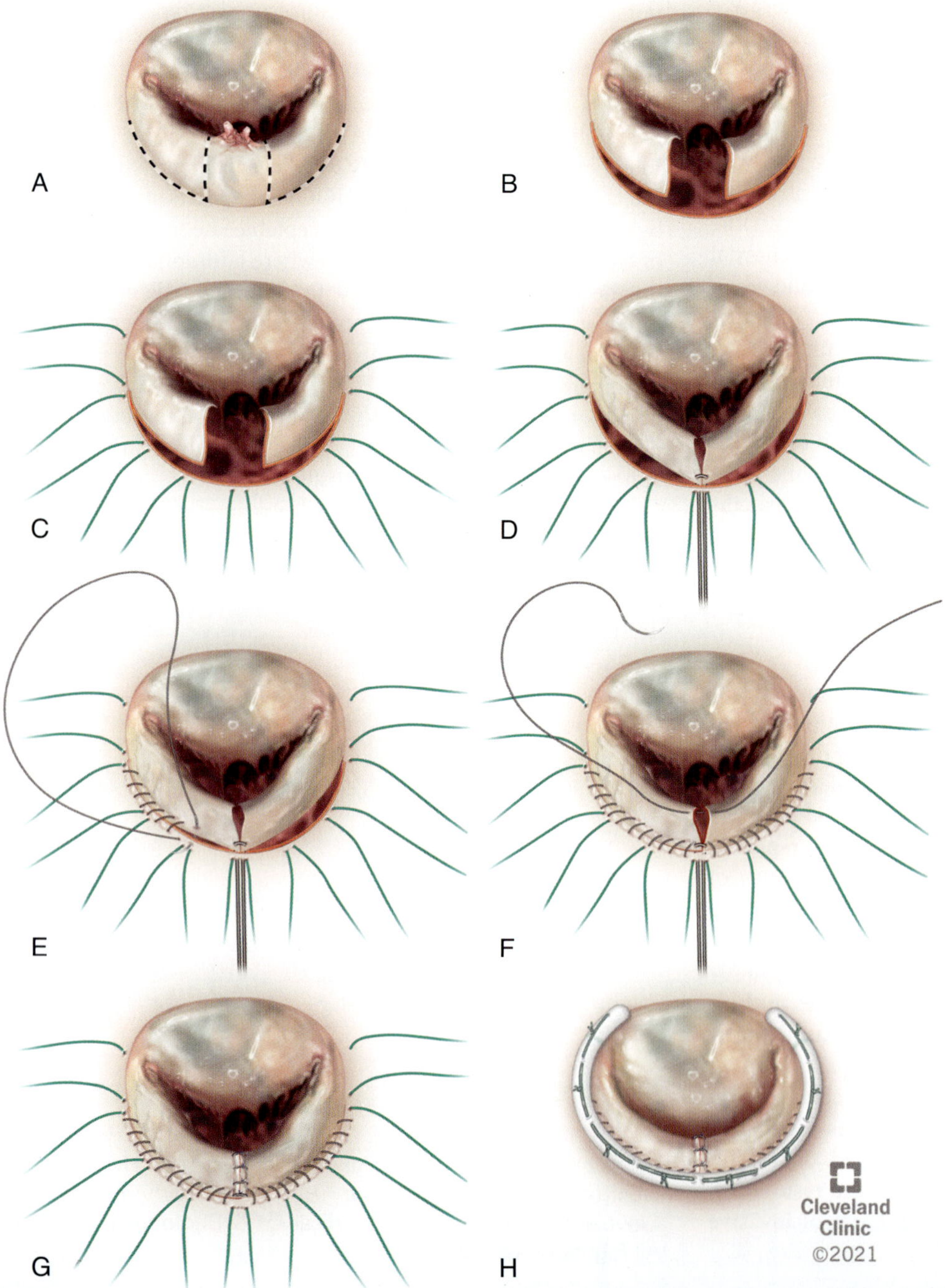

Fig. 19.3 Quadrangular Resection With Sliding Plasty. (A and B) Excision of the prolapsing leaflet segment and mobilization of the remaining leaflet tissue along the posterior annulus. (C and D) Reattachment of remnant leaflet tissue to the annulus, anchored at the midline. (E–G) Approximation of remaining leaflet edges directly with suture. (H) Annuloplasty placement to complete repair. *Reprinted with permission*, Cleveland Clinic Center for Medical Art & Photography ©2021. All Rights Reserved.

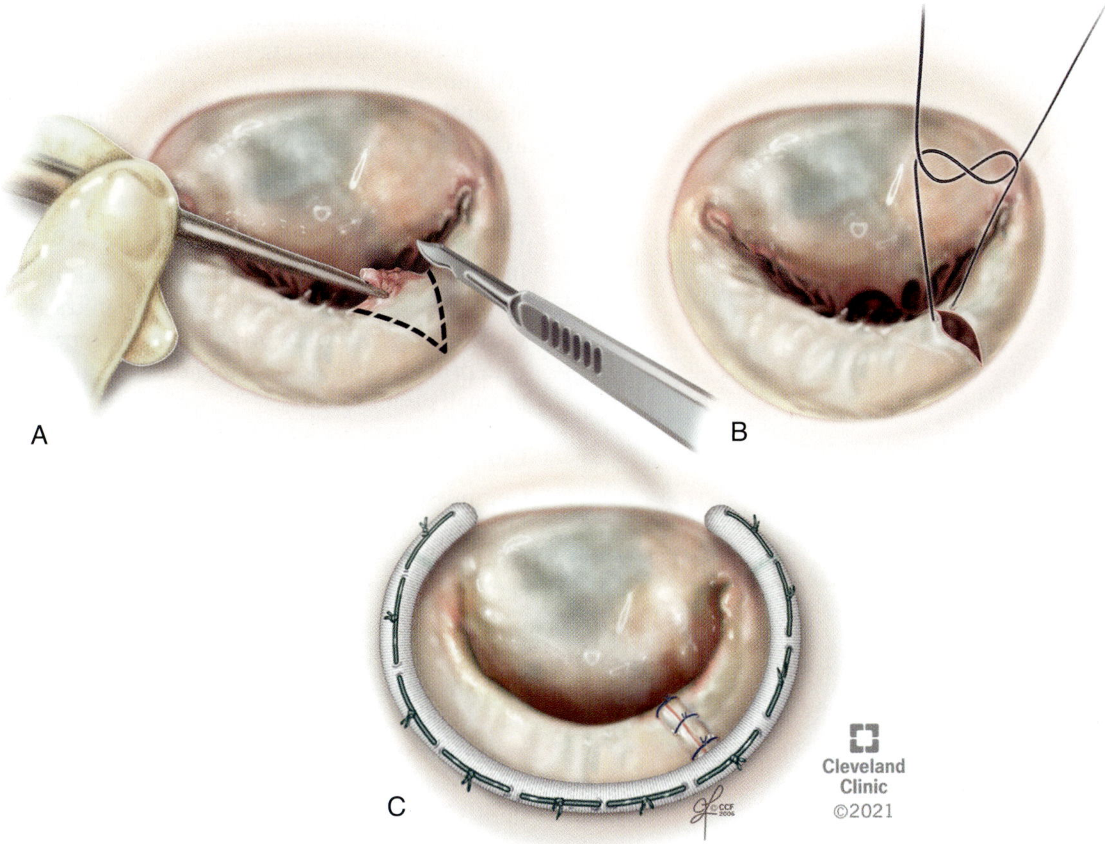

Fig. 19.4 Triangular Resection. (A) A triangular-shaped segment of the prolapsing leaflet tissue is excised with its apex towards the annulus. (B) The defect is closed directly with suture. (C) Repair is completed with an annuloplasty ring. *Reprinted with permission,* Cleveland Clinic Center for Medical Art & Photography ©2021. All Rights Reserved.

resection is performed. This allows for a more physiologic valve repair. The diseased leaflet segment is excised in a triangular fashion, with its apex towards the annulus and its base towards the free edge. After excision, the leaflet is directly approximated with suture (Fig. 19.4). The repair is completed with an annuloplasty band.

Artificial Chord Repair

Since Frater and David introduced the technique in 1989,[43–45] the use of artificial chordae to repair and reconstruct the mitral valve has provided a novel opportunity to repair the mitral valve while avoiding resection of leaflet tissue. Other limitations of classic resectional techniques avoided by repair with artificial chordae include the deformation of the left ventricle (LV)subannular region, risk of circumflex artery injury, and risk of LVOT due to SAM.[46] Using 4-0 or 5-0 expanded polytetrafluoroethylene (ePTFE), the artificial chordae are constructed using either a free-hand technique or with premeasured loops and have been shown to provide equivalent outcomes when compared with classic resectional techniques.[47]

Free-hand technique

After passing through the fibrous region of a papillary muscle head adjacent to the area of prolapse, each end of the suture is brought up to the leaflet edge and passed twice through leaflet tissue from the ventricular to atrial side. The chordal length is adjusted to a level that optimizes leaflet coaptation, using A1–P1 as a reference point, and tied on the atrial side of the valve (Fig. 19.5).

Pre-measured loops: Determining the appropriate length of neochordae can be difficult. Mohr and von Oppell developed the technique of measuring normal chordae near the area of prolapse with calipers to guide creation of premeasured chordal loops.[48] The loops are attached to the papillary muscle and then to the leaflet edge using separate suture, taking care not to cross the middle of the valve (Fig. 19.6).

Artificial chord techniques have broad applicability and can be applied across the spectrum of mitral valve disease. In cases involving large prolapsing segments (e.g., Barlow valve) or in the setting of endocarditis where otherwise prohibitive tissue destruction has occurred, the use of artificial chordae can be particularly beneficial.[20] Artificial chordae can also be used for leaflet support in cases where a pericardial patch has been used to reconstruct the mitral leaflet after extensive resection. It is important to adjust the chordal height to a level that optimizes leaflet coaptation and to direct the zone of coaptation well posteriorly to reduce the risk of LVOT due to SAM.

Pericardial Patch Repair

Mitral valve repair can also be achieved by pericardial patch repair using either autologous or bovine pericardium. This is often used to repair perforations or clefts of the mitral valve, as often encountered in the setting of endocarditis or with mitral calcification. In cases where valve pathology involves the leaflet free margin, or where extensive posterior leaflet resection

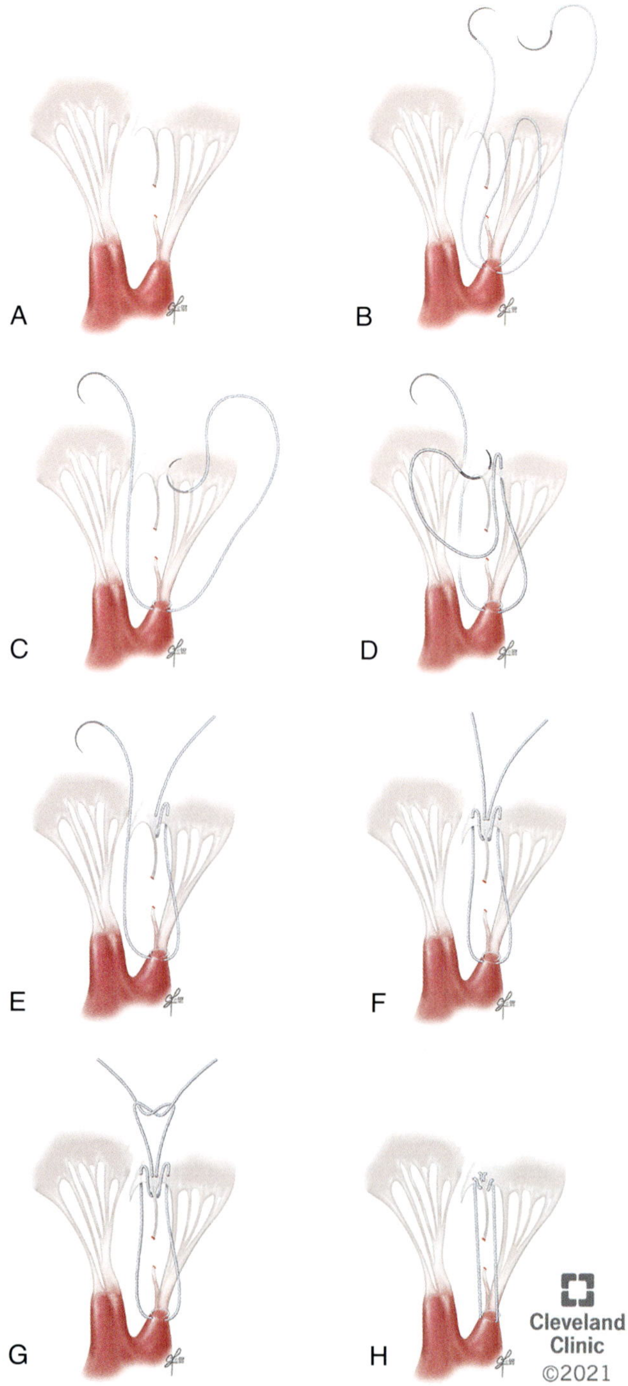

Fig. 19.5 Free-Hand Technique for Artificial Chord Placement. After identification of the prolapsing segment (A) the neochordae is passed through a papillary muscle head corresponding to the area of prolapse (B). Each end of the neochordae is brought up to the leaflet edge (C) and passed twice through the leaflet tissue in the region of the prolapse (D and E). The needles pass from the ventricular side to the atrial side, finishing adjacent to one another (F). The chordal length is adjusted, and the knot is secured on the atrial side of the valve (G and H). *Reprinted with permission*, Cleveland Clinic Center for Medical Art & Photography ©2021. All Rights Reserved.

is required, this technique can be employed to reconstruct the valve leaflets, supporting the free edge of the repair with artificial chords (Fig. 19.7). Patch repair can also be used to reconstruct the mitral annulus or mitral commissures in cases where extensive debridement is required (e.g., mitral annular calcification [MAC], annular abscess).

Primary Debridement With Direct Suture Repair

In cases where lesions contributing to mitral valve dysfunction are confined to the leaflet body or the mitral annulus, as in the setting of endocarditis or MAC, valve repair can be achieved with primary debridement and direct suture repair of any clefts or small perforations.

Commissuroplasty

Commissural prolapse is often due to the elongation or rupture of chordae at the commissure. This can happen to chordae belonging to either the anterior or posterior leaflet. Simple suture closure of the commissure can achieve a reliable repair, while more traditional techniques may be difficult to employ in this area (Fig. 19.8).[49] By obliterating the commissure with mattress sutures, the need for resection and reconstruction of the commissure is eliminated.[47] This is particularly useful in patients with degenerative prolapse and a large mitral orifice.[50] While commissural closure does reduce the mitral orifice area, studies have demonstrated good freedom from MR and mitral stenosis using this technique.[49]

Edge-to-Edge Repair

Originally described by Alfieri in 1991, an edge-to-edge repair can be performed by anchoring the free edge of the prolapsing leaflet to the free edge of the opposite leaflet, creating a double orifice valve (Fig. 19.9).[51] The rationale behind this approach is to achieve a functional repair rather than an anatomic one, where an annuloplasty completes the repair.[52,53] This technique has proven particularly useful in patients with isolated anterior leaflet prolapse or bi-leaflet prolapse due to Barlow disease.[51,54] While the results for this technique have been acceptable in patients with degenerative mitral valve prolapse, we generally avoid this approach due to the inevitable development of varying degrees of mitral stenosis, especially in patients with a small mitral orifice.

Annuloplasty Placement

Functioning to increase leaflet coaptation, restore annular size and shape, reduce tension on suture lines, and prevent future annular dilatation, we invariably use a prosthetic annuloplasty for all cases of mitral valve repair. A number of annuloplasty devices are available and include complete rings or partial bands that are structured as rigid, semi-rigid, or flexible. The ring/band size is determined by measuring the height of the anterior leaflet with appropriate sizers. Studies comparing annuloplasty devices have shown no significant difference in outcomes in degenerative mitral valve disease,[55–57] and the choice is ultimately left up to the surgeon. We generally employ a flexible band as it allows for dynamic movement of the mitral annulus throughout the cardiac cycle and has been associated with lower mitral valve gradients.[58]

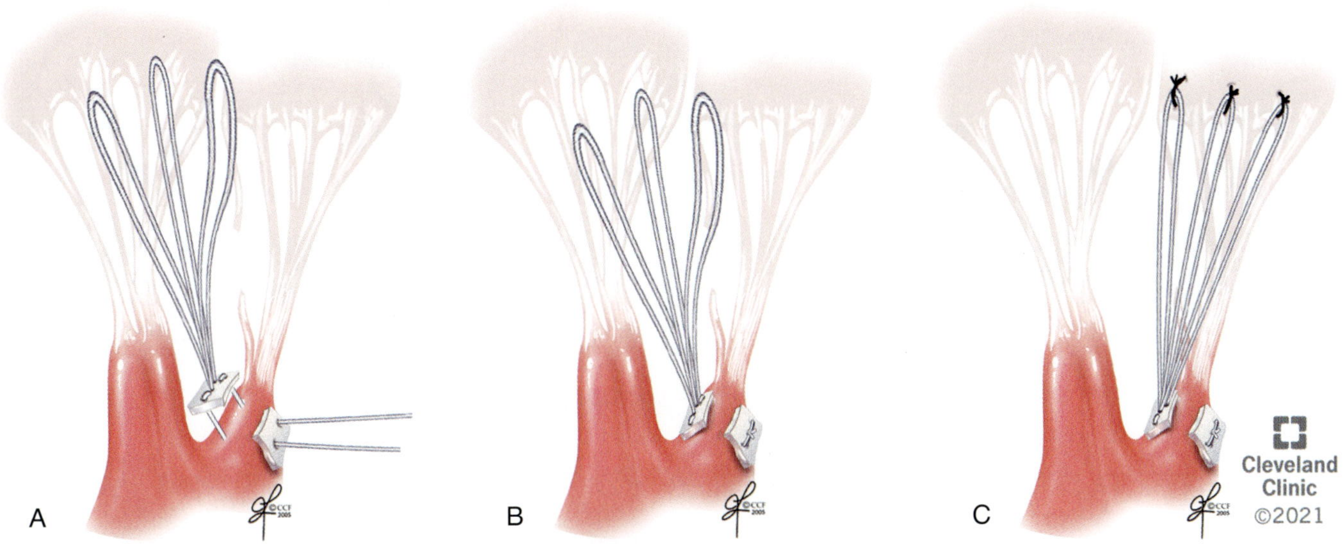

Fig. 19.6 Remeasured Technique for Artificial Chord Placement. A normal chord adjacent to the area of prolapse is measured with a caliper, establishing the desired length of the neochord loops. The premeasured chordal loops are attached to the papillary muscle (A and B). Separate sutures are used to attach the loops to the leaflet edge in the area of the prolapse (C). *Reprinted with permission*, Cleveland Clinic Center for Medical Art & Photography ©2021. All Rights Reserved.

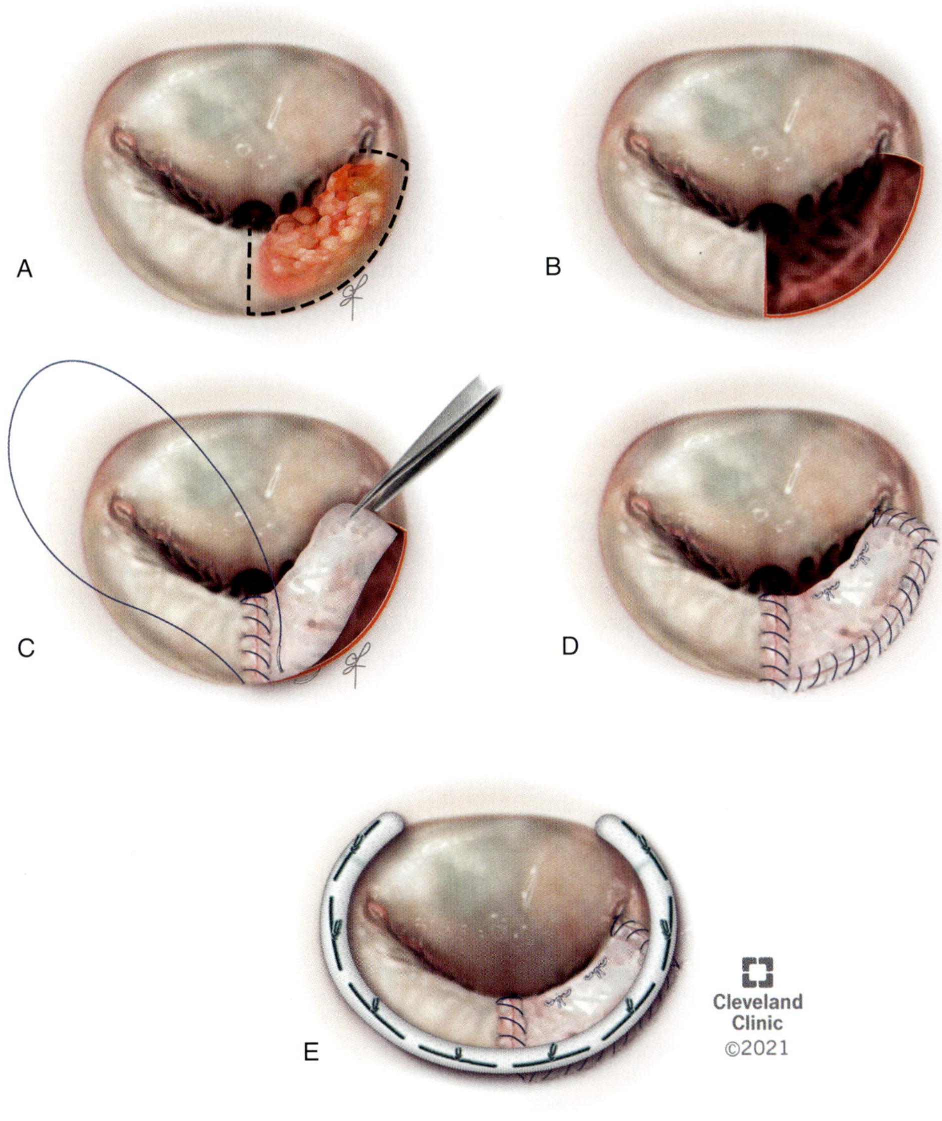

Fig. 19.7 Pericardial Patch Repair With Leaflet Reconstruction. (A and B) The diseased valve segment is excised. (C) A pericardial patch is used to reconstructing the mitral leaflet, secured directly with suture. (D) Artificial chordae are placed to support the free edge of the patch repair. (E) The repair is completed with an annuloplasty. *Reprinted with permission*, Cleveland Clinic Center for Medical Art & Photography ©2021. All Rights Reserved.

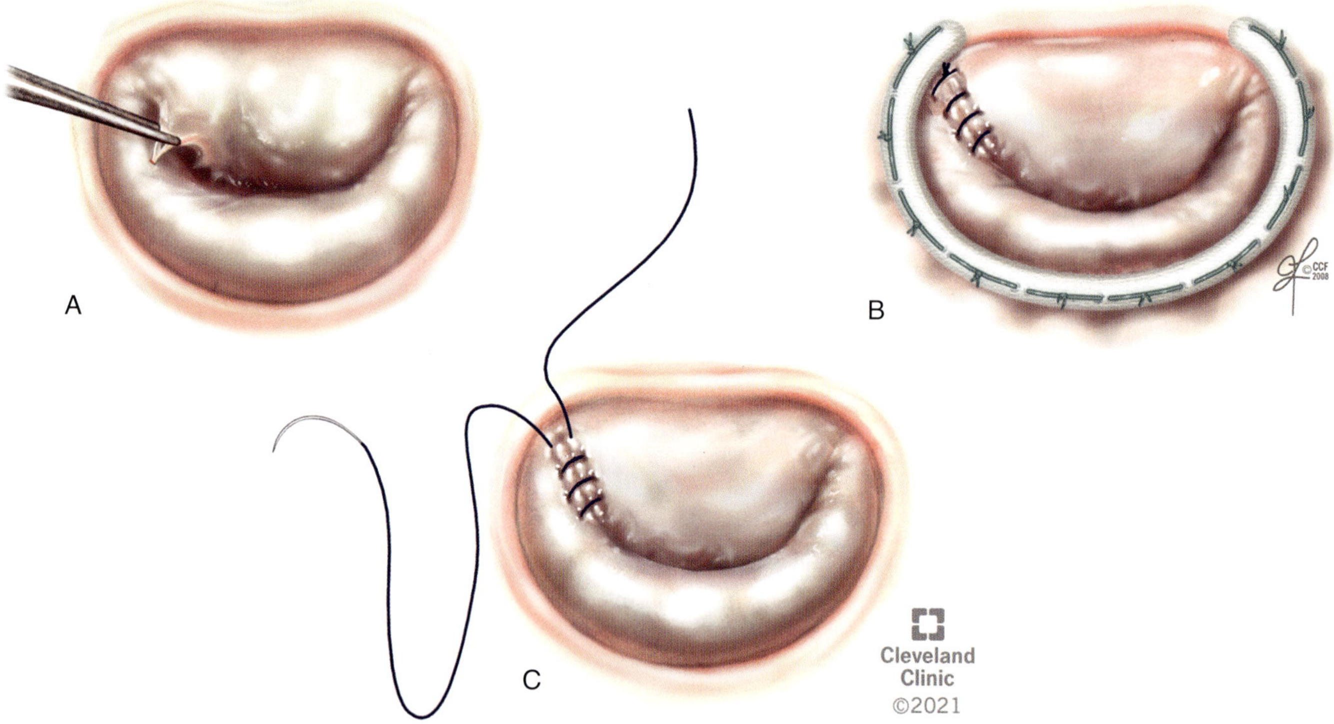

Fig. 19.8 Simple Commissuroplasty. (A and B) The commissural prolapse is identified and repaired by obliterating the commissure with mattress sutures avoiding resection and reconstruction of the commissure. (C) The repair is completed with an annuloplasty ring. *Reprinted with permission*, Cleveland Clinic Center for Medical Art & Photography ©2021. All Rights Reserved.

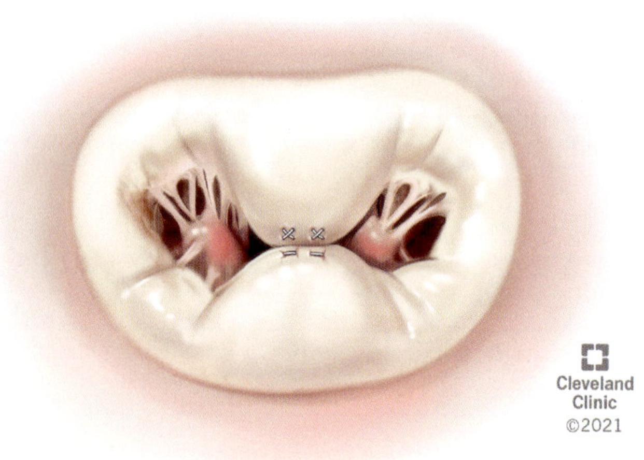

Fig. 19.9 Edge-to-Edge Repair of the Mitral Valve. *Reprinted with permission*, Cleveland Clinic Center for Medical Art & Photography ©2021. All Rights Reserved.

OUR PHILOSOPHY FOR MITRAL VALVE REPAIR

With a suite of repair techniques at the surgeon's disposal, mitral valve repair is possible in nearly all patients with degenerative disease/mitral valve prolapse. Whether the leaflet is managed by resection or creation of artificial chordae, all repairs include an annuloplasty. The majority of patients with isolated degenerative disease can be treated with minimally invasive or robotic chest wall approaches. Patients with endocarditis should also be approached with the goal of mitral valve repair. In contrast, when treating patients with severe functional MR associated with left ventricular dysfunction, we generally favor valve replacement. While valve repair is feasible in such patients, repair durability is poor.

SUMMARY

- Across most etiologies of mitral regurgitation, valve repair has performed favorably to valve replacement concerning overall survival, and freedom from reoperation.
- Thorough preoperative assessment of patient history and preoperative echocardiography are fundamental to determining likelihood of successful valve repair.
- The etiology of mitral regurgitation has technical implications that influence the decision to attempt valve repair or valve replacement at the time of surgery.
- When attempting valve repair, surgeons have a wide array of techniques at their disposal to restore valve integrity and function.
- As techniques for valve repair continue to evolve, its application should continue to broaden and should be encouraged in patients for whom it is expected to provide benefits over valve replacement.

CASE-BASED ASSESSMENT

A 65-year-old man with a past medical history of hypertension and hyperlipideemia presents to his cardiologist with shortness of breath and dyspnea on exertion. Echocardiography shows a flail segment in the middle of his posterior mitral leaflet. The cardiologist refers him to your office to consider surgical intervention and his discussion with you raises the following questions:

1. What is the most likely etiology of this patient's mitral valve prolapse?
   A. Rheumatic
   B. Congenital
   C. Endocarditis
   D. Degenerative
   E. HOCM
2. Which of the following is the most common chest wall approach to repairing the mitral valve, owing to optimal exposure and greater operative control?
   A. Sternotomy
   B. Right Thoracotomy
   C. Partial Sternotomy
   D. Robotic-assisted approach
3. When considering mitral valve repair, what is the rate of repairability for patients with degenerative prolapse?
   A. Greater than >60%
   B. Greater than >75%
   C. Greater than >80%
   D. Greater than >85%
   E. Greater than >95%
4. Traditional resectional techniques, as described by Dr. Carpentier in 1983, include which of the following?
   A. Artificial chord repair
   B. Pericardial patch repair
   C. Quadrangular and triangular resection
   D. Primary debridement
   E. Edge-to-edge repair
5. Which of the following, along with artificial chord repair, has broadened the applicability of nonresectional mitral valve repair, particularly in cases where otherwise prohibitive tissue destruction has occurred?
   A. Commissuroplasty
   B. Pericardial patch repair
   C. Quadrangular and triangular resection
   D. Primary debridement
   E. Edge-to-edge repair

See page 318 for the answers.

REFERENCES

1. Mick S, Keshavamurthy SGM. Mitral valve repair versus replacement. *Ann Cardiothorac Surg*. 2015;4(3):230–237.
2. Suri RM, Schaff HV, Dearani JA, et al. Survival advantage and improved durability of mitral repair for leaflet prolapse subsets in the current era. *Ann Thorac Surg*. 2006;82(3):819–826.
3. David TE, Armstrong S, McCrindle BW, et al. Late outcomes of mitral valve repair for mitral regurgitation due to degenerative disease. *Circulation*. 2013;127(14):1485–1492.
4. Daneshmand MA, Milano CA, Rankin JS, et al. Mitral valve repair for degenerative disease: a 20 years experience. *Ann Thorac Surg*. 2009;88(6):1828–1837.
5. Lazar HL. Robotic mitral valve repair for degenerative mitral valve regurgitation is it for everyone? *Circulation*. 2000;132:1941–1942.
6. Mohty D, Orszulak TA, Schaff HV, et al. Very long-term survival and durability of mitral valve repair for mitral valve prolapse. *Circulation*. 2001;104(12 suppl 1):I1–I7.
7. Coutinho GF, Antunes MJ. Mitral valve repair for degenerative mitral valve disease: surgical approach, patient selection and long-term outcomes. *Heart*. 2017;103(21):1663–1669.
8. Castillo JG, Anyanwu AC, Fuster V, et al. A near 100% repair rate for mitral valve prolapse is achievable in a reference center: implications for future guidelines. *J Thorac Cardiovasc Surg*. 2012;144(2):308–312.
9. Gillinov AM, Cosgrove DM, Blackstone EH, et al. Durability of mitral valve repair for degenerative disease. *J Thorac Cardiovasc Surg*. 1998;116(5):734–743.
10. Carpentier A, Relland J, Deloche A, et al. Conservative management of the prolapsed mitral valve. *Ann Thorac Surg*. 1978;26:294–302.
11. Carpentier A. Cardiac valve surgery—the "French correction". *J Thorac Cardiovasc Surg*. 1983;86(3):323–337.
12. Del Forno B, De Bonis M, Agricola R, et al. Mitral valve regurgitation: a disease with a wide spectrum of therapeutic options. *Nat Rev Cardiol*. 2020, Dec;17(12):807–827. Epub 2020 Jun 29. https://doi.org/10.1038/s41569-020-0395-7. PMID: 32601465.
13. El Sabbagh A, Reddy YNV, Nishimura RA. Mitral Valve Regurgitation in the Contemporary Era: Insights Into Diagnosis, Management, and Future Directions. *JACC Cardiovasc Imaging*. 2018;11(4):628–643. doi:10.1016/j.jcmg.2018.01.009. PMID: 29622181.
14. Gillinov AM, Mihaljevic T, Javadikasgari H, et al. Early results of robotically assisted mitral valve surgery: analysis of the first 1000 cases. *J Thorac Cardiovasc Surg*. 2018;155(1):82–91. e2. doi:10.1016/j.jtcvs.2017.07.037. Epub Aug 1, 2017. PMID: 28893396.
15. Javadikasgari H, Suri RM, Tappuni B, et al. Robotic mitral valve repair for degenerative posterior leaflet prolapse. *Ann Cardiothorac Surg*. 2017, jan;6(1):27–32. doi:10.21037/acs.2017.01.07. PMID: 28203538; PMCID: PMC5293624.
16. Suri RM, Dearani JA, Mihaljevic T, et al. Mitral valve repair using robotic technology: safe, effective, and durable. *J Thorac Cardiovasc Surg*. 2016;151(6):1450–1454. doi:10.1016/j.jtcvs.2016.02.030 Epub 2016 Feb 24. PMID: 27012453.
17. Javadikasgari H, Suri RM, Gillinov AM. Robotic mitral valve repair: algorithmic approach in degenerative mitral valve disease. *Ann Cardiothorac Surg*. 2016;5(6):586–588. doi:10.21037/acs.2016.11.07. PMID: 27942493; PMCID: PMC5135547.
18. Enriquez-Sarano M, Akins CW, Vahanian A. Mitral regurgitation. *Lancet*. 2009;373(9672):1382–13894. doi:10.1016/S0140-6736(09)60692-9. Epub 2009 Apr 6. PMID: 19356795.
19. De Bonis M, Alfieri O, Dalrymple-Hay M, et al. Mitral Valve Repair in Degenerative Mitral Regurgitation: State of the Art. *Prog Cardiovasc Dis*. 2017;60(3):386–393. doi:10.1016/j.pcad.2017.10.006. Epub 2017 Nov 5. PMID: 29117502.
20. Chemtob RA, Mick S, Gillinov M, et al. Repair of bileaflet prolapse in Barlow syndrome: the 4-chord technique. *J Card Surg*. 2019;34(7):605–609. doi:10.1111/jocs.14078. Epub 2019 May 17. PMID: 31102304.
21. Castillo JG, Anyanwu AC, Fuster V, et al. A near 100% repair rate for mitral valve prolapse is achievable in a reference center: implications for future guidelines. *J Thorac Cardiovasc Surg*. 2012;144(2):308–312. doi:10.1016/j.jtcvs.2011.12.054. Epub 2012 Jun 12. PMID: 22698565.

22. Gillinov AM, Cosgrove DM, Blackstone EH, et al. Durability of mitral valve repair for degenerative disease. *J Thorac Cardiovasc Surg*. 1998;116(5):734–743. doi:10.1016/S0022-5223(98)00450-4. PMID: 9806380.
23. Suri RM, Schaff HV, Dearani JA, et al. Survival advantage and improved durability of mitral repair for leaflet prolapse subsets in the current era. *Ann Thorac Surg*. 2006;82(3):819–826. doi:10.1016/j.athoracsur.2006.03.091. PMID: 16928491.
24. David TE, Armstrong S, Sun Z, et al. Late results of mitral valve repair for mitral regurgitation due to degenerative disease. *Ann Thorac Surg*. 1993;56(1):7–12; discussion 13–14. doi:10.1016/0003-4975(93)90396-y. PMID: 8328879.
25. Muehrcke DD, Cosgrove DM, Lytle BW, et al. Is there an advantage to repairing infected mitral valves? *Ann Thorac Surg*. 1997;63:1718–1724.
26. Pagani FD, Monaghan HL, Deeb GM, et al. Mitral valve reconstruction for active and healed endocarditis. *Circulation*. 1996;94:II133–II138.
27. Hendren WG, Morris AS, Rosenkranz ER, et al. Mitral valve repair for bacterial endocarditis. *J Thorac Cardiovasc Surg*. 1992;103:124–128; discussion 128–129.
28. Dreyfus G, Serraf A, Jebara VA, et al. Valve repair in acute endocarditis material and methods patient population. *Ann Thorac Surg*. 1990;49:706–713.
29. Toyoda N, Itagaki S, Egorova NN, et al. Real-world outcomes of surgery for native mitral valve endocarditis. *J Thorac Cardiovasc Surg*. 2017;154(6):1906–1912.e9. doi:10.1016/j.jtcvs.2017.07.077 Epub 2017 Sep 1. PMID: 28942975.
30. Solari S, De Kerchove L, Tamer S, et al. Active infective mitral valve endocarditis: is a repair-oriented surgery safe and durable?. *Eur J Cardiothorac Surg*. 2019;55(2):256–262. doi:10.1093/ejcts/ezy242. PMID: 30085002.
31. Lamas GA, Mitchell GF, Flaker GC, et al. Clinical significance of mitral regurgitation after acute myocardial infarction. *Circulation*. 1997;96:827–833.
32. Grigioni F, Enriquez-Sarano M, Zehr KJ, et al. Ischemic mitral regurgitation: long-term outcome and prognostic implications with quantitative Doppler assessment. *Circulation*. 2001;103:1759–1764.
33. Acker MA, Parides MK, Perrault LP, et al. Mitral-valve repair versus replacement for severe ischemic mitral regurgitation. *N Engl J Med*. 2014;370(1):23–32. doi:10.1056/NEJMoa1312808. Epub 2013 Nov 18. PMID: 24245543; PMCID: PMC4128011.
34. Maron MS, Olivotto I, Betocchi S, et al. Effect of left ventricular outflow tract obstruction on clinical outcome in hypertrophic cardiomyopathy. *N Engl J Med*. 2003;348:295–303.
35. Ommen SR, Maron BJ, Olivotto I, et al. Long-term effects of surgical septal myectomy on survival in patients with obstructive hypertrophic cardiomyopathy. *J Am Coll Cardiol*. 2005;46:470–476.
36. Schoendube FA, Klues HG, Reith S, et al. Long-term clinical and echocardiographic follow-up after surgical correction of hypertrophic obstructive cardiomyopathy with extended myectomy and reconstruction of the subvalvular mitral apparatus. *Circulation*. 1995;92(suppl 9):II122–II127.
37. Yu EH, Omran AS, Wigle ED, et al. Mitral regurgitation in hypertrophic obstructive cardiomyopathy: relationship to obstruction and relief with myectomy. *J Am Coll Cardiol*. 2000;36:2219–2225.
38. Bogachev-Prokophiev A, Afanasyev AV, Zheleznev S, et al. Septal myectomy with vs without subvalvular apparatus intervention in patients with hypertrophic obstructive cardiomyopathy: a prospective randomized study. *Semin Thorac Cardiovasc Surg*. 2019;31(3):424–431. doi:10.1053/j.semtcvs.2019.01.011. Epub 2019 Jan 11. PMID: 30641129.
39. Afanasyev A, Bogachev-Prokophiev A, Lenko E, et al. Myectomy with mitral valve repair versus replacement in adult patients with hypertrophic obstructive cardiomyopathy: a systematic review and meta-analysis. *Interact Cardiovasc Thorac Surg*. 2019;28(3):465–472. doi:10.1093/icvts/ivy269. PMID: 30184144.
40. Cui B, Wang S, Xu J, et al. The surgical management of hypertrophic obstructive cardiomyopathy with the concomitant mitral valve abnormalities. *Interact Cardiovasc Thorac Surg*. 2015;21(6):722–726. doi:10.1093/icvts/ivv257. Epub 2015 Sep 15. PMID: 26374266.
41. Bogachev-Prokophiev A, Afanasyev A, Zheleznev S, et al. Mitral valve repair or replacement in hypertrophic obstructive cardiomyopathy: a prospective randomized study. *Interact Cardiovasc Thorac Surg*. 2017;25(3):356–362. doi:10.1093/icvts/ivx152. PMID: 28575282.
42. Hong JH, Schaff HV, Nishimura RA, et al. Mitral regurgitation in patients with hypertrophic obstructive cardiomyopathy: implications for concomitant valve procedures. *J Am Coll Cardiol*. 2016;68(14):1497–1504. doi:10.1016/j.jacc.2016.07.735. PMID: 27687190.
43. Tirone D. Replacement of chordae tendineae with expanded polytetrafluoroethylene sutures. *J Card Surg*. 1989;4(4):286–290.
44. Frater RW. 10th Goretex chorda anniversary. *J Heart Valve Dis*. 1996;5(4):348–351.
45. David TE. Artificial chordae. *Semin Thorac Cardiovasc Surg*. 2004;16(2):161–168.
46. Perier P, Hohenberger W, Lakew F, et al. Prolapse of the posterior leaflet: resect or respect. *Ann Cardiothorac Surg*. 2015;4(3):273–277.
47. Chemtob RA, Wierup P, Mick S, et al. Choosing the "Best" surgical techniques for mitral valve repair: lessons from the literature. *J Card Surg*. 2019;34:717–727.
48. von Oppell UO, Mohr FW. Chordal replacement for both minimally invasive and conventional mitral valve surgery using premeasured Gore-Tex loops. *Ann Thorac Surg*. 2000;70(6):2166–2168.
49. Gillinov AM, Shortt KG, Cosgrove DM. Commissural closure for repair of mitral commissural prolapse. *Ann Thorac Surg*. 2005;80(3):1135–1136.
50. Cohn LH, Couper GS, Aranki SF, et al. Long- term results of mitral valve reconstruction for regurgitation of the myxomatous mitral valve. *J Thorac Cardiovasc Surg*. 1994;107(1):143–150.
51. Alfieri O, Maisano F. An effective technique to correct anterior mitral leaflet prolapse. *Echocardiography*. 1985;2(6):468–470.
52. Nielsen SL, Timek TA, Lai DT, et al. Edge-to-edge mitral repair: tension on the approximating suture and leaflet deformation during acute ischemic mitral regurgitation in the ovine heart. *Circulation*. 2001, Sept 18;104(suppl 1): I-29–I-35. 87. PMID: 11568026.
53. De Bonis M, Alfieri O. The edge-to-edge technique for mitral valve repair. *HSR Proc Intensive Care Cardiovasc Anesth*. 2010;2(1):7–17.
54. Maisano F, Schreuder JJ, Oppizzi M, et al. The double-orifice technique as a standardized approach to treat mitral regurgitation due to severe myxomatous disease: surgical technique. *Eur J Cardiothorac Surg*. 2000;17(3):201–205.

55. Chang BC, Youn YN, Ha JW, et al. Long-term clinical results of mitral valvuloplasty using flexible and rigid rings: a prospective and randomized study. *J Thorac Cardiovasc Surg.* 2007;133(4):995–1003.
56. Kunzelman KS, Reimink MS. Flexible versus rigid ring annuloplasty for mitral valve annular dilatation: a finite element model. *J Heart Valve Dis.* 1998;7(1):108–116.
57. Chee T, Haston R, Togo A, et al. Is a flexible mitral annuloplasty ring superior to a semi-rigid or rigid ring in terms of improvement in symptoms and survival? *Interact Cardiovasc Thorac Surg.* 2008;7(3):477–484.
58. Sharony R, Saunders PC, Nayar A, et al. Semirigid partial annuloplasty band allows dynamic mitral annular motion and minimizes valvular gradients: an echocardiographic study. *Ann Thorac Surg.* 2004;77(2):518–522.

20

Surgical Replacement of the Mitral Valve

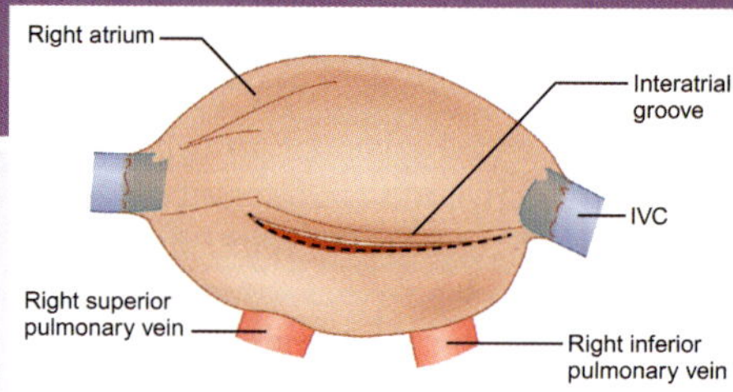

Benjamin Smood, Mark R. Helmers, Jason J. Han, Pavan Atluri

CHAPTER OUTLINE

LEARNING OBJECTIVES

1. Summarize the indications of mitral valve replacement.
2. Individualize prosthetic valve selection for mitral valve replacement.
3. Describe the most common complications associated with mitral valve replacement.
4. Explain and differentiate three techniques for chordal preservation during mitral valve replacement.

INTRODUCTION

When the decision is made to operate on a patient's mitral valve, mitral valve repair (MVr) is typically preferred over replacement whenever possible.[1] However, surgeons must be prepared to either repair or replace any mitral valve encountered, as intraoperative findings may alter the anticipated surgical plan. Additionally, there are many scenarios in which the primary treatment modality will involve direct mitral valve replacement (MVR). As such, this chapter serves as an introduction to the foundations of surgical MVR that all cardiac surgeons should be familiar with. However, this chapter should not be considered a comprehensive review of the technical details and perioperative care that surgeons must master to adequately and effectively care for patients who require MVR. Rather, essential concepts have been selected to underscore common surgical indications, key aspects of prosthetic valve selection, surgical techniques that are ubiquitously used, and important considerations in postoperative care and management after MVR in adult cardiac surgery to complete direct training.

INDICATIONS FOR SURGICAL MITRAL VALVE REPLACEMENT

Extensive diagnostic and management algorithms have been developed for mitral valve disease, which are helpful when considering if a patient should be treated with further medical optimization, percutaneous interventions, and/or cardiac surgery.[1–4] Once it has been decided that a surgical intervention is warranted, several factors must be weighed to determine if a patient would be better served by surgical MVr or MVR.

Alongside evolving operative techniques, perioperative and long-term outcomes after MVr have greatly improved over the years,[5] and in most circumstances, MVR should be reserved for individuals in whom adequate MVr appears unlikely to be successful. Thus, when attempting to identify which patients would be better suited by MVR, surgeons must have a masterful understanding of the prognosticators for successful MVr.[3,6–10]

In any case, the concept of the pathophysiologic triad is often used to relate underlying etiologies, valvular lesions, and the resulting dysfunction that develops in mitral valve disease.[11] These relationships help define unique indications for surgical intervention on the mitral valve. With this context, select preoperative and intraoperative findings will be reviewed in order to highlight instances in which MVR may be preferred over MVr in settings of mitral stenosis (MS) and/or mitral regurgitation (MR).

Mitral Stenosis: Indications for Mitral Valve Repair or Replacement

MS may arise from any number of underlying diseases,[12,13] but is most often caused by rheumatic fever.[14,15] Although the prevalence of rheumatic disease has been drastically reduced in developed nations; it continues to impose a substantial burden worldwide.[16,17] MS may also develop as degenerative calcific disease, usually in elderly populations, and specifically those with cardiovascular comorbidities or renal disease.[1,2,18]

The pathophysiology of varying etiologies of MS often results in distinct valvular lesions with unique patient presentations.[19,20] For example, rheumatic MS is often characterized as an indolent disease that progresses to severe fibrosis and calcification of the valve apparatus, with fusion of the chordal structures and commissures and gradual onset of symptoms. In contrast, degenerative MS is often characterized by leaflet and mitral annular calcification rather than chordal and commissural fusion.[21] Developing symptoms may be delayed, but when symptoms manifest, deterioration may occur relatively acutely. In this respect, surgeons should be familiar with the American Heart Association/American College of Cardiology (AHA/ACC) guidelines for staging the severity of MS disease and symptoms, as these are often sufficient for determining when surgical intervention is indicated.[1,2]

To briefly summarize some common recommendations, mitral valve surgery (i.e., MVr/commissurotomy or MVR) is recommended for patients with severe symptoms and severe MS who have either failed percutaneous intervention and/or those who are not candidates for percutaneous intervention. Among other indications, mitral valve surgery is also indicated in asymptomatic patients with severe MS or severely symptomatic patients who are undergoing cardiac surgery for other reasons.

It is important to recognize that the guidelines rarely mention MVR specifically. Rather, they are broadly phrased in terms of "mitral valve surgery," or more specifically MVr, and it is worth reiterating that whenever possible, MVr is usually preferred to MVR.[1–4] However, some preoperative and intraoperative findings may indicate that MVR is favored over MVr, including the presence of severe leaflet and/or annular calcification, significant subvalvular apparatus involvement (i.e., chordae tendinae and papillary muscles), and/or coexistent MS with MR, which is often unamenable to MVr.[22]

It is also worth noting that although there are some cases in which asymptomatic and/or less-symptomatic patients may meet criteria for MVr when a surgeon concludes that MVR will likely be necessary for MS, it may be preferential to delay surgical intervention until symptoms become more severe if cardiac function is preserved, due to the inherent risks associated with prosthetic valve implantation in MVR (see "Valve Selection" below).[22]

Mitral Regurgitation: Indications for Mitral Valve Repair or Replacement

Because of the myriad disease states that may lead to MR, deciding when and how to intervene in MR is often more complicated than in stenotic lesions. Nevertheless, MR is most often caused by degenerative valvopathy, with mitral valve prolapse accounting for ~50% of cases in the United States.[23,24] However, MR can also be caused by rheumatic, ischemic, or infectious etiologies, among others.[25] Proper preoperative evaluation of disease etiology, severity of valvular lesions and/or resulting ventricular dysfunction, and patient symptoms is essential to determining when surgical intervention is indicated.[1–4] In developing recommendations for surgical intervention, the AHA/ACC guidelines have broadly categorized MR into two classes, either primary or secondary MR.[1,2]

Primary Mitral Regurgitation

Primary MR (often referred to degenerative or organic MR) can be defined as mitral incompetence resulting from an intrinsic abnormality of some part of the valve apparatus (i.e., the annulus, leaflets, chordae, papillary muscles, and/or the underlying myocardium).[26] Depending on the presence or absence of symptoms, either MVr or MVR may be indicated (or reasonably considered) in patients with severe primary MR.[1]

Of note, MVr is usually attempted in all cases of degenerative MR, specifically in cases of mitral valve prolapse, where the rate of successful repair may approach 90%.[27–29] Nevertheless, meticulous preoperative and intraoperative evaluation can help elucidate circumstances when MVR might be the preferred surgical strategy, for example, in patients with chronic arrhythmias, severe pulmonary hypertension, and/or significant atrial and ventricular dilation.[30–34]

Secondary Mitral Regurgitation

In contrast to primary MR, secondary MR (often referred to as functional MR) typically spares the components of the valve apparatus itself and instead arises from diseases associated with ventricular dysfunction.[1–4,35] Functional MR most often develops as sequelae of ischemic cardiomyopathies but can develop from nonischemic cardiomyopathies as well. Regardless, it is important to understand that restoring mitral valve competence in secondary MR does not cure the underlying pathology. Therefore outcomes after MVr/MVR in secondary MR are typically worse than in cases of primary MR.[36–39]

As a result, consensus is lacking regarding the preferred strategy for mitral valve surgery in secondary MR.[1] For example, recent trials have suggested that MVr has a higher incidence of significant MR recurrence compared to MVR despite similar survival outcomes, particularly in cases of ischemic MR.[1,37,39,40] Therefore current guidelines state that it is reasonable to consider MVR over MVr in patients with severe ischemic MR who are severely symptomatic.[1] However, some still argue that MVr is preferred over MVR in select patients with appropriate anatomy for the beneficial effects of ventricular remodeling and to avoid potential complications associated with prosthesis degeneration or anticoagulation (see "Valve Selection" below).[22]

Consideration of Ventricular Function in Timing Mitral Valve Surgery

Particular attention must be paid to the function of the left ventricle when considering surgical interventions on the mitral valve. For example, although an ejection fraction less than 40% is often cited as an index of severe left ventricular dysfunction that confers a poorer prognosis in cardiac surgery,[41–43] regurgitant flow through an incompetent mitral valve makes ejection fraction a poor metric for assessing the true degree of ventricular dysfunction in the presence of MR.[28,43,44] In fact, patients with severe MR are likely to have developed some degree of ventricular dysfunction even when ejection fraction appears preserved near 60%.[28,43,44] Therefore some have advocated that left ventricular end-systolic dimensions greater than 40 mm may be more reliable for identifying early ventricular dysfunction in patients with MR.[1,28,43,45–49] In any case, because chronic volume overload in the setting of MR perpetuates a cycle of cardiac dysfunction and irreversible damage, and because ventricular dysfunction is a consequential prognosticator of early- and long-term surgical outcomes, it is imperative to understand the derivation and nuances of the AHA/ACC guidelines regarding indications for mitral valve surgery concerning ventricular function.[1,2,22,50–53]

Other Indications: Mixed Lesions, Concomitant Procedures, and Endocarditis

Although MS and MR are often dichotomized, mitral valve disease etiologies, valvular lesions, and their resulting dysfunction often overlap. Surgeons will certainly encounter patients with mitral valve disease encompassing aspects of both primary and secondary MR and/or MS.[1,22,43] In fact, only about 25% of patients with MS have isolated disease, whereas an additional 40% have some degree of MR.[25,43] In such cases, one might seriously consider MVR, as successful MVr may be likely to be successful in such complicated lesions with additional concerns for durability of repair depending on disease severity.[22]

Meanwhile, guidelines exist for evaluating when mitral valve surgery may be considered when other procedures are the primary indication for cardiac surgery and vice versa.[1] For example, in some cases, MVr/MVR may be reasonably considered at the time of coronary artery bypass grafting. On the other hand, when mitral valve surgery is the primary indication for cardiac surgery, prophylactic repair or replacement of other valves may not necessarily be indicated, such as when there is concomitant aortic stenosis that is unlikely to progress.[1,22] In any case, when multiple procedures are planned, important consideration should be given to preoperative planning that will optimize the order of component procedures, thereby minimizing operative times and reducing the risk of associated complications (see "Concomitant Procedures" below).

Lastly, it should be no surprise that MVr is again preferred over MVR in cases of endocarditis to minimize the amount of foreign material implanted and the subsequent risk for prosthesis infection (see "Prosthetic Valve Endocarditis and Prophylaxis" below). Still, there are circumstances in which MVR may be warranted, particularly when extensive debridement is required without any chance for valve preservation. When MVR is required in endocarditis, normal criteria should be used to decide whether to implant a mechanical or biologic prosthesis.[54]

VALVE SELECTION

As with any valve replacement surgery, bioprosthetic heart valves (BHVs) or mechanical prostheses are most frequently used for MVR. Because no prosthesis is ideal for all patients, valve selection must often be considered along a spectrum of compromises with respect to the patient's age, the durability of the prosthesis, and requirements for anticoagulation.[1,55–60] However, prosthetic valve selection must be individualized to each patient by strategically considering a multitude of other factors, including preexisting comorbidities, risks associated with potential future reinterventions, and a patient's projected survival after MVR.

Importantly, patients must be well-informed of the associated risks and benefits of each type of prosthetic valve, as the ultimate decision of whether to implant a BHV or mechanical valve should be theirs.[1,56–58,61–63] Thus, cardiac surgeons must not only be familiar with guidelines regarding which type of prosthesis is generally recommended,[1,2] but they must also be able to clearly and simply articulate the evidence supporting the development of these recommendations so that they can adequately inform patients of their choice in a process of shared decision-making.[1,56,60–65]

Age-Related Guidelines for Prosthesis Selection: Considering Valve Durability and Anticoagulation Requirements

After a prosthetic valve is implanted, some degree of tissue overgrowth around the prosthesis is expected as the heart heals itself from the insult of open-heart surgery. In fact, this is important in developing a nonthrombogenic surface at the suture line.[66–68] However, pathologic overgrowth can occur, particularly in BHVs, often referred to as structural valve degeneration (SVD). Although the precise mechanisms of SVD are unclear, it appears to be an age-related phenomenon that likely results from differences in immunity and calcium metabolism.[66,69–71]

Some studies suggest that the risk for SVD at 15-years after BHV implantation exceeds 20% among patients less than 50 years of age,[1,60–62,65,72,73] whereas others estimate the incidence to be ~65% in patients less than 40 years of age, compared to just 10% in those 70 years or older.[43,74–76] Regardless, SVD remains the most common cause of BHV failure, and generally speaking, it can be expected that BHVs implanted into patients younger than 60 years of age will eventually need to be replaced.[43,43,76–80] Therefore when determining whether or not to implant a BHV, one must consider the patient's individual risk for reoperation and the potential morbidity and mortality associated with surgical reintervention.

In contrast, mechanical valves offer excellent durability and have the potential to last the entirety of a patient's lifetime, regardless of age. Thus, mechanical valves are particularly well-suited for younger patients whose primary concern is the avoidance of reoperation.[22,43] However, because mechanical valves are especially thrombogenic, all patients who receive a mechanical prosthesis require lifelong anticoagulation (see "Anticoagulation Guidelines" below), which carries additional risks for significant bleeding complications, specifically among the elderly.[1,56,58,61] Of course, this means that mechanical valves should be avoided in all patients with any contraindication to anticoagulation and/or those who are unable to adequately monitor their therapeutic levels. Each of these considerations can significantly impact long-term outcomes after MVR, underscoring that prosthetic valve selection must be individualized for each.[1]

Nevertheless, for patients 50 to 69 years of age, it has been repeatedly demonstrated that long-term survival is similar after MVR when implanting either a BHV or mechanical valve.[1,56,58,61] On the other hand, increasing evidence suggests that a long-term survival advantage persists up to 70 years of age after MVR with a mechanical prosthesis compared to a BHV.[1,61,62,64] Therefore, the recently updated AHA/ACC guidelines have lowered the recommended age for mechanical MVR from 60 to 50 years, noting that it is reasonable to implant either a BHV or mechanical prosthesis in patients 50 to 70 years of age.[1] These guidelines have continued to recommend that BHVs should be implanted in patients over 70 years of age.

It is important to note that evolving technology in MVR is promising but remains uncertain. Specifically, the potential for transcatheter valve-in-valve replacement therapy after surgical MVR may ultimately impact future guidelines such that the minimum age recommended for BHV implantation could be reduced to patients younger than 70 years of age. These existing uncertainties regarding the future of mitral valve surgery underscore the importance of strategic decision-making when determining which type of prosthesis to implant during MVR and highlight that additional factors beyond just the patient's age should be considered when deciding whether to implant a BHV or mechanical prosthesis.[1,69]

Additional Considerations for Prosthetic Valve Selection

Any patient factor that might favorably reduce the risk for complications associated with either a BHV or mechanical valve should be carefully considered when determining which type of prosthesis to implant. For example, although BHVs are usually avoided in patients <50 years of age, there are circumstances in which BHVs may be preferred in younger individuals.[61,81–83] For example, a relatively young, middle-aged patient (~50 years of age) with significant comorbidities might be unlikely to outlive a BHV, in which case the associated risks of SVD, valve failure, and subsequent reoperation may be relatively diminished.[84] In this respect, some evidence suggests that BHVs may be preferred in patients with end-stage renal disease, regardless of age, in part because of their attenuated life span and also because of their potentially increased risk for bleeding complications with systemic anticoagulation.[85,86] On the other hand, a similarly aged patient with chronic atrial fibrillation who is compliant with taking an oral anticoagulant prior to MVR might reasonably choose a mechanical prosthesis, as the improved durability could prove beneficial, whereas many of the risks associated with lifelong anticoagulation would not be newly introduced.[87]

Prosthesis Design and Performance

Decisions regarding prosthetic valve selection do not stop after deciding whether to implant a BHV or mechanical valve, and surgeons must be familiar with the nuanced differences of valve design that exist for both types of prostheses, which can significantly affect hemodynamic performance after MVR.[69]

Although several mechanical prostheses have been developed over the years, contemporary mechanical prostheses are bileaflet valves, of which two extant models are routinely used in MVR.[61,69] The St. Jude mechanical valve (St. Jude Medical, Saint Paul, MN) is the most common mechanical prosthesis implanted in the mitral position, owing to its relative ease of implantation and reliable long-term performance. More recently, the On-X Valve (CryoLife, Kennesaw, GA) has gained early enthusiasm due to its potential advantage for lower anticoagulation requirements.[88] However, this promise remains to be validated with clinical trials, specifically in the mitral position.

Meanwhile, there are multiple models to choose from when selecting a BHV for MVR.[22,61,69] Most often, these xenografts are assembled from porcine aortic valve leaflets or fabricated from sheets of bovine pericardium, which are mounted on a metallic or polymer stent.[69] BHVs are usually treated with glutaraldehyde and/or other proprietary solutions throughout sterilization, processing, and storage to reduce immunogenicity and improve durability with respect to SVD.[61,69] Although a detailed analysis of each valve model is beyond the scope of this chapter, suffice it to say that not all biologic valves are created equally, and debate remains regarding which models offer optimal durability and hemodynamics in MVR.

It is worth noting that other biologic valves have been used in the mitral position, including stentless xenografts, cryopreserved homografts (particularly in cases of endocarditis), as well as autologous pulmonary valves.[22,43,89–95] However, to date, there is no convincing evidence that these biologics are superior to traditional BHVs, as study populations and follow-up remain quite limited, raising questions as to the utility of the added complexity.[22,43,93,96] It is important to recognize that even as newer-generation prosthetic valves are developed, convincing evidence to demonstrate one model's superiority over established models will lag while awaiting definitive long-term clinical results.[1]

Valve Sizing and Prosthesis-Patient Mismatch

Despite advances in BHV and mechanical valve design, prosthesis-patient mismatch (PPM) has remained a significant challenge in MVR.[69,97,98] In the simplest of terms, PPM occurs when an implanted prosthesis is too small for a patient's body size. Ultimately, PPM results in higher postoperative gradients and is associated with persisting pulmonary hypertension, congestive heart failure, and overall mortality.[69,98–100] Although the risk for PPM is higher among younger patients, appropriate valve sizing is essential to minimizing its risk among all patients. However, adequate valve sizing can be challenging in part because the configuration of prosthetic valve leaflets, struts, and other components can vary drastically.[43,69] Each prosthesis model may have a varying ability to accommodate the hemodynamic demands of an individual's cardiac output. As such, when choosing which BHV model or mechanical prosthesis to implant, it is imperative to evaluate the risk of PPM preoperatively. Continued surveillance is necessary at each interval of postoperative follow-up (see "Routine Follow-Up" below).

A common formula for evaluating PPM is to divide the effective orifice area (EOA) of the prosthetic valve by the patient's body surface area, which is termed the index EOA.[69,99] Mild PPM (index EOA >1.2 cm^2/m^2) is considered clinically insignificant, whereas moderate (index EOA >0.9–1.2) and severe PPM (index EOA ≤0.9) have been associated with worse outcomes, as mentioned above. Perhaps surprisingly, PPM is not uncommon, and depending on the size and/or model of the prosthesis implanted, the incidence of moderate and severe PPM after valve implantation may be as high as 30% to 70% and 2–10%, respectively.[69,98–100]

In part, this is a result of the fact that there are fewer low-profile prosthetic valves available for MVR compared to the number of prostheses that can be used in other valvular operations, namely aortic valve replacement. Similarly, MVR is not amenable to annular enlargement due to the risk of atrioventricular groove disruption.[69,101] As such, particular attention must be placed on preoperative evaluation and intraoperative assessment to reduce the risk of PPM during MVR. Therefore the surgeon should calculate index EOA during the preoperative evaluation so that they can enter the operation with a plan for which prosthesis models and sizes would be appropriate.

It is important to recognize that although manufacturer-provided sizing charts are useful, they may use different definitions for grading PPM and may not adequately reflect the true risk of PPM for any given size of a specific prosthesis. Moreover, although surgeons should attempt to maximize the index EOA by implanting the largest valve possible, this must be done safely with respect to the patient's size and cardiac anatomy. Oversized prostheses (i.e., usually >31 mm) may interfere with valvular-ventricular coordination during systole, leading to a progressive decline in ventricular function and worse long-term outcomes. In this respect, there are some circumstances in which a mechanical valve may be preferred to a BHV in MVR due to their lower profile and reduced risk for PPM, particularly in younger and smaller patients.

OPERATIVE STEPS AND SURGICAL APPROACH TO MITRAL VALVE REPLACEMENT

Multiple approaches have been described in detail for nearly every aspect of MVR, including patient positioning, cannulation strategies for cardiopulmonary bypass, exposure of the mitral valve, and technical components for prosthesis implantation, among others.[22,61,102–105] However, because adequate visualization of the mitral valve is paramount to a successful operation, it is strongly encouraged that surgeons first master an open approach to MVR via median sternotomy using bicaval cannulation and both antegrade and retrograde cardioplegia before attempting alternative and/or less-invasive surgical techniques.[11,105] With this understanding, important operative steps that are required and/or commonly used in MVR will be briefly reviewed, emphasizing the technical aspects of prosthetic valve implantation.

Dissection, Cannulation, and Myocardial Protection

After median sternotomy and adequate dissection of the mediastinum is completed, the pericardium is opened and tacked to the right chest wall to elevate the posterior heart for improved exposure during MVR.[22,27,43,105] The heart should be inspected for anatomic abnormalities, specifically pulmonary vein anomalies and/or a persistent left superior vena cava (SVC), which can have important consequences when using retrograde cardioplegia.[106–109] Cardiopulmonary bypass is established via central aortic and bicaval venous cannulation. Avoiding electrocautery that can injure the phrenic nerve, the posterior inferior vena cava (IVC) is freed by incising the pericardial reflection to the level just below the inferior right pulmonary vein, taking care to avoid hepatic veins.[11,22,43] Of note, critically ill patients may not tolerate a compromise in cardiac function while retracting the right atrium to expose the IVC, in which case partial cardiopulmonary bypass using the SVC may be required before completing dissection of the IVC. Nevertheless, purse-string sutures are placed on the anterior SVC (making sure to avoid the sinoatrial node) and low in the atrium at the entrance of the IVC. A small plastic or metal-tipped right angle cannula is secured in the SVC, with a larger straight or angled cannula in the IVC.[22,27,43,105,110]

Antegrade and potentially retrograde cardioplegia lines are placed in the aorta (with suction for later deairing) and coronary sinus, respectively. With the widespread adoption of delNido or Custodiol cardioplegia, the retrograde coronary sinus catheter can be eliminated in these cases. Once the bypass is established, tepid hypothermia (28°C to 34°C) can be considered for myocardial protection. With the aortic cross-clamp applied, antegrade cardioplegia delivery for cardiac arrest can be initiated. The field should be flooded with CO_2 in preparation for cardiac incision and mitral valve exposure.[22,27,43,105,110] Similar minimally invasive approaches can also be incorporated to avoid sternotomy.

Mitral Valve Exposure and Intraoperative Analysis

A variety of incisions have been described to expose the mitral valve, which may be particularly useful when adequate visualization is challenging.[22,43,105,111–114] Thus, cardiac surgeons should be comfortable using multiple techniques for mitral valve exposure, recognizing that different approaches may risk injury to unique cardiac structures. Nevertheless, perhaps the most common incision for exposing the mitral valve is via a vertical left atriotomy at or near the fatty interatrial junction by developing the interatrial (Sondergaard) groove (Fig. 20.1). This approach provides excellent exposure and minimizes direct cardiac damage, which some evidence suggests may reduce the risk of postoperative arrythmias.[11,105,115]

With the table rotated to the left, the superior aspect of the left atrium is dissected away from the right pulmonary artery before developing the Sondergaard groove and uncovering the roof of the left atrium. A vertical left atriotomy is made 2 to 4 cm from to the interatrial septum, with an incision that begins 4 to 6 cm anterior to the right superior pulmonary vein (depending on the size of the atrium) and posterior to the interatrial septum. As the incision is extended along the left atrial roof to ~1 cm behind the level of the SVC, care is taken to avoid injuring the right pulmonary artery. The incision is continued inferiorly into the oblique fissure until the midpoint between the right inferior pulmonary vein and the IVC (see Fig. 20.1).[11,22,43]

Upper/anterior and lateral blades are placed to expose the mitral valve using a variety of handheld or self-retaining retractors (Fig. 20.2). Additional retractors can be placed as needed. If

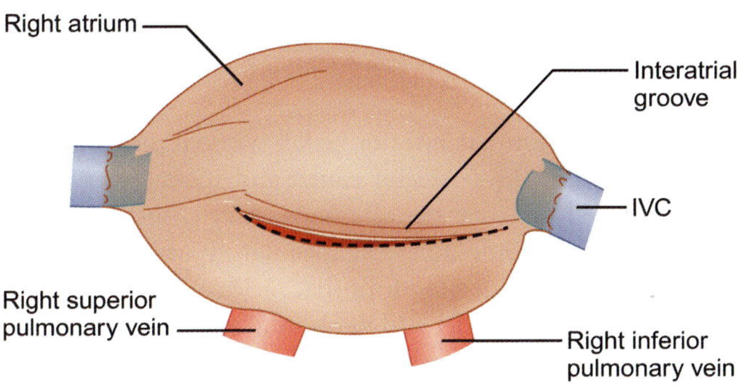

Fig. 20.1 Vertical Left Atriotomy for Exposure of the Mitral Valve. The superior aspect of the left atrium is dissected away from the right pulmonary artery before developing the Sondergaard groove and uncovering the roof of the left atrium. A vertical left atriotomy is made 2 to 4 cm posterior to the interatrial septum, beginning 4 to 6 cm anterior to the right superior pulmonary vein (depending on the size of the atrium). The incision is extended along the left atrial roof to ~1 cm behind the level of the superior vena cava. The incision continues inferiorly into the oblique fissure until the midpoint between the right inferior pulmonary vein and the inferior vena cava *(IVC)*. (Adapted from Kouchoukos NT, Blackstone EH, Hanley FL, et al. Mitral valve disease with or without tricuspid valve disease. In: Kirklin J, Blackstone E. *Kirklin/Barratt-Boyes Cardiac Surgery*. 4th ed. Philadelphia: Elsevier/Saunders; 2013:473–540; Kaneko T, Yammine M, Loberman D, et al. Mitral valve replacement. In: Cohn LH, Adams DH, eds. *Cardiac Surgery in the Adult*. 5th ed. New York:. McGraw-Hill Education; 2017.)

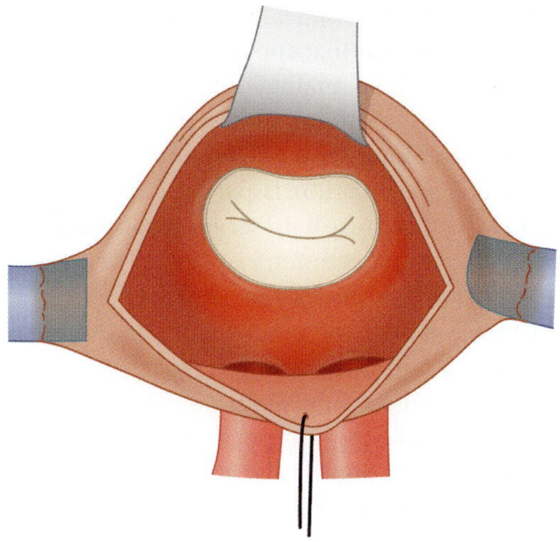

Fig. 20.2 Exposure of the Mitral Valve. Upper/anterior and lateral blades are placed to expose the mitral valve. Additional retractors can be placed as needed. Of note, these retractors may distort the aorta and prohibit adequate delivery of antegrade cardioplegia, underscoring the importance of intermittent retrograde cardioplegia or longer-acting cardioplegic solutions. A weighted drop sucker should be placed through the left atriotomy near the level of the superior pulmonary vein to keep the field clear and dry. (Adapted from Kouchoukos NT, Blackstone EH, Hanley FL, et al. Mitral valve disease with or without tricuspid valve disease. In: Kirklin J, Blackstone E. *Kirklin/Barratt-Boyes Cardiac Surgery*. 4th ed. Philadelphia: Elsevier/Saunders; 2013:473–540; Kaneko T, Yammine M, Loberman D, et al. Mitral valve replacement. In: Cohn LH, Adams DH, eds. *Cardiac Surgery in the Adult*. 5th ed. New York: McGraw-Hill Education; 2017.)

necessary, the chest wall may be further retracted for improved exposure, but this should be done slowly and carefully to ensure that the IVC is not avulsed and avoid rib fractures that increase the risk for postoperative bleeding and/or paresthesia. Recognize that these retractors may distort the aorta and prohibit adequate delivery of antegrade cardioplegia, underscoring the importance of intermittent retrograde cardioplegia or longer-acting cardioplegic solutions. A weighted drop sucker should be placed through the left atriotomy near the level of the superior pulmonary vein to keep the field clear and dry.[22,43,105,110]

Inspect the cardiac chambers and atrial appendage for any thrombus, and conduct a thorough valve analysis, which should be completed with every mitral valve operation.[11] Note areas of endocardial thickening or heavy calcification, evaluate for evidence of degenerative disease, including annular asymmetry or dilation, and assess the extent of disease involving the chordae and papillary muscles. Although in situ valve analysis often confirms the surgeon's preoperative assessment and prior imaging findings, unrecognized but important aspects of disease etiology and severity may be discovered, which can alter the course of the operation, and specifically which techniques can be used for MVR.[11,22,43]

Surgical Techniques for Mitral Valve Replacement

In 1964, Lillehei and colleagues first demonstrated that at least partial preservation of the valvular apparatus, specifically the posterior leaflet and its chordal attachments, improves outcomes after MVR compared to total leaflet excision.[116,117] Since then, it has been well-established that complete preservation of papillo-annular continuity (i.e., maintaining the subvalvular apparatus of both the anterior and posterior leaflets) during MVR improves early- and long-term outcomes.[15,43,118–120]

Total chordal preservation is particularly beneficial in lesions of MR, in part because it preserves myocardial function by maintaining the natural geometry of the left ventricle.[15,43,118–120] However, some have suggested that chordal preservation is less important in MS where the contractility of the mitral tensor apparatus may be diminished.[121–123] Regardless, preserving the posterior leaflet and its subvalvular apparatus all but eliminates the risk of catastrophic postoperative atrioventricular groove disruption and ventricular rupture.[43,117,121,124–126] Therefore every effort should be made to maintain at least the posterior leaflet and its chordal attachments during MVR whenever possible.

However, it must be noted that merely preserving diseased leaflets, chordae, and papillary muscles may not be sufficient to improve outcomes after MVR. Rather, consideration must be given to the integrity and functionality of the subvalvular apparatus during MVR. That is, the surgeon must ensure that the preserved papillo-annular continuity has sufficient length to accommodate changes in both ventricular distension and tension during diastole and systole, respectively. Chordae that are too short may compromise ventricular and valvular function and even lead to papillary muscle rupture.[121,127,128] Meanwhile, attachments left too long may become entangled in the prosthetic valve, resulting in obstruction and disruption in valvular or ventricular function.[22,117,121,127,129]

Thus, a variety of surgical techniques for partial and total leaflet and/or chordal preservation have evolved over the years, which can accommodate an adequately sized prosthetic valve.[117,121,127,130] Here, three commonly used methods for chordal preservation will be described, including partial (posterior) leaflet preservation, and two techniques for total chordal preservation, which may be used in MR and/or MS.[22,43,117,121,127]

Partial (Posterior) Chordal Preservation

In the classic partial leaflet/chordal preservation technique, the posterior leaflet and its ventricular attachments are entirely preserved, and the anterior leaflet is completely excised. To begin, a scalpel is used to make the initial incision 2 to 3 mm from the annulus at the midpoint of the anterior leaflet (i.e., segment A2).[22,117,121,127] While extending the incision towards both commissures, a similar distance is maintained from the central fibrous body of the annulus (Fig. 20.3). However, at the commissures, the anterior leaflet should be excised closer to the annulus (making sure not to incise the annulus itself) to separate the anterior and posterior leaflets while preserving the latter's valvular apparatus.[22,121,130,131] The anterior leaflet should be retracted from the base to expose the underlying chordae to complete the intraoperative valve analysis and determine if complete excision of the anterior leaflet and/or its chordal structures is necessary. When it is determined appropriate, the anterior leaflet can be removed by transecting the tip of the papillary muscle that contains its chordal attachments.[22,127] Only a minimal rim of residual anterior leaflet tissue remains attached to the annulus. If the posterior leaflet and subvalvular apparatus are severely fused or stenotic, secondary chordae that connect the posterior leaflet to the ventricular myocardium may be carefully excised, understanding that at least partial preservation of the posterior leaflet and its chordal attachments is always preferred when implanting the prosthetic valve (see "Prosthetic Valve Implantation" below).[22,43,127]

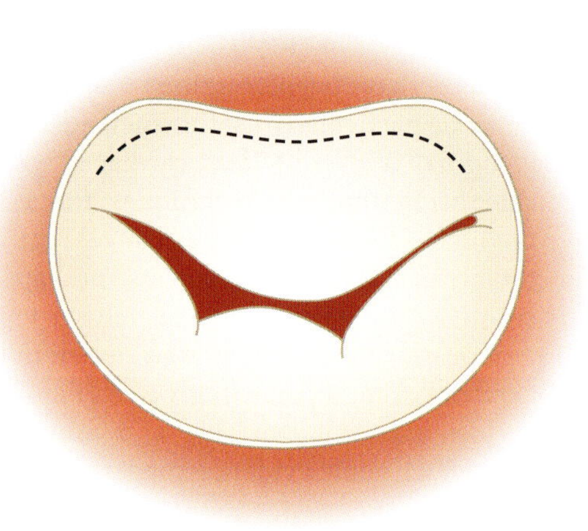

Fig. 20.3 Partial (Posterior) Chordal Preservation. A scalpel is used to make an incision 2 to 3 mm from the annulus at the midpoint of the anterior leaflet, which is extended towards both commissures. At the commissures, the anterior leaflet should be excised closer to the annulus (making sure not to incise the annulus itself) to separate the anterior and posterior leaflets while preserving the latter's valvular apparatus. The anterior leaflet can be removed by transecting the tip of the papillary muscle that contains its chordal attachments. Only a minimal rim of residual anterior leaflet tissue remains attached to the annulus. (Adapted from Kaneko T, Yammine M, Loberman D, et al. Mitral valve replacement. In: Cohn LH, Adams DH, eds. *Cardiac Surgery in the Adult*. 5th ed. New York: McGraw-Hill Education; 2017; Talwar S, Jayanthkumar H, Kumar PS. Chordal preservation during mitral valve replacement: basis, techniques and results. *Indian J Thorac Cardiovasc Surg*. 2005;21:45–52; Miki S, Kusuhara K, Ueda Y, et al. Mitral valve replacement with preservation of chordae tendineae and papillary muscles. *Ann Thorac Surg*. 1988;45[1]:28–34.)

Total Chordal Preservation Techniques

To reiterate, total chordal preservation is preferred whenever possible, and a number of techniques have been described that have repeatedly demonstrated superior surgical outcomes in MVR compared to isolated posterior leaflet/chordal preservation.[117,121,127,130,132] However, leaving both the anterior and posterior leaflets entirely intact may increase the risks of outflow tract and/or prosthesis obstruction. Therefore many routinely used techniques describe some method of dividing and/or resecting a small portion of the anterior and/or posterior leaflets while preserving their subvalvular apparatus. Using proper technique, these methods permit implantation of an appropriately sized valve without additional risks for obstruction.[121,127]

Here, the David and Miki techniques are described for total chordal preservation, both of which are commonly used and can be adapted with relative ease from the partial (posterior) leaflet preservation technique described above.[121,127,132] Although both techniques permit successful MVR across a broad range of mitral valve etiologies and lesions, the Miki and David techniques may prove particularly useful in cases of MS and MR, respectively.

The Miki Technique for Total Chordal Preservation. In rheumatic or degenerative MS, where the leaflets and/or the subvalvular apparatus are thickened, fibrotic, fused, and/or calcified, it can be challenging to implant an adequately sized prosthesis while preserving chordal attachments. Similar challenges may be encountered in specific lesions that present with MR, for example, when chordae or papillary muscles are scarred from infarction.[22,43,133–135] In such cases, the Miki technique for total chordal preservation can be an optimal technique for MVR.[127,132]

The initial incision begins 2 to 3 mm from the annulus at the center of the anterior leaflet and is extended towards the commissures, as described above for the posterior preservation technique (see Fig. 20.3).[132] However, rather than excising the anterior leaflet and its chordal attachments, the anterior leaflet is instead divided centrally into two segments to preserve the papillo-annular continuity (Fig. 20.4). The middle portions of the divided anterior leaflet segments are then excised where they are free from chordal attachments. At this point, the remaining leaflet segments can be mobilized and resecured to their respective commissures using pledgeted sutures.

A vertical incision is then made centrally in the posterior leaflet, and thickened leaflets may be thinned by carefully slicing calcified or diseased tissue off the atrial surface of the valve.[127,132] Similarly, when chordae are excessively fused and/or shortened, most of the subvalvular apparatus can still be preserved by carefully excising small chordal segments with the leaflet attached.[22,127,132]

It must be underscored that aggressive decalcification should be avoided, as this can injure the left circumflex artery and/or increase the risk of atrioventricular groove disruption and ventricular rupture.[22,132,136] Thus, minimal and conservative decalcification should only be attempted when it can be reasonably and safely completed without disrupting the integrity of the annulus or myocardium. Occasionally, severe disease may require artificial chordal reconstruction, which can be completed using techniques that have been described elsewhere.[127,137–139]

With portions of the leaflets incised and/or appropriately resected with preservation of subvalvular apparatus, sutures for the prosthetic valve may be placed (see "Prosthetic Valve Implantation" below).[127,132]

The David Technique for Total Chordal Preservation. The David technique for total chordal preservation during MVR is particularly useful in cases of severe, myxomatous MR where leaflets may be billowing, and chordae can be excessively elongated. Nevertheless, this technique has certainly been used with demonstrated success in other etiologies and lesions of the mitral valve, including MS.[121,127]

To begin, the anterior leaflet is once again incised at the A2 segment, 2 to 3 mm from the annulus. However, the incision is angled and continued in a triangular, trapezoidal, or rectangular fashion along the borders of the A2 segment to permit its resection.[22,43,121,127] The lateral and medial segments (i.e., A1 and A3) are preserved, as are their chordal attachments (Fig. 20.5). The remaining free edges of the anterior leaflet can then be resuspended to the annulus when the mitral prosthesis is sutured into place (see "Prosthetic Valve Implantation" below).[22,43,121,127]

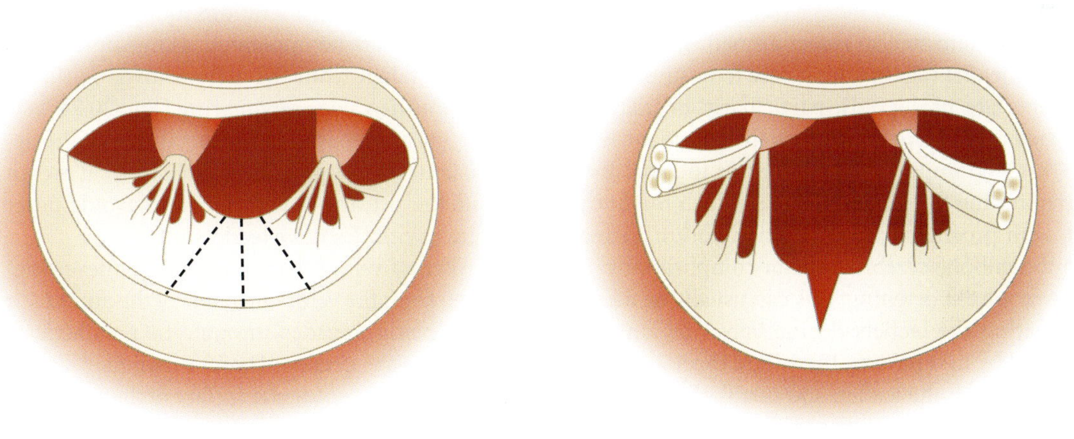

Fig. 20.4 The Miki Technique for Total Chordal Preservation. For the Miki technique for total chordal preservation, the initial incision begins at the center of the anterior leaflet and is extended towards the commissures. Rather than excising the anterior leaflet, it is divided centrally into two segments to preserve the papillo-annular continuity *(left)*. The middle portions of the divided anterior leaflet segments are then excised where they are free from chordal attachments *(right)*. At this point, the remaining leaflet segments can be mobilized and resecured to their respective commissures using pledgeted sutures, and a vertical incision is made centrally in the posterior leaflet. (Adapted from Kaneko T, Yammine M, Loberman D, et al. Mitral valve replacement. In: Cohn LH, Adams DH, eds. *Cardiac Surgery in the Adult*. 5th ed. New York: McGraw-Hill Education; 2017; Miki S, Kusuhara K, Ueda Y, et al. Mitral valve replacement with preservation of chordae tendineae and papillary muscles. *Ann Thorac Surg*. 1988;45[1]:28–34.)

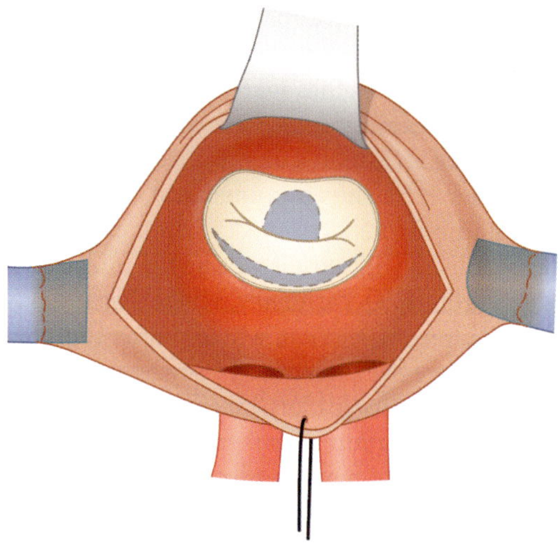

Fig. 20.5 The David Technique for Total Chordal Preservation. The David technique for total chordal preservation during mitral valve repair (MVR) is particularly useful in cases of severe, myxomatous MR where leaflets may be billowing, and chordae can be excessively elongated. The anterior leaflet is centrally incised 2 to 3 mm from the annulus. The incision continues in an angled trajectory to create a triangular, trapezoidal, or rectangular shape for resection of the A2 segment of the leaflet. The lateral and medial segments (i.e., A1 and A3) are preserved, as are their chordal attachments. It is also important to resect a small elliptical portion of the posterior leaflet, particularly in lesions of severe myxomatous MR where there is often redundant tissue. (Adapted from Kaneko T, Yammine M, Loberman D, et al. Mitral valve replacement. In: Cohn LH, Adams DH, eds. *Cardiac Surgery in the Adult*. 5th ed. New York: McGraw-Hill Education; 2017; David TE. Mitral valve replacement with preservation of chordae tendinae: rationale and technical considerations. *Ann Thorac Surg*. 1986;41[6]:680–682.)

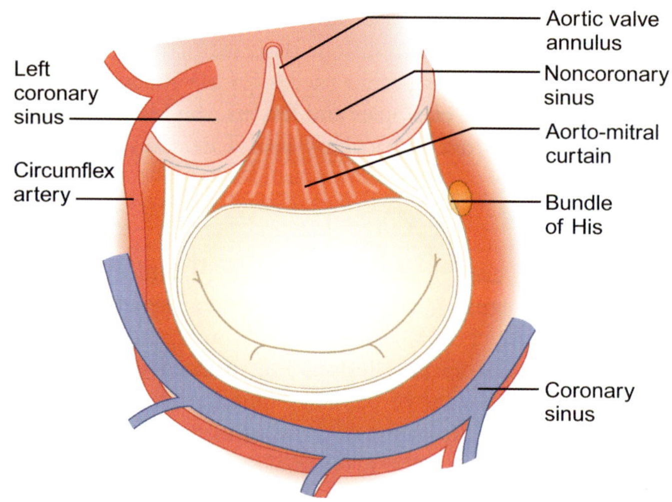

Fig. 20.6 Important Anatomic Relationships During Mitral Valve Surgery. When replacing the mitral valve, one must be careful to avoid distortion of the aortic leaflets, and injury to the conduction system, left circumflex coronary artery, and coronary sinus. Adapted from Carpentier A, Adams DH, Filsoufi F. Carpentier's Reconstructive Valve Surgery. Philadelphia: Saunders; 2010. p31.

However, it is important to also resect a small elliptical portion of the posterior leaflet (again taking care to ensure that the chordal attachments are preserved), particularly in lesions of severe myxomatous MR where there is often redundant tissue (see Fig. 20.5). This step importantly minimizes the amount of excess tissue surrounding the mitral annulus, which might otherwise interfere with prosthetic valve function and/or increase the risk of thromboembolic cerebrovascular complications.[121]

If the chordae require shortening, this can usually be accomplished by imbricating the leaflets during valve implantation. This is accomplished by first passing the suture through the mitral annulus, then through the leaflet, and finally the prosthesis, leaving the pledgets on the atrial side of the annulus.[22,121,127]

Prosthetic Valve Implantation

Prior to valve implantation, the annulus should be sized in situ with respect to the considerations described earlier in this chapter (see "Valve Sizing and Prosthesis-Patient Mismatch" above).[130] When ready to suture the prosthesis into place, the surgeon must anticipate the trajectory and depth of their needle at all times, executing each bite of every stitch with precision. Failure to do so risks injury to critical structures surrounding the mitral annulus (Fig. 20.6). In addition, when securing a mechanical valve, care must be taken to ensure that hinges of the leaflets are oriented in a vertical position (i.e., 12 and 6 o'clock) to minimize risks of tissue interference and obstruction. In any case, a variety of suturing techniques can be used for securing the prosthesis to the annulus during MVR.[22,43] However, interrupted horizontal mattress sutures are usually preferred. Pledgeted sutures are frequently used to buttress the suture line, which may be particularly valuable when implanting mechanical valves with smaller sewing rings.[43] Typically, all sutures are first placed through the annulus in series before attaching them to the sewing ring of the prosthesis.[22,43]

With these considerations, both bioprosthetic and mechanical valves may be implanted using supraannular (i.e., everting) stitches taken from the atrium towards the ventricle and then through the valve's sewing ring (Fig. 20.7). With this technique, pledgets are secured to the atrial side of the annulus, which can be useful when implanting a mechanical prosthesis, as this positions the prosthesis centrally and avoids potential tissue interference with the valve leaflets.[22,43]

Alternatively, subannular (i.e., noneverting) sutures can be placed from the ventricular side of the annulus towards the atrium before being threaded through the prosthetic sewing ring, as described in the original David technique.[43,121,124] Here, pledgets are secured to the ventricular surface of the annulus (see Fig. 20.7). This method is the strongest way to secure a prosthetic mitral valve and significantly reduces the risk of prosthesis dehiscence and atrioventricular groove disruption.[22,43,121] Thus, this suturing method can be particularly valuable when securing the prosthesis is complicated by a heavily calcified annulus or difficult exposure. Of note, some advocate that the subannular suturing method should be reserved for when BHVs are implanted in MVR, in part because there may be less risk for obstruction compared to when a mechanical prosthesis is implanted.[43] However, when properly performed, this technique can be used in nearly all etiologies and lesions warranting MVR, regardless of the type of prosthesis used.[121]

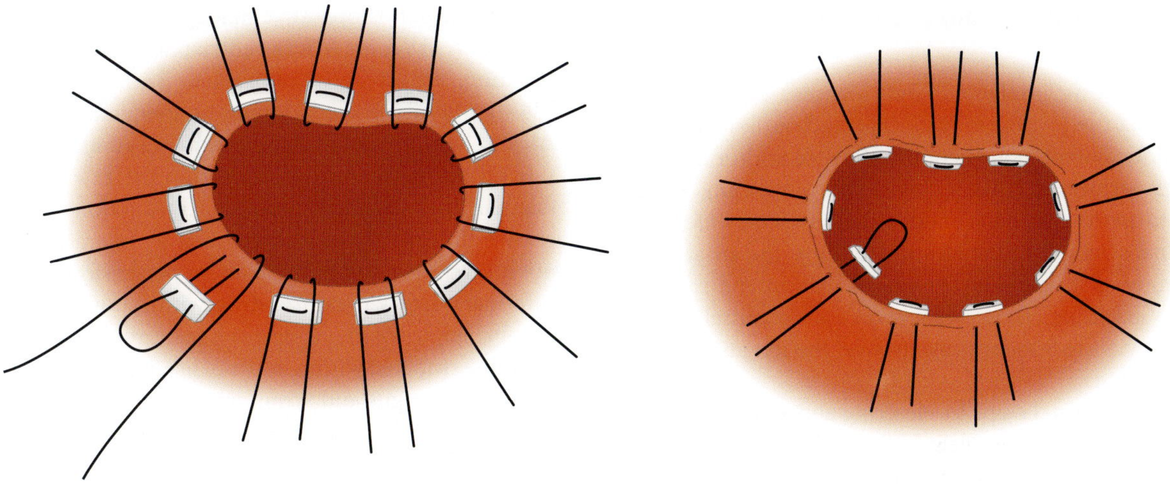

Fig. 20.7 Mitral Valve Prosthesis Implantation Using Supraannular and Subannular Sewing Techniques. Both bioprosthetic and mechanical valves may be implanted using supraannular (i.e., everting) stitches taken from the atrium towards the ventricle and then through the valve's sewing ring so that pledgets are secured to the atrial side of the annulus *(left).* Alternatively, subannular (i.e., noneverting) sutures can be placed from the ventricular side of the annulus towards the atrium before being threaded through the prosthetic sewing ring so that pledgets are secured to the ventricular surface of the annulus *(right).* This method is the strongest way to secure a prosthetic mitral valve and significantly reduces the risk of prosthesis dehiscence and atrioventricular groove disruption. When properly performed, this technique can be used in nearly all mitral valve replacements regardless of the type of prosthesis used. (Adapted from Kaneko T, Yammine M, Loberman D, et al. Mitral valve replacement. In: Cohn LH, Adams DH, eds. *Cardiac Surgery in the Adult.* 5th ed. New York: McGraw-Hill Education; 2017; David TE. Mitral valve replacement with preservation of chordae tendinae: rationale and technical considerations. *Ann Thorac Surg.* 1986;41[6]:680–682; Miki S, Kusuhara K, Ueda Y, et al. Mitral valve replacement with preservation of chordae tendineae and papillary muscles. *Ann Thorac Surg.* 1988;45[1]:28–34.)

Whichever suturing technique is used, the posterior suture line is usually completed first, commencing at the anterolateral commissure and progressing counterclockwise. The anterior suture line follows, advancing in a clockwise direction. Once all sutures are secured to the annulus and sewing ring of the prosthesis (usually ~12 sutures in total), the valve can be lowered into position and tied into place. Each stitch should be carefully ligated, as excessively long suture tails have the potential to damage the delicate leaflets of BHVs.[22]

Concomitant Procedures

After a BHV or mechanical valve is secured in place, one should refrain from lifting or manipulating the heart with the rigid prosthesis in place to minimize the risk of atrioventricular groove disruption.[22,124] Therefore when additional concomitant procedures are indicated (see "Other Indications: Mixed Lesions, Concomitant Procedures, and Endocarditis" above), the order of component procedures must be strategically planned. This preparation also improves the efficiency of the operation, thereby reducing the risks associated with prolonged cardiopulmonary bypass times and myocardial ischemia.

Coronary bypass grafting is the most common concomitant procedure performed during MVR, and one should complete the distal anastomoses before implanting the prosthetic valve. Failure to do so makes it extremely challenging to access the posterior coronary. This can also improve myocardial protection by permitting direct cardioplegia delivery through the grafts after the distal anastomoses are completed.[22,43,124]

Meanwhile, when multivalve procedures are planned, alternative methods for mitral valve exposure might be beneficial. For example, if the tricuspid valve requires intervention during MVR, it may be preferentially to expose the mitral valve using a biatrial and/or transseptal incision, as is described elsewhere.[22] Not surprisingly, MVR should be completed prior to intervening on the tricuspid valve.[43,140] In addition, when multiple valves require surgical intervention, an effort should be made to minimize the number of valves replaced, as dual-valve replacement has been associated with poorer outcomes than combined repair and replacement.[1,141] Nevertheless, there are instances in which multiple valve replacements are required. In these circumstances, one must consider the sequence of valvular intervention. For example, when both MVR and aortic valve replacement are necessary, the aortic valve is typically excised first, as exposing the anterior mitral annulus can be quite challenging with an aortic prosthesis in place.[43,124]

As a final note, many antiarrhythmic procedures may be reasonable to consider at the time of MVR (i.e., Maze procedure, pulmonary vein isolation, etc.). At a minimum, the left atrial appendage should be either ligated or occluded in patients with chronic atrial fibrillation.[1,43]

Closing and Weaning From Cardiopulmonary Bypass

With the prosthesis implanted and secured, retractors are removed so that the prosthesis, ventricle, and outflow tract can be inspected for potential areas of interference and/or obstruction. The left atriotomy is then closed with a running suture, taking care to approximate the endocardial surfaces, which provides maximal strength to the closure. Of note, the atrial tissue is often thinner as it nears the interatrial septum and carries a higher risk of bleeding. Thus, when access to the mitral valve is accomplished via the Sondergaard groove, the left atriotomy is typically oversewn.[22,105,124,132]

In any case, the usual steps for deairing and exiting from the left side of the heart are completed.[22] Note, if a sump sucker is advanced into the ventricle for venting prior to closing the left atriotomy, care must be taken to avoid entrapping the catheter within the suture line of the atriotomy. In addition, it is important to ensure that prosthetic leaflets are not torn when the catheter is finally removed.[142] Nevertheless, as volume is gradually added to the heart, pulmonary artery pressures should be monitored. With the atriotomy closed, the heart resuscitated, and the patient rewarming, a final and thorough assessment of the heart should be performed with transesophageal echocardiography (TEE). In the absence of significant aortic valve distortion, outflow tract obstruction, prosthesis dysfunction, paravalvular leak, or other alarming findings, the patient may be weaned off cardiopulmonary bypass as tolerated.[11,22,43,124]

Rarely (1% to 2% of patients), a moderate-to-severe periprosthetic (paravalvular) leak will be identified, which typically warrants immediate return to cardiopulmonary bypass to fix the lesion.[69] In contrast, clinically insignificant paravalvular leaks are not uncommon immediately after MVR and may be present in as many as 10% to 25% of patients prior to weaning from cardiopulmonary bypass.[69,143–145] Most of these jets usually resolve once protamine is administered or early in the postoperative period (days to weeks). Few (1% to 2%) will progress and require subsequent intervention within 1 to 2 years after surgery. Even then, about half of these paravalvular leaks can be adequately repaired using percutaneous techniques.[69,145] In any case, when a paravalvular leak is identified, close follow-up is warranted to monitor for persisting or progressive symptoms as well as prosthesis and/or ventricular dysfunction.

POSTOPERATIVE MANAGEMENT AND EARLY COMPLICATIONS

In the immediate postoperative period after MVR, the primary goal is restoring cardiac output and pulmonary function. Therefore pulmonary artery catheters should be left in place when exiting the operating room. It is important to recognize that when MVR is performed in the setting of MR, a parallel circuit of low resistance that had been provided by the incompetent valve is eliminated almost immediately, and thus resistance to ventricular myocardial fiber shortening (i.e., afterload) rises drastically.[22] As a result, myocardial contractile reserve is diminished, and myocardial oxygen consumption rises.[146] Therefore a cornerstone of postoperative management in patients who have undergone MVR for MR is ventricular unloading via afterload reduction, especially in individuals with low cardiac output. This should be initiated as soon as adequate volume resuscitation and hemodynamic stabilization are attained.[11,22,43]

In addition, removal of fluid from the extracellular space is essential to normalizing pulmonary function after MVR. Aggressive diuresis should be pursued as tolerated, especially in patients with severe pulmonary hypertension. In most cases, pulmonary artery pressures drop within hours after MVR, and these principles of management permit most patients to be successfully extubated within hours of leaving the operating room.[43]

Of course, signs and symptoms of common complications in cardiac surgery that occur early in the postoperative period should always be monitored after MVR. Specifically, postoperative supraventricular arrhythmias are more often seen than not.[129,147,148] These can usually be controlled with pharmacologic agents, though unstable tachyarrhythmias warrant immediate cardioversion, whereas temporary or permanent pacemakers are occasionally required for bradyarrhythmias. There should be a high index of suspicion for ischemia and/or coronary entrapment when ventricular arrhythmias are identified or if a patient shows new electrocardiogram changes suggestive of infarction, especially in the distribution of the left circumflex coronary artery. Perhaps the most dreaded complication after MVR is atrioventricular groove disruption. This complication must be identified quickly if the patient has any chance of surviving, and even then, surgical repair is challenging and carries a very high-risk of mortality.[149–151]

LONG-TERM CARE AND FOLLOW-UP

Although most patients can expect a relatively uncomplicated hospital course, roughly 20% will be readmitted within 30 days of discharge.[152] Therefore close monitoring after discharge is essential, and routine, longitudinal follow-up should be maintained for important surveillance, diagnosis, and prompt treatment of potential complications that may arise late after MVR.

Routine Follow-Up

Patients are typically seen 4 weeks and 12 months postoperatively. Transthoracic echocardiography (TTE) should be obtained immediately prior to hospital discharge (or within 30 days), and again at 6 and 12 months, and then annually thereafter. It is important to recognize that indirect signs of cardiac dysfunction seen on TTE often provide the first signs of prosthetic valve dysfunction, including atrial enlargement, persistent or progressive ventricular dysfunction, and/or pulmonary hypertension, among others.[69] Therefore surgeons should be familiar with basic metrics and normal reference ranges used for interpreting prosthetic MVR function on echocardiography.[69,153–155] However, one must recognize that not all findings outside of normal reference ranges are pathologic. For example, one must be able to discern if an elevated transprosthetic valve gradient (mean >5 to 7 mm Hg after MVR) is the result of physiologic high-flow conditions, or pathologic PPM, valve obstruction, etc.[69] Nevertheless, a thorough evaluation should be conducted for every patient any time clinical signs and/or symptoms suggest the potential for prosthetic valve dysfunction. Because TTE images may be obfuscated by sonographic shadowing from the prosthetic valve, there should be a low threshold for additional diagnostic imaging, specifically with TEE, which is more sensitive to detecting valve lesions and dysfunction.[1,69,156,155]

Anticoagulation Guidelines

As described above, all patients who receive a mechanical mitral valve require lifelong anticoagulation with a vitamin K inhibitor. The target INR after mechanical MVR is 3.0 (range 2.5 to 3.5), and all patients should also take low-dose daily aspirin (75 to 100 mg).[1] Although the risk for prosthesis-related thrombotic and embolic events are significantly higher in patients with a mechanical prosthesis, patients with BHVs are at an increased risk for these complications as well, even if to a lesser degree.[1,157,158] This is thought to be related to incomplete reendothelialization of the suture line in the early postoperative period, which is supported by the fact that these risks are highest within 3 months after MVR.[1,69,157]

Therefore patients who undergo MVR with a BHV typically receive anticoagulation for 3 to 6 months after surgery with a goal INR of 2.5 (range 2.0 to 3.0).[1] Antiplatelet therapy after MVR with a BHV is a reasonable consideration, as evidence suggests that this reduces stroke rates, the incidence of valve thrombosis, and cardiovascular mortality without significantly increasing the risk of bleeding complications.[1,159] However, postoperative anticoagulation and/or antiplatelet strategies after MVR with a BHV vary widely among institutions. Some estimate that ~30% of centers routinely treat patients with only aspirin after MVR with a BHV, at least in part because there have been mixed results regarding the risks of bleeding in patients with BHVs who receive both antiplatelet therapy and oral anticoagulation compared to aspirin alone.[69,160]

Bleeding Complications

The annual risk of hemorrhagic events with the use of long-term anticoagulation is ~1% per patient-year.[65,69,161,162] Significant bleeding events after MVR are most often related to supratherapeutic anticoagulation. Thus, when a significant bleeding event occurs, oral anticoagulation should be held, and serial assays of anticoagulation levels should be monitored. Individualized assessment is needed to determine how and when to restart anticoagulation with respect to the risks of recurrent bleeding compared to potential thrombotic and/or embolic complications while holding anticoagulation.[69]

Of note, there may be times when patients on oral anticoagulation after MVR may need an invasive procedure that increases their risk for significant bleeding. In such circumstances, careful consideration must be given to the procedure's necessity, particularly among individuals with a mechanical valve who are at high risk of valve thrombosis and/or thromboembolic complications.[1,2,51,69] When there is no alternative, oral anticoagulation may be temporarily held for several hours before and after the procedure. However, it is imperative to carefully monitor patients and follow established guidelines for holding anticoagulation, which may include bridging patients with intravenous heparin.[1,2,51,69,163] As soon as it is safe, therapeutic anticoagulation should be restarted, as the risk of thrombotic and/ or embolic can have devastating complications.

Thrombotic, Embolic, and Obstructive Complications

Thrombotic and embolic complications after MVR are relatively uncommon. The incidence of stroke and valve thrombosis ranges from 0.2% to 3.3% and 0.3% to 1.3% per patient-year, respectively.[157–159,164] Although there is some evidence to suggest that these complications are similar among patients with either a BHV or mechanical valve, these risks are likely higher among those with mechanical valves, particularly when other comorbidities are present, including atrial fibrillation, ventricular dysfunction (ejection fraction ≤35%), and/or left atrial dilation (diameter ≥50 mm).[a]

Regardless, any cerebrovascular or systemic thromboembolic event that occurs in a patient with either a BHV or mechanical valve must be considered a consequence of their prosthesis until proven otherwise. Similarly, any patient with sudden or progressive decline in functional status (i.e., dyspnea, fatigue, etc.) should be evaluated for prosthesis dysfunction resulting from thrombotic obstruction. This is particularly true in patients who have recently stopped anticoagulation, and those who have trouble maintaining a therapeutic level of anticoagulation, as a highly variable INR may be the strongest prognosticator of survival after mechanical MVR.[69,165]

When a patient presents with findings concerning for systemic emboli or prosthetic valve obstruction, it is imperative to evaluate their level of anticoagulation while preparing for urgent imaging assessment, usually with TEE. If thrombus is confirmed and the patient is adequately anticoagulated, the target international normalized ratio (INR) may be adjusted to the higher end of the recommended range. If anticoagulation is clearly subtherapeutic, intravenous heparin should be initiated and titrated to a therapeutic level immediately. If not already prescribed, aspirin should be started.[1,2,51,69]

However, it is important to note that one must thoroughly evaluate further anticoagulation with respect to concomitant bleeding risks. Specifically, with ischemic strokes that are at a high risk for hemorrhagic transformation (i.e., ~35% of cerebral hemisphere involvement and/or occurring in the setting of uncontrolled hypertension), it may be preferential to hold oral anticoagulation for up to 5 days while bridging with intravenous heparin to allow for tighter therapeutic control.[69,166]

In any case, if a thrombus is large (5 to 10 mm) or continues to enlarge despite adequate anticoagulation, surgical reintervention via thrombectomy or redo MVR may be warranted, especially if symptoms persist or progress. Prompt recognition and early intervention are imperative to improving operative outcomes in obstructive valve thrombosis, with some studies suggesting that operative mortality increases from 5% to 20% when a patient's functional status declines from NYHA class III

[a] References 1, 2, 65, 69, 159, 161.

to class IV at the time of reintervention.[51,69,167–169] In select cases, such as in patients who are too frail for reoperation, alternative interventions may be considered, including targeted pharmacologic thrombolysis.

Non-thrombotic Prosthetic Valve Obstruction

It is important to recognize that prosthetic valve obstruction is not always caused by thrombus formation, and mechanical valves may fail for a number of reasons (see "Valve Sizing and Prosthesis-Patient Mismatch" above).[157–159,164] Meanwhile, as previously described, SVD remains the most common cause of prosthetic valve failure and reoperation after MVR with a BHV (see "Age-Related Guidelines for Prosthesis Selection: Considering Valve Durability and Anticoagulation Requirements" above). Just as early intervention in mechanical valve obstruction is key to improving operative outcomes, once SVD develops, it appears that early reintervention with redo MVR should be completed before ventricular dysfunction develops and/or symptoms deteriorate.[69]

Early subclinical signs of prosthesis obstruction may include progressive or significant hemolysis, which should be monitored with routine measurements of lactate dehydrogenase and complete blood counts. Some degree of hemolysis resulting in mild-to-moderate anemia is not uncommon in patients with mechanical valves (50% to 90%).[69,170] Isolated hemolysis resulting in the absence of prosthetic valve dysfunction rarely requires surgical intervention and can usually be treated conservatively with a combination of folate, erythropoietin, and/or beta-blockers. In contrast, severe hemolysis with significant, refractory anemia usually suggests significant prosthetic valve dysfunction.[69,170]

Prosthetic Valve Endocarditis

When a vegetation is observed on a prosthetic valve, clinicians must attempt to discern if it represents thrombus, a fibroelastoma, or infective endocarditis using established guidelines. To minimize the risk of prosthetic valve infection after MVR, the clinician should administer prophylactic antibiotics for any procedure that could lead to bacterial seeding of the prosthetic valve, specifically dental work or endoscopic procedures.[1,2] However, even with appropriate prophylaxis, prosthetic valve endocarditis still occurs at a rate of ~0.5% per patient-year, which holds quite a morbid prognosis with mortality ranging from 30% to 50%.[69,166,170] Therefore any patient who becomes febrile after MVR or who has a suspicious vegetation identified on TTE should have blood cultures drawn in addition to closer evaluation with TEE, specifically looking for evidence of abscess formation or prosthesis regurgitation.[69,155]

In some cases, prompt administration of appropriate antibiotics can successfully treat prosthetic valve endocarditis and avoid the need for reoperation. However, surgery should be seriously considered in patients who fail to improve with early antibiotics and/or those who have evidence of intracardiac abscesses and/or fistulas.[1,2,171] Similarly, surgery is usually indicated when prosthetic valve dysfunction is hemodynamically significant or when valvular and/or ventricular dysfunction progressively deteriorates. In contrast to the mild and clinically insignificant periprosthetic leaks commonly observed immediately after MVR (see "Closing and Weaning from Cardiopulmonary Bypass" above), new or acutely progressive paravalvular leaks may suggest prosthesis dehiscence in the setting of endocarditis, which should be treated as a surgical emergency.[69,171]

CONCLUSIONS/SUMMARY

Surgical replacement of the mitral valve requires a masterful understanding of all aspects of perioperative, intraoperative, and postoperative care in cardiac surgery. Surgeons must recognize when MVR is preferred to mitral valve repair and consider many factors related to prosthesis selection and the optimal surgical technique. Surgical decisions regarding MVR must be tailored to each patient with respect to their personal preferences and the underlying etiology of their valvular disease.

CASE-BASED ASSESSMENT

A middle-aged male is diagnosed with severe rheumatic mitral stenosis. Repeated balloon valvuloplasty has been ineffective, and the patient remains severely symptomatic.

1. The patient is 58 years old. According to current AHA/ACC guidelines, which type of prosthetic valve is usually preferred in a patient of his age?
   A. Mechanical valve
   B. Bioprosthetic valve
   C. Either mechanical or bioprosthetic valve, depending on the patient's preference and other considerations regarding chronic arrhythmias, comorbidities, etc.
2. According to current AHA/ACC guidelines, what age is mitral valve replacement with a *bioprosthetic* prosthetic valve usually indicated?
   A. Younger than 50 years of age
   B. Younger than 60 years of age
   C. Younger than 70 years of age
   D. Younger than 80 years of age
   E. Older than 50 years of age
   F. Older than 60 years of age
   G. Older than 70 years of age
   H. Older than 80 years of age
3. According to current AHA/ACC guidelines, what age is mitral valve replacement with a *mechanical* prosthetic valve usually indicated?
   A. Younger than 50 years of age
   B. Younger than 60 years of age
   C. Younger than 70 years of age
   D. Younger than 80 years of age
   E. Older than 50 years of age
   F. Older than 60 years of age
   G. Older than 70 years of age
   H. Older than 80 years of age
4. What is the strongest way to suture in a prosthetic mitral valve?
   A. Subannular (i.e., noneverting) sutures
   B. Supraannular (i.e., everting) sutures

See page 318 for the answers

REFERENCES

1. Nishimura RA, Otto CM, Bonow RO, et al. 2017 AHA/ACC Focused Update of the 2014 AHA/ACC Guideline for the Management of Patients With Valvular Heart Disease: A Report of the American College of Cardiology/American Heart Association Task Force on Clinical Practice Guidelines. *Circulation.* 2017;135(25):e1159–e1195.
2. Nishimura RA, Otto CM, Bonow RO, et al. 2014 AHA/ACC guideline for the management of patients with valvular heart disease: a report of the American College of Cardiology/American Heart Association Task Force on Practice Guidelines. *J Am Coll Cardiol.* 2014;63(22):e57–185.
3. O'Gara PT, Grayburn PA, Badhwar V, et al. 2017 ACC Expert Consensus Decision Pathway on the Management of Mitral Regurgitation: A Report of the American College of Cardiology Task Force on Expert Consensus Decision Pathways. *J Am Coll Cardiol.* 2017;70(19):2421–2449.
4. Baumgartner H, Falk V, Bax JJ, et al. 2017 ESC/EACTS Guidelines for the management of valvular heart disease. *Eur Heart J.* 2017;38(36):2739–2791.
5. David TE, Armstrong S, McCrindle BW, et al. Late outcomes of mitral valve repair for mitral regurgitation due to degenerative disease. *Circulation.* 2013;127(14):1485–1492.
6. Wilkins GT, Weyman AE, Abascal VM, et al. Percutaneous balloon dilatation of the mitral valve: an analysis of echocardiographic variables related to outcome and the mechanism of dilatation. *Heart.* 1988;60(4):299–308.
7. Kamperidis V, van Wijngaarden SE, van Rosendael PJ, et al. Restrictive Mitral Valve Annuloplasty: Prognostic Implications of Left Ventricular Forward Flow. *Ann Thorac Surg.* 2017;104(5):1464–1470.
8. Abdelnoor M, Fjeld NB, Vaage K, et al. Risk factors for morbidity and mortality in mitral valve replacement. *Eur J Cardiothorac Surg.* 1990;4(8):425–430.
9. Rey Meyer M-A, von Segesser LK, Hurni M, et al. Long-term outcome after mitral valve repair: a risk factor analysis. *Eur J Cardiothorac Surg.* 2007;32(2):301–307.
10. Turina J, Stark T, Seifert B, et al. Predictors of the Long-Term Outcome After Combined Aortic and Mitral Valve Surgery. *Circulation.* 1999;100(suppl_2):48 II–.
11. Carpentier A, Adams DH, Filsoufi F. *Carpentier's Reconstructive Valve Surgery.* Philadelphia: Saunders; 2010.
12. Hakim FA, Kendall CB, Alharthi M, et al. Parachute mitral valve in adults-a systematic overview. *Echocardiography.* 2010;27(5):581–586.
13. Hull MC, Morris CG, Pepine CJ, et al. Valvular dysfunction and carotid, subclavian, and coronary artery disease in survivors of Hodgkin lymphoma treated with radiation therapy. *JAMA.* 2003;290(21):2831–2837.
14. Olson LJ, Subramanian R, Ackermann DM, et al. Surgical pathology of the mitral valve: a study of 712 cases spanning 21 years. *Mayo Clin Proc.* 1987;62(1):22–34.
15. Horstkotte D, Niehues R, Strauer BE. Pathomorphological aspects, aetiology and natural history of acquired mitral valve stenosis. *Eur Heart J.* 1991;12(suppl B):55–60.
16. Gordis L. The virtual disappearance of rheumatic fever in the United States: lessons in the rise and fall of disease. T. Duckett Jones memorial lecture. *Circulation.* 1985;72(6):1155–1162.
17. Zühlke L, Engel ME, Karthikeyan G, et al. Characteristics, complications, and gaps in evidence-based interventions in rheumatic heart disease: the Global Rheumatic Heart Disease Registry (the REMEDY study). *Eur Heart J.* 2015;36(18):1115–1122a.
18. Pressman GS, Agarwal A, Braitman LE, Muddassir SM. Mitral annular calcium causing mitral stenosis. *Am J Cardiol.* 2010;105(3):389–391.
19. Abramowitz Y, Jilaihawi H, Chakravarty T, et al. Mitral Annulus Calcification. *J Am Coll Cardiol.* 2015;66(17):1934–1941.
20. Marcus RH, Sareli P, Pocock WA, et al. The spectrum of severe rheumatic mitral valve disease in a developing country. Correlations among clinical presentation, surgical pathologic findings, and hemodynamic sequelae. *Ann Intern Med.* 1994;120(3):177–183.
21. Joint Task Force on the Management of Valvular Heart Disease of the European Society of Cardiology (ESC), European Association for Cardio-Thoracic Surgery (EACTS), Vahanian A, et al. Guidelines on the management of valvular heart disease (version 2012). *Eur Heart J.* 2012;33(19):2451–2496.
22. Kouchoukos NT, Blackstone EH, Hanley FL, et al. Mitral Valve Disease with or without Tricuspid Valve Disease. *Kirklin/Barratt-Boyes Cardiac Surgery.* 4th ed.: Philadelphia, PA: Elsevier/Saunders; 2013:473–540.
23. Ancona R, Pinto SC. Mitral valve incompetence: epidemiology and causes. *E-Journal of Cardiology Practice.* 2018;16(11).
24. Freed LA, Levy D, Levine RA, et al. Prevalence and Clinical Outcome of Mitral-Valve Prolapse. *N Engl J Med.* 1999;341(1):1–7. doi:10.1056/NEJM199907013410101.
25. Libby P, Bonow RO, Mann DL. *Braunwald's Heart Disease: A Textbook of Cardiovascular Medicine.* 12th ed. Philadelphia: Elsevier; 2022.
26. Apostolidou E, Maslow AD, Poppas A. Primary mitral valve regurgitation: update and review. *Glob Cardiol Sci Pract.* 2017(1):e201703.
27. Yarboro LT, Kron IL. How I teach mitral valve surgery. *Ann Thorac Surg.* 2016;101(5):1641–1643.
28. Enriquez-Sarano M, Tajik AJ, Schaff HV, et al. Echocardiographic prediction of left ventricular function after correction of mitral regurgitation: results and clinical implications. *J Am Coll Cardiol.* 1994;24(6):1536–1543.
29. Harris KM, Pastorius CA, Duval S, et al. Practice variation among cardiovascular physicians in management of patients with mitral regurgitation. *Am J Cardiol.* 2009;103(2):255–261.
30. Braunberger E, Deloche A, Berrebi A, et al. Very long-term results (more than 20 years) of valve repair with carpentier's techniques in nonrheumatic mitral valve insufficiency. *Circulation.* 2001;104(12 suppl 1):I8–I11.
31. Cohn LH, Allred EN, Cohn LA, et al. Early and late risk of mitral valve replacement. A 12 year concomitant comparison of the porcine bioprosthetic and prosthetic disc mitral valves. *J Thorac Cardiovasc Surg.* 1985;90(6):872–881.
32. Cohn LH, Couper GS, Aranki SF, et al. The long-term results of mitral valve reconstruction for the "floppy" valve. *J Card Surg.* 1994;9(suppl 2):278–281.
33. Cosgrove DM, Chavez AM, Lytle BW, et al. Results of mitral valve reconstruction. *Circulation.* 1986;74(3 Pt 2):I82–I87.
34. el Asmar B, Perier P, Couetil JP, Carpentier A. Failures in reconstructive mitral valve surgery. *J Med Liban.* 1991;39(1):7–11.
35. Asgar AW, Mack MJ, Stone GW. Secondary mitral regurgitation in heart failure: pathophysiology, prognosis, and therapeutic considerations. *J Am Coll Cardiol.* 2015;65(12):1231–1248.
36. Acker MA, Parides MK, Perrault LP, et al. Mitral-valve repair versus replacement for severe ischemic mitral regurgitation. *N Engl J Med.* 2014;370(1):23–32.
37. Goldstein D, Moskowitz AJ, Gelijns AC, et al. Two-year outcomes of surgical treatment of severe ischemic mitral regurgitation. *N Engl J Med.* 2016;374(4):344–353.

38. Smith PK, Puskas JD, Ascheim DD, et al. *Surgical Treatment of Moderate Ischemic Mitral Regurgitation.* http://dx.doi.org/10.1056/NEJMoa1410490.
39. Michler RE, Smith PK, Parides MK, et al. Two-year outcomes of surgical treatment of moderate ischemic mitral regurgitation. *N Engl J Med.* 2016;374(20):1932–1941.
40. Nishimura RA, Otto CM, Bonow RO, et al. 2017 AHA/ACC Focused Update of the 2014 AHA/ACC Guideline for the Management of Patients With Valvular Heart Disease: A Report of the American College of Cardiology/American Heart Association Task Force on Clinical Practice Guidelines. *J Am Coll Cardiol.* 2017;70(2):252–289.
41. Nakano S, Sakai K, Taniguchi K, et al. Relation of impaired left ventricular function in mitral regurgitation to left ventricular contractile state after mitral valve replacement. *Am J Cardiol.* 1994;73(1):70–74.
42. Kontos GJ, Schaff HV, Gersh BJ, Bove AA. Left ventricular function in subacute and chronic mitral regurgitation. Effect on function early postoperatively. *J Thorac Cardiovasc Surg.* 1989;98(2):163–169.
43. Kaneko T, Yammine M, Loberman D, et al. Mitral Valve Replacement. In: Cohn LH, Adams DH, eds. *Cardiac Surgery in the Adult.* 5th ed.: New York, NY: McGraw-Hill Education; 2017.
44. Timmis SB, Kirsh MM, Montgomery DG, Starling MR. Evaluation of left ventricular ejection fraction as a measure of pump performance in patients with chronic mitral regurgitation. *Catheter Cardiovasc Interv.* 2000;49(3):290–296.
45. Wisenbaugh T, Skudicky D, Sareli P. Prediction of outcome after valve replacement for rheumatic mitral regurgitation in the era of chordal preservation. *Circulation.* 1994;89(1):191–197.
46. Matsumura T, Ohtaki E, Tanaka K, et al. Echocardiographic prediction of left ventricular dysfunction after mitral valve repair for mitral regurgitation as an indicator to decide the optimal timing of repair. *J Am Coll Cardiol.* 2003;42(3):458–463.
47. Tribouilloy C, Rusinaru D, Szymanski C, et al. Predicting left ventricular dysfunction after valve repair for mitral regurgitation due to leaflet prolapse: additive value of left ventricular end-systolic dimension to ejection fraction. *Eur J Echocardiogr.* 2011;12(9):702–710.
48. Quintana E, Suri RM, Thalji NM, et al. Left ventricular dysfunction after mitral valve repair–the fallacy of "normal" preoperative myocardial function. *J Thorac Cardiovasc Surg.* 2014;148(6):2752–2760.
49. Suri RM, Schaff HV, Dearani JA, et al. Determinants of early decline in ejection fraction after surgical correction of mitral regurgitation. *J Thorac Cardiovasc Surg.* 2008;136(2):442–447.
50. Corin WJ, Sütsch G, Murakami T, et al. Left ventricular function in chronic mitral regurgitation: preoperative and postoperative comparison. *J Am Coll Cardiol.* 1995;25(1):113–121.
51. Bonow Robert O, Carabello Blase A, Chatterjee Kanu, et al. ACC/AHA 2006 guidelines for the management of patients with valvular heart disease. *Circulation.* 2006;114(5):e84–e231.
52. Schuler G, Peterson KL, Johnson A, et al. Temporal response of left ventricular performance to mitral valve surgery. *Circulation.* 1979;59(6):1218–1231.
53. Ross J. Afterload mismatch in aortic and mitral valve disease: implications for surgical therapy. *J Am Coll Cardiol.* 1985;5(4):811–826.
54. Pettersson GB, Hussain ST. Current AATS guidelines on surgical treatment of infective endocarditis. *Ann Cardiothorac Surg.* 2019;8(6):630–644.
55. Glaser N, Jackson V, Holzmann MJ, et al. Aortic valve replacement with mechanical vs. biological prostheses in patients aged 50–69 years. *Eur Heart J.* 2016;37(34):2658–2667.
56. Chikwe J, Chiang YP, Egorova NN, et al. Survival and outcomes following bioprosthetic vs mechanical mitral valve replacement in patients aged 50 to 69 years. *JAMA.* 2015;313(14):1435–1442.
57. McClure RS, McGurk S, Cevasco M, et al. Late outcomes comparison of nonelderly patients with stented bioprosthetic and mechanical valves in the aortic position: a propensity-matched analysis. *J Thorac Cardiovasc Surg.* 2014;148(5):1931–1939.
58. Chiang YP, Chikwe J, Moskowitz AJ, et al. Survival and long-term outcomes following bioprosthetic vs mechanical aortic valve replacement in patients aged 50 to 69 years. *JAMA.* 2014;312(13):1323–1329.
59. Bourguignon T, Bouquiaux-Stablo A-L, Candolfi P, et al. Very long-term outcomes of the Carpentier-Edwards Perimount valve in aortic position. *Ann Thorac Surg.* 2015;99(3):831–837.
60. Bourguignon T, Bouquiaux-Stablo A-L, Loardi C, et al. Very late outcomes for mitral valve replacement with the Carpentier-Edwards pericardial bioprosthesis: 25-year follow-up of 450 implantations. *J Thorac Cardiovasc Surg.* 2014;148(5):2004–2011.e1.
61. Kaneko T, Aranki S, Javed Q, et al. Mechanical versus bioprosthetic mitral valve replacement in patients <65 years old. *J Thorac Cardiovasc Surg.* 2014;147(1):117–126.
62. Badhwar V, Ofenloch JC, Rovin JD, et al. Noninferiority of closely monitored mechanical valves to bioprostheses overshadowed by early mortality benefit in younger patients. *Ann Thorac Surg.* 2012;93(3):748–753.
63. Kulik A, Bédard P, Lam B-K, et al. Mechanical versus bioprosthetic valve replacement in middle-aged patients. *Eur J Cardiothorac Surg.* 2006;30(3):485–491.
64. Goldstone AB, Chiu P, Baiocchi M, et al. Mechanical or Biologic Prostheses for Aortic-Valve and Mitral-Valve Replacement. *N Engl J Med.* 2017;377(19):1847–1857.
65. Hammermeister K, Sethi GK, Henderson WG, et al. Outcomes 15 years after valve replacement with a mechanical versus a bioprosthetic valve: final report of the Veterans Affairs randomized trial. *J Am Coll Cardiol.* 2000;36(4):1152–1158.
66. Smood B, Hara H, Cleveland DC, Cooper DKC. Search of the Ideal Valve: Optimizing Genetic Modifications to Prevent Bioprosthetic Degeneration. *Ann Thorac Surg.* 2019;108(2):624–635.
67. Siddiqui RF, Abraham JR, Butany J. Bioprosthetic heart valves: modes of failure. *Histopathology.* 2009;55(2):135–144.
68. Soares JS, Feaver KR, Zhang W, et al. Biomechanical Behavior of Bioprosthetic Heart Valve Heterograft Tissues: Characterization, Simulation, and Performance. *Cardiovasc Eng Technol.* 2016;7(4):309–351.
69. Philippe P, Jean DG. Prosthetic heart valves. *Circulation.* 2009;119(7):1034–1048.
70. Carpentier A, Lemaigre G, Robert L, et al. Biological factors affecting long-term results of valvular heterografts. *J Thorac Cardiovasc Surg.* 1969;58(4):467–483.
71. Carpentier A, Deloche A, Relland J, et al. Six-year follow-up of glutaraldehyde-preserved heterografts. With particular reference to the treatment of congenital valve malformations. *J Thorac Cardiovasc Surg.* 1974;68(5):771–782.
72. van Geldorp MWA, Eric Jamieson WR, Kappetein AP, et al. Patient outcome after aortic valve replacement with a mechanical or biological prosthesis: weighing lifetime anticoagulant-related event risk against reoperation risk. *J Thorac Cardiovasc Surg.* 2009;137(4):881–886, 886e1–886e5.
73. Weber A, Noureddine H, Englberger L, et al. Ten-year comparison of pericardial tissue valves versus mechanical prostheses for aortic valve replacement in patients younger than 60 years of age. *J Thorac Cardiovasc Surg.* 2012;144(5):1075–1083.

74. Cohn LH, Collins JJ, DiSesa VJ, et al. Fifteen-year experience with 1678 Hancock porcine bioprosthetic heart valve replacements. *Ann Surg.* 1989;210(4):435–442; discussion 442–443.
75. Pupello DF, Bessone LN, Hiro SP, et al. Bioprosthetic valve longevity in the elderly: an 18-year longitudinal study. *Ann Thorac Surg.* 1995;60(2 suppl):S270–S274; discussion S275.
76. Burdon TA, Miller DC, Oyer PE, et al. Durability of porcine valves at fifteen years in a representative North American patient population. *J Thorac Cardiovasc Surg.* 1992;103(2):238–251; discussion 251–252.
77. Cohn LH, Collins JJ, Rizzo RJ, et al. Twenty-year follow-up of the Hancock modified orifice porcine aortic valve. *Ann Thorac Surg.* 1998;66(6 Suppl):S30–S34.
78. Corbineau H, Du Haut Cilly FB, et al. Structural durability in Carpentier Edwards Standard bioprosthesis in the mitral position: a 20-year experience. *J Heart Valve Dis.* 2001;10(4):443–448.
79. van Doorn CA, Stoodley KD, Saunders NR, et al. Mitral valve replacement with the Carpentier-Edwards standard bioprosthesis: performance into the second decade. *Eur J Cardiothorac Surg.* 1995;9(5):253–258.
80. Khan SS, Chaux A, Blanche C, et al. A 20-year experience with the Hancock porcine xenograft in the elderly. *Ann Thorac Surg.* 1998;66(6 Suppl):S35–S39.
81. Jamieson WR, Miller DC, Akins CW, et al. Pregnancy and bioprostheses: influence on structural valve deterioration. *Ann Thorac Surg.* 1995;60(2 Suppl):S282–S286; discussion S287.
82. Badduke BR, Jamieson WR, Miyagishima RT, et al. Pregnancy and childbearing in a population with biologic valvular prostheses. *J Thorac Cardiovasc Surg.* 1991;102(2):179–186.
83. Mihaljevic T, Paul S, Leacche M, et al. Valve replacement in women of childbearing age: influences on mother, fetus and neonate. *J Heart Valve Dis.* 2005;14(2):151–157.
84. Grunkemeier GL, Jamieson WR, Miller DC, Starr A. Actuarial versus actual risk of porcine structural valve deterioration. *J Thorac Cardiovasc Surg.* 1994;108(4):709–718.
85. Williams ML, Bavaria JE, Acker MA, et al. Valve Selection in End-Stage Renal Disease: Should It Always Be Biological? *Ann Thorac Surg.* 2016;102(5):1531–1535.
86. Brinkman WT, Williams WH, Guyton RA, et al. Valve replacement in patients on chronic renal dialysis: implications for valve prosthesis selection. *Ann Thorac Surg.* 2002;74(1):37–42.
87. Jamieson WRE, von Lipinski O, Miyagishima RT, et al. Performance of bioprostheses and mechanical prostheses assessed by composites of valve-related complications to 15 years after mitral valve replacement. *J Thorac Cardiovasc Surg.* 2005;129(6):1301–1308.
88. Puskas J, Gerdisch M, Nichols D, et al. Reduced anticoagulation after mechanical aortic valve replacement: interim results from the prospective randomized on-X valve anticoagulation clinical trial randomized Food and Drug Administration investigational device exemption trial. *J Thorac Cardiovasc Surg.* 2014;147(4):1202–1210; discussion 1210–1211.
89. Gulbins H, Kreuzer E, Uhlig A, et al. Mitral valve surgery utilizing homografts: early results. *J Heart Valve Dis.* 2000;9(2): 222–229.
90. Brown JW, Ruzmetov M, Turrentine MW, et al. Mitral valve replacement with the pulmonary autograft: Ross II procedure with Kabanni modification. *Semin Thorac Cardiovasc Surg Pediatr Card Surg Annu.* 2004;7:107–114.
91. Athanasiou T, Cherian A, Ross D. The Ross II procedure: pulmonary autograft in the mitral position. *Ann Thorac Surg.* 2004;78(4):1489–1495.
92. Lehmann S, Walther T, Kempfert J, et al. Stentless mitral valve implantation in comparison to conventional mitral valve repair or replacement at five years. *Thorac Cardiovasc Surg.* 2006;54(1):10–14.
93. Ali M, Iung B, Lansac E, et al. Homograft replacement of the mitral valve: eight-year results. *J Thorac Cardiovasc Surg.* 2004;128(4):529–534.
94. Deac RF, Simionescu D, Deac D. New evolution in mitral physiology and surgery: mitral stentless pericardial valve. *Ann Thorac Surg.* 1995;60(2 Suppl):S433–S438.
95. Kumar AS, Choudhary SK, Mathur A, et al. Homograft mitral valve replacement: five years' results. *J Thorac Cardiovasc Surg.* 2000;120(3):450–458.
96. Mohr FW, Lehmann S, Falk V, et al. Clinical Experience With Stentless Mitral Valve Replacement. *Ann Thorac Surg.* 2005;79(3):772–775.
97. Walther T, Rastan A, Falk V, et al. Patient prosthesis mismatch affects short- and long-term outcomes after aortic valve replacement. *Eur J Cardiothorac Surg.* 2006;30(1):15–19.
98. Lam B-K, Chan V, Hendry P, et al. The impact of patient-prosthesis mismatch on late outcomes after mitral valve replacement. *J Thorac Cardiovasc Surg.* 2007;133(6):1464–1473.
99. Pibarot P, Dumesnil JG. Prosthesis-patient mismatch: definition, clinical impact, and prevention. *Heart Br Card Soc.* 2006;92(8):1022–1029.
100. Magne J, Mathieu P, Dumesnil JG, et al. Impact of Prosthesis-Patient Mismatch on Survival After Mitral Valve Replacement. *Circulation.* 2007;115(11):1417–1425.
101. Castro LJ, Arcidi JM, Fisher AL, Gaudiani VA. Routine enlargement of the small aortic root: a preventive strategy to minimize mismatch. *Ann Thorac Surg.* 2002;74(1):31–36; discussion 36.
102. Coutinho GF, Antunes MJ. Mitral valve repair for degenerative mitral valve disease: surgical approach, patient selection and long-term outcomes. *Heart Br Card Soc.* 2017;103(21):1663–1669.
103. Imanaka K, Kyo S, Ogiwara M, et al. Mitral valve surgery under perfused ventricular fibrillation with moderate hypothermia. *Circ J Off J Jpn Circ Soc.* 2002;66(5):450–452.
104. Takami Y, Tajima K, Terazawa S, et al. Safer aortic crossclamping during short-term moderate hypothermic circulatory arrest for cardiac surgery in patients with a bad ascending aorta. *J Thorac Cardiovasc Surg.* 2009;137(4):875–880.
105. Pezzella AT, Effler DB, Levy IE. Operative Approaches to the Left Atrium and Mitral Valve Apparatus. *Tex Heart Inst J.* 1983;10(2):119–123.
106. Winter FS. Persistent left superior vena cava; survey of world literature and report of thirty additional cases. *Angiology.* 1954;5(2):90–132.
107. Horrow JC, Lingaraju N. Unexpected persistent left superior vena cava: diagnostic clues during monitoring. *J Cardiothorac Anesth.* 1989;3(5):611–615.
108. Choudhry AK, Conacher ID, Hilton CJ, et al. Persistent left superior vena cava. *J Cardiothorac Anesth.* 1989;3(5):616–619.
109. Yokota M, Kyoku I, Kitano M, et al. Atresia of the coronary sinus orifice. Fatal outcome after intraoperative division of the drainage left superior vena cava. *J Thorac Cardiovasc Surg.* 1989;98(1):30–32.
110. Pezzella AT, Utley JR. Vander Salm TJ. operative approaches to the left atrium and mitral valve: an update. *Oper Tech Thoracic Cardiovasc Surg.* 1998;3(2):74–94.
111. Barner HB. Combined superior and right lateral left atriotomy with division of the superior vena cava for exposure of the mitral valve. *Ann Thorac Surg.* 1985;40(4):365–367.

112. Kon ND, Tucker WY, Mills SA, et al. Mitral valve operation via an extended transseptal approach. *Ann Thorac Surg.* 1993;55(6):1413–1416; discussion 1416–1417.
113. Selle JG. Temporary division of the superior vena cava for exceptional mitral valve exposure. *J Thorac Cardiovasc Surg.* 1984;88(2):302–304.
114. Kyger ER, Coselli M, Kalchoff WP. A method for improved exposure of the mitral valve: cannulation of innominate vein and division of superior vena cava for extended left atriotomy in mitral valve operations. *J Thorac Cardiovasc Surg.* 1986;91(1):143–146.
115. Larbalestier RI, Chard RB, Cohn LH. Optimal approach to the mitral valve: dissection of the interatrial groove. *Ann Thorac Surg.* 1992;54(6):1186–1188.
116. Lillehei CW, Levy MJ, Bonnabeau RC. Mitral valve replacement with preservation of papillary muscles and chordae tendineae. *J Thorac Cardiovasc Surg.* 1964;47:532–543.
117. Guo Y, He S, Wang T, et al. Comparison of modified total leaflet preservation, posterior leaflet preservation, and no leaflet preservation techniques in mitral valve replacement—a retrospective study. *J Cardiothorac Surg.* 2019;14(1):102.
118. Okita Y, Miki S, Ueda Y, et al. Mid-term results of mitral valve replacement combined with chordae tendineae replacement in patients with mitral stenosis. *J Heart Valve Dis.* 1997;6(1):37–42.
119. Sugita T, Matsumoto M, Nishizawa J, et al. Long-term outcome after mitral valve replacement with preservation of continuity between the mitral annulus and the papillary muscle in patients with mitral stenosis. *J Heart Valve Dis.* 2004;13(6):931–936.
120. Cohn LH, Couper GS, Kinchla NM, Collins JJ. Decreased operative risk of surgical treatment of mitral regurgitation with or without coronary artery disease. *J Am Coll Cardiol.* 1990;16(7):1575–1578.
121. David TE. Mitral valve replacement with preservation of chordae tendinae: rationale and technical considerations. *Ann Thorac Surg.* 1986;41(6):680–682.
122. Roberts WC, Perloff JK. Mitral valvular disease. A clinicopathologic survey of the conditions causing the mitral valve to function abnormally. *Ann Intern Med.* 1972;77(6):939–975.
123. Miller DW, Johnson DD, Ivey TD. Does Preservation of the Posterior Chordae Tendineae Enhance Survival during Mitral Valve Replacement? *Ann Thorac Surg.* 1979;28(1):22–27.
124. Huddleston SJ, Yuh DD. Mitral Valve Replacement. In: Yuh DD, Vricella LA, Yang SC, Doty JR, eds. *Johns Hopkins Textbook of Cardiothoracic Surgery*: McGraw-Hill Education; 2014.
125. Yun KL, Sintek CF, Miller DC, et al. Randomized trial comparing partial versus complete chordal-sparing mitral valve replacement: effects on left ventricular volume and function. *J Thorac Cardiovasc Surg.* 2002;123(4):707–714.
126. David TE, Armstrong S, Sun Z. Left ventricular function after mitral valve surgery. *J Heart Valve Dis.* 1995;4(Suppl 2):S175–S180.
127. Talwar S, Jayanthkumar H, Kumar PS. Chordal Preservation during mitral valve replacement: basis, techniques and results. *Indian J Thorac Cardiovasc Surg.* 2005;21:45–52.
128. Trites PN, Kiser JC, Johnson C, et al. Occlusion of Medtronic Hall mitral valve prosthesis by ruptured papillary muscle and chordae tendineae. *J Thorac Cardiovasc Surg.* 1984;88(2):301–302.
129. Hsieh WC, Aboud A, Henry BM, et al. Mitral Valve Replacement Using Subvalvular Apparatus: A Systematic Review and Meta-Analysis. *Heart Surg Forum.* 2020;23(3):E385–E392.
130. Ozdemir AC, Emrecan B, Baltalarli A. Bileaflet versus posterior-leaflet-only preservation in mitral valve replacement. *Tex Heart Inst J.* 2014;41(2):165–169.
131. Goor DA, Mohr R, Lavee J, et al. Preservation of the posterior leaflet during mechanical valve replacement for ischemic mitral regurgitation and complete myocardial revascularization. *J Thorac Cardiovasc Surg.* 1988;96(2):253–260.
132. Miki S, Kusuhara K, Ueda Y, et al. Mitral valve replacement with preservation of chordae tendineae and papillary muscles. *Ann Thorac Surg.* 1988;45(1):28–34.
133. Byrne JG, Aranki SF, Cohn LH. Repair versus replacement of mitral valve for treating severe ischemic mitral regurgitation. *Coron Artery Dis.* 2000;11(1):31–33.
134. Cohn LH, Rizzo RJ, Adams DH, et al. The effect of pathophysiology on the surgical treatment of ischemic mitral regurgitation: operative and late risks of repair versus replacement. *Eur J Cardiothorac Surg.* 1995;9(10):568–574.
135. Grossi EA, Goldberg JD, LaPietra A, et al. Ischemic mitral valve reconstruction and replacement: comparison of long-term survival and complications. *J Thorac Cardiovasc Surg.* 2001;122(6):1107–1124.
136. McEnany MT. Mitral valve replacement in the presence of severe valvular and annular calcification. *J Card Surg.* 1993;8(2): 117–124.
137. Borger MA, Yau TM, Rao V, et al. Reoperative mitral valve replacement: importance of preservation of the subvalvular apparatus. *Ann Thorac Surg.* 2002;74(5):1482–1487.
138. Soga Y, Nishimura K, Ikeda T, et al. Chordal-sparing mitral valve replacement using artificial chordae tendineae for rheumatic mitral stenosis: experience of the "oblique" method. *Artif Organs.* 2002;26(9):802–805.
139. Lafci G, Cagli K, Cicek OF, et al. Papillary Muscle Repositioning as a Subvalvular Apparatus Preservation Technique in Mitral Stenosis Patients with Normal Left Ventricular Systolic Function. *Tex Heart Inst J.* 2014;41(1):33–39.
140. Cohn LH. Tricuspid regurgitation secondary to mitral valve disease: when and how to repair. *J Card Surg.* 1994;9(2 Suppl):237–241.
141. Gillinov AM. Mitral valve replacement after late failure of mitral valve repair. *Oper Tech Thorac Cardiovasc Surg.* 2003;8(1):42–50.
142. Karuppiah S, George G, Chacko B, Philip MA. Entrapped left atrial pressure monitoring catheter in a prosthetic mitral valve. *Ann Card Anaesth.* 2015;18(2):276–277.
143. Akins CW, Bitondo JM, Hilgenberg AD, et al. Early and late results of the surgical correction of cardiac prosthetic paravalvular leaks. *J Heart Valve Dis.* 2005;14(6):792–799; discussion 799–800.
144. Dávila-Román VG, Waggoner AD, Kennard ED, et al. Prevalence and severity of paravalvular regurgitation in the Artificial Valve Endocarditis Reduction Trial (AVERT) echocardiography study. *J Am Coll Cardiol.* 2004;44(7):1467–1472.
145. O'Rourke DJ, Palac RT, Malenka DJ, et al. Outcome of mild periprosthetic regurgitation detected by intraoperative transesophageal echocardiography. *J Am Coll Cardiol.* 2001;38(1):163–166.
146. Grossman W, Braunwald E, Mann T, et al. Contractile state of the left ventricle in man as evaluated from end-systolic pressure-volume relations. *Circulation.* 1977;56(5):845–852.
147. Gandhavadi M, Cox EJ. Prevalence of intra-atrial reentrant tachycardia following mitral valve surgery: Relationship to surgical approach. *J Card Surg.* 2020;35(8):1871–1876.
148. Izzat MB, Aljasem H, Alsharabi M, et al. Comparison of safety and outcomes with two approaches to the mitral valve. *J Card Surg.* 2020;35(7):1458–1463.
149. Dobrilovic N, Raman J, Fingleton JG, et al. Long-term outcomes of external repair as a rescue operation for atrioventricular groove disruption. *Ann Thorac Surg.* 2017;103(2):491–496.

150. Sersar SI, Jamjoom AA. Left ventricular rupture post mitral valve replacement. *Clin Med Cardiol.* 2009;3:101–113.
151. Zacharias A. Repair of spontaneous rupture of the posterior wall of the left ventricle after mitral valve replacement. *Oper Tech Thorac Cardiovasc Surg.* 2003;8(1):36–41.
152. Goel NJ, Iyengar A, Kelly JJ, et al. Causes, Risk Factors, and Costs of 30-Day Readmissions After Mitral Valve Repair and Replacement. *Ann Thorac Surg.* 2019;108(6):1729–1737.
153. Fernandes V, Olmos L, Nagueh SF, et al. Peak early diastolic velocity rather than pressure half-time is the best index of mechanical prosthetic mitral valve function. *Am J Cardiol.* 2002;89(6):704–710.
154. Zoghbi WA, Enriquez-Sarano M, Foster E, et al. Recommendations for evaluation of the severity of native valvular regurgitation with two-dimensional and Doppler echocardiography. *J Am Soc Echocardiogr.* 2003;16(7):777–802.
155. Bach DS. Transesophageal echocardiographic (TEE) evaluation of prosthetic valves. *Cardiol Clin.* 2000;18(4):751–771.
156. Jamieson WRE, Cartier PC, Allard M, et al. Surgical management of valvular heart disease 2004. *Can J Cardiol.* 2004;20 (suppl E):7E–120E.
157. Heras M, Chesebro JH, Fuster V, et al. High risk of thromboemboli early after bioprosthetic cardiac valve replacement. *J Am Coll Cardiol.* 1995;25(5):1111–1119.
158. Whitlock RP, Sun JC, Fremes SE, et al. *Antithrombotic and thrombolytic therapy for valvular disease: Antithrombotic Therapy and Prevention of Thrombosis.* 9th ed. American College of Chest Physicians Evidence-Based Clinical Practice Guidelines. *Chest.* 2012;141(2 Suppl):e576S–e600S.
159. Carnicelli AP, O'Gara PT, Giugliano RP. Anticoagulation after heart valve replacement or transcatheter valve implantation. *Am J Cardiol.* 2016;118(9):1419–1426.
160. Colli A, Verhoye J-P, Heijmen R, et al. Antithrombotic therapy after bioprosthetic aortic valve replacement: ACTION Registry survey results. *Eur J Cardiothorac Surg.* 2008;33(4):531–536.
161. Bloomfield P, Wheatley DJ, Prescott RJ, et al. Twelve-year comparison of a Bjork-Shiley mechanical heart valve with porcine bioprostheses. *N Engl J Med.* 1991;324(9):573–579.
162. Vesey JM, Otto CM. Complications of prosthetic heart valves. *Curr Cardiol Rep.* 2004;6(2):106–111.
163. Kovacs MJ, Kearon C, Rodger M, et al. Single-arm study of bridging therapy with low-molecular-weight heparin for patients at risk of arterial embolism who require temporary interruption of warfarin. *Circulation.* 2004;110(12):1658–1663.
164. Cohn LH, Mudge GH, Pratter F, Collins JJ. Five to eight-year follow-up of patients undergoing porcine heart-valve replacement. *N Engl J Med.* 1981;304(5):258–262.
165. Butchart EG, Payne N, Li H-H, et al. Better anticoagulation control improves survival after valve replacement. *J Thorac Cardiovasc Surg.* 2002;123(4):715–723.
166. Butchart EG, Gohlke-Bärwolf C, Antunes MJ, et al. Recommendations for the management of patients after heart valve surgery. *Eur Heart J.* 2005;26(22):2463–2471.
167. Vahanian A, Baumgartner H, Bax J, et al. Guidelines on the management of valvular heart disease: The Task Force on the Management of Valvular Heart Disease of the European Society of Cardiology. *Eur Heart J.* 2007;28(2):230–268.
168. Bonow RO, Carabello BA, Chatterjee K, et al. 2008 Focused update incorporated into the ACC/AHA 2006 guidelines for the management of patients with valvular heart disease: a report of the American College of Cardiology/American Heart Association Task Force on Practice Guidelines (Writing Committee to Revise the 1998 Guidelines for the Management of Patients With Valvular Heart Disease): endorsed by the Society of Cardiovascular Anesthesiologists, Society for Cardiovascular Angiography and Interventions, and Society of Thoracic Surgeons. *Circulation.* 2008;118(15):e523–e661.
169. Roudaut R, Serri K, Lafitte S. Thrombosis of prosthetic heart valves: diagnosis and therapeutic considerations. *Heart Br Card Soc.* 2007;93(1):137–142.
170. Vesey JM, Otto CM. Complications of prosthetic heart valves. *Curr Cardiol Rep.* 2004;6(2):106–111.
171. Baddour LM, Wilson WR, Bayer AS, et al. Infective Endocarditis in Adults: Diagnosis, Antimicrobial Therapy, and Management of Complications: A Scientific Statement for Healthcare Professionals From the American Heart Association. *Circulation.* 2015;132(15):1435–1486.

21

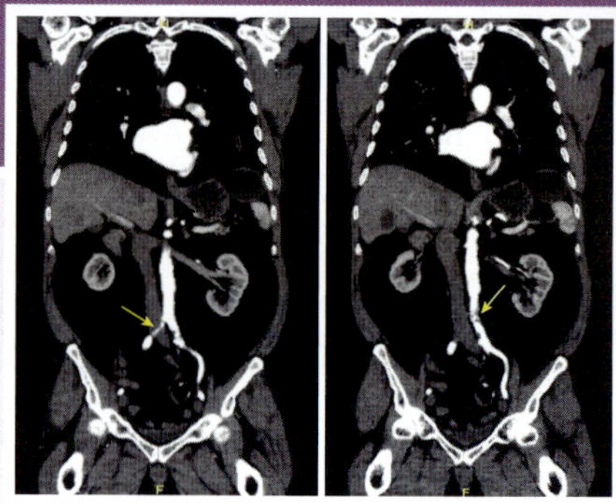

Evaluation, Common Pitfalls, and Complications

Robert L. Smith II, Lee Hafen, John J. Squiers

CHAPTER OUTLINE

LEARNING OBJECTIVES

1. Understand the separate preoperative and intraoperative phases of surgical evaluation of mitral valve (MV) disease.
2. Understand evaluation of MV disease in the preoperative phase of care to include indications for surgery, patient suitability for surgery, and determination of surgical approach.
3. Understand intraoperative evaluation of MV disease to include anatomic features of the MV as well as anatomical and hemodynamic assessment of the adequacy of the completed procedure.

INTRODUCTION

Surgical evaluation of the patient with mitral valve (MV) pathology involves an algorithmic analysis oriented to the objectives of the relevant phase of care. Preoperatively, evaluation is centered on determining patient suitability for surgery, whether guideline indications for MV surgery and any other necessary procedures are present, and the surgical approach and general surgical planning. Intraoperatively, the evaluation focuses primarily on anatomical features of the valve that will affect the conduct of the procedure, as well as an anatomic and hemodynamic assessment of the adequacy of the completed procedure or need for revision. Thorough evaluation of the patient, their MV pathology, and adequacy of the operation, as well as avoidance of common pitfalls throughout the process, will yield the highest likelihood of a successful outcome while minimizing risks. This chapter reviews strategies for comprehensive evaluation of patients with surgical MV disease, including common pitfalls and potential complications that may be avoided by careful preparation and planning.

PREOPERATIVE EVALUATION

During the preoperative evaluation, an appropriate workup includes the collection of a thorough history, performance of a detailed physical examination, and completion of diagnostic tests/studies that will facilitate planning a successful operation. There are several important questions the surgeon must consider when evaluating the patient preoperatively. Whether the patient has mitral stenosis (MS) or mitral regurgitation (MR), each of these questions must be addressed:

1. Does the patient meet current guideline criteria for MV surgery?
2. Are any concomitant procedures indicated?
3. What operative approach is most appropriate?
4. Is the valve repairable, or is replacement necessary?
5. Is the patient medically optimized for cardiac surgery?

Mitral Valve Surgery Guidelines

In patients of suitable surgical risk, MV surgery should be contemplated when a guideline-based indication for surgery is present. Complete guidelines can be obtained elsewhere.[1–3] However, it is worth noting specific subtleties relevant to MR where errors in decision-making are more common. Differentiating between primary and functional MR is critical, as not only do the indications for surgery differ based on the presence or absence of symptoms and the degree of heart failure, but the repair techniques also differ, including the decision to place a ring versus a band, band sizing, and leaflet interventions.

- MV surgery is a Class I recommendation for **symptomatic** patients with chronic, severe **primary** MR and left ventricular ejection fraction (LVEF) greater than 30%.
- MV surgery is a Class I recommendation for **asymptomatic** patients with chronic, severe **primary** MR and LVEF 30% to 60% and/or left ventricular end-systolic diameter (LVESD) at least 40 mm (45 mm, European guidelines).
- MV surgery is reasonable (Class IIa recommendation) for **asymptomatic** patients with chronic, severe **primary** MR and LVEF at least 60% and LVESD less than 40 mm if the likelihood of repair is at least 95%, mortality risk is less than 1%, and operation is performed at a center of excellence.
    - European guidelines more specifically modify this subset to asymptomatic patients with preserved LV function who also have new-onset atrial fibrillation (AF) and pulmonary hypertension at rest, without the stipulation for the likelihood of durable repair or mortality/risk. Also, a specific category is included for asymptomatic, severe MR with preserved LV function in those with flail leaflet, with the stipulation for the likelihood of repair with low mortality/risk.
- MV surgery may be considered (Class IIb recommendation) for **severely symptomatic** patients (New York Heart Association [NYHA] Class III or IV) with chronic, severe **secondary** MR with persistent symptoms despite guideline-directed medical therapy for heart failure.

The fastest-growing segment of the United States population is the elderly, and the prevalence of valvular disease increases with age. The diagnostic and therapeutic complexity of valvular heart disease increases in conjunction with the costs to provide this care as the number of medical and procedural therapies grow. However, these advances expand the cohort of patients with valvular disease who may benefit from evaluation by a valve-specific team at a center of excellence. For these reasons, those of prohibitive surgical risk or patients who may currently lack a clear indication for surgery still benefit from evaluation by a heart team who will ensure guideline-directed diagnostic studies, medical treatment, follow-up, and pursue alternative therapies. A recently published expert consensus statement outlines minimum requirements for centers offering valvular interventions, with a focus on the capabilities of centers offering MV surgery and transcatheter MV interventions in the setting of a valvular heart disease system of care.[4]

A gap analysis related to the care of MV regurgitation was published in 2016 and highlights several of the pitfalls associated with MV surgery guidelines.[5]

PITFALL

Misclassification of Primary/Secondary Mitral Regurgitation

Primary MR is due to the pathology of the mitral annulus, leaflets, chordae tendineae, or papillary muscles. Secondary (or functional) MR is due to restricted leaflet mobility and poor coaptation of otherwise normal leaflets. Rarely, a mixed etiology may complicate classification. Additionally, specific findings such as anterior leaflet pseudoprolapse in chronic ischemic MR must be recognized to avoid misclassification, emphasizing the need for an experienced, multidisciplinary heart team. In general, this first step of correctly classifying the predominant mechanism will guide the appropriate type and timing of therapy.

PITFALL

Delaying Surgical Therapy

Between 19% and 24% of cardiologists delayed surgical referral due to a lack of understanding of the LVESD and pulmonary hypertension indications for surgery in asymptomatic patients with chronic, severe primary MR.[6,7] Careful assessment of cardiac limitation to physical activity or a change from a previous level of activity are symptoms that are likely attributable to MR and stresses the importance of close follow-up and thorough history to avoid incorrectly classifying symptomatic patients as asymptomatic. Failure to offer surgery when an indication to operate is present may result in higher operative risk associated with the delayed surgery as well as irreversible pulmonary hypertension, atrial fibrillation, and left ventricular systolic dysfunction.

PITFALL

Access to High-Quality Mitral Valve Interventions

A recent expert consensus statement has outlined a proposal for the designation of comprehensive and primary valve surgery centers to balance optimization of outcomes with sufficient access to valve experts.[8] This document suggests that surgeons at primary valve centers have sufficient expertise regarding MV repair for posterior leaflet primary MR and MV replacement. Any other MV interventions should be performed at comprehensive valve centers, according to expert recommendations.

Concomitant Procedures

In patients referred for MV surgery, a transthoracic echocardiogram (TTE) has almost certainly been performed. This TTE, and any prior available echocardiograms, should be reviewed in detail by the surgeon. If the quality of the TTE is insufficient to evaluate the function of all cardiac valves, other structural anatomy, and biventricular function, a repeat TTE or transesophageal echocardiogram (TEE) should be obtained. We have a low threshold for obtaining a TEE whenever any additional valvular abnormality is identified on TTE. We also obtain TEE when the process responsible for MV pathology is not obvious. For example, a TEE is warranted in cases of restrictive valve disease that appears functional but is without any underlying ventricular dysfunction, with consideration of valvulitis or amyloid disease if ventricular walls are thickened in an elderly patient.

The aortic valve should be evaluated for aortic stenosis (AS) or aortic insufficiency (AI), and if present at more than a mild degree, TEE is warranted. It is more common to diagnose significant MR while working up AS (present in 15% to 20% and primary in about 50%) than to find AS while working up primary MR. However, in the setting of classical low-flow, low-gradient AS, where the severity of AS may not be appreciated, the patient may be sent initially for evaluation due to MR. It is important to consider the effect of MR when evaluating AS, as the severity of MR is a major determinant of a low-flow state, which may underestimate the degree of AS and result in one or both valve lesions being observed rather than intervened upon. Aortic valve surgery, concomitant with MV surgery, is recommended for severe AS or AI (Class I) and considered reasonable for moderate AS or AI (Class IIa). However, simultaneous aortic and MV surgery is associated with increased mortality. Therefore, after assessment of individual patient risk, consideration may be given to staged procedures, that is, MV repair followed by transcatheter aortic valve replacement (TAVR) or, alternatively, surgical aortic valve replacement (SAVR) or TAVR with a period of observation for improvement in functional MR, followed by percutaneous MV intervention if necessary.[9,10,11]

Another scenario that warrants thoughtful consideration is the presence of simultaneous AS and MS, which may be due to degenerative disease or, less commonly, rheumatic disease. In fact, this scenario is not uncommon, as up to 17% of concomitant aortic valve-MV operations are for AS/MS, suggesting the need for particular mention.[12] The physiology of the combined lesions can complicate echocardiographic diagnosis, and suspicion of combined AS/MS based on the appearance of significant calcification or thickening may indicate invasive hemodynamic pressure measurements for sound diagnosis. Although both the American and European valvular heart disease guidelines address concomitant aortic and MV surgery for respective stenoses, in conjunction with other cardiac surgeries, they do not specifically address this challenging combined lesion set. Double valve surgery for combined degenerative stenotic disease has nearly twice the mortality rate of isolated surgery based on Society of Thoracic Surgeons (STS) data.[13] The presence of both AS and MS is historically associated with 40% to 50% mortality over a 10 to 20 year period, and patients with AS are more likely to have NYHA class IV heart failure, dialysis dependence, and associated valve insufficiency when MS is present compared to when it is not. TAVR has been increasingly used in this high-risk scenario; in fact, about 10% of TAVR valves are placed in patients with MS, with a resultant increased incidence of 1-year adverse outcomes.[14] The emergence of more transcatheter MV options has expanded the possibilities of managing this problem through a totally percutaneous route, although data is lacking.[15] Though currently under formal clinical trial investigation, we have implemented surgical implantation of a transcatheter valve in native mitral annular calcification (SITRAL) concomitantly with TAVR for aortic stenosis with some early success.[16]

Functional tricuspid regurgitation is common in the setting of MR, with at least moderate tricuspid regurgitation (TR) occurring in up to 20% of patients. Although multiple studies show improvement in the grade of TR after the reduction in volume overload that occurs with MV surgery, the long-term effect is not optimal. TR is found in up to 74% of patients followed long term after left side valve surgery. Additionally, reoperation for tricuspid valve disease confers operative mortality up to 37%. The challenge in cases of functional tricuspid regurgitation is determining which patients will have a long-term favorable improvement in TR due to right ventricle (RV) remodeling and volume overload reduction by MV surgery alone and which patients require concomitant TV surgery.

Fortunately, there are prospective, randomized trials in progress to address this question, but these are not completed as of yet. There are, however, multiple retrospective studies that evaluate small cohorts of patients at single centers, comparing outcomes in MV surgery patients who have or have not undergone concomitant tricuspid valve repair.[17,18] Clearly, selection bias is inevitable with this design. Additionally, the criteria to opt for tricuspid valve surgery vary by study, some basing the decision on the grade of TR, annulus size, RV dysfunction, or a combination, making a meta-analysis or systematic review difficult. All current guidelines related to tricuspid valve surgery have a "C" level of evidence. Concomitant tricuspid surgery is recommended for patients with severe tricuspid regurgitation at the time of left-side valve surgery (Class I). Concomitant tricuspid valve repair can be beneficial (Class IIa) for any grade TR when there is tricuspid annular dilation (annulus greater than 40 mm on TTE, greater than 21 mm/m^2 indexed to body surface area, or greater than 70 mm on direct intraoperative measurement) or prior evidence of right-sided heart failure. Concomitant tricuspid repair may be considered (Class IIb) in patients with pulmonary artery hypertension. A best-evidence review found that the downside to concomitant tricuspid valve surgery was prolonged clamp, cardiopulmonary bypass, and total operative times, but this effect on surgical times did not result in an increase in perioperative complications or mortality.[19] A study following postoperative patients by echocardiographic imaging found improved right ventricular function and geometry if TV annuloplasty was performed.[20] With median 7-year follow-ups, two studies have shown that if mild-moderate TR in the setting of tricuspid annular dilation or RV dysfunction was left untreated during MV surgery, patients had persistent or worsened TR long-term and freedom from moderate-severe TR, or TR progression declined over long-term follow-up.[21,22] A recent study from 2020 showed that aggressive adherence to guideline recommendations in 171 consecutive patients was safe, with a low mortality rate, pacemaker rate equivalent to isolated MV surgery, and high freedom from moderate or worse TR at 14 months.[23] The conclusions of most of these studies are a recommendation for more aggressive adherence to guidelines regarding concomitant TR at the time of MV surgery.

Hypertrophic cardiomyopathy (HCM) is the most common inherited myocardial disease, with wide phenotypic expression, frequently occurring in conjunction with MR. The mechanism for MR can be multifactorial, complicating operative planning. Septal hypertrophy narrows the left ventricular outflow tract (LVOT), which can create a dynamic outflow tract obstruction during systole, especially with any abnormality in the MV. In most cases, septal myectomy alone will eliminate the pressure gradient, resolving both the systolic anterior motion (SAM) of the anterior mitral leaflet and the associated SAM-related MR. However, there are phenotypic variations of HCM with anatomic abnormalities of the MV/subvalvular apparatus favoring SAM by anteriorly shifting coaptation. These abnormalities include elongation of the anterior leaflet, anterior displacement and abnormal insertion of papillary muscles, and abnormal attachment of chordae. Typical primary etiologies for MR may coexist as well, such as flail or prolapsing leaflets. In these situations, concomitant MV repair is required to relieve LVOT obstruction and address valvular abnormalities causing MR, in addition to myectomy. There also exist phenotypes where MV abnormalities are present in association with little to no septal hypertrophy. It is important to recognize the possibility of HCM when SAM is present on preoperative TTE, even if there is minimal septal hypertrophy, because a limited myectomy may ultimately be required to alleviate LVOT.[24]

Diagnosing concomitant coronary artery disease (CAD) with degenerative MV disease has implications on the approach to the operation, eliminating the option for typical minimally invasive techniques if present and warranting bypass. In a single-institution review of a 20-year experience with degenerative MV disease, 26% of MV operations for degenerative disease included coronary artery bypass grafting (CABG).[25] In contrast to ischemic functional MR, where a diagnosis of CAD is mandated and thus workup is aimed at defining its severity, in patients with degenerative MR, the incidence of concomitant CAD should mimic the general population. Therefore, a standardized system for coronary clearance should be routinely followed in these patients based on risk factor analysis. Importantly, there is better long-term survival when MV repair is performed over replacement in patients with degenerative MR undergoing MV surgery with concomitant coronary artery bypass.[26] In individualized cases, minimally invasive MV surgery may be staged with percutaneous coronary intervention (PCI) though this requires careful planning and thoughtful consideration by the heart team.

At the patient encounter, any arrhythmias should be specifically elucidated on history, physical exam, and electrocardiogram. As previously discussed, the presence of any arrhythmias, particularly AF, has implications on timing and indications for MV surgery. Guidelines for the surgical management of AF divide indications into concomitant and stand-alone ablation.[27] Guidelines for concomitant surgical ablation are further separated into two scenarios—symptomatic patients who are intolerant to at least one Class 1 or 3 antiarrhythmic and symptomatic patients who have yet to start a Class 1 or 3 antiarrhythmic. In both cases, concomitant ablation is a Class IIa recommendation for all categories of AF (paroxysmal, persistent, long-standing persistent) except in long-standing persistent AF where an antiarrhythmic has not been started, in which case the recommendation is Class IIb. The guidelines conclude that a more extensive ablation is superior to pulmonary vein isolation (PVI) and that a biatrial procedure should be considered in symptomatic patients and those with long-standing persistent AF. Intervention has also been recommended in the literature for asymptomatic patients to improve quality of life and survival while decreasing the risk of stroke or heart failure; however, these indications were not included in the most recent guidelines.

Prior to MV surgery, computed tomography (CT) of the chest is routinely obtained, with the mandatory addition of abdomen and pelvis imaging with contrast if a minimally invasive approach is under consideration. The most common findings that alter our planned operative approach are proximal aortic or peripheral arterial disease, as these affect clamping and cannulation strategies. Details are discussed later in this chapter. Additional findings on CT that may impact the operation are concomitant aneurysms of the aortic root, ascending aorta, or aortic arch. Even when cardiac surgery is planned, the recommendation for replacement of the thoracic aorta remains dilation of at least 5.5 cm in the absence of connective tissue disorders, including bicuspid aortic valve, which may otherwise mandate a lower threshold for repair.

Operative Approach

The surgical approach to the MV can be broadly divided into sternotomy or sternum-sparing techniques. A sternum-sparing approach involves access to the MV through the right chest, whether by mini-anterolateral thoracotomy or robotic-assisted surgery. The decision regarding which approach to pursue depends on multiple factors, some of which are objective, based on preoperative imaging studies and patient characteristics, while others depend on surgeon experience and judgment as well as patient preference.

Sternotomy is clearly the approach of choice when certain concomitant procedures are indicated, including aortic valve replacement, aortic aneurysm repair, or Coronary artery bypass grafting (CABG). However, alternative treatment modalities to address concomitant pathologies, such as TAVR or PCI, may be more appropriate options in individualized patient scenarios. This determination is based on patient and pathology factors, such as age, frailty, and expected benefit to the patient's recovery by accessing the MV in a minimally invasive manner rather than sternotomy. In particular, the surgeon must consider the presence of a hostile mediastinum due to prior surgery or radiation and patent bypass grafts under the sternum or around the right atrium in patients with a prior history of CABG. In these situations, entry to the pericardium and left atrium may be simplified by approaching the mediastinum from the right chest, and alternative treatments for concomitant pathology may be advantageous.

Any patient being considered for a minimally invasive approach to MV surgery requires a CT-angiogram of the chest, abdomen, and pelvis. Our preferred site for peripheral cardiopulmonary bypass cannulation is the right common femoral artery and right femoral vein. CT-angiography allows evaluation of the extent of calcification at the cannulation site and vessel size, either of which may preclude utilization of the femoral artery for cannulation (Fig. 21.1). Likewise, the presence of extensive

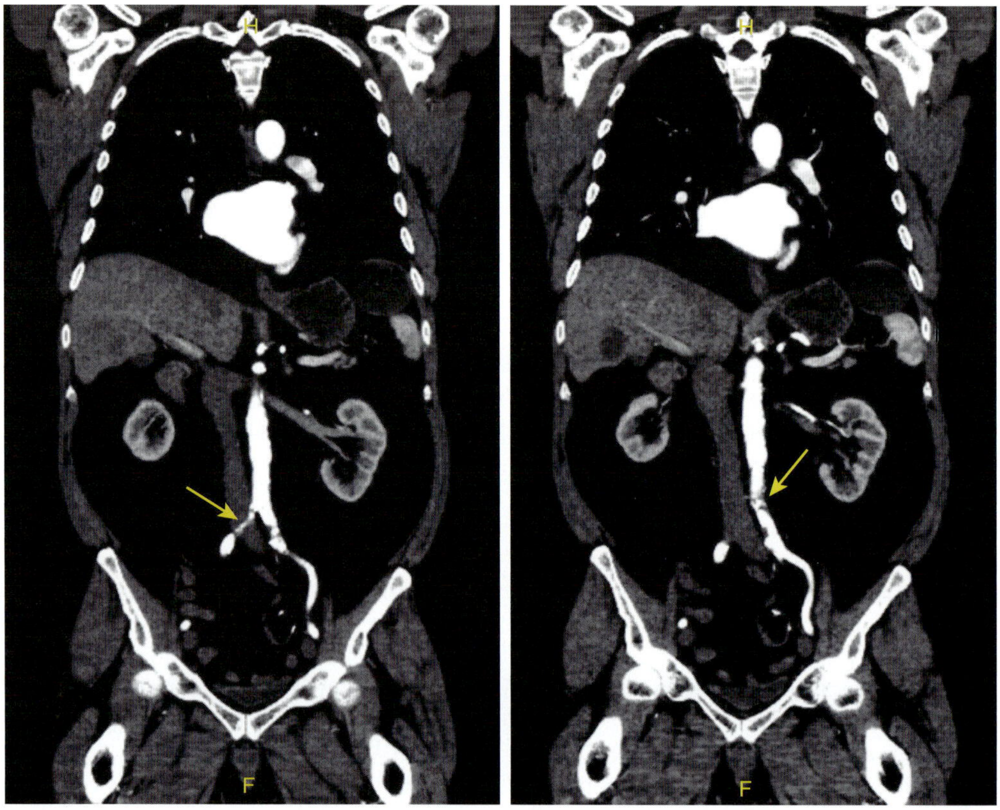

Fig. 21.1 Coronal computed tomography angiography of chest, abdomen, and pelvis revealing severe aortoiliac atherosclerotic disease *(yellow arrows)* that was not present more distally in the femoral vessels. In this case, axillary cannulation was selected.

calcification or plaque within the aorta is a contraindication to the use of retrograde flow due to the risk of embolic stroke, which is two to three times more likely with peripheral cannulation than central.[28,29] When any of these findings are present, we must decide whether to persist in the minimally invasive route by finding an alternative cannulation site, such as the right axillary artery, or to adjust plans and proceed with sternotomy. This decision is often made by determining the relative benefit we expect a patient to derive from a minimally invasive approach, which includes less blood utilization, shorter ICU length of stay, and a faster return to work and driving.

Additional information that should be gleaned from the preoperative CT scan includes the presence of ascending aorta calcification that would preclude the placement of an aortic cross-clamp. In such cases, when a minimally invasive approach is planned, either an aortic balloon occlusion device is required, or the operation must be performed with cold fibrillatory arrest. A dilated ascending aorta and/or aortic root is a relative contraindication to balloon occlusion due to the tendency for balloon migration. Balloon migration can hinder exposure of the MV and may cause AI by distorting the root, altering the delivery of cardioplegia and causing left ventricular distention, both of which impair adequate cardioprotection.

Lung windows must also be evaluated on the preoperative CT. Severe chronic obstructive pulmonary disease (COPD) is a relative contraindication to accessing the MV valve from the thorax due to the risk of prolonged ventilator dependence as a result of longer clamp and cardiopulmonary bypass times. In patients with severe COPD, it may be safer to perform MV surgery through sternotomy to limit these times.[30]

In our experience, robotic-assisted surgery is the preferred approach in cases where MV repair is likely and anatomy favors peripheral cannulation. Robotic-assisted surgery provides the advantages of a clear, magnified, 3D view of the MV and subvalvular structures. The degrees of freedom allowed by wristed robotic instruments facilitate annulus suture placement. An assistant who is facile with suture organization and tying knots extracorporeally is essential to expedite these portions of the procedure. In patients where the likelihood of MV replacement is high, we prefer a port-access mini-anterolateral thoracotomy approach simply because prosthetic valves are too large to fit through the incision used for the assistant port in robotic cases.

Other considerations in planning the MV approach include patient size factors, such as the height of the thorax, amount of the chest occupied by the heart, and severe elevation of the right hemidiaphragm. Despite the use of diaphragm and pericardial retraction sutures and proper patient positioning, space restrictions may limit the ability to adequately expose the MV to safely and efficiently complete the operation minimally invasively (Fig. 21.2).

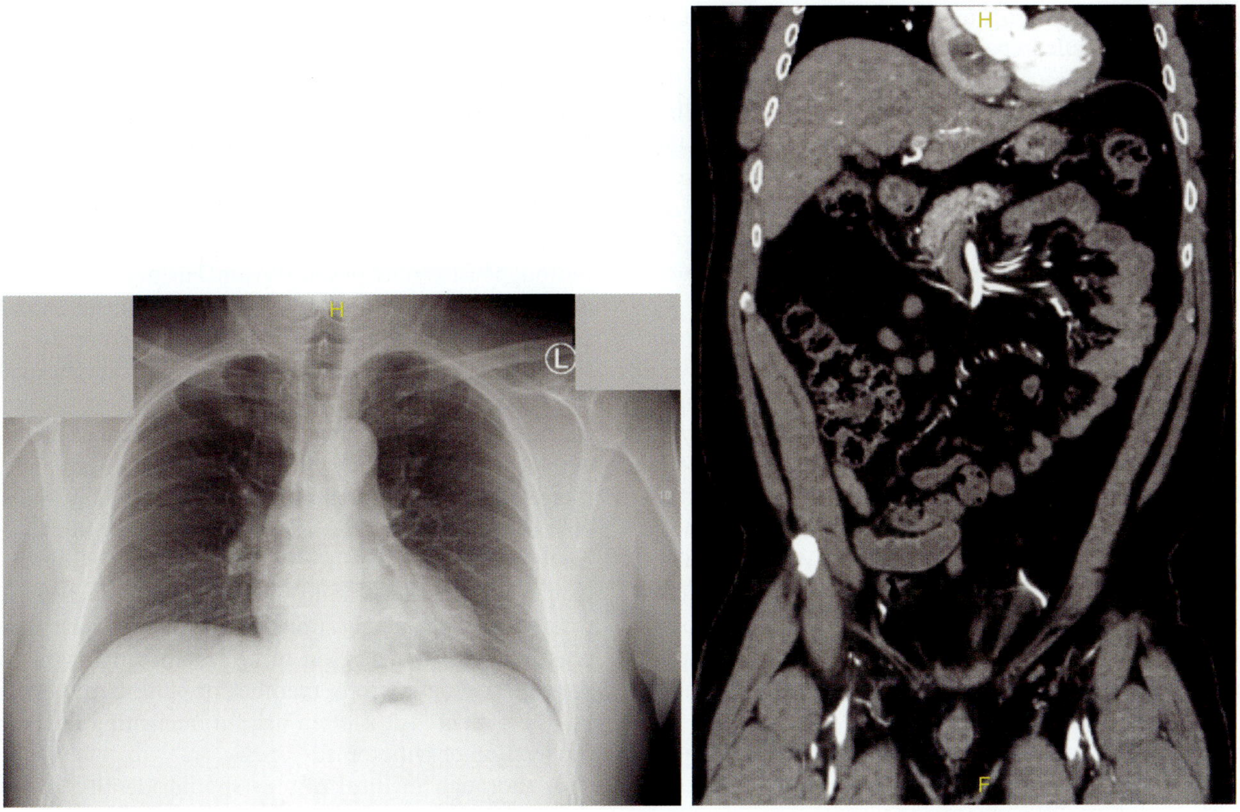

Fig. 21.2 Chest radiography and computed tomography of the abdomen revealing elevated right hemidiaphragm in patient planned for robot-assisted port-access mitral valve surgery. Entry was modified to the third interspace rather than the standard approach through the fourth interspace. Intraoperatively, a diaphragm stitch was placed to pull the diaphragm down to clear space for surgical instruments.

Once the minimally invasive approach has been chosen, avoidance of conversion to sternotomy is critical, though this still occurs in about 1% of cases in the hands of experts. In one study, conversion to sternotomy is associated with a host of poor outcomes, including increased cardiopulmonary bypass time, increased likelihood of postoperative low cardiac output syndrome with the need for aortic balloon pump or extracorporeal membrane oxygenation, increased postoperative renal failure, respiratory failure, stroke, multisystem organ failure, and increased 30-day mortality.[31]

Repair or Replacement?

With few exceptions, the determination of whether to repair or replace the MV should be made preoperatively based on a review of the TTE. In nearly all cases of primary MR, the valve can be repaired, and repair is the default intervention of expert surgeons. When the etiology is due to a prolapsed or flail leaflet segment(s), the affected segment(s) can usually be determined on TTE based on the trajectory of the regurgitant jet and the medial/lateral location on the annulus where the raised leaflet is seen. This information informs planning regarding the extensiveness of MV repair maneuvers that will be required. When repair is undertaken in secondary MR, placement of a reducing annuloplasty ring may be all that is required. Preoperative TTE does not provide an accurate estimate of annulus sizing and should be based on intraoperative measurement. However, the TTE is useful to note whether any predictors of postrepair LVOT obstruction are present that will need to be addressed during the procedure and which may alter the decision whether to downsize versus true-size the annuloplasty ring. MV replacement is acceptable when the following findings are present on TTE:

- *Mitral stenosis or regurgitation caused by rheumatic disease where leaflets and/or chordae are thickened, fused, and motion restricted.* Although in some cases of rheumatic disease, repair may be technically possible, progression of the disease is likely, so replacement is typically chosen. In many cases, chordae are thickened and shortened to the point where even a chordal-sparing technique is not possible.
- *Significant mitral annular calcification (MAC) is present.* In these cases, 4-dimensional cardiac CT is helpful to evaluate the extent of calcification and annular involvement. There are multiple techniques for replacement, including debridement of calcification, but when MAC is so extensive that it limits traditional MV replacement, we favor placement of a balloon-expandable valve into native MAC under direct and thoracoscopic vision.[32,57] This technique negates the need for annulus debridement, limiting the risk of groove disruption. These complicated techniques need to be performed at centers of excellence by surgeons with extensive experience. In cases with limited MAC, repair may still be feasible with

calcium debridement, resection of the affected portion of the valve leaflet, and leaflet repair with annuloplasty.

- *Mitral regurgitation caused by a short anterior leaflet.* In this case, although a repair may be technically possible by pulling in the free edge of the posterior leaflet, the coaptation height is likely to be too short for durable long-term repair. Also, by shifting the coaptation point anteriorly, the risk of LVOT obstruction by SAM of the anterior leaflet is created. When this scenario is present, a standard chordal sparing replacement is our preferred choice.
- *Significant leaflet or annulus destruction by infectious endocarditis.* TEE, and in some cases cardiac CT, is required to determine the extent of annulus destruction. When endocarditis is secondary to intravenous drug use, every attempt to repair the MV should be made to avoid implantation of prosthetic material that will be at increased risk of reinfection with continued drug use and at increased risk of thrombosis due to noncompliance with anticoagulation. When the infection involves either the left noncommissural aortic annulus or the anterior mitral annulus, involvement of the aortomitral curtain must be carefully ruled out, as this finding may require replacement of both the aortic valve and MV with a reconstruction of the aortomitral curtain.
- *Ischemic mitral regurgitation (IMR) is present.* This diagnosis portends a poor prognosis, and patients are often high-risk surgical candidates. When we encounter this problem, we obtain cardiac MRI to evaluate left ventricular dysfunction and viability before proceeding with surgical decision-making. Guidelines favor optimal medical therapy for heart failure along with cardiac resynchronization therapy (CRT) for severe MR with reduced ejection fraction (EF) and left ventricular (LV) dyssynchrony, with randomized controlled trials (RCTs) showing improvement in rehospitalization and survival. However, this improvement may only manifest in about half of patients. In those who do not have improved symptoms or quality of life with progressive LV remodeling and increased LV dysfunction (end-stage heart failure), transplantation or left ventricular assist device (LVAD) is a more effective treatment. In those with continued symptoms despite optimal medical and device therapy, without end-stage heart failure, with viable areas of the myocardium and high-grade proximal coronary lesions, surgery may be indicated. Due to a lack of evidence showing a survival benefit to concomitant MV surgery, indications are limited. There is a Class IIa recommendation for MV repair by reduction annuloplasty or replacement for chronic severe IMR when CABG or aortic valve surgery is being performed. Despite several studies, including three RCTs (Randomised Ischaemic Mitral Evaluation (RIME) Trial,[33] POINT,[34] and Cardiothoracic Surgical Trials Network [CTSN][35]) showing no survival benefit to MV repair in chronic moderate IMR, concomitant MV surgery in chronic moderate IMR with CABG is a Class IIb recommendation due to the proven improvement in reverse LV remodeling, LVEF, NYHA class, and MR grade. Another CTSN RCT showed similar survival comparing isolated reduction annuloplasty repair and replacement groups at 2 years for severe IMR with reduced MR recurrence and heart failure readmissions in the replacement group.[36] Therefore, surgical decision-making remains controversial in IMR and should be made in collaboration with an experienced heart team. When indications for surgery are met, proceeding with MV replacement is an acceptable option.[37]

Preoperative Medical Optimization

Evaluation of any patient with MV pathology must begin with a thorough history and physical exam. History should focus on the severity and progression of symptoms. While chest pain solely as a result of MV disease is possible, a chief complaint of angina should elicit a more complete workup for an alternate cause. Heart failure symptoms are more common and are sometimes subtle or progress so slowly that patients adjust their lifestyle without recognizing any change. Careful questioning can elicit these subtle points, specifically with regard to any limitations in physical activity that may be attributable to heart disease that has been compensated for by exertion modifications. In particular, the surgeon should probe for small changes since any prior visits. Specific questions about tiredness or daytime napping may clue the surgeon to symptoms unrecognized by the patient. Having a family member or close friend present during the patient visit is often helpful in eliciting the presence or progression of symptoms.

A thorough medical history should identify any problems that require optimization preoperatively. Taking into consideration medical comorbidities in conjunction with heart failure severity will render a prohibitive patient risk for MV surgery in some cases. These patients will be best managed with optimal guideline-directed medical therapy directed by the heart team. In some cases, the patient may be eligible for consideration for transcatheter MV interventions. This decision-making process can be guided by the use of the surgical risk calculator provided by the Society of Thoracic Surgeons.[38]

An accurate medication history is also crucial. Many patients whose heart failure regimen is optimized will experience improvement in symptoms, ventricular function, and in turn, the severity of MR. Similarly, patients with pacemakers may experience improvement in symptoms and function by optimizing pacer timing.

Antiplatelet and anticoagulant medications must be noted, and an appropriate preoperative plan regarding when and whether to hold these medications should be made.

Physical exam should focus on signs of volume overload. The lungs should be auscultated for signs of edema. The abdomen should be assessed for ascites or hepatomegaly. Extremities, including feet and ankles, should be examined to determine the extent of peripheral edema. Careful examination of the extremities will also alert to the presence of wounds as a result of arterial occlusive disease, venous stasis, or diabetes.

Basic laboratory studies, including nutritional markers and serum chemistry, should be ordered. All patients should have two-view plain films of the chest to evaluate for cardiomegaly and pulmonary edema or signs of pulmonary disease.

Based on the above evaluations, additional functional assessments and/or frailty evaluations may be warranted. Such evaluations include a 6-minute walk test, sit-to-stand test, and a mini-mental status exam. Each of these studies may further elucidate whether a patient has sufficient baseline resilience to withstand the surgical insult and recover well following MV intervention.[39]

After taking into consideration all of these factors, certain high-risk surgical candidates benefit from preadmission prior to MV surgery. They should be evaluated by a heart failure cardiology team to establish a plan for medical optimization, including intravenous diuretic therapy with or without the aid of inotropes and monitoring for organ dysfunction if at risk during this process. Preadmission also allows for bridging of anticoagulation, if necessary. Finally, preadmission also facilitates continuity of care with the appropriate specialist consultants if a complicated postoperative course is anticipated, particularly the nephrologists.

INTRAOPERATIVE EVALUATION

Intraoperatively, there are multiple critical junctures where accurate analysis of available information leads to a favorable outcome and avoidance of common pitfalls in patients with MV disease. The key decision-making points intraoperatively include:

1. Preincision TEE
2. Inspection of valvular structures
3. Testing and determination of the suitability of repair
4. Postcardiopulmonary bypass TEE and hemodynamic assessment

Preincision Transesophageal Echocardiogram

In most cases, a TEE will not have been obtained preoperatively. Although a general surgical plan should already be in place based on the preoperative TTE, the TEE performed by the anesthesiologist before an incision is crucial for refining the finer details of the operative plan. A thorough understanding of echocardiography by the surgeon is essential to jointly evaluate the structure and function of the heart with the anesthesiologist before commencing the operation. Careful attention to the TEE will ensure that no surprises are encountered, the operation may be conducted as efficiently as possible, and clamp time can be minimized.

We specifically and algorithmically evaluate each of the following items during preincision TEE before every operation.

Annulus Size

The intertrigone distance is measured to determine annuloplasty band sizing for degenerative MR. We attempt to obtain the measurement in diastole, but often it is obtained in systole. Sizing is also determined based on anterior leaflet length.

Leaflet Function

Each leaflet segment is evaluated in multiple planes and in three dimensions to confirm which segment is prolapsed, flail, or restricted. This determination is aided by noting the location and direction of regurgitant jets. Clefts between segments should also be identified. This evaluation allows for an accurate preincision estimate of the number and location of NeoChords that will be placed and whether a cleft will need to be closed. Any leaflet restriction is noted, and an anatomical search for its cause, such as the presence of second- or third-order chordae, is performed.

Chordal Assessment

The chordae and papillary muscles are evaluated to assess for thickening and/or fusion that may preclude successful repair. A search is made for second-order or third-order chords that may need to be excised. For example, restriction of the anterior leaflet secondary to sclerosis of the strut chords may result in a plan to divide those chords to improve anterior leaflet mobility.

Predictors of Left Ventricular Outflow Tract Due to Systolic Anterior Motion

The risk of postrepair LVOT obstruction due to SAM of the anterior leaflet is analyzed. Criteria that increase risk include:[40,41]

Major predictors

- C-sept length (shortest distance from coaptation point at end-systole to the interventricular septum) less than 2.5 cm (Fig. 21.3).
- Anterior leaflet length to posterior leaflet length ratio less than 1.3.
- Aortomitral angle less than 120 degrees or override of A2 over LVOT greater than 20 degrees.

Minor predictors

- Posterior leaflet length greater than 15 mm.
- LV end-diastolic diameter less than 45 mm.
- Basal-interventricular septal diameter in diastole greater than 15 mm.
- Presence of pre-bypass SAM.
- Lateral A2 height minus medial A2 height greater than 5 mm.

Coronary Artery Location

The distance of the circumflex artery from the MV annulus is noted. Close proximity requires caution when placing annular sutures, beginning at the lateral trigone, moving through the P1 segment to the P2 segment. If there is any difficulty coming off bypass, notably if there is considerable posterolateral wall motion abnormality, the possibility of circumflex artery obstruction should be at the forefront of the surgeon's differential.

Mitral Annulus Calcification

The presence and extent of any MAC are noted and should not be a surprise if encountered intraoperatively. Any significant amount of MAC should have been recognized on the workup TTE and left heart catheterization, prompting cardiac CT. Mitigating the risk of groove disruption while achieving a leak-free replacement in the setting of MAC was discussed previously.

Mitral Annular Disjunction

The rate of mitral annulus disjunction (MAD) is ~50% in patients with myxomatous MV disease[42] and ~33% in patients with MV prolapse.[43] Evidence suggest that MAD is associated with ventricular arrhythmias and possibly cardiac arrest. Experience notes that these are generally more involved repairs. It is important to get deep annular sutures to secure a band into

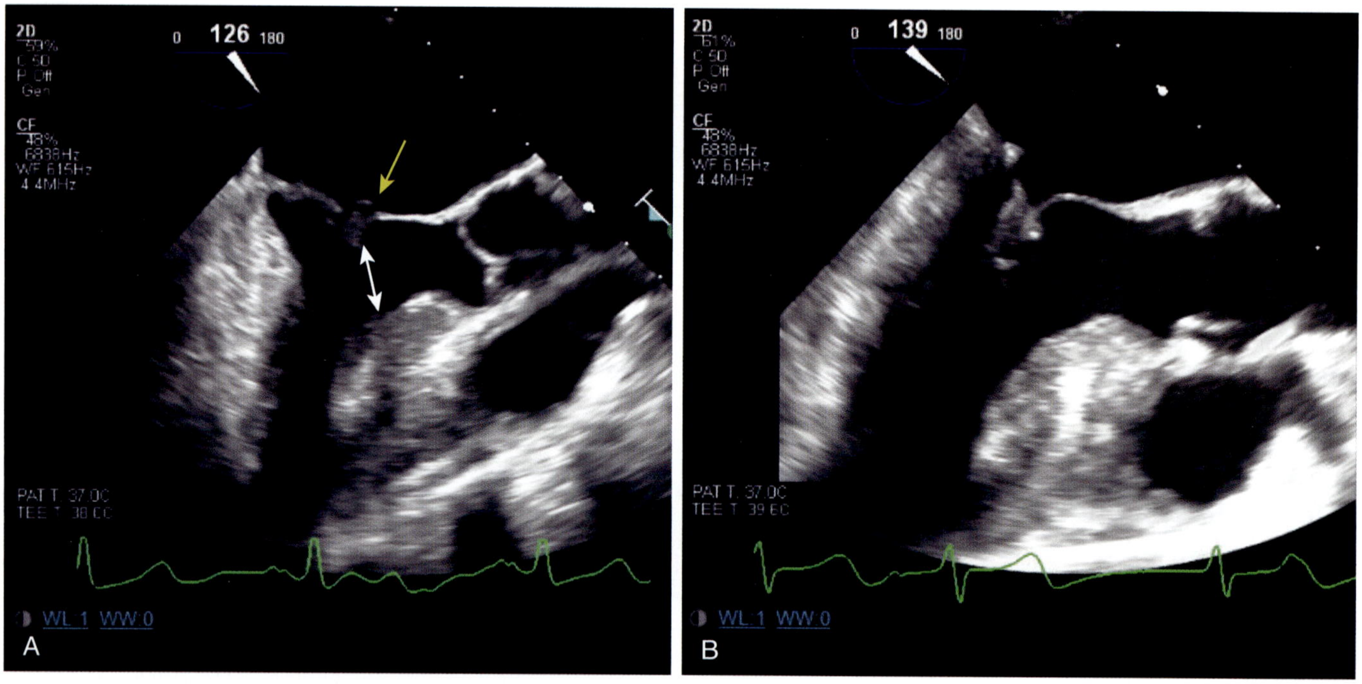

Fig. 21.3 Intraoperative transesophageal echocardiography demonstrating (A) short anterior leaflet, short C-sept *(white double-arrow)*, and anterior leaflet hinging *(yellow arrow)* due to a second-order chord and (B) a long, arching anterior leaflet without hinging after repair. The prerepair image also demonstrates a septal knob that narrows the left ventricular outflow tract (in a patient without true hypertrophic cardiomyopathy); a limited myectomy was performed through the annulus, and postrepair, the outflow tract is no longer narrowed.

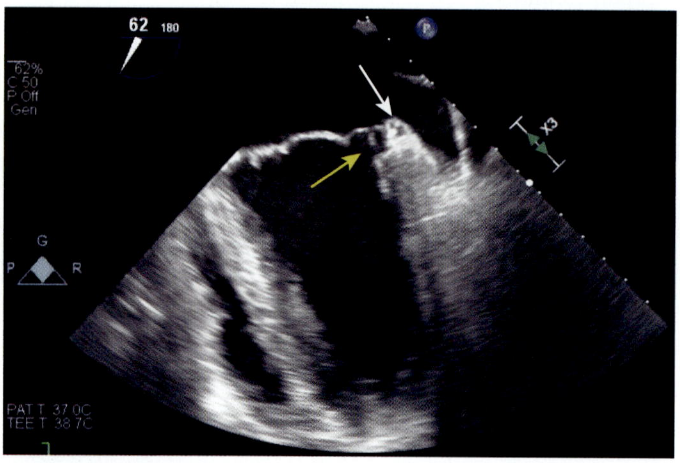

Fig. 21.4 Intraoperative transesophageal echocardiography demonstrated mitral annular disjunction *(yellow arrow)* and a very close left circumflex artery *(white arrow)*.

position. In these areas, overlapping sutures are helpful to assure annular support with minimizing skipped areas. Additionally, these valves are frequently associated with longer posterior leaflet lengths, which get back to SAM risk (Fig. 21.4).[44]

Left Ventricular Function

Left ventricular dimensions, global function, regional wall motion abnormalities, and ejection fraction are noted. These observations provide a baseline for comparison when separating from cardiopulmonary bypass. This also provides an opportunity to compare function to the initial TTE performed at workup, keeping in mind function on TEE under general anesthesia and with mechanical ventilation often appears worse than on preoperative TTE. In rare circumstances, an unexpectedly poor function may result in aborting the operation in favor of medical optimization before proceeding with surgery. A very large ventricle has implications on NeoChord length if these are a planned part of the repair. Remodeling of the left ventricle can result in a previously competent repair becoming regurgitant due to prolapse from NeoChords that are now too long for the ventricle size. Additionally, depressed ventricular function prerepair alerts to the possible need for chemical support postbypass.

Right Ventricular Function

The stress of cardiopulmonary bypass and cardiac arrest is significant. Preexisting right ventricular dysfunction should cause a pause in the workup of these patients for surgical MV repair. The degree of RV dysfunction is a spectrum, and there are multiple factors at play. It is not the goal of this chapter to review all of this. However, it is essential in evaluating a patient for surgical MV repair to have evaluated the RV, and if there is a concern for significant dysfunction that a multidisciplinary team approach to evaluating and optimizing the RV function is taken. If there are factors that are not reversible, or unlikely to be reversed, it may determine that the patient is of prohibitive risk for surgery, and other treatment strategies should be evaluated.

Left Atrial Appendage

The appendage is evaluated for thrombus. If present, manipulation is avoided at all costs, to the point that a procedure planned via right chest approach may be converted to sternotomy to avoid the risk of embolization during clamp placement. Alternatively, utilization of a balloon occlusion device instead of cross-clamping may be considered.

Aortic Insufficiency

The presence of moderate or worse AI may limit the ability to achieve good antegrade cardioplegia delivery, resulting in a distended, poorly protected ventricle. It requires the placement of a retrograde coronary sinus catheter, necessitating sternotomy if a percutaneous catheter is not available or cannot be placed. During the administration of antegrade cardioplegia, the aortic root and left ventricle should be viewed on TEE so these problems can be rapidly identified. This is additionally true when aortic balloon occlusion is used, as malposition or migration of the balloon can distort the aortic annulus, creating AI that was not necessarily present on the initial TEE. If one chooses not to replace the aortic valve with moderate AI, there must be a functioning LV vent and pacing options already in place at clamp removal when the heart is not ejecting.

Tricuspid Regurgitation

Management of tricuspid regurgitation in the setting of MV disease was discussed at length in the concomitant procedures section of this chapter. Importantly, what was judged to be mild-moderate TR on preoperative TTE may appear worse on pre-incision TEE performed by anesthesia and deserves thoughtful consideration before committing to repair.

Inspection of Valvular Structures After Atriotomy

Exposure of the MV is critical for intraoperative evaluation. Once adequate exposure has been achieved, a segmental analysis of the MV and subvalvular apparatus should be performed to confirm TEE findings. The leaflets are examined for perforations, clefts, thickening, restricted mobility, or shortening. The location of a regurgitant jet is noted, as this is a clue as to the etiology of the leak. The trigones are identified. Leaflets are retracted, and chords are examined for thickening and fusion. If there is a restriction of leaflet motion and tenting of the leaflet, a search is made to identify the offending secondary or tertiary chord for excision. In the case of a flail segment, the location of the avulsed chord on the appropriate papillary muscle is identified, and the placement of NeoChords should be done in a way that restores the original geometry and functionality. If the preoperative echocardiographic assessment was thorough, no surprises should be encountered. While leaflets are retracted, the aortic valve is noted to ensure that annulus suture placement does not inadvertently incorporate an aortic valve leaflet, causing iatrogenic AI.

Prior to any repair maneuvers, the MV is tested with saline. Although the saline test is performed during diastolic arrest, this maneuver does give an accurate representation of MV competency.[45] It also provides visual feedback on whether the pattern of MR coincides with the expectation based on all prior evaluations. A final decision is made at this point whether MV repair is possible. A sizer is introduced to confirm the intertrigonal distance as measured on TEE. The shape and asymmetry of the distorted annulus are noted, as well as an assessment for MAD. This allows for the planning of appropriate suture spacing on both the annulus and the annuloplasty ring/band/sewing ring and to anticipate deep, ventricular-directed sutures when MAD is present. The annulus from mid P2 stretching to the medial commissure tends to be the most distorted region, and proper suture planning will allow for a symmetric annuloplasty without bunching of the band or overplasty of a relatively normal segment of the annulus.

Testing and Determination of the Suitability of Repair

Following each step of the repair, a saline test is performed. Multiple chordal length adjustments may be necessary, and a saline test should be performed after each adjustment until the surgeon is satisfied with both the length of coaptation and the anteroposterior location of coaptation. The goal of the saline test is not necessarily to achieve no leaks but to ensure coaptation occurs posterior enough to avoid SAM while still achieving adequate coaptation height, which is essential for a long-term durable repair. In fact, we have found optimal predischarge TTE results when leaflets have been pulled in slightly past the point where no leak is seen, in effect creating a tiny central regurgitant jet during the intraoperative saline test. By postoperative day 3 to 4, some degree of stretching will have occurred, which, when combined with the absence of the immediate postcardiopulmonary bypass hyperdynamic state, results in an MV repair with trivial to no residual regurgitation. While a postrepair central leak is often observed, anything more than trivial residual regurgitation after the repair is usually not tolerated intraoperatively. A reassessment of the MV should be made, and additional repair measures taken. When using NeoChords, it is also important to consider what is the current LV functional state and dimensions compared to the optimal state and dimensions. In a ventricle that is significantly dilated, but where there will be marked changes in the remodeled ventricle, it may be necessary to overcorrect the leaflets by pulling the chords shorter to achieve a mild central leak with the anticipation that in the postremodeled state, the chordal lengths are appropriate. This is not a very common issue, but it is important to think that a mild prolapse can occur if the ventricle remodels and the NeoChords were not shortened enough. The concern is that with the creation of prolapse, the leaflet will be under further degenerative strain that may reduce the durability of a repair. Another issue that occurs during saline testing is when the anterior leaflet is prolapsing after leaflet repair despite not prolapsing on the preoperative echocardiogram. In these cases, it is important to trust the echocardiogram—if there was no anterior leaflet prolapse on TEE, then there is no anterior leaflet prolapse in the arrested state, and additional NeoChords should not be placed, and an assessment on the beating heart should be made on intraoperative TEE. Remember that saline testing in a ventricle arrested in diastole is not a perfect representative

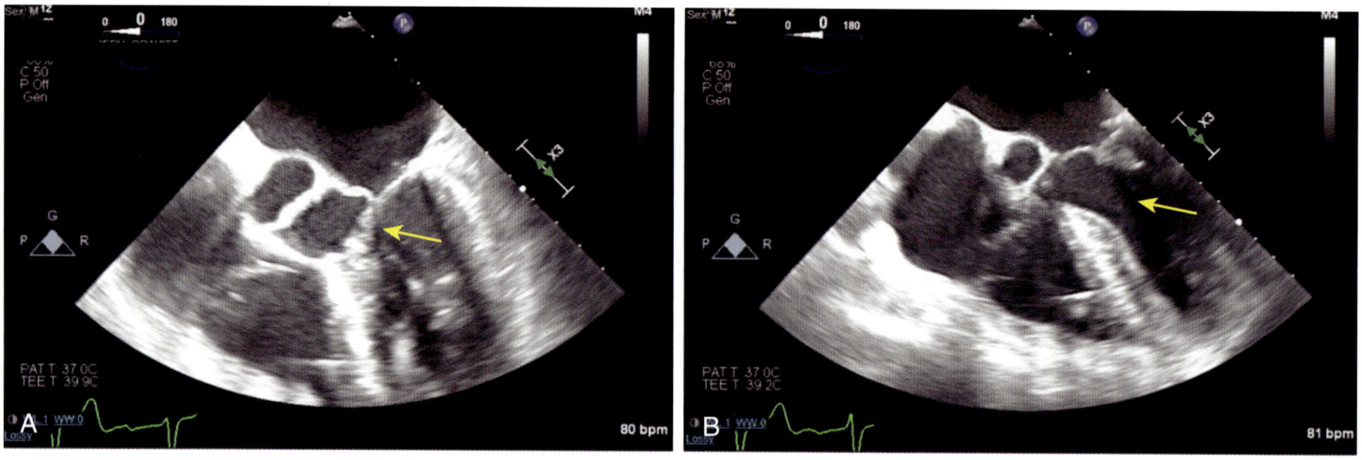

Fig. 21.5 Intraoperative transesophageal echocardiography demonstrating (A) severe systolic anterior motion (SAM) after mitral valve repair and (B) resolution of SAM after giving the patient volume and weaning inotropic medications.

of what will happen in the beating heart. To minimize some of the issues in testing, we release any tension retractors that are putting stress on the aortic root as it would push into the LA roof and, in doing so, drive the anterior MV annulus atrially. We test until the MV leaflets retract into the ventricle and the aortic root can be seen filling and is no longer collapsed by the root vent, and the vent is off during testing. It is helpful to have a videoscope to see the valve better as the LA chamber is usually reduced in size with these maneuvers and makes direct visualization difficult at times.

Postcardiopulmonary Bypass Evaluation: Transesophageal Echocardiogram and Hemodynamic Assessment

After separation from cardiopulmonary bypass, TEE is again performed. An initial, rapid assessment of valve competency is made while the LV vent is still crossing the valve to grossly determine whether reinstitution of CPB will be needed due to a failed repair. Assuming the valve function appears grossly reasonable, an evaluation for SAM is made, including an LVOT gradient. The relatively empty, immediate postbypass heart is often hyperdynamic. Some degree of SAM may be present due to these factors, and appropriate measures should be implemented to resolve it, including weaning of inotropes, volume administration, and lastly, beta-blocker administration to slow the rate and allow for more LV filling time (Fig. 21.5). If the SAM cannot be resolved medically and it is resulting in LVOT obstruction with or without severe MR, then reinstitution of CPB, rearresting, and rerepair of the MV is required. Once satisfied, SAM/LVOT obstruction is not an issue, and an assessment of biventricular function is made, including posterolateral wall motion. The presence of depressed LV function with a regional wall dysfunction, particularly in the circumflex distribution, must not be oversupported just to get to the ICU. A decision must be made on how much additional clamp time the patient can tolerate—informing whether to rerepair/rereplace the valve or bypass the circumflex artery. Once satisfied with the LVOT and biventricular function and that most of the air is out of the LV, the vent is pulled into the left atrium. At this point, a thorough assessment of the valve repair is made, focusing on many of the points previously discussed. Again, a small central leak in the immediate postbypass heart is acceptable. The other valves are assessed for any new dysfunction. When everything checks out, protamine is administered, and cannulas are removed.

COMPLICATIONS AFTER MITRAL VALVE SURGERY

Proper pre- and intraprocedural evaluation of the MV in patients undergoing surgical intervention is key in avoiding complications in both the short term and long term postoperatively. Operative mortality reported in the STS database ranges between 1% and 8% for MV repair and 4% to 15% for MV replacement depending on the etiology of MV disease, with degenerative MV carrying the lowest risk and acute IMR carrying the highest operative risk.[46] Risk for operative mortality has been reported at even lower rates at expert referral centers and when surgery is performed by high-volume mitral valve surgeons.[55,56] With hospital mortality after valve surgery approaching zero over time, many factors must be considered to determine the success of MV surgery, including long-term survival, MV function, and need for reintervention.

Failure of MV repair is categorized into three intervals: immediate (intraoperative), early (<2 years), and late (>2 years). Our approach to immediate MV repair failure has been described in the previous section and must be addressed intraoperatively because residual MR greater than trace is predictive of the need for reoperation over the long term.[47] Early MV repair failure is typically related to technique. Early failure is typically caused by rupture of a repaired chordae or suture line dehiscence and, more commonly, though still rarely, occurs after repair of a degenerative MV. Late failure is typically due to the progression of valvular pathology over time and most commonly, though again rarely, occurs in patients with rheumatic

MV disease. MV repair failure requiring reoperation occurs in approximately 5% to 20% of patients between 10- and 20-years of follow-up at expert centers.[48,49]

After MV replacement, failure can occur through structural valve deterioration (SVD) or periprosthetic leakage. SVD is uncommon in the first 5 years after replacement, but the risk increases substantially thereafter in patients with bioprosthetic valves.[50] SVD is extremely rare after mechanical MV replacement. Due to the risks associated with reoperation in failed bioprosthetic valves, mechanical valves afford a survival benefit to patients as old as 70-years at the time of index MV replacement.[51] Periprosthetic leakage is also extremely rare in the modern era, and when it does occur is typically associated with prosthetic valve endocarditis.

Besides a clear short- and long-term survival benefit associated with MV repair over replacement in patients with degenerative disease, MV repair offers several other distinct advantages when it can be successfully performed. Stroke and other thromboembolic events are rare after MV repair, occurring at a rate of 0.1% per patient-year.[46] On the other hand, MV prostheses are associated with a 1% to 2% per patient-year risk of thromboembolism, with a slightly lower incidence in biologic as compared to mechanical valves.[52] In patients that are noncompliant with their anticoagulation, acute valve thrombosis is another devastating complication of MV replacement. In addition, patients with supratherapeutic anticoagulation are exposed to a risk of serious hemorrhagic events, which occur at a rate of 1% to 2% per patient-year after MV replacement.[53] Infective endocarditis is rare after MV repair or replacement but is more much more common after replacement than after repair.[54]

SUMMARY

Expert surgeons must evaluate patients with MV disease in a systematic way throughout all phases of care. Preoperative evaluation of all available data is essential to ensure each patient meets criteria for intervention and, when they do, for procedural planning that will ensure successful surgery without any unexpected findings in the operating theater. Intraoperatively, rigorous evaluation of the key anatomy and hemodynamic performance of the MV and related structures will ensure that a proper repair can be, and ultimately was, performed. Because MV repair has distinct short- and long-term advantages over MV replacement, every effort should be made to achieve excellent, durable repair of the MV. In this chapter, we have strategies for comprehensive evaluation of patients with MV disease, including common pitfalls and potential complications that may be avoided by careful preparation and planning.

SELF-ASSESSMENT QUESTIONS

1. Which of the following is not a consideration during the preoperative evaluation of a patient with MV disease?
   A. Does the patient meet current guideline criteria for MV intervention?
   B. Are any concomitant procedures indicated?
   C. Does the patient have medical insurance?
   D. What operative approach is most appropriate?
   E. Is the valve repairable, or is replacement necessary?
2. In which scenario would a minimally invasive approach for mitral valve surgery be most appropriate?
   A. Isolated MV regurgitation with pathology limited to the posterior leaflet
   B. MV regurgitation with concomitant CAD requiring surgical revascularization
   C. MV regurgitation with aortic aneurysm requiring repair
   D. MV and aortic valve endocarditis
3. In which scenario would MV replacement not be the treatment of choice?
   A. Mitral stenosis
   B. Mitral regurgitation caused by rheumatic disease
   C. Significant MAC
   D. Primary mitral regurgitation due to posterior leaflet prolapse
   E. Mitral regurgitation caused by short anterior leaflet

See page 318 for the answers.

REFERENCES

1. Nishimura RA, Otto CA, Bonow RO, et al. 2014 AHA/ACC Guideline for the management of patients with valvular heart disease: executive summary. *Circulation*. 2014;129:2440–2492.
2. Nishimura RA, Otto CM, Bonow RO, et al. 2017 AHA/ACC focused update on the 2014 AHA/ACC guideline for the management of patients with valvular heart disease. *Circulation*. 2017;135:e1159–e1195.
3. Baumgartner H, Falk V, Bax JJ, et al. 2017 ESC/EACTS guidelines for the management of valvular heart disease. *Eur Heart J*. 2017;38:2739–2791.
4. Nishimura RA, O'Gara PT, Bavaria JE, et al. 2018 AATS/ACC/ASE/SCAI/STS expert consensus systems of care document: A proposal to optimize care for patients with valvular heart disease. *J Am Coll Cardiol*. 2019;73:2609–2635.
5. Wang A, Grayburn P, Foster JA, et al. Practice gaps in the care of mitral valve regurgitation: insights from the American College of Cardiology mitral regurgitation gap analysis and advisory panel. *Am Heart J*. 2016;172:70–79.
6. Bach DS, Awais M, Gurm HS, et al. Failure of guideline adherence for intervention in patients with severe mitral regurgitation. *J Am Coll Cardiol*. 2009;54:860–865.
7. Iung B, Delgado V, Lazure P, et al. Educational needs and application of guidelines in the management of patients with mitral regurgitation. A European mixed-methods study. *Eur Heart J*. 2018;39:1295–1303.
8. Nishimura RA, O'Gara PT, Bavaria JE, et al. 2019 AATS/ACC/ASE/SCAI/STS expert consensus systems of care document: a proposal to optimize care for patients with valvular heart disease. *J Am Coll Cardiol*. 2019;73:2609–2635. doi:10.1016/j.jacc.2018.10.007.
9. Sannino A, Grayburn PA. Mitral regurgitation in patients with severe aortic stenosis: diagnosis and management. *Heart*. 2018;104:16–22.

10. Benfari G, Clavel MA, Nistri S, et al. Concomitant mitral regurgitation and aortic stenosis: one step further to low-flow preserved ejection fraction aortic stenosis. *Eur Heart J Cardiovasc Imaging*. 2018;19:569–573.
11. Freitas-Ferraz AB, Lerakis S, Ribeiro HB, et al. Mitral regurgitation in low-flow, low-gradient aortic stenosis patients undergoing TAVR: Insights from the TOPAS-TAVI registry. *JACC Cardiovasc Interv*. 2020;13:567–579.
12. Unger P, Lancellotti P, de Canniere D. The clinical challenges of concomitant aortic and mitral valve stenosis. *Acta Cardiol*. 2016;71:3–6.
13. Lee R, Li S, Rankin JS, et al. Fifteen-year outcome trends for valve surgery in North America. *Ann Thorac Surg*. 2011;91:677–684.
14. Joseph L, Bashir M, Xiang Q, et al. Prevalence and outcomes of mitral stenosis in patients undergoing transcatheter aortic valve replacement: findings from the Society of Thoracic Surgeons/ American College of Cardiology transcatheter valve therapies registry. *JACC Cardiovasc Interv*. 2018;11:693–702.
15. Settergren M, De Palma R. Combined severe aortic and mitral stenosis: an expanding potential for transcatheter therapies? *JACC Cardiovasc Interv*. 2020;11:703–734.
16. Hamandi M, Lanfear AT, Squiers JJ, et al. Double valve replacement in patients with mitral annular calcification and aortic stenosis. *Ann Thorac Surg*. 2021;111(e311):e313. in press.
17. Pfannmueller B, Verevkin A, Borger MA, et al. Role of tricuspid valve repair for moderate tricuspid regurgitation during minimally invasive mitral valve surgery. *Thorac Cardiovasc Surg*. 2013;61:386–391.
18. Van De Veire NR, Braun J, Delgado V, et al. Tricuspid annuloplasty prevents right ventricular dilatation and progression of tricuspid regurgitation in patients with tricuspid annular dilatation undergoing mitral valve repair. *J Thorac Cardiovas Surg*. 2011;141:1431–1439.
19. Zhu TY, Wang JG, Meng X. Does concomitant tricuspid annuloplasty increase perioperative mortality and morbidity when correcting left-sided valve disease. *Interact Cardiovasc Thorac Surg*. 2015;20:114–118.
20. Bertrand PB, Koppers G, Verbrugge FH, et al. Tricuspid annuloplasty concomitant with mitral valve surgery: effects on right ventricular remodeling. *J Thorac Cardiovasc Surg*. 2014;147:1256–1264.
21. Kusajima K, Fujita T, Hata H, et al. Long-term echocardiographic follow-up of untreated 2+ functional tricuspid regurgitation in patients undergoing mitral valve surgery. *Interact Cardiovasc Thorac Surg*. 2016;23:96–103.
22. De Bonis M, Lapenna E, Pozzoli A, et al. Mitral valve repair without repair of moderate tricuspid regurgitation. *Ann Thorac Surg*. 2015;100:2206–2212.
23. Brescia AA, Ward ST, Watt TMF, et al. Outcomes of guideline-directed concomitant annuloplasty for functional tricuspid regurgitation. *Ann Thorac Surg*. 2020;109:1227–1232.
24. Teekakirikul P, Wong TC. *MR in patients with hypertrophic cardiomyopathy referred for septal reduction therapy*: American College of Cardiology Latest in Cardiology; 2018. January 10. Access at. https://www.acc.org/latest-in-cardiology/articles/2018/01/10/07/00/mr-in-patients-with-hypertrophic-cardiomyopathy-referred-for-srt.
25. Daneshmand MA, Milano CA, Rankin JS, et al. Mitral valve repair for degenerative disease: a 20-year experience. *Ann Thorac Surg*. 2009;88:1828–1837.
26. Javadikasgari H, Gillinov AM, Idress JJ, et al. Valve repair is superior to replacement in most patients with coexisting degenerative mitral valve and coronary artery disease. *Ann Thorac Surg*. 2017;103:1833–1841.
27. Dunning J, Nagendran M, Alfieri OR, et al. Guideline for the surgical treatment of atrial fibrillation. *Eur J Cardiothorac Surg*. 2013;44:777–791.
28. Murzi M, Cerillo AG, Gasbarri T, et al. Antegrade and retrograde perfusion in minimally invasive mitral valve surgery with transthoracic aortic clamping: a single-institution experience with 1632 patients over 12 years. *Interact Cardiovasc Thorac Surg*. 2017;24:363–368.
29. Cheng DCH, Martin J, Lal A, et al. Minimally invasive versus conventional open mitral valve surgery: a meta-analysis and systematic review. *Innovations (Phila)*. 2011;6:84–103.
30. Muuler L, Hofer D, Holfeld J, et al. Indications and contraindications for minimally invasive mitral valve surgery. *J Vis Surg*. 2018;4:255.
31. Vollroth M, Seeburger J, Garbade J, et al. Conversion rate and contraindications for minimally invasive mitral valve surgery. *Ann Cardiothorac Surg*. 2013;2:853–854.
32. Baumgarten H, Squiers JJ, Brinkman WT, et al. Implantation of transcatheter aortic prosthesis in 3 patients with mitral annular calcification. *Ann Thorac Surg*. 2016;102:e433–e435.
33. Chan KMJ, Pnjabi PP, Flather M, et al. Coronary artery bypass surgery with or without mitral valve annuloplasty in moderate functional ischemic mitral regurgitation: final results of the randomized ischemic mitral evaluation (RIME) trial. *Circulation*. 2012;126:2502–2510.
34. Fattouch K, Guccione F, Sampognaro R, et al. POINT: efficacy of adding mitral valve restrictive annuloplasty to coronary artery bypass grafting in patients with moderate ischemic mitral valve regurgitation: a randomized trial. *J Thorac Cardiovasc Surg*. 2009;138:278–285.
35. Michler RE, Smith PK, Parides MK, et al. Two-year outcomes of surgical treatment of moderate ischemic mitral regurgitation. *N Engl J Med*. 2016;374:1932–1941.
36. Acker MA, Parides MK, Perrault LP, et al. Mitral-valve repair versus replacement for severe ischemic mitral regurgitation. *N Engl J Med*. 2014;370:23–32.
37. Nappi F, Singh SSA, Padala M, et al. The choice of treatment in ischemic mitral regurgitation with reduced left ventricular function. *Ann Thorac Surg*. 2019;108:1901–1912.
38. O'Brien SM, Feng L, He X. The Society of Thoracic Surgeons 2018 adult cardiac surgery risk models: Part 2—Statistical methods and results. *Ann Thorac Surg*. 2018;105:1419–1428.
39. Iyengar A, Goel N, Kelly JJ, et al. Effects of frailty on outcomes and 30-day readmissions after surgical mitral valve replacement. *Ann Thorac Surg*. 2020;109:1120–1126.
40. Varghese R, Itagaki S, Anyanwu AC, et al. Predicting systolic anterior motion after mitral valve reconstruction: using intraoperative transesophageal echocardiography to identify those at greatest risk. *Eur J Cardiothorac Surg*. 2014;45:132–137.
41. Maslow AD, Regan MM, Haering JM, et al. Echocardiographic predictors of left ventricular outflow tract obstruction and systolic anterior motion of the mitral valve after mitral valve reconstruction for myxomatous valve disease. *J Am Coll Cardiol*. 1999;34:2096–2104.
42. Bennett S, Thamman R, Griffiths T, et al. Mitral annular disjunction: a systematic review of the literature. *Echocardiography*. 2019;36:1549–1558.
43. Konda T, Tani T, Suganuma N, et al. Mitral annular disjunction in patients with primary severe mitral regurgitation and mitral valve prolapse. *Echocardiography*. 2020;37:1716–1722.

44. Putnam AJ, Kebet K, Mor-Avi V, et al. Prevalence of mitral annular disjunction in patients with mitral valve prolapse and severe regurgitation. *Int J Cardiovasc Imaging*. 2020;36:1363–1370.
45. Watanabe T, Arai H. Leakage test during mitral valve repair. *Gen Thorac Cardiovasc Surg*. 2014;62:645–650.
46. Rankin JS, Grau-Sepulveda M, Shahian DM, et al. The impact of mitral disease etiology on operative mortality after mitral valve operations. *Ann Thorac Surg*. 2018;106:1406–1413.
47. Gillinov AM, Cosgrove DJ, Blackstone EH, et al. Durability of mitral valve repair for degenerative disease. *J Thorac Cardiovasc Surg*. 1998;116:734–743.
48. David TE, David CM, Tsang W, et al. Long-term results of mitral valve repair for regurgitation due to leaflet prolapse. *J Am Coll Cardiol*. 2019;74:1044–1053.
49. Mohty D, Orszulak TA, Schaff HV, et al. Very long-term survival and durability of mitral valve repair for mitral valve prolapse. *Circulation*. 2001;104:I1–I7.
50. Beute TJ, Goehler M, Parker J, et al. Long-term outcomes of mosaic versus perimount mitral replacements: 17-year follow-up of 940 implants. *Ann Thorac Surg*. 2020;110:508–515.
51. Goldstone AB, Chiu P, Baiocchi M, et al. Mechanical or biologic prostheses for aortic-valve and mitral-valve replacement. *N Engl J Med*. 2017;377:1847–1857.
52. Chikwe J, Chiang YP, Egorova NN, et al. Survival and outcomes following bioprosthetic vs mechanical mitral valve replacement in patients aged 50 to 69 years. *JAMA*. 2015;313:1435–1442.
53. Russo A, Grigioni F, Avierinos JF, et al. Thromboembolic complications after surgical correction of mitral regurgitation: incidence, predictors, and clinical implications. *J Am Coll Cardiol*. 2008;51:1203–1211.
54. Manne MB, Shrestha NK, Lytle BW, et al. Outcomes after surgical treatment of native and prosthetic valve infective endocarditis. *Ann Thorac Surg*. 2012;93:489–493.
55. Badhwar V, Vemulapalli S, Mack M, et al. Volume-outcome association of mitral valve surgery in the United States. *JAMA Cardiol*. 2020;5(10):1092–1101.
56. Chikwe J, Toyoda N, Anyanwu AC, et al. Relation of mitral valve surgery volume to repair rate, durability, and survival. *Am Coll Cardiol*. 2017;69(2397):2506.
57. Smith RL, Hamandi M, Ailawadi G, et al. Surgical implantation of balloon-expandable heart valves for the treatment of mitral annular calcification. *J Thorac Cardiovasc Surg*. 2022; in press. doi:10.1016/j.jtcvs.2021.08.047.

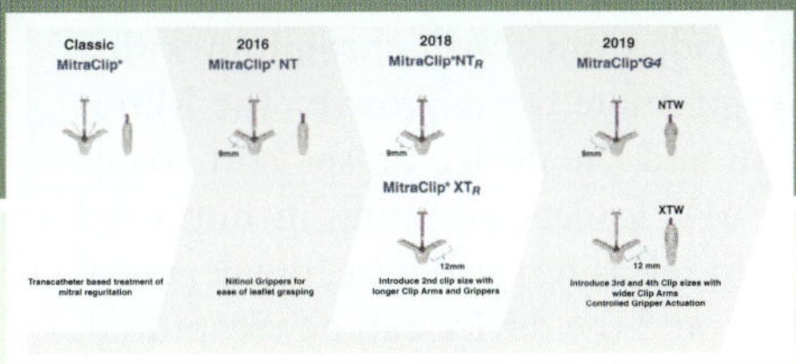

22

Transcatheter Mitral Valve Repair

Clarence M. Findley, Molly Szerlip

CHAPTER OUTLINE

LEARNING OBJECTIVES

1. The mitral valve is a complex anatomical structure that can be difficult to treat from a percutaneous standpoint. In-depth anatomic knowledge is essential to procedural success.
2. Currently approved therapies for percutaneous mitral valve repair are based on surgical approaches. We explore the surgical approaches and provide an in-depth description of the procedures and the data behind their approval in both the United States and Europe.
3. Guideline-directed medical therapy must be optimized prior to moving forward with any transcatheter-based mitral valve repair procedure.

Kollaborate link: https://www.kollaborate.tv/link?id=614b20249c495

INTRODUCTION

In previous chapters, the discussion of mitral valve (MV) anatomy, pathology, and pathophysiology have been undertaken. This chapter focuses on current percutaneous MV repair therapies. We briefly discuss surgical therapies for mitral regurgitation (MR) and transition to an in-depth discussion of the development of recent percutaneous approaches and their derivation from established surgical approaches. We discuss some device mechanics and focus on the specific trials that contributed to either the Federal Drug Administration (FDA) or the Conformitè Europëenne (CE) mark approval. It should be noted that current guidelines emphasize the importance of implementing optimal guideline-directed medical therapy (GDMT) prior to moving forward with any form of catheter-based therapies, and this directive should be heavily underscored in the treatment of patients with transcatheter MV repair approaches.

CURRENT SURGICAL THERAPIES AND THEIR ASSOCIATION WITH CATHETER-BASED METHODS

Patients with severe MV disease can be treated surgically. Surgical repair and replacement are invasive therapies aimed at significantly improving MR. Surgical repair has become the preferred mode of treatment for patients with primary MR and is noted to have better outcomes relative to MV replacement.[1] Repair of MR can be achieved by targeting different aspects of the mitral apparatus. Quadrangular or triangular resection of an isolated P2 segment with reapproximation of the P1 and P3 leaflets can be performed. The excision is paired with an annuloplasty ring, which is used to stabilize the annulus and prevent further annular dilatation. Another technique often used is replacement of the chordae tendineae, or surgical chordoplasty.[2] In scenarios where the chordae tendineae are ruptured or elongated, artificial sutures can be used to substitute for the abnormal chordae and restore valvular function. Lastly, the Alfieri stitch technique (or edge-to-edge repair) involves sewing the anterior and posterior leaflets together in the P2 and A2 segments to correct prolapse and restructure the valve into a double orifice.[3]

Percutaneous approaches to repairing the MV mimic commonly used surgical techniques. In the MV surgical repair space, there are devices aimed at (a) indirect or direct annuloplasty ring insertion, (b) chordal implantation, and (c) leaflet edge-to-edge repair. Transcatheter MV replacement apparatus have also been devised; however, these therapies are investigational at this time.

DISCUSSION OF FDA-APPROVED THERAPIES: INDICATIONS

This section will focus on FDA-approved MV therapies in the United States. At the time of writing this chapter, there is only one FDA-approved device in the mitral space. MitraClip (Abbott Laboratories, Abbott Park, IL, USA) carries an indication for primary (degenerative MR) and secondary (functional MR). The MitraClip Delivery System is indicated for the reduction of significant symptomatic mitral regurgitation (MR ≥ 3+) due to primary MR in patients who have been determined to be at prohibitive risk for MV surgery by a heart team. Additionally, the MitraClip System is indicated for the treatment of symptomatic, moderate-to-severe or severe secondary MR in patients with a left ventricular ejection fraction (LVEF) 20% to 50% and a left ventricular end systolic dimension (LVESD) ≤ 70 mm whose symptoms and MR severity persist, despite maximally tolerated GDMT. Often, these patients are evaluated in a multidisciplinary heart team setting and deemed appropriate to move forward with percutaneous intervention by a cardiac surgeon and a structural interventionalist. Pursuing MitraClip implantation in patients who cannot tolerate anticoagulant or antiplatelet regimens, have active MV endocarditis, rheumatic MV disease or evidence of intracardiac, inferior vena cava, or femoral vein thrombus is contraindicated.

DISCUSSION OF FDA-APPROVED THERAPIES: PROCEDURAL DESCRIPTION

The MitraClip Delivery System consists of two major components, the steering guide catheter and the clip delivery system. The steering guide catheter is 80 cm with a 24 Fr outer diameter. The clip delivery system consists of a steerable sleeve and a delivery catheter for clip placement. Following right femoral vein access, transseptal puncture is performed at a height sufficient to maneuver in the left atrium and reach the MV. This tends to be in the superior-posterior position on the interatrial septum. The ideal location of transseptal puncture is 3.5 to 4.0 cm above the mitral annular plane or 4.0 to 4.5 cm to the coaptation site for the valve pathology.[4] The steering guide catheter is then introduced into the body via the femoral vein and positioned across the interatrial septum and angled inferiorly toward the MV. Once the steering guide catheter has been placed, the clip delivery system is inserted and used to accurately position the clip. The use of transesophageal echo (TEE) is integral to guiding transseptal puncture, maneuvering within the left atrium (i.e., avoiding the left atrial appendage) and through the MV. The steerable guide catheter and clip delivery system are then manipulated to position the device through the MV. On the end of the steerable guide catheter exists a clip made from cobalt chromium with a polyester cover designed to promote tissue growth. The MitraClip is positioned with TEE and the device grasps and coapts the anterior and posterior MV leaflets, resulting in improved coaptation of the MV. Prior to releasing the device, the degree of MR can be assessed via TEE, and the device can be recaptured, repositioned, and redeployed until the best site for minimizing regurgitation is identified. At times, more than one device may be necessary to adequately address the degree of MR. The newer version of the MitraClip system, G4, comes with four clip sizes (Fig. 22.1). The XT and XTW clip lengths are 12 mm, but they vary by grasping width (4 mm and 6 mm, respectively). The NT and NTW clip lengths are 9 mm and vary by grasping width (4 mm and 6 mm, respectively). In general, the XT clips feature longer clip arms that aid in easier leaflet grasping and wider reach to facilitate clip deployment, while the NT clips are smaller and designed to be more precise. The NT clips are favored in scenarios where chord entanglement and smaller leaflet lengths are of concern, such as commissural anatomy. Additionally, in smaller valves (mitral valve area [MVA] < 4.0 cm^2), the risk for mitral stenosis is increased after clip implantation; thus, the use of NT clips may be preferred. The G4 system also provides the added luxury of both simultaneous and independent leaflet grasping, which was not available on earlier versions of the device.

When looking at data from the early investigator experience (2006 to 2008), 5-year results from the Everest II trial provide a glimpse into the complications associated with this procedure.[5] Single leaflet device detachment (SLDA) was observed in 5.8% of patients within the first year of follow-up. After the first year, only one additional patient experienced late SLDA at 14 months post-MitraClip implantation. All patients with SLDA subsequently underwent MV surgery (5 replacement, 5 repair). No cases of device embolization through the 5-year follow-up were observed. The percutaneous approach proved to be safe during follow-up with only one case of late (>1 year) SLDA (0.6%) and no reported episodes of device embolization. A single case of mitral stenosis (0.6%) was observed after the index procedure but before discharge; the patient subsequently underwent MV replacement surgery. As the technology and operator experience matured, complications decreased. More recently, a review of data from the COAPT (Cardiovascular Outcomes Assessment of the MitraClip Percutaneous Therapy for Heart Failure Patients With Functional Mitral Regurgitation) trial reveals a relatively low device-related complication rate of 3.4% at 12 months. Specifically, SLDA occurred at 0.7%, device embolization at 0.3%, left ventricular assist device implantation at 1.2%, and heart transplant at 0.8%. Other potential complications such as endocarditis requiring surgery or mitral stenosis requiring surgery were not observed.

Approval of this device for primary MR was based on the EVEREST II trial.[6] This study was a randomized trial that compared MitraClip-based leaflet repair versus surgical repair. In the EVEREST II trial, 279 patients with moderate-to-severe or severe MR were included in a 2:1 ratio to undergo either percutaneous repair

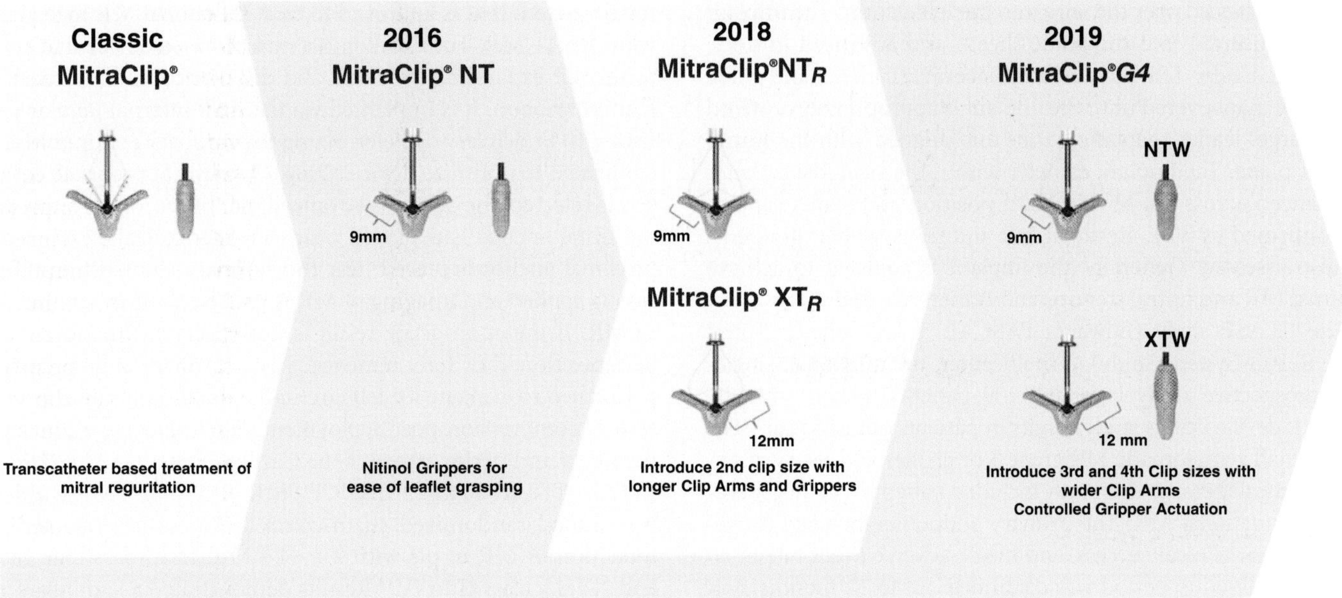

Fig. 22.1 Evolution of MitraClip technology. (Abbot Laboratories, Abbott Park, IL. Tendyne is a trademark of Abbott or its related companies. Reproduced with permission of Abbott, © 2021. All rights reserved.)

or conventional surgery for repair or replacement of the MV. The majority of study patients had heart failure at baseline and 73% of patients had primary MR. The primary composite endpoint for efficacy was freedom from death, from surgery for mitral valve dysfunction, and from grade 3+ or 4+ MR at 12 months. The primary safety endpoint was a composite of major adverse events within 30 days. At 12 months, both groups had improved left ventricular size, New York Heart Association functional class, and quality-of-life measures, as compared with baseline. Although percutaneous repair was less effective at reducing MR than conventional surgery, the procedure was associated with a better safety profile and similar improvements in clinical outcomes.

At 12 months, the rates of the primary endpoint for efficacy were reduced in the percutaneous repair group (55%) relative to the surgery group (73%) ($P = .007$). This difference was primarily driven by the higher rate of surgery required for patients in the percutaneous repair group (20% vs. 2%). Similar mortality rates were noted in both the percutaneous and surgical repair groups. Major adverse event rates at 30 days were lower in the percutaneous group relative to the surgical group, and this difference was primarily driven by the higher rate of blood transfusions in the surgical patient population. At 4-year follow-up, moderate-to-severe/severe regurgitation (21.9% vs. 24.7%) and mortality rates (17.4% vs. 17.8%) were similar in both the percutaneous and surgical groups.[6]

MitraClip approval for secondary MR is based on the COAPT trial.[7] In the COAPT trial, high surgical risk patients with moderate-to-severe/severe MR and heart failure were randomized to either percutaneous mitral repair or the control group with standard medical therapy. Patients who remained symptomatic despite the use of maximal doses of guideline-directed medical therapy were enrolled in the trial. The primary effectiveness endpoint was all hospitalizations for heart failure within 24 months of follow-up. The primary safety endpoint was freedom from device-related complications at 12 months. In total, 302 patients were assigned to the device group and 312 patients were assigned to the control group. The annualized rate of all hospitalizations for heart failure within 24 months was 35.8% per patient-year in the device group as compared with 67.9% per patient-year in the control group (hazard ratio, 0.53; 95% confidence interval [CI], 0.40 to 0.70; $P < .001$). Death from any cause within 24 months occurred in 29.1% of the patients in the device group as compared with 46.1% in the control group (hazard ratio, 0.62; 95% CI, 0.46 to 0.82; $P < .001$). The MitraClip is the only approved percutaneous mitral repair device in the United States and has been employed in numerous patients with great success. Recently CMS (Centers for Medicare and Medicaid Services) has approved reimbursement for MitraClip in functional MR, allowing more patients to be treated with this therapy.

APPROVED THERAPIES IN EUROPE

Leaflet Therapy

MitraClip technology received CE mark approval in 2008. It is a well-established technology and has been implanted in over 10,000 patients worldwide.[8] See the above section for details specific to the MitraClip technology.

The PASCAL transcatheter MV repair system (Edwards Lifesciences, Irvine, CA, USA) also exploits leaflet edge-to-edge therapy. Similar to the MitraClip, the PASCAL device received CE mark approval in 2019. The PASCAL device differs from the design of the MitraClip and is characterized by larger clasps to grip larger amounts of leaflet surface and the presence of a spacer, allowing for better coaptation and independent articulation of both arms. Similar to the MitraClip procedure, access is obtained via the right femoral vein. Transeptal puncture is performed to gain access to the left atrium. A wire is placed in the left atrium. A guidewire/

sheath is advanced over the wire into the left atrium. The implant system is inserted into the guide sheath and advanced into the left atrium. Under TEE guidance, the steerable catheter and guide sheath are maneuvered until the implant is appropriately centered in the target leaflet coaptation zone and aligned with the mitral annular plane. The implant catheter within the steerable catheter is advanced across the MV. Implant position and leaflet capture are confirmed by TEE. Residual MR and transvalvular gradients are also assessed. Generally, the implant is adjusted to achieve minimal MR and mitral stenosis and is then released.

The CLASP study (Edwards PASCAL TrAnScatheter Mitral Valve RePair System Study), a multicenter, multinational, single-arm, prospective study involving 109 patients treated with the PASCAL device details study results in patients out to 1 year.[9] The patients had symptomatic MR grade 3 or greater and received optimal medical therapy. This study included patients with degenerative and functional MR. The primary endpoints included procedural success, clinical success, and major adverse event rate at 30 days. The follow-up period was continued out to 12 months. MR severity was ≤1 in 82% of patients (79% functional mitral regurgitation [FMR], 86% degenerative mitral regurgitation [DMR]) and ≤2 in 100% of patients. Eighty-eight percent of patients were NYHA functional class I or II, and their Kansas City Cardiomyopathy Questionnaire (KCCQ) score improved. Notably, patients with either degenerative or functional MR derived favorable clinical and echocardiographic improvement. The results with the PASCAL repair system in the CLASP study demonstrate favorable clinical and echocardiographic results in a heterogeneous population of patients with FMR and DMR. Complications of the therapy include leaflet detachment, stroke, and bleeding. At the time of this chapter, the CLASP 2-year data were submitted for publication. This device is now in a pivotal trial (CLASP IID/IIF) and should be reporting outcomes in the near future.

Indirect Annuloplasty

The benefit of surgical annuloplasty, particularly in high-risk patients, has not been demonstrated despite a reduction in MR.[10] However, annuloplasty-based technology has also taken hold in Europe. Specifically, the Carillon Mitral Contour System (Cardiac Dimension, Inc., Kirkland, WA, USA) takes advantage of indirect annuloplasty technology by using the proximity of the coronary sinus to the postural and lateral mitral annuli. A device is introduced into the coronary sinus and advanced to the lateral wall of the LV along the lateral portion of the MV. Once in position, the device creates tension, which is transmitted to the mitral annulus and results in decreased annular circumference. These changes result in improved leaflet coaptation and a reduction in MR. Interestingly, there are some data that suggest leaflet edge-to-edge therapy is not as good as annuloplasty in patients with functional MR. Specifically, a registry study looked at 123 consecutive patients treated with Cardioband (annuloplasty) versus 455 consecutive patients treated with the MitraClip and demonstrated effective reduction in MR and heart failure (HF) symptoms in both groups; however, a more pronounced improvement in NYHA functional class, rehospitalization rates, and mortality rates were observed in the Cardioband cohort.[11]

The Carillon device received CE mark approval in 2011.[12] The Carillon Mitral Contour System is a transcatheter MV repair system that is approved to treat functional MR in patients with 2 to 4+ MR. The Carillon is a nitinol-based device that comprises self-expanding proximal and distal anchors connected by a nitinol ribbon. It is implanted via the right internal jugular vein with a 10 Fr delivery catheter. Sizing the coronary ostium must be confirmed to optimize device sizing. Once the appropriate device size is selected, the device is advanced into the coronary sinus and the distal anchor is deployed near the anterior leaflet, while the proximal anchor is placed near the coronary sinus ostium. Tension is applied and imaging of MR is used to confirm a reduction in MR. If the appropriate result is not observed, the device can be repositioned or fully removed. Also, coronary angiography is performed to evaluate for left circumflex/obtuse marginal arterial system compression post deployment. Four trials have evaluated the safety and performance of the Carillon System—AMADEUS, TITAN, TITAN II, and REDUCE FMR. REDUCE FMR is a double-blinded, randomized, sham-controlled trial that evaluated the reduction in MR in pts with 2 + −4 + MR, LVEF less than 50%, and NYHA class II to IV.[13] Results demonstrated a significant reduction in MV regurgitant volume and favorable LV remodeling as determined by changes in left ventricular end diastolic and end systolic volumes. The results demonstrate that FMR patients treated with the Carillon System experience a significant reduction in left ventricular end diastolic volume (LVEDV) and left ventricular end systolic volume (LVESV). They also have favorable long-term (3-year) survival and reduction in total/recurrent HF admissions. The device has a favorable safety profile; however, limitations of the device include difficulty cannulating the coronary sinus (dissection and perforation), ineffective reduction in MR or compression of a coronary artery.[13] Presumably, difficulty with coronary sinus cannulation is a function of operator experience and will improve. Wire ribbon fracture was a concern with earlier versions of the device but has improved with the most current iteration.

Another device, the Edwards Cardioband Mitral Reconstruction System (Edwards Lifesciences, Irvine, CA, USA) is a transcatheter device designed to reduce MR through annular reduction and is an approved direct annuloplasty device.[14] It received CE mark approval in 2015. The Cardioband is available in six lengths to cover a wide range of annular circumference sizes. The length of the implant is chosen based on the mitral annulus perimeter measured using CT. The delivery system includes an implant catheter, guide catheter, a steerable sheath, and a size adjustment tool. After femoral vein access, transseptal puncture is performed to gain access to the left atrium. Once access to the left atrium (LA) is obtained, the delivery system is introduced over a wire and the device is maneuvered to align with an optimal position near the anterior lateral trigone under TEE guidance. A steerable catheter helps to direct the device to the appropriate supra-annular position. The Cardioband implant is a polyester sleeve with radiopaque markers spaced 8 mm apart containing a premounted contraction wire. A series of stainless steel anchors are advanced through the implant fabric and into the annular tissue, resulting in anchoring of the Cardioband along the posterior annulus of the MV from the posteromedial commissure to the anterolateral commissure. For each anchor implantation and before release, a pull test is performed under TEE and fluoroscopic guidance to ensure proper anchoring. A coronary angiography is recommended before releasing the first set of anchors to rule out potential circumflex coronary artery injury/compression. When the last anchor is deployed in the trigone near the posterior medial commissure, the implant is disconnected from the device and the size adjustment tool is used to reduce implant length. Under fluoroscopic and transesophageal guidance, the Cardioband implant is contracted to achieve targeted annular constraint and optimal reduction in mitral valvular regurgitation.

The Cardioband device received CE mark approval in 2015 based upon data from a single-arm, multicenter, prospective trial that enrolled 31 patients from five institutions in Europe.[15] Thirty-one patients (71.8 ± 6.9 years of age; 83.9% male) with moderate-to-severe FMR, symptomatic heart failure, and depressed left ventricular function (LVEF 34 ± 11%) were prospectively enrolled. There were no periprocedural deaths and the mortality rate at 1 month or prior to hospital discharge and at 7 months was 5% and 9.7% respectively. Patients with New York Heart Association (NYHA) functional class III/IV decreased from 95.5% to 18.2% after 7 months. Exercise capacity, as assessed by the 6-minute walk test improved, and the quality of life, as assessed by the Minnesota Living With Heart Failure Questionnaire (MLHFQ), were also significantly improved. Cinching of the Cardioband implant reduced the annular septo-lateral dimension by greater than 30% from baseline. Lastly, the percentage of patients with moderate-to-severe or worse FMR was reduced from 77.4% to 13.6% at 7 months.

In a more recent Cardioband trial, 61 patients with moderate-to-severe functional MR on GDMT were treated at 11 European institutions.[16] At 1 year, overall survival was 87%. Survival rates free of readmission for heart failure at 1 year was 66% (16 patients were readmitted within the first year for congestive heart failure). Survival free of secondary procedures at 1 year was 78% (six patients underwent a secondary transcatheter procedure with another device for recurrent/persistent significant MR). At 12 months, 61% of patients presented with moderate or less MR. MR worsening over time was noted in 22% of patients at 12 months. Septo-lateral diameter reduction was maintained out to 12 months. Functional parameters, such as NYHA and 6-minute walk test, remained improved at the 12-month mark. Complications included two in-hospital deaths (nondevice and nonprocedure related) and five additional deaths (three cardiac and two noncardiac causes). There was also one stroke, one tamponade, and two coronary artery complications. Anchor disengagement was observed in 10 patients. The trial in the United States for this device has been put on hold until a newer iteration of the device is available.

Direct Annuloplasty

The Mitralign system (Mitralign, Inc., Tewksbury, MA) received CE mark approval in 2016. The Mitralign Percutaneous Annuloplasty System (MPAS), which mimics surgical annuloplasty, aims to approximate the dilated posterior MV annulus in patients with FMR.[17]

The deflectable 12.5 Fr guide catheter is inserted in the femoral artery and is designed to direct all subsequent procedural catheters toward the posterior mitral annulus. The wire-delivery catheter is an 8 Fr steerable catheter, which is used to access points of interest on the ventricular side of the posterior mitral annulus and deliver the crossing wires. The radiofrequency (RF) crossing wire is a guidewire with polyester insulation and a hydrophilic coating. It is connected to an RF generator and advanced across the mitral annulus and into the left atrium. The delivery catheter is then tracked over the crossing wire and deploys half of the pledget on the atrial side and the other half on the ventricular side of the annulus. The polyester pledget incorporates two platinum–iridium radiopaque markers to aid deployment and annulus plication. The pledget and attached suture serve as a buttressed anchor for plication of the annulus. To plicate the annulus, a pair of pledgets has to be delivered and cinched together. The plication catheter is preloaded with a stainless steel locking implant. It is tracked to the annulus over the two sutures and provides a means for plication of the mitral annulus by pulling the two pledgets together. Once plication is achieved, the plication catheter deploys the lock onto the sutures, thereby securing the plication. The suture cutter performs the final suture cut following deployment of the lock.

Subvalvular Apparatus Therapies

Thus far, many of the therapies discussed focus on annular therapy. However, as discussed earlier, several components of the MV apparatus can become dysfunctional and may be optimal targets for minimizing valve dysfunction.[18] In particular, chordoplasty-based therapies have also been developed and approved. The NeoChord (NeoChord Inc, St. Louis Park, MN) received CE mark approval in 2013. The NeoChord System is indicated for use in patients with moderate-to-severe degenerative MV regurgitation and specifically intended for use when the native chordae tendineae have become elongated or ruptured.[18] The NeoChord procedure is performed via left mini-thoracotomy access at the fifth-intercostal space with TEE guidance and under general anesthesia. The puncture site tends to be about 2 to 4 cm postero-lateral from the real apex in order to obtain a perfect posterior and symmetrical alignment with the papillary muscles.[19] Using 2D and 3D echo guidance, the system is positioned near the mitral annular plane. The prolapsing segment of the MV leaflet is then grasped and pierced, and the expanded polytetrafluoroethylene (ePTFE) chord is passed through the leaflet and retrieved together with the device from the LV. Three to four artificial chordae are placed along the free edge of the MV leaflet to resuspend the prolapsed segment. Using TEE, the level of MV regurgitation is reduced by adjusting the length of the artificial chordae. Once regurgitation has been reduced to the desired level, the artificial chordae are secured to a pledget on the epicardium of the heart.

To date, the most robust published experience comes from registry data. A total of 213 patients were enrolled in the NeoChord Independent International Registry, which is a retrospective multicenter study between February 2013 and July 2016 in seven hospitals in Europe.[20] All patients presented with severe MR due to flail/prolapse of one or both leaflets. The successful placement of two or more NeoChords was achieved in 96.7% of patients and resulted in a significant reduction of MR severity. The composite primary endpoint was composed of procedural success, freedom from mortality, stroke, reintervention, recurrence of severe MR, rehospitalization, and decrease of at least one NYHA functional class at 1-year follow-up. At 30 days, of the 205 patients who reached this follow-up time, MR was absent/trace in 84 (41%) patients, mild in 73 (35.6%) patients, moderate in 35 (17.1%) patients, and severe in 13 (6.3%) patients. At 1-year follow-up, MR was absent/trace in 60 (31.4%) patients, mild in 84 (44%) patients, moderate in 32 (16.7%) patients, and severe in 15 (7.9%) patients. They also compared outcomes according to the anatomical classification (Type A: isolated central posterior leaflet disease; Type B: posterior multisegment disease; Type C: anterior, bi-leaflet, para-commissural disease with/without leaflet/annular calcifications), which demonstrated achievement of the primary endpoint 94 ± 2.6%, 82.6 ± 3.8%, and 63.6 ± 8.4% in Type A, Type B, and Type C patients, respectively. This trend suggests that specific anatomical selection criteria are necessary to achieve stable results. The major complications associated with the procedure are leaflet perforation and NeoChord dehiscence. Five-year durability data in 5 patients demonstrated good long-term data without the recurrence of MV prolapse, regurgitation, or annular dilatation.[21]

Another device aimed at transcatheter chordal repair is the Harpoon.[18] The Harpoon received CE mark approval. The harpoon system consists of a hemostatic introducer and a delivery system. The delivery system contains a preformed ePTFE knot wrapped on a 21-gauge needle and is designed to securely anchor artificial ePTFE cords on targeted locations on a prolapsed MV leaflet. The procedure is performed under general anesthesia. Transthoracic echocardiography is used to identify the optimal intercostal space (usually, the fourth-intercostal space) and location for an incision on the left chest. A small thoracotomy is made, the pericardium is opened, and a location on the epicardium approximately 3 cm basal to the true apex and 1 cm lateral to the left anterior descending coronary artery is identified for insertion of the hemostatic introducer. TEE assessment is performed to ensure that the entrance site is immediately apical to the base of the anterolateral papillary muscle. Two pledgeted purse-string sutures are placed in the myocardium, and the delivery system is advanced through the introducer and guided to the target on the prolapsed segment of the mitral leaflet using TEE guidance. The tip of the delivery system shaft is positioned on the targeted segment of the mitral leaflet with echocardiographic guidance, and the device is deployed resulting in penetration of the leaflet tissue by the needle and ePTFE wrap. The needle is rapidly withdrawn and the coil of ePTFE is tightened to form a double-helix knot on the atrial surface of the leaflet. After each knot deployment, the delivery system is withdrawn from the heart, leaving two ePTFE strands exteriorized through the introducer lumen. One delivery system is used for each knot deployment. This sequence is repeated for the desired number of knots (usually 4 to 6), then the introducer is withdrawn, and the purse-string sutures are tied. The ePTFE suture pairs are then threaded individually through a stiff ePTFE pledget and are tightened simultaneously and incrementally by using TEE guidance to optimize coaptation and minimize MR. Once the optimal length of the artificial cords is achieved, each pair is tied over the pledget.

A recent study evaluated 12-month outcomes in 65 patients treated with the Harpoon system. Sixty-five patients were enrolled from two prospective multicenter studies.[22] Technical success was achieved in 62 patients (95%). Two patients required conversion to open surgery, and one procedure was terminated. The primary performance endpoint was successful implantation of ≥1 ePTFE cord on the prolapsed leaflet with a reduction of MR to ≤ moderate after the procedure and after 30 days. The primary endpoint was met in 59/65 (91%) patients. Through discharge, there were no deaths, strokes, or renal failure events. At 12 months, 2 of the 62 patients died (3%) and 8 (13%) others required reoperations. At 12 months, 98% of the patients with Harpoon cords were New York Heart Association class I or II, and MR was none/trace in 52% (n = 27), mild in 23% (n = 12), moderate in 23% (n = 12), and severe in 2% (n = 1). Of note, at the time of discharge, the MR grade was none/trace in 74% (43/58), mild in 21% (12/58), moderate in 3% (2/58), and severe in 2% (1/58). Favorable cardiac remodeling outcomes at 1 year included decreased end-diastolic left ventricular volume and diameter and the mean transmitral gradient was 1.4 ± 0.7 mm Hg. Complications associated with this therapy include leaflet perforation, reprolapse of the leaflet, and ePTFE cord rupture.

! TIPS AND TRICKS

Percutaneous Mitral Valve Repair

This section will focus on the only approved device for percutaneous mitral valve (MV) therapies in the United States, MitraClip. Proper patient selection and procedure planning is key for the MitraClip procedure:

1. Risk factors for mitral stenosis include patients with small MVAs (<4.0 cm^2) at baseline, use of a larger device (XTR vs. NTR), and the use of multiple Mitral Clips.
2. The location of the defect is important. Commissural disease will require a smaller clip, as there tends to be crowding of chordae in that location, which can result in clip entrapment and torn chordae. Also, the treatment of commissural disease is less likely to cause significant mitral stenosis as compared to treating A2-P2 pathology because the resultant orifice area will be larger than in the A2-P2 pathology.
3. Large flail gaps may require more than one clip with the first clip used to pull the leaflet down and the second clip to reduce the mitral regurgitation (MR) appropriately.
4. The arms of the XTR are longer and may carry a higher risk for mitral stenosis and potential damage to subvalvular structures in certain scenarios.
5. In the event of elevated transmitral gradients, multiple grasps may have to be attempted to obtain the best balance between reduction in MR and the presence of mitral stenosis (MS). In some instances, mitral stenosis can be reduced by reducing the amount of leaflet tissue grasped, thereby reducing the tension on the leaflets. This can be done by releasing and grasping at a slightly medial or lateral position. This maneuver can also be done to optimize the leaflet grasp. If more leaflet is needed, the gripper can be raised independently, the device rotated anterior or posterior depending on which leaflet is being optimized and the grippers reclosed. These maneuvers should be performed with caution and not at the expense of precipitating single leaflet device detachment.
6. At the time of MitraClip deployment, the patient is under general anesthesia. This can result in artificially tachycardic, bradycardic, hypotensive, or hypertensive scenarios. In borderline cases, it is recommended to use pharmacologic means of mimicking physiologic conditions to generate measurements that are more reflective of what the patient will experience during everyday life. This includes raising the blood pressure to greater than 120/80 post deployment to get an accurate gradient across the MV, holding respiration to stabilize leaflet grasping, or giving adenosine during leaflet grasp to stabilize the grasp and optimize clip position.

CASE-BASED ASSESSMENT

An 85-year-old-man with hx of DM, HTN, HLD, CRI, AF, CAD s/p CABG presented with a progressively worsening SOB and fatigue for several months, worsening over the past 2 weeks. A TTE demonstrated severe MR with a flail posterior leaflet. A TEE confirmed a flail P2 segment with severe MR. Flail gap was 14 mm and had a flail width of 2 cm. The proximal isovelocity surface area (PISA) was 2.2 cm, reconfirming severe MR (see Videos 22.1 through 22.3). The MV area was 7.0 cm^2 with a mean gradient of 2 mm Hg (Fig. 22.2). He was optimized on GDMT without improvement in symptoms. Two MitraClip XTr devices were implanted in the A2–P2 segment with a reduction in MR to 1+ (see Video 22.4 and Video 22.5). The total resulting MVA was 3.5cm^2 post-leaflet repair. Follow-up mean MV gradient was 2 mm Hg (Fig. 22.3).

1. A 76-year-old man with history of atrial fibrillation and coronary artery disease with a stent in an unknown coronary artery presents to the hospital with shortness of breath and a BNP of 1500. Pt undergoes echo and is shown to have EF 30%, large left atrium, moderately dilated LV, and severe mitral regurgitation. The posterior leaflet is restricted. Pts medications include carvedilol twice a day, spironolactone once a day, and Lasix twice a day. Initial treatment in the hospital includes:
   - A. IV diuresis with Mitral Clip placement
   - B. Initiation of Entresto with IV diuresis and clinic follow-up
   - C. BiV-ICD placement and clinic follow-up
   - D. IV diuresis and palliative care consult
2. A 75-year-old woman presents to the emergency room with new onset shortness of breath. Her history included a diagnosis of mitral valve prolapse. Pt has HTN that is under control, normal renal function, and normal EF. She is a 70-kg woman who is 165 cm. Her BNP is 1000. Pt is admitted with new onset heart failure. Echocardiogram shows flail P2 of the mitral valve. Treatment includes:
   - A. Surgical repair of the mitral valve
   - B. Surgical replacement of the mitral valve
   - C. Percutaneous mitral valve repair
   - D. Percutaneous mitral valve replacement
3. Which device is approved for the treatment of functional mitral regurgitation in the United States?
   - A. Cardioband
   - B. Carillion
   - C. Mitralign
   - D. MitraClip
4. True or False: MitraClip has independent grippers to grasp leaflet?
5. Which is NOT a risk factor for mitral stenosis post-MitraClip placement?
   - A. Commissural disease
   - B. Small valve area
   - C. A2P2 pathology
   - D. Multiple clips used

See page 318 for the answers.

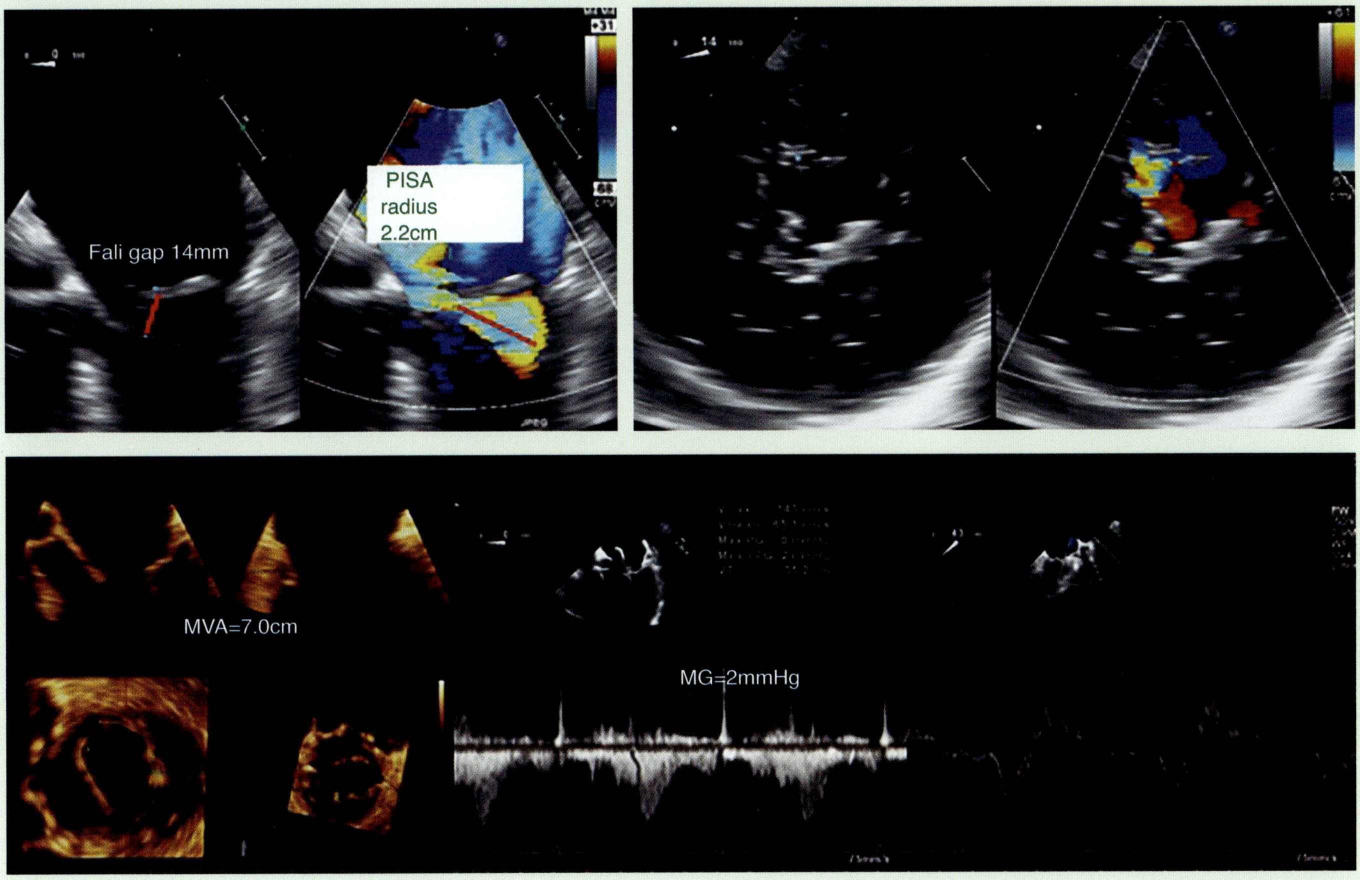

Fig. 22.2 Measurements From Baseline Transesophageal Echo Images.

(*Continued*)

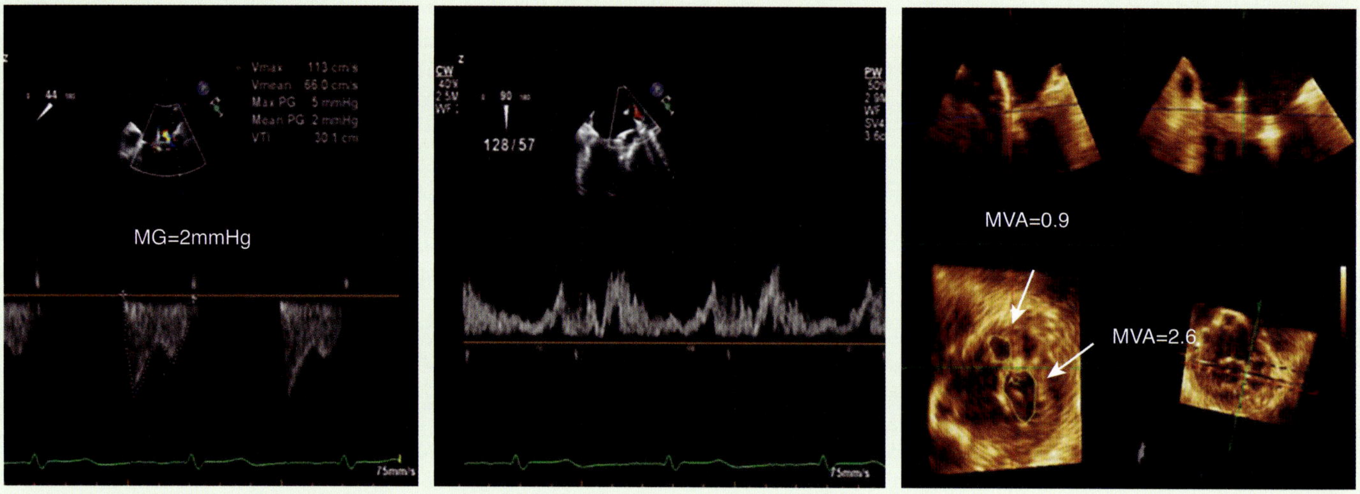

Fig. 22.3 Measurement From Post-MitraClip Transesophageal Echo Images.

REFERENCES

1. Enriquez-Sarano M, Schaff HV, Orszulak TA, et al. Valve repair improves the outcome of surgery for mitral regurgitation. A multivariate analysis. *Circulation*. 1995;91(4):1022–1028.
2. Perier P, Hohenberger W, Lakew F, et al. Toward a new paradigm for the reconstruction of posterior leaflet prolapse: midterm results of the "respect rather than resect" approach. *Ann Thorac Surg*. 2008;86(3):718–725. discussion 718–725.
3. Alfieri O, Maisano F, De Bonis M, et al. The double-orifice technique in mitral valve repair: a simple solution for complex problems. *J Thorac Cardiovasc Surg*. 2001;122(4):674–681.
4. Muller DWM, Farivar RS, Jansz P, et al. Transcatheter mitral valve replacement for patients with symptomatic mitral regurgitation: A global feasibility trial. *J Am Coll Cardiol*. 2017;69(4):381–391.
5. Feldman T, Kar S, Elmariah S, et al. Randomized comparison of percutaneous repair and surgery for mitral regurgitation: 5-year results of EVEREST II. *J Am Coll Cardiol*. 2015;66(25):2844–2854.
6. Mauri L, Foster E, Glower DD, et al. 4-year results of a randomized controlled trial of percutaneous repair versus surgery for mitral regurgitation. *J Am Coll Cardiol*. 2013;62(4):317–328.
7. Stone GW, Lindenfeld J, Abraham WT, et al. Transcatheter Mitral-Valve Repair in Patients with Heart Failure. *N Engl J Med*. 2018;379(24):2307–2318.
8. Stewart MH, Jenkins JS. The Evolving Role of Percutaneous Mitral Valve Repair. *Ochsner J*. 2016;16(3):270–276.
9. Webb JG, Hensey M, Szerlip M, et al. 1-Year Outcomes for Transcatheter Repair in Patients With Mitral Regurgitation From the CLASP Study. *JACC Cardiovasc Interv*. 2020;13(20):2344–2357.
10. Wu AH, Aaronson KD, Bolling SF, et al. Impact of mitral valve annuloplasty on mortality risk in patients with mitral regurgitation and left ventricular systolic dysfunction. *J Am Coll Cardiol*. 2005;45(3):381–387.
11. Weber M, Ozturk C, Taramasso M, et al. Leaflet edge-to-edge treatment versus direct annuloplasty in patients with functional mitral regurgitation. *EuroIntervention*. 2019;15(10):912–918.
12. Schofer J, Siminiak T, Haude M, et al. Percutaneous mitral annuloplasty for functional mitral regurgitation: results of the CARILLON Mitral Annuloplasty Device European Union Study. *Circulation*. 2009;120(4):326–333.
13. Witte KK, Lipiecki J, Siminiak T, et al. The REDUCE FMR trial: A Randomized Sham-Controlled Study of Percutaneous Mitral Annuloplasty in Functional Mitral Regurgitation. *JACC Heart Fail*. 2019;7(11):945–955.
14. Miller M, Thourani VH, Whisenant B. The Cardioband transcatheter annular reduction system. *Ann Cardiothorac Surg*. 2018;7(6):741–747.
15. Nickenig G, Hammerstingl C, Schueler R, et al. Transcatheter Mitral Annuloplasty in Chronic Functional Mitral Regurgitation: 6-Month Results With the Cardioband Percutaneous Mitral Repair System. *JACC Cardiovasc Interv*. 2016;9(19):2039–2047.
16. Messika-Zeitoun D, Nickenig G, Latib A, et al. Transcatheter mitral valve repair for functional mitral regurgitation using the Cardioband system: 1 year outcomes. *Eur Heart J*. 2019;40(5):466–472.
17. Mandinov L, Asch FM, Grube E. Mitralign Percutaneous Annuloplasty System for the Treatment of Functional Mitral Regurgitation. *Eur Cardiol*. 2010;6(2):67–70.
18. Fiocco A, Nadali M, Speziali G, et al. Transcatheter Mitral Valve Chordal Repair: Current Indications and Future Perspectives. *Front Cardiovasc Med*. 2019;6:128.
19. Francesco Maisano, Paolo Denti, Hugo K Vanermen, Joerg Seeburger, Volkmar Falk, Friedrich Wilhelm Mohr, Michael J Mack, Ottavio R Alfieri, Neochordae implantation made easy with an adjustable device: early report of acute and chronic animal experiments, *Innovations (Phila)*. Jul-Aug 2010;5(4):287–90. doi: 10.1097/IMI.0b013e3181ee865d.
20. Colli A, Manzan E, Aidietis A, et al. An early European experience with transapical off-pump mitral valve repair with NeoChord implantation. *Eur J Cardiothorac Surg*. 2018;54(3):460–466.
21. Kiefer P, Meier S, Noack T, et al. Good 5-Year Durability of Transapical Beating Heart Off-Pump Mitral Valve Repair With Neochordae. *Ann Thorac Surg*. 2018;106(2):440–445.
22. Gammie JS, Bartus K, Gackowski A, et al. Safety and performance of a novel transventricular beating heart mitral valve repair system: 1-year outcomes. *Eur J Cardiothorac Surg*. 2021;59(1):199–206.

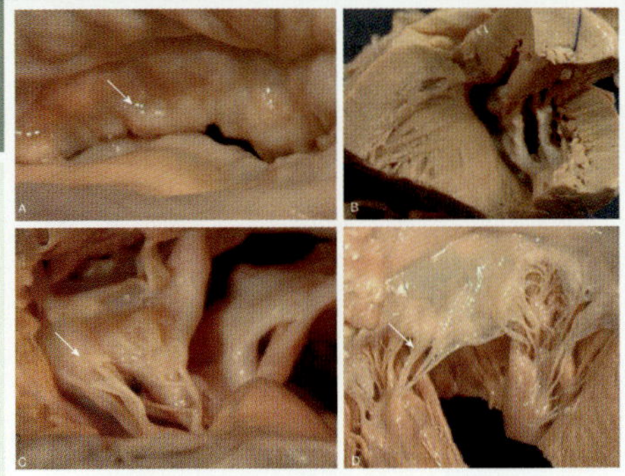

23

Transcatheter Valvuloplasty

Vinayak Nagaraja, Samir Kapadia

CHAPTER OUTLINE

LEARNING OBJECTIVES

1. Patient selection based on anatomical features for percutaneous mitral commissurotomy.
2. Procedural steps of percutaneous mitral commissurotomy.
3. To identify complications of percutaneous mitral commissurotomy and management.
4. Long-term results of percutaneous mitral commissurotomy
   Kollaborate link: https://www.kollaborate.tv/link?id=614b9325b57d4.

INTRODUCTION

Mitral stenosis (MS) continues to be the most common valvular heart disease in the developing and underdeveloped nations. Globally the most common cause of MS is rheumatic heart disease and the prevalence of rheumatic heart disease ranges between 0.6% and 14% across Asia and Africa.[1,2] The other causes of MS include mitral annular calcification, and rarely congenital MS or infiltrative conditions. Percutaneous mitral commissurotomy (PMC) was first described in 1984 by Inoue and his colleagues.[3] This first case series consisted of five patients that had marked reduction in transmitral gradients along with improvement in clinical status.[3] Before the advent of PMC, closed surgical commissurotomy was the only treatment option available for MS. Over the last 36 years, a large number of patients have been treated with this procedure.[4]

PATIENT SELECTION

After holistic evaluation of the patient (that includes the history, quality of life, functional status and physical examination), transthoracic echocardiography (TTE) is the key next step in evaluating eligibility for PMC suitability. TTE evaluates the mitral valve area, transmitral gradient, pulmonary pressure, and the right ventricular function. PMC is considered for patients with a mitral valve area of less 1.5 cm^2. Other aspects that need to be taken into account include clinical status, transmitral gradient and body mass index. In addition to mitral valve area and gradient, TTE also assesses leaflet thickening/calcification/pliability, commissural fusion, subvalvular pathology especially calcification. PMC is not suited for patients with severe subvalvular pathology and minimal commissural fusion. Fig. 23.1 is pathological specimen demonstrating rheumatic MS. Mitral valve morphology based on TTE have been well described and the most important contemporary scores are Wilkins/Cormier score. Wilkins score of 8 or lower or a Cormier class 1 is considered suitable for PMC.[5] The scoring systems are limited by a lack of reproducibility and often underestimate subvalvular pathology. Off-axis parasternal views to visualize papillary muscles and chordal structure can be very useful (Table 23.1).

Transesophageal echocardiography (TEE) can be performed to confirm the diagnosis in patients with poor acoustic windows and exclude a left atrial thrombus, which is an absolute contraindication for PMC; however, patients with organized thrombus deep into the left atrial appendage (LAA) can be treated with careful manipulation of catheter by avoiding entry into LAA. Other relative contraindications for PMC include severe thoracic deformity, bleeding diathesis, moderate mitral regurgitation (MR), concomitant severe coronary artery disease/aortic valve disease, and severe commissural mitral valve calcification. Severe MS is the class I indication for PMC and is an attractive option for all individuals where mitral valve replacement can be avoided, leading to multiple surgeries, especially in young patients. The burden of mitral prosthesis, and anticoagulation, especially in the case of

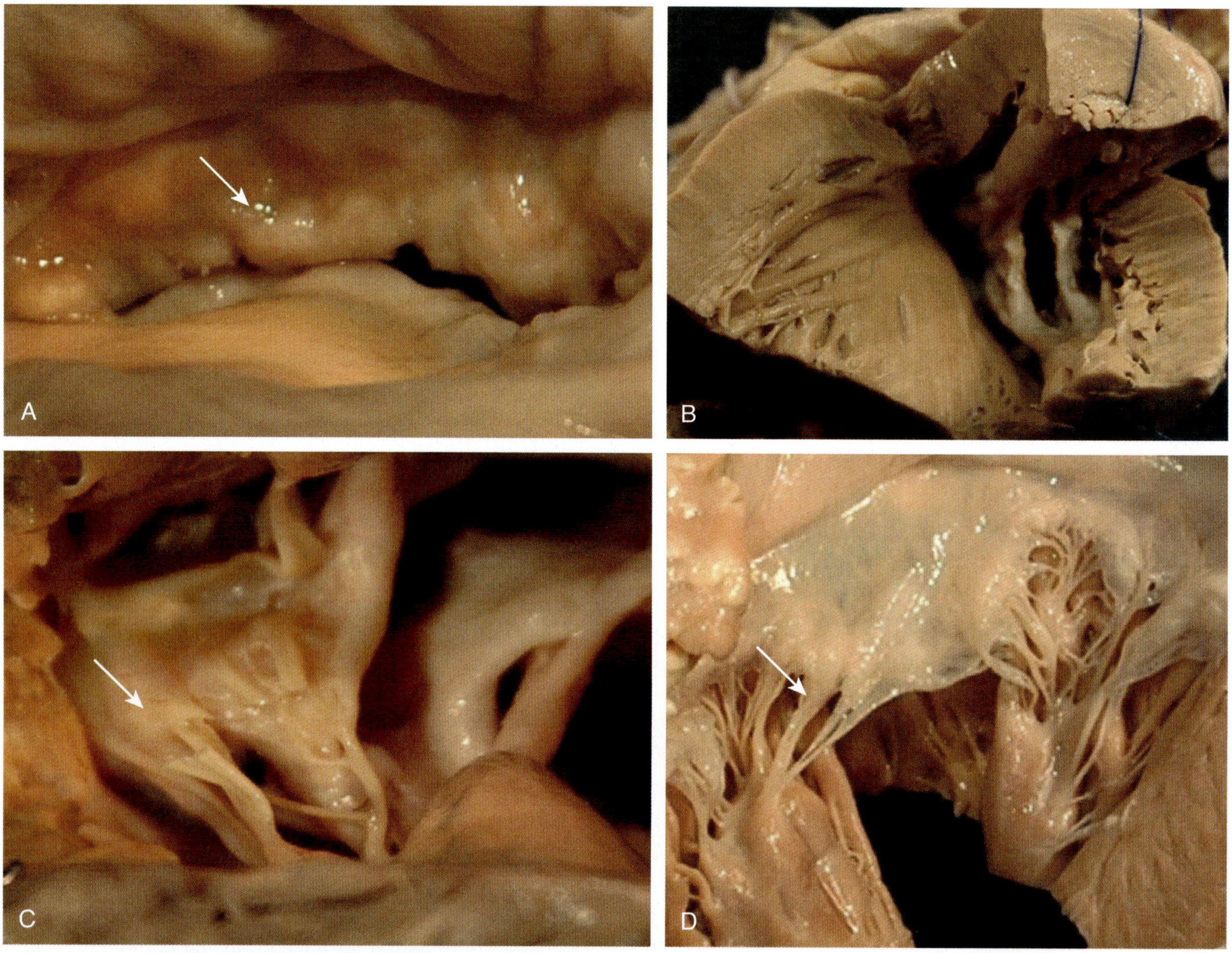

Fig. 23.1 Pathologic specimens demonstrating rheumatic mitral stenosis from the (A) atrial and (B) ventricular sides. (C) Thick, fused, shortened subvalvular apparatus is seen. (D) Normal anatomy. (From Chandrashekhar Y, Westaby S, Narula J. Mitral stenosis. *Lancet.* 2009;374[9697]:1271–1283.)

mechanical mitral valve, cannot be underestimated. This is particularly a useful strategy in women of childbearing age so that they can complete their families and reduce complications during pregnancy. In patients with symptomatic MS and unsuitable anatomy for PMC, the decision to perform PMC must be individualized, taking into account the surgical risks and long-term demerits of a mitral prostheses. PMC is an appealing option in young patients with sinus rhythm and unfavorable anatomy. PMC can be considered in asymptomatic patients to allow pregnancy in young women or undergo urgent noncardiac surgery. PMC is also appropriate in asymptomatic patients with resting pulmonary hypertension or individuals who are at a higher risk of embolic events or hemodynamic decompensation. Exercise echocardiography can sometimes help delineate the asymptomatic from the symptomatic patients. A pulmonary pressure of more than 60 mm Hg during exercise can be considered an indication for PMC.

SPECIAL POPULATIONS

A cautious approach is essential while performing PMC in patients with severe pulmonary hypertension. The limited literature in this genre suggests that PMC is feasible in individuals with MS and severe pulmonary hypertension.[6] PMC reduces pulmonary pressure by improving transmitral flow and, hence, reducing the patient's surgical risk. PMC can also be used as a bridge to surgery or as a palliative procedure in critically ill as well as elderly patients. PMC in previous surgical commissurotomy has been evaluated.[7–10] PMC is feasible in patients with previous surgical commissurotomy; however, it is particularly challenging in "funnel-shaped" stenosis that is common postsurgery. PMC in surgical commissurotomy patients reduces the transmitral gradient short term and has satisfactory long-term results.[8]

TABLE 23.1 Scoring Systems Based on Echocardiography for Mitral Valve Intervention

Wilkins or Abascal Score				
Grade	**SCORED MITRAL VALVE CHARACTERISTICS**			
	Leaflet Mobility	**Leaflet Thickening**	**Leaflet Calcification**	**Involvement of Subvalvular Apparatus**
1	Highly mobile with only leaflet tips restricted	Leaflet near normal in thickness (45 mm)	Single area of increased echo brightness	Minimal thickening just below the MV leaflets
2	Leaflet mid and base portions have normal mobility	Midleaflets normal, considerable thickening of leaflet margins (58 mm)	Scattered areas of brightness confined to leaflet margins	Thickening of chordal structures extending to one-third of the chordal length
3	Valve continues to move forward in diastole, mainly from the base	Thickening extending through the entire leaflets (5 8 mm)	Brightness extending into midportions of the leaflets	Thickening extended to distal third of the chords
4	No or minimal forward movement of the leaflets in diastole	Considerable thickening of all leaflet tissue (>810 mm)	Extensive brightness throughout much of the tissue leaflet	Extensive thickening and shortening of all chordal structures extending down to the papillary muscle
Interpretation of result	Score range: 4–16. A score >8 suggests the MV may not be suitable to PMBC and is associated with poor short- and long-term results.			
Group assignment according to anatomical characteristics of the MV and the MV apparatus as assessed by 2D echocardiography and fluoroscopy (Cormier score)				
	Group 1	**Group 2**	**Group 3**	
Anatomical characteristics	Pliable, noncalcified anterior mitral leaflet and midsubvalvular disease, that is, thin chordate 10 mm or longer.	Pliable noncalcified anterior mitral leaflet and severe subvalvular disease, that is, thickened chordate <10 mm long..	Calcification of mitral valve of any extent as assessed by fluoroscopy, whatever the state of the subvalvular apparatus is..	
Interpretation of result	In a subset of 40 patients a Wilkins score in the range of 7–9 correlated with the echocardiographic group 1, a Wilkins score range 8–12 correlated with the echocardiographic group 2, and a Wilkins score range 10–15 with group. An echocardiographic grouping score of 2 or higher is associated with poor long-term results.			

Continued

TABLE 23.1 Scoring Systems Based on Echocardiography for Mitral Valve Intervention—cont'd

Wilkins or Abascal Score						
Grade	**SCORED MITRAL VALVE CHARACTERISTICS**					
Assessment of commissural calcium This method quantifies the extent of calcification in both commissures by giving a half commissure of each commissure a score of 1 with the detection of intensive bright echoes as seen by 2D TTE						
Grade 1	**Grade 2**	**Grade 3**	**Grade 4**			
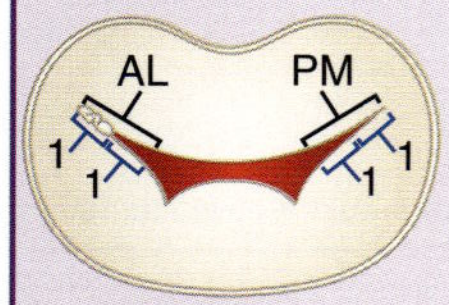	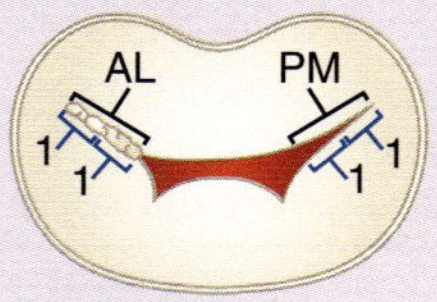	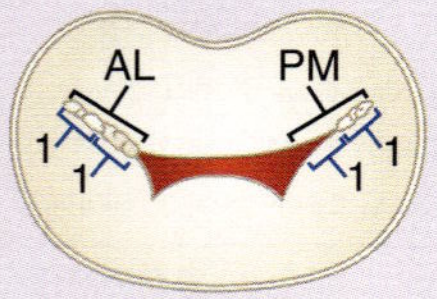	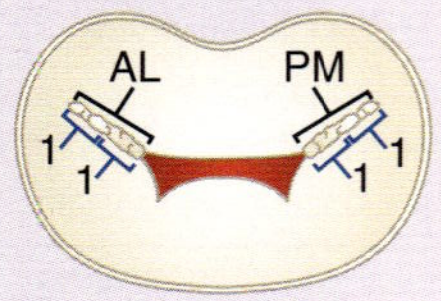			
Interpretation of result	Patients with a commissural calcium score grade 0–1were found to have larger MVA and an improvement in symptoms than those with grade 2–3 after PMBC. Commissural calcification is one of the strongest predictors of outcome of PMBC and may also predict severe MR as a major complication of PMBC. A commissural calcium grade of 2 or higher is a predictor of poor immediate results					
Real-time transthoracic 3D echocardiographic score						
Leaflets	**AML**			**PML**		
Leaflet segments	**A1**	**A2**	**A3**	**P1**	**P2**	**P3**
Leaflet thickness (0–6) (0 = normal, 1 = thickened)[a]	0–1	0–1	0–1	0–1	0–1	0–1
Leaflet mobility (0–6) (0 = normal, 1 = thickened)[a]	0–1	0–1	0–1	0–1	0–1	0–1
Leaflet calcification (0–10)(0 = no, 1–2 = calcified)[b]	0–2	0–1	0–2	0–2	0–1	0–2

Subvalvular mitral apparatus[b]			
Affected part of the subvalvular apparatus	**Proximal third**	**Middle third**	**Distal third**
Thickness (0–3) (0 = normal, 1 = thickened)	0–1	0–1	0–1
Separation (0–6) (0 = normal, 1 = partial, 2 = no)	0, 1, 2	0, 1, 2	0, 1, 2
Interpretation of result	[a]Normal = 0, mild = 1–2, moderate 3–4, severe 5–6 [b]Normal = 0, mild = 1–2, moderate 3–5, severe = 6 The individual score points are added up, with the calculated total score ranging from 0–31 points. Mild MV involvement is defined as <8 points, moderate MV involvement 8–13, and severe MV involvement >14 points.		
Echo score "Revisited" (to predict immediate outcome)			
Echocardiographic variables	**Points for score (0–11)**		
MVA ≤1 cm^2	2		
Maximum leaflet displacement ≤12 mm	3		
Commissural area ratio ≥1.25	3		
Subvalvular involvement	3		
Interpretation of result	3 risk groups are defined: low (score 0–3); intermediate (score 4–5); high (score 6–11). This score is more predictive than the Wilkins score and is particularly useful for predicting outcomes for patients categorized in the intermediate-risk group		

AL, Anterolateral; *AML,* anterior mitral leaflet; *MR,* mitral regurgitation; *MV,* mitral valve; *MVA,* mitral valve area; *PM,* posteromedial; *PML,* posterior mitral leaflet; *TTE,* transthoracic echocardiography.

(Modified from Wunderlich NC, Dalvi B, Ho SY, et al. Rheumatic mitral valve stenosis: diagnosis and treatment options. *Curr Cardiol Rep.* 2019;21(3):14.)

Severe MS carries a bad prognosis among pregnant women and is a common clinical scenario in developing countries. Untreated severe MS during pregnancy is often associated with maternal and fetal mortality.[11] Surgery during pregnancy has adverse outcomes on fetus especially when extracorporeal circulation is needed. PMC during pregnancy has been shown to be feasible and safe.[12,13] PMC can be performed after 20 weeks' of gestation and ideally performed in the third trimester. To avoid radiation to the fetus, a lead shield is laid over the patient's abdomen. If PMC results in a complication (e.g., MR) requiring urgent cardiac surgery, a cesarean section should be performed prior to surgery if MR can be tolerated. The stakes are high during pregnancy. PMC should be performed by skilled experienced operators with short inflation-deflation cycles.

PROCEDURE

PMC's mechanism of action is similar to surgical commissurotomy where the fused commissures are opened. PMC can be performed via the anterograde transvenous/transseptal or retrograde/transarterial approach. Technically, PMC can be performed using the Inoue or double-balloon technique. The transseptal approach can be performed via the jugular vein or femoral vein. The atrial anatomy is considerably different to normal given the enlarged atria as well the exaggerated convex septum. The ideal puncture site is the midpoint of the fossa ovalis. Often, assistance for the transseptal puncture can be gained by placing a pigtail in the noncoronary cusp of the aortic valve. If transseptal puncture is not guided by TEE, transseptal puncture should not be performed with an INR greater than 2. Special care should be taken in patients with previous cardiac surgery. We recommend that full-dose heparin be administered before transseptal puncture to reduce the risk of left atrial thrombus formation. We routinely use and recommend the TEE echocardiography during PMC to exclude left atrial/appendage thrombus, guide transseptal puncture, and optimize results. The Inoue technique is the most popular technique for PMC. It is a low-profile balloon that measures around 4.5 mm and its diameter ranges between 24 and 30 mm. The diameter is chosen based on patient's height (balloon diameter equals 0.1 times height [cm] plus 10). In very severe MS with a valve area of less than 0.5 cm^2 or extreme commissural calcification, it would be reasonable to undersize the balloon by 1 to 2 mm.

PROCEDURAL STEPS

CASE REPORT

A 75-year-old gentleman of Southeast Asian heritage with a long-standing history of rheumatic heart disease with aortic sclerosis without stenosis and mild-to-moderate mitral stenosis, minimal coronary artery disease. He had noticed reduction in exercise tolerance. On further evaluation, he was found to have severe mitral stenosis caused by doming and restricted opening. There was trace mitral valve regurgitation with a peak transmitral valve gradient of 20 mm Hg and a mean of 10 mm Hg. The pressure half-time was 222 ms with a mitral valve area 0.64 cm^2 (0.37 cm^2/m^2). His left and right ventricular size and systolic function were normal. There was severe left atrial enlargement, and right ventricular systolic pressure is 32 mm Hg—consistent with normal pulmonary artery pressures. His coronary angiogram revealed mild coronary artery disease.

A 4/5 Glidesheath Slender sheath (Terumo Corporation, Shibuya City, Tokyo, Japan) was placed in the right radial, a preclosed (Perclose ProGlide [Abbott Vascular, Santa Clara, CA, USA]) 8 Fr sheath in the right common femoral vein (RCFV) and 7Fr sheath in the left common femoral vein (LCFV). We advanced a Swan-Ganz catheter and (Edwards Lifesciences, Irvine, CA, USA) took hemodynamic measurements obtaining the following: mean right atrium 12 mm Hg, mean pulmonary artery 37 mm Hg, cardiac output of 3.13 L/min, and cardiac index of 1.81 L/min using Fick principle.

We advanced a pigtail catheter into the left ventricle (LV) obtaining an LV pressure of 170/20. We performed a power injection of the LV showing trace MR. We exchanged the 8 Fr RCFV sheath for 16 Fr sheath (Cook Medical, Bloomington, IN, USA) in the right femoral vein. Through this sheath, a Mullins sheath (Medtronic, Minneapolis, MN, USA) was advanced for transseptal puncture. The echocardiography team inserted a TEE probe to rule out (r/o) LAA thrombus and help with location of puncture. The interatrial septum was crossed using a Brockenbrough needle (Medtronic, Minneapolis, MN, USA), guided by fluoroscopy, TEE, and hemodynamics. It is important to perform the puncture posteriorly and somewhat inferiorly. Too anterior or superior of a puncture should be avoided.

We obtained simultaneous left atrium (LA)/LV pressures to obtain a mean LA pressure of 28 and preprocedural transmitral gradient of 10 at a heart rate (HR) of 63 beats/min. We advanced a Toray wire (Toray Industries, Tokyo, Japan) into the left atrial cavity through the Mullins sheath. The atrial septum was dilated using a Toray rigid dilator (14 Fr). This step facilities the introducing the Inoue into the LA.

The Inoue balloon (Toray Industries, Tokyo, Japan) is first inflated fully outside the body and after cautiously expelling all the air from the Inoue balloon (to avoid air embolism in case of balloon rupture) was exchanged for the Mullins sheath. The Inoue balloon is chronologically inflated in the right anterior oblique view. Initially, the distal portion is inflated with 1 to 2 mL of diluted contrast. We advanced the balloon across the mitral valve and performed serial inflations.

We repeated our LA/LV gradients through the Inoue balloon and took repeated hemodynamics through the Swan-Ganz catheter obtaining the following: the mean LA pressure was 18 mm Hg, with a mitral gradient of 2 mm Hg at a HR of 64 beats/min, the LV end-diastolic pressure was 14 mm Hg, mean pulmonary artery 28 mm Hg, cardiac output of 3.13 L/min, and cardiac index of 1.81 L/min using Fick principle. TEE showed trace MR and confirmed our hemodynamic gradient.

The RCFV and LCFV were closed with a Perclose and the radial sheath removed, and hemostasis was achieved with a TR Band (Terumo Corporation, Shibuya City, Tokyo, Japan). Video 23.1 illustrates the case sequentially. The final therapeutic outcome ideally to be achieved by PMC is a valve area of greater than 1 cm^2/m^2, commissural opening of both commissures with some commissural MR. The procedure should be stopped if there is evidence of injury to mitral leaflets with flail segments causing new MR or increase in MR, which is greater than mild-moderate. Kollaborate link: https://www.kollaborate.tv/link?id=614b9325b57d4

COMPLICATIONS

Complications during the procedure are often a result of a combination of factors that include the patient's clinical anatomical features and operator experience.[14,15] Operator experience and volume have been well recognized to improve outcomes in structural intervention.[16] The incidence rates of complications related to transseptal puncture reduced with greater operator experience.[17] Mortality as a result of PMC ranges between 0% and 3%. This is commonly due to pericardial tamponade (which is completely avoidable) or frailty. Hemopericardium is commonly related to transseptal puncture or left ventricular wire perforation and its incidence ranges between 0.5% and 1%. The hardly used metallic commissurotome has a higher incidence of hemopericardium compared to the Inoue technique. Pericardial tamponade should be promptly treated with emergency pericardiocentesis under echocardiographic guidance and reversal of anticoagulation using protamine. Systemic embolism is another complication that operators should be vigilant about, and its incidence ranges between 0.5% and 5%. Systemic embolism could be due to established left atrial/atrial appendage thrombus prior to the start of the case or air embolism after balloon rupture. Systemic embolism can manifest as a stroke or transient ST segment elevation due to coronary embolism.

Acute severe MR[17,18] is a rare but a dreaded complication of PMC, with an incidence ranging between 2% and 4%. The findings during surgery[18] include noncommissural leaflet tearing, chordal rupture and rarely papillary muscle rupture. Severe MR rarely occurs due to excessive commissural splitting and majority of severe MR cases happen because of unfavorable anatomical characteristics leading to tearing of anterior mitral leaflet. This scenario commonly requires valve replacement, and timing surgery can be determined based on the clinical state, surgical risk, pulmonary pressure, and mechanism of MR. In patients with severe MR, normal blood pressure, and pulmonary hypertension, early surgery should be considered. Insertion of intraaortic balloon pump/mechanical support might be necessary before open-heart surgery in patients with cardiogenic shock. Acute severe MR post-PMC carries a poor prognosis and is largely unpredictable. This dreaded complication can be avoided by stepwise Inoue technique along with echocardiography. Other rare indications of open-heart surgery post-PMC include left ventricular perforation. Interatrial shunts can occur because of PMC, which can result in hypoxemia in patients with severe pulmonary hypertension because of right to left shunt. Other complications include atrial fibrillation and vascular injury.

SHORT- AND LONG-TERM OUTCOMES

The definition of hemodynamic success post-PMC is variable across literature. Commonly used criteria include a mitral valve area greater than 1.6 cm^2 and a 25% increase in valve area compared to baseline along with minimal MR. The independent predictors of procedural failure and worse long-term outcomes include unfavorable anatomy, older age, history of surgical commissurotomy, poor functional class, very small mitral valve area, presence of MR, and severe pulmonary hypertension.[19,20] Long-term follow-up (over 20 year) post-PMC is available.[7] The long-term, event free chance of survival post-PMC (composite of survival and lack of valvular reintervention) is estimated to be around 35% to 70%.[20] Procedural features associated with poor long-term outcomes include higher residual gradient, small final valve area, inadequate commissural opening, and presence of MR.[20] Repeat valvuloplasty accounts for 10% to 30% of all PMC, and the incidence of restenosis ranges between 2% and 40%.[7] The outcomes of repeat valvuloplasty appear to be favorable in a select group of patients with commissural refusion. Most interatrial shunts tend to close over time, however, clinically and hemodynamically significant shunts with a Qp/Qs of greater than 1.5 warrant closure. Some claim that PMC improves left atrial function and could potentially reduce the rate of atrial fibrillation as well as systemic embolism.[7,21] Short- and long-term outcomes post-PMC are similar to surgical commissurotomy (Table 23.2).[22-26]

TABLE 23.2 Randomized Trials Comparing Percutaneous Mitral Balloon Commissurotomy and Surgical Commissurotomy

First author	Patel et al.[25]		Turi et al.[26]		Arora et al.[27]		Reyes et al.[24]		Ben Farhat et al.[23]		
Year	1991		1991		1993		1994		1998		
Mean follow-up	Immediate		7 months		22 months		3 years		7 years		
Procedure	Percutaneous mitral commissurotomy	Closed commissurotomy	Percutaneous mitral commissurotomy	Closed commissurotomy	Percutaneous mitral commissurotomy	Closed commissurotomy	Percutaneous mitral commissurotomy	Open commissurotomy	Percutaneous mitral commissurotomy	Open commissurotomy	Closed commissurotomy
Number of patients	23	22	20	20	100	100	30	30	30	30	30
Age (years, Mean ± SD)	30 ± 11	26 ± 26	27 ± 8	28 ± 1	19 ± 5	20 ± 6	30 ± 9	31 ± 9	29 ± 12	27 ± 9	28 ± 10

Continued

TABLE 23.2 Randomized Trials Comparing Percutaneous Mitral Balloon Commissurotomy and Surgical Commissurotomy—cont'd

First author		Patel et al.[25]		Turi et al.[26]		Arora et al.[27]		Reyes et al.[24]		Ben Farhat et al.[23]		
Mean score		6	6	7.2	8.4	—	—	6.7	7	6	6	6
Mitral valve area (Mean ± SD)	Pre	0.8 ± 0.3	0.7 ± 0.2	0.8 ± 0.2	0.9 ± 0.4	0.8 ± 0.3	0.8 ± 0.2	0.9 ± 0.3	0.9 ± 0.3	0.9 ± 0.2	0.9 ± 0.2	0.9 ± 0.2
	Post	2.1 ± 0.7	1.3 ± 0.3	1.6 ± 0.2	1.7 ± 0.2	2.3 ± 0.1	2.1 ± 0.4	2.4 ± 0.6*	1.8 ± 0.4	1.8 ± 0.4	1.8 ± 0.3	1.3 ± 0.3
Restenosis rate		—	—	—	—	5%	4%	10%	13%	—	—	—
Freedom from reintervention		—	—	—	—	—		—	—	90%	93%	50%
New York Heart Association functional class I (%)		91%	—	—	—	—		72%	57%	87%	90%	33%

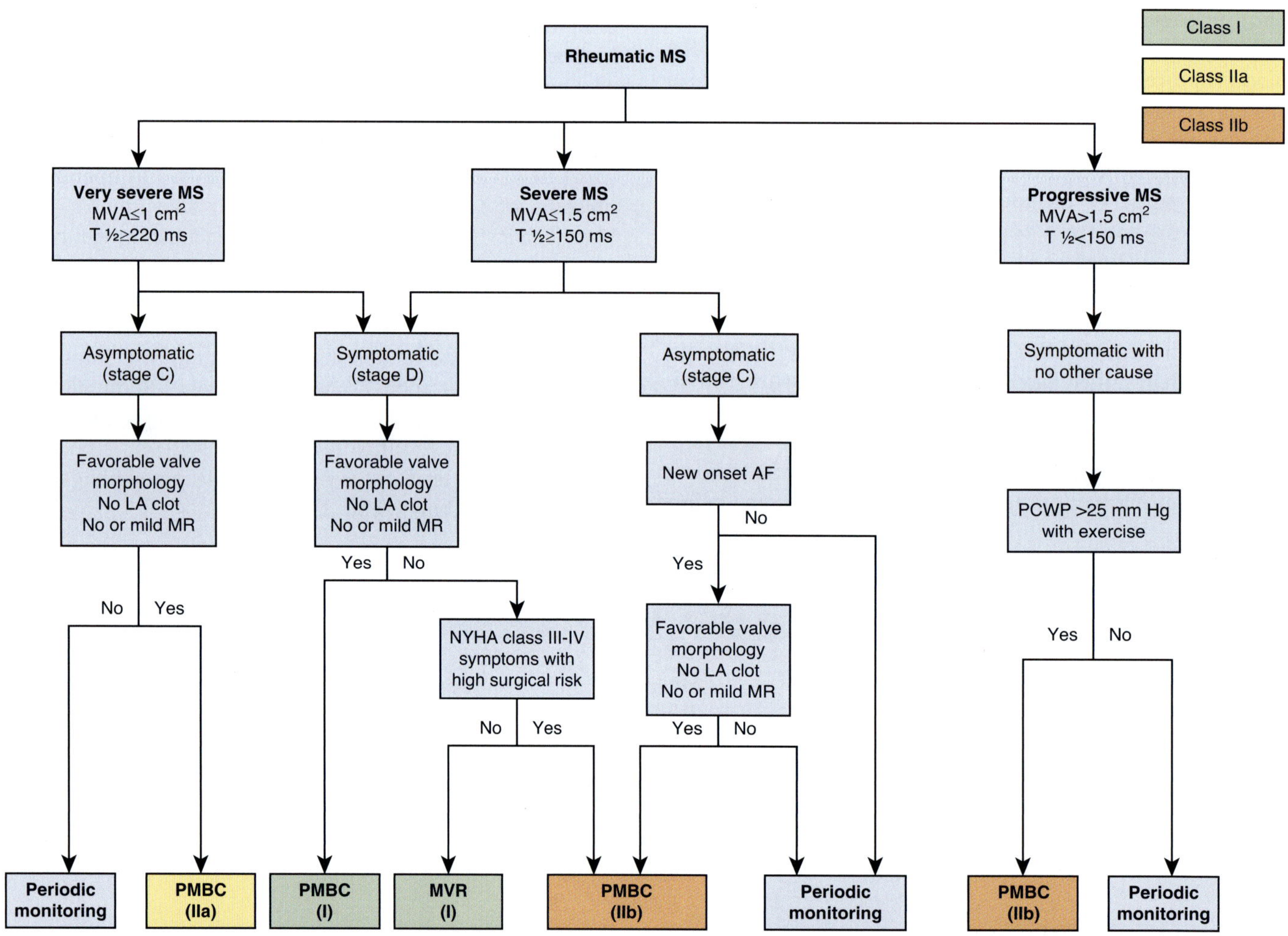

Fig. 23.2 Rheumatic MS Stages and Management Options. *AF*, Atrial fibrillation; *LA*, left atrial; *MR*, mitral regurgitation; *MS*, mitral stenosis; *MVA*, mitral valve area; *MVR*, mitral valve surgery (repair or replacement); *NYHA*, New York Heart Association; *PCWP*, pulmonary capillary wedge pressure; *PMBC*, percutaneous mitral balloon commissurotomy; and *T1/2*, pressure half-time. (From Nishimura RA, Otto CM, Bonow RO, et al. 2014 AHA/ACC guideline for the management of patients with valvular heart disease: executive summary: a report of the American College of Cardiology/American Heart Association Task Force on Practice Guidelines. *J Am Coll Cardiol.* 2014;63[22]:2438–2488.)

SUMMARY

Since its inception over three decades ago, PMC has dramatically changed the way rheumatic MS has been managed. PMC mimics surgical commissurotomy, and it is an attractive option especially for young individuals. PMC helps postpone valve replacement and avoids the burden of anticoagulation/mitral prosthesis. Eventually, PMC can be succeeded by surgical valve replacement. The key to achieving an ideal result is patient selection and choosing the appropriate anatomy for PMC. The management of MS should be individualized. requires a multidisciplinary team approach that includes an imaging cardiologist, an interventional cardiologist, and a cardiac surgeon. Fig. 23.2 demonstrates an algorithm for the management of MS. The management of MS in pregnancy is challenging, and PMC should be performed meticulously by an experienced operator using short inflation-deflation cycles. Long-term results with PMC are comparable to surgical commissurotomy, and it has completely replaced surgery.

CASE-BASED ASSESSMENT

The following questions are based on the above Case Report:

1. What anatomical feature is not suitable for PMC?
   A. Severe subvalvular calcification and minimal commissural fusion
   B. Severe commissural fusion and no subvalvular calcification
   C. No mitral regurgitation
   D. None of the above
2. What is the ideal of site of the transseptal puncture site for PMC?
   A. Midpoint of the fossa ovalis
   B. Anterior and superior
   C. Posterior and inferior
   D. None of the above
3. When should be the Inoue balloon be undersized?
   A. A valve area of less than 0.5 cm^2
   B. Extreme commissural calcification
   C. A and B
   D. None of the above
4. What is the most common cause of mitral stenosis across the globe?
   A. Rheumatic heart disease
   B. Mitral annular calcification
   C. Congenital mitral stenosis
   D. Infiltrative cardiomyopathy
5. When should the PMC procedure be stopped?
   A. New significant mitral regurgitation (MR)
   B. Valve area less than 1 cm^2/m^2
   C. Incomplete commissural opening
   D. None of the above

See page 318 for the answers

REFERENCES

1. Chandrashekhar Y, Westaby S, Narula J. Mitral stenosis. *Lancet.* 2009;374(9697):1271–1283.
2. Iung B, Vahanian A. Epidemiology of acquired valvular heart disease. *Can J Cardiol.* 2014;30(9):962–970.
3. Inoue K, Owaki T, Nakamura T, et al. Clinical application of transvenous mitral commissurotomy by a new balloon catheter. *J Thorac Cardiovasc Surg.* 1984;87(3):394–402.
4. Marijon E, Iung B, Mocumbi AO, et al. What are the differences in presentation of candidates for percutaneous mitral commissurotomy across the world and do they influence the results of the procedure? *Arch Cardiovasc Dis.* 2008;101(10):611–617.
5. Palacios IF, Sanchez PL, Harrell LC, et al. Which patients benefit from percutaneous mitral balloon valvuloplasty? *Circulation.* 2002;105(12):1465–1471.
6. Maoqin S, Guoxiang H, Zhiyuan S, et al. The clinical and hemodynamic results of mitral balloon valvuloplasty for patients with mitral stenosis complicated by severe pulmonary hypertension. *Eur J Intern Med.* 2005;16(6):413–418.
7. Bouleti C, Iung B, Himbert D, et al. Long-term efficacy of percutaneous mitral commissurotomy for restenosis after previous mitral commissurotomy. *Heart.* 2013;99(18):1336–1341.
8. Bouleti C, Iung B, Himbert D, et al. Reinterventions after percutaneous mitral commissurotomy during long-term follow-up, up to 20 years: the role of repeat percutaneous mitral commissurotomy. *Eur Heart J.* 2013;34(25):1923–1930.
9. Tuzcu EM, Kapadia SR. Long-term efficacy of percutaneous mitral commissurotomy for recurrent mitral stenosis. *Heart.* 2013;99(18):1307.
10. Jang IK, Block PC, Newell JB, et al. Percutaneous mitral balloon valvotomy for recurrent mitral stenosis after surgical commissurotomy. *Am J Cardiol.* 1995;75(8):601–605.
11. Hameed A, Karaalp IS, Tummala PP, et al. The effect of valvular heart disease on maternal and fetal outcome of pregnancy. *J Am Coll Cardiol.* 2001;37(3):893–899.
12. Esteves CA, Munoz JS, Braga S, et al. Immediate and long-term follow-up of percutaneous balloon mitral valvuloplasty in pregnant patients with rheumatic mitral stenosis. *Am J Cardiol.* 2006;98(6):812–816.
13. de Souza JAM, Martinez EE, Ambrose JA, et al. Percutaneous balloon mitral valvuloplasty in comparison with open mitral valve commissurotomy for mitral stenosis during pregnancy. *J Am Coll Cardiol.* 2001;37(3):900.
14. Krishnamoorthy KM, Dash PK, Radhakrishnan S, et al. Response of different grades of pulmonary artery hypertension to balloon mitral valvuloplasty. *Am J Cardiol.* 2002;90(10):1170–1173.
15. Badheka AO, Shah N, Ghatak A, et al. Balloon Mitral Valvuloplasty in the United States: A 13-Year Perspective. *Am J Med.* 2014;127(11) 1126.e1–e12.
16. Vemulapalli S, Carroll JD, Mack MJ, et al. Procedural Volume and Outcomes for Transcatheter Aortic-Valve Replacement. *N Engl J Med.* 2019;380(26):2541–2550.
17. Iung B, Nicoud-Houel A, Fondard O, et al. Temporal trends in percutaneous mitral commissurotomy over a 15-year period. *Eur Heart J.* 2004;25(8):701–707.
18. Varma PK, Theodore S, Neema PK, et al. Emergency surgery after percutaneous transmitral commissurotomy: operative versus echocardiographic findings, mechanisms of complications, and outcomes. *J Thorac Cardiovasc Surg.* 2005;130(3):772–776.
19. Iung B, Cormier B, Ducimetière P, et al. Immediate results of percutaneous mitral commissurotomy. A predictive model on a series of 1514 patients. *Circulation.* 1996;94(9):2124–2130.
20. Cruz-Gonzalez I, Sanchez-Ledesma M, Sanchez PL, et al. Predicting success and long-term outcomes of percutaneous mitral valvuloplasty: A multifactorial score. *Am J Med.* 2009;122(6) 581.e11–e19.

21. Chiang CW, Lo SK, Ko YS, et al. Predictors of systemic embolism in patients with mitral stenosis. A prospective study. *Ann Intern Med.* 1998;128(11):885–889.
22. Singh AD, Mian A, Devasenapathy N, et al. Percutaneous mitral commissurotomy versus surgical commissurotomy for rheumatic mitral stenosis: a systematic review and meta-analysis of randomised controlled trials. *Heart.* 2020;106(14):1094–1101.
23. Ben Farhat M, Ayari M, Maatouk F, et al. Percutaneous balloon versus surgical closed and open mitral commissurotomy: seven-year follow-up results of a randomized trial. *Circulation.* 1998;97(3):245–250.
24. Reyes VP, Raju BS, Wynne J, et al. Percutaneous balloon valvuloplasty compared with open surgical commissurotomy for mitral stenosis. *N Engl J Med.* 1994;331(15):961–967.
25. Patel JJ, Shama D, Mitha AS, et al. Balloon valvuloplasty versus closed commissurotomy for pliable mitral stenosis: a prospective hemodynamic study. *J Am Coll Cardiol.* 1991;18(5):1318–1322.
26. Turi ZG, Reyes VP, Raju BS, et al. Percutaneous balloon versus surgical closed commissurotomy for mitral stenosis. A prospective, randomized trial. *Circulation.* 1991;83(4):1179–1185.
27. Arora R, Nair M, Kalra GS, et al. Immediate and long-term results of balloon and surgical closed mitral valvotomy: a randomized comparative study. *Am Heart J.* 1993;125(4):1091–1094.

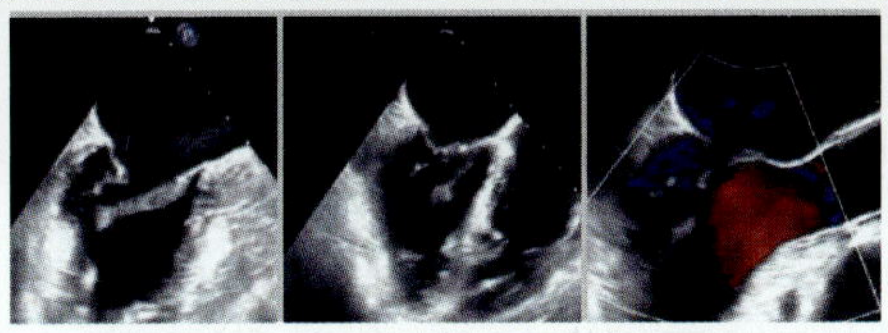

24

Transcatheter Mitral Valve Replacement

Justin Johannesen, Chunguang Chen, Mark J. Russo

CHAPTER OUTLINE

LEARNING OBJECTIVES

- While a transcatheter approach has become ubiquitous for aortic valve replacement, transcatheter mitral valve replacement has been slower to gain traction.
- The more complex anatomy and pathophysiology of mitral valve disease, in comparison to the aortic valve, complicates device design and deployment technique of transcatheter replacement for the mitral valve.
- TMVR is most likely to gain use in the near future as an alternative for prohibitively high-risk surgical patients with severe mitral regurgitation who are not suitable for repair with MitraClip.

INTRODUCTION

While surgical mitral valve repair or replacement remains the standard of care for symptomatic, severe mitral regurgitation, nearly 50% of these patients are not referred for conventional surgical mitral valve replacement (MVR) due to significant comorbidities and high surgical risk. Over the past few years, transcatheter mitral valve interventions using edge-to-edge repair have helped to address some of these high-risk patients. However, a significant group of patients are not candidates for this technique because of unsuitable mitral anatomy for clip repair. In addition, a substantial group of patients (10% to 20%) continue to have significant, moderate or severe, residual regurgitation after the clip repair. Transcatheter mitral valve replacement (TMVR) is a niche for those patients that are not currently served with the existing treatment options (Table 24.1).

CURRENT INDICATIONS AND USE

TMVR is a novel option to treat both severe mitral regurgitation and mitral stenosis without the need for surgery. TMVR valves can be classified broadly based on whether the patient has had prior mitral valve intervention into valve-in-valve or native valve replacement. Valve-in-valve TMVR involves implanting a catheter expandable valve (usually an Edwards S3 valve) inside an existing prosthetic valve. This technique has gained food and drug administration (FDA) approval for patients with failing bioprosthetic valves who are too high risk for a surgical re-do MVR. Valve-in-valve TMVR has also been used for patients with prior mitral rings presenting with worsening mitral regurgitation (MR) or mitral stenosis (MS). Conversely, native TMVR involves replacement in patients with native mitral valve disease without prior interventions. As of today, TMVR for native mitral valve disease has not gained FDA approval.

TABLE 24.1 Considerations Favoring Transcatheter Mitral Valve Replacement Versus Repair

TMVR	Edge-to-Edge Repair (MitraClip)
Diffuse, broad MR jet	Central MR jet
Small, non-coapting leaflets	Large leaflets with coaptation length >2 mm
Excessive flail	Flail gap <10 mm, width <15 mm
Valve area <3.5 cm^2	Adequate valve area to accommodate clipping
Central leaflet calcification	No calcification at grasping zone
Concomitant mitral stenosis	No mitral stenosis

TMVR, Transcatheter mitral valve replacement.

TMVR can be done either via a transseptal or transapical approach. For native TMVR, the vast majority, over 80%, of valves implanted thus far today have been via the transapical approach. This approach is the most direct route to the mitral valve. Valve-in-valve TMVR has been performed mostly via the transseptal approach. A transseptal approach is also usually preferred in patients with extensive annular calcification.

While TMVR is a promising alternative option for mitral valve disease, it remains in a very early stage with many different types of valves, via both approaches, in development.[9] The first dedicated device for TMVR was the CardiAQ self-expanding valve that was first used in 2014. This valve helped establish the feasibility of both transseptal and transapical delivery of a transcatheter mitral valve. Piggybacking on the success of transcatheter aortic valve replacement (TAVR), a modified Edwards SAPIEN 3 was then investigated via a transseptal approach for use in the mitral position. Early feasibility results first published in 2018 in 15 patients with severe 3+ native valve MR, New York Heart Association (NYHA) 2 symptoms, and high surgical risk showed 86.7% technical success and 0% 30-day mortality.[1] There are now several different transseptal delivered valves in various stages of clinical investigation.

The Tendyne valve (Abbot Laboratories, Abbott Park, IL), likely the valve with the most clinical data thus far, is a transapically delivered TMVR that can be repositioned after initial deployment (Fig. 24.1). It consists of a porcine trileaflet valve fixed to a one-size inner stent that maintains an effective orifice area of at least 3.2 cm^2. The outer stent is designed to match the D-shape of the native mitral annulus. Attached to the valve prosthesis is a tether that is secured to a pad resting on the apical epicardial surface.[2] The system is delivered through a transapical sheath, accessed via a small left anterior thoracotomy. The device received the world's first CE mark for transcatheter mitral valve implantation in Europe in January 2020.

Currently, several pivotal trials to assess long-term outcomes of TMVRs are underway (Table 24.2). The APOLLO Trial is investigating a self-expanding, transapically delivered valve from Medtronic in patients with severe, symptomatic mitral regurgitation. Initial results in 50 patients published in 2019 showed a technical success rate of 96% with 14% 30-day mortality. The SUMMIT Trial is investigating the Abbott Tendyne valve for patients with symptomatic mitral regurgitation. Initial results in 100 patients demonstrated technical success in 96% with 6% 30-day mortality. Full results of this trial are expected in 2024.[1]

TMVR has emerged as an alternative treatment option for patients with degenerated bioprosthetic mitral valves who are at high surgical risk for a re-do. A recent prospective cohort study

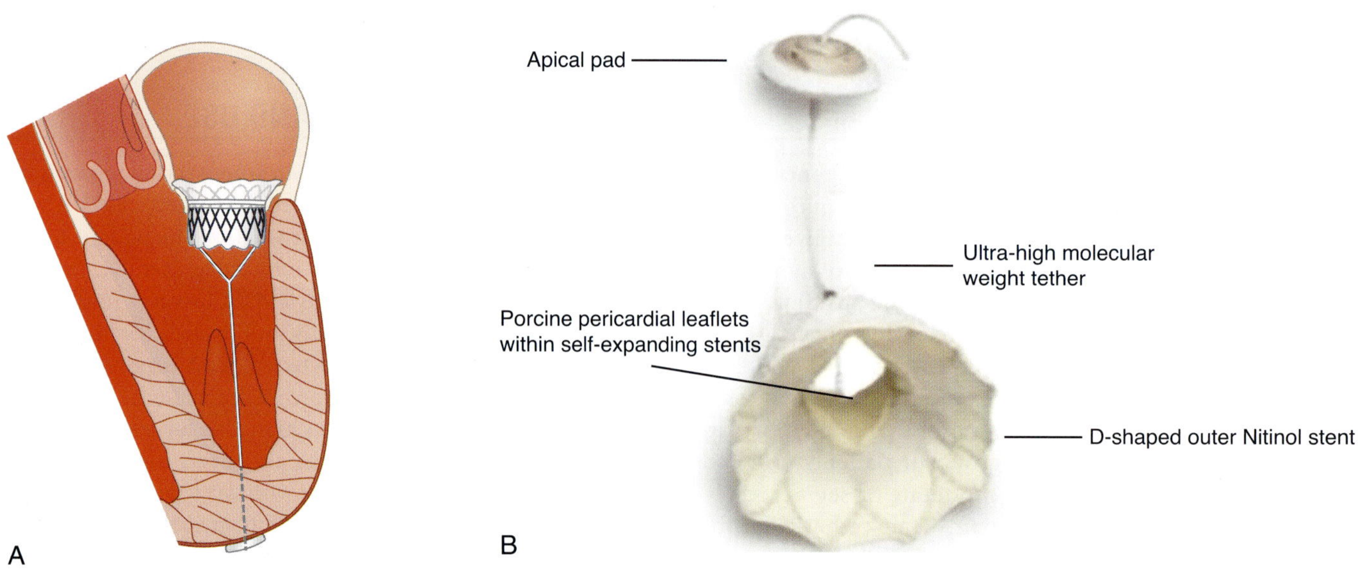

Fig. 24.1 (A and B) Tendyne valve with tethering via epicardial pad. The Tendyne valve is a transapically delivered valve, which is secured using resistance between the mitral annulus and an epicardial pad, which is placed outside the apex of the left ventricle. (Abbot Laboratories, Abbott Park, IL. Tendyne is a trademark of Abbott or its related companies. *Reproduced with permission* of Abbott, © 2021. All rights reserved)

TABLE 24.2 **Current Published Clinical Trials Evaluating Transcatheter Mitral Valve Replacement**

	Intrepid	Tendyne	Tiara	Evoque	SAPIEN M3
Manufacturer	Medtronic	Abbott	Neovasc	Edwards	Edwards
No. patients	50	100	79	14	45
Delivery	Transapical	Transapical	Transapical	Transseptal	Transseptal
Age	72.6	75.4	74.1	80.9	75.2
STS score	6.4 ± 5.5	7.8 ± 5.7	7.9 ± 6.7	5.3 ± 2.8	6.4 ± 3.9
NYHA III/IV	43/50	66/100	70/79	9/14	43/45
Technical success	48/49	96/100	73/79	14/14	40/45
Greater than mild MR	0/48	1/97	1/48	1/14	NA
Follow-up					
Mean follow-up (days)	173	416	30	30	30
Mortality	11/50	26/100	7/57	1/14	1/45
HF hospitalization	12/50	31/100	NA	0/14	NA
Greater than mild MR	0/42	0/62	1/38	0/12	1/41
Mean gradient	4.1	3.0	1.0	5.7	5.7
NYHA III/IV	9/43	7/86	19/39	2/12	16/42

assessing 1529 patients with failed surgical bioprosthetic mitral valves who underwent either transseptal or transapical SAPIEN 3 valve-in-valve replacement found all-cause mortality was low, with 5.4% at 30 days and 16.7% at 1 year. Patients at 1 year had a significant reduction in heart failure symptoms, with only 9.7% of patients being NYHA Class III/IV versus 87.1% prior to intervention. Of note, transseptal access was associated with lower 1-year mortality than transapical access (15.8% vs 21.7%).[3]

Patients with significant mitral annular calcification represent one of the more challenging subsets of mitral disease to treat and are traditionally considered poor surgical candidates. A multicenter retrospective review of 116 patients with prohibitive surgical risk with severe mitral annular calcification (MAC) who underwent TMVR found high mortality (25% at 30 days and 53.7% at 1 year); however, patients had significant symptomatic improvement. Patients at 1 year were functionally improved with 71.8% improving to NYHA Class I or II. Seventy five percent of patients had zero or trace MR after the procedure.[4] This is likely a group of patients who will be well suited with TMVR techniques in the future.

There are currently no large-scale randomized studies comparing TMVR with surgical MVR. Future studies will hopefully reveal improved long-term outcomes of prosthetic mitral valve replacements either percutaneously or with innovative surgical techniques and further define the role of TMVR in patients with mitral valve disease.[11]

CHALLENGES WITH TRANSCATHETER MITRAL VALVE REPLACEMENT

The success of transcatheter valve replacement for aortic disease has paved the way for the use of this technique on other valvular pathology. However, while TAVR has become the standard of care for aortic stenosis, significant challenges still exist for the clinical adoption of TMVR for mitral regurgitation. The complicated pathophysiology and anatomy of the mitral valve render mitral valve replacement a much more difficult endeavor than transcatheter aortic valve replacement. The mitral valve, as described in earlier chapters, is a more intricate three-dimensional (3D) apparatus with several components, including valve leaflets, mitral annulus, chordal and papillary muscles, and a more variable size secondary to changes in the geometry of the left ventricle and atrium. All components of the apparatus may contribute to mitral regurgitation. Valve pathologies involving the structural integrity of the mitral leaflets, papillary muscle, or chords are considered primary. In contrast, secondary etiologies include mitral annular dilation, left ventricular (LV) dilatation, and papillary muscle and/or LV dysfunction. Left atrial dilatation due to chronic atrial fibrillation leading to mitral regurgitation is likely a third classification that has yet to be fully characterized. The heterogeneity of conditions that result in mitral regurgitation make a more challenging proposition for uniform treatment with valve replacement. All aspects of the mitral valve anatomy and adjacent chambers must be considered in TMVR.

While the aortic annulus is a rigid, elliptical structure, the mitral annulus is a much more variable and dynamic structure. The annulus is much larger, requiring larger valves with larger introduction devices. It is D-shaped and asymmetric and lacks a complete fibrous ring for prosthesis attachment. Achieving a uniform seal around the valve is thus very challenging with just a simple stenting structure like a TAVR valve. This could lead to a much higher incidence of paravalvular leak and migration than the TAVR valve if the same valve design was used in the mitral position. Furthermore, unlike aortic stenosis, which is primarily a calcific lesion, mitral regurgitation typically is not accompanied by extensive leaflet or annular calcification to hold a valve in place. These factors require different designs and implantation techniques for transcatheter mitral valves.

Outcomes research in regard to mitral valve replacement is more challenging than with aortic valve replacement as the patient population is more heterogeneous with more comorbidity and cardiac dysfunction. Aortic stenosis tends to be an isolated lesion in patients with either an intact ejection fraction or a reduced ejection fraction that can improve post-valve replacement. Severe mitral regurgitation, conversely, is often seen in sicker remodeled left ventricles with significant concurrent valvular dysfunction in other locations. Furthermore, the timing of mitral valve intervention is still evolving as early intervention on severe mitral regurgitation in asymptomatic patients has been shown to have better outcomes.[5] Finally, while surgical mitral valve repair has been shown to have better outcomes than surgical valve replacement with favorable anatomy, whether replacement is better than repair with transcatheter options has yet to be determined.

PATIENT SELECTION AND PRE-PROCEDURE PLANNING

There are currently more than a dozen different transcatheter-delivered mitral valves in various stages of clinical trials. Patient selection and pre-procedural planning differ slightly for each type of valve. Planning is also different for native mitral valves compared to patients with prior bioprosthetic valves or rings.

Transcatheter Mitral Valve Replacement for Native Mitral Valve

Generally, the initial workup for TMVR candidates should include confirming the patient's mitral regurgitation-related clinical symptoms and NYHA Class. B type natriuretic peptide (BNP) or pro B type natriuretic peptide (proBNP), in addition to basic blood work, should be obtained. Patients should have an electrocardiogram, chest X-ray, transthoracic echocardiogram (TTE), transesophageal echocardiogram (TEE), and multidetector computed tomography (MDCT). Cardiac magnetic resonance imaging (MRI) can be helpful in quantifying the severity of MR in some patients. In addition to assessing the severity of MR, imaging should focus on the etiology of mitral valve dysfunction with careful attention to valve morphology, the presence of previous repairs or replacement, mitral annular dimension, annular calcification, and an assessment of adjacent structures such as the left atrium, left ventricle, and left ventricular outflow tract (LVOT). A detailed anatomic assessment of each of the mitral apparatus components contributing to MR is important in deciding on which treatment option to pursue: transcatheter repair/replacement or surgical repair/replacement.

- **Mitral leaflets.** A determination by a surgeon with a cardiac imager as to whether a leaflet can be surgically repaired needs to be done prior to mitral valve replacement. If the valve can be repaired, mitral valve repair, whether it is surgical or transcatheter, should be the treatment of choice. Mitral valve replacement (transcatheter or surgical) should only be considered when a valve is not feasible for repair. A high-quality transthoracic echocardiogram is required for accurately assessing the degree of MR, the mitral valve anatomy, and the structural basis for mitral regurgitation. A transesophageal echocardiography (TEE) is often needed for the anatomic details related to the MR, particularly for vegetation, perforation, or cleft. Generally, a simple posterior mitral leaflet flail or prolapse at mid scallop (P2) with fibrotic deficiency has a successful repair rate of greater than 95%. In contrast, significant calcification of the leaflets or annulus or significant vegetation with leaflet perforation is not typically favorable for repair, and patients are likely better served with replacement. Mitral regurgitation due to shortening and diastolic restriction of the leaflets, often seen with mitral stenosis, is also a contraindication for transcatheter mitral valve repair with MitraClip and favors valve replacement.
- **Mitral annulus.** An assessment of the mitral annular dimension is important for valve size selection (Fig. 24.2 through 24.4). Severe mitral annular calcification associated with mitral stenosis or regurgitation is a difficult entity to treat. Generally, transcatheter mitral valve repair is contraindicated with severe MAC. Surgical correction, however, is technically challenging with the risk of atrioventricular dissociation. TMVR may play an important role in treating these patients. The degree and extent of mitral annular calcification can typically be assessed by echocardiography; however, there are often excessive artifacts due to acoustic shadowing from the calcium. Cardiac CT is often the tool of choice for annular sizing in mitral annular calcification.[10]
- **LV and LVOT.** One of the major differences between TMVR and surgical replacement is that TMVR does not remove the native mitral leaflets. The anterior mitral leaflet is pushed toward the LVOT, and a part of the TMVR strut/stent and native leaflet can protrude into the LVOT, which can result in a smaller "neo" LVOT after implanting the valve (Fig. 24.5). A small neo-LVOT is at risk for LVOT obstruction. Thus, TMVR is generally contraindicated in patients with a small LV cavity or LVOT obstruction at baseline. TMVR should be avoided in IHSS patients since it can cause more severe LVOT obstruction. In some circumstances, alcohol septal ablation can be performed to reduce LVOT obstruction prior to valve replacement. A neo-LVOT smaller than $\leq$150 mm^2 is generally considered not suitable for TMVR, with a size $\geq$180 to 200 mm^2 being favorable.[6] Currently, a pre-procedural neo-LVOT assessment (Fig. 24.6) is required using 4D dynamic cardiac CT. 3D TEE may also provide similar information, but it needs further investigation and validation against CT and clinical outcomes.
- **Left atrium.** The left atrium is typically dilated in patients with chronic, severe mitral regurgitation. A small atrium may pose a problem in manipulating and positioning the valve. The presence of a left atrium or left atrial appendage thrombus is a contraindication for TMVR. A course of anticoagulation and demonstration of thrombus resolution must be demonstrated prior to attempting valve replacement.
- **Right ventricle (RV) and Pulmonary artery (PA) pressure.** Right-side cardiac catheterization can be performed for the measurement of PA pressure. An estimation of right-sided

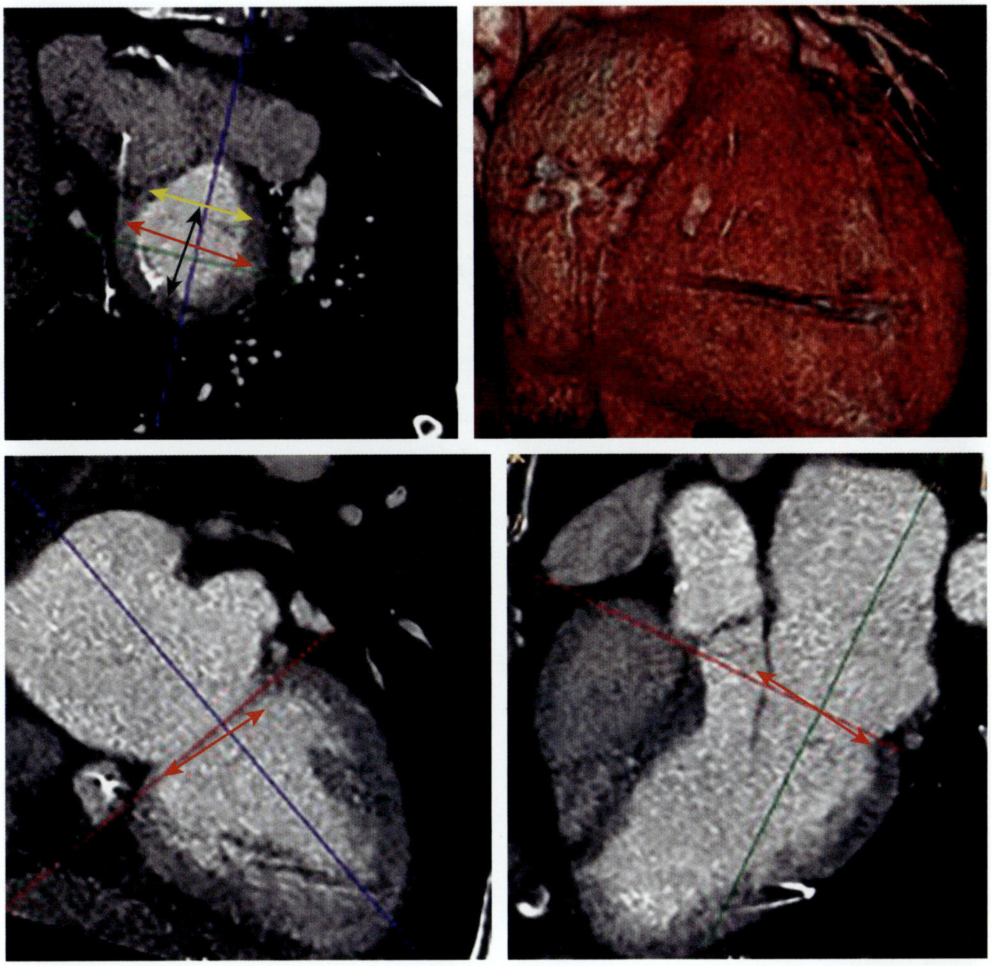

Fig. 24.2 *(Top)* CT-based assessment and sizing of the mitral annulus. All dimensions of the mitral annulus should be assessed: trigone to trigone distance *(yellow arrow line)*, septal-lateral diameter *(black arrow line)*, and inter-commissural diameter *(red arrow line)*. *(Bottom)* Long axis orientations for proper mitral annular segmentation.

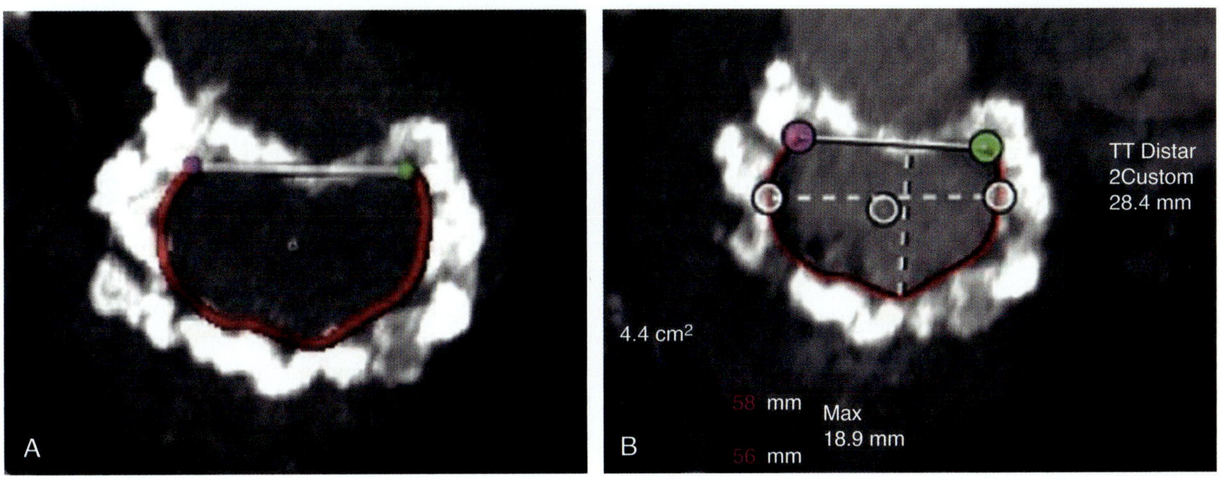

Fig. 24.3 (A) Mitral annulus circumference. (B) Measurement of trigone to trigone *(solid line)*, septal-lateral and intercommissural diameters *(dotted lines)*.

pressures using the tricuspid regurgitant velocity profile can be obtained by TTE or TEE. Severe pulmonary hypertension with a severely dilated RV and severe RV dysfunction portends a poor prognosis for any valve intervention. Severe TR also increases mortality with any valvular heart disease, even postsurgical intervention.[7]

- **Concurrent valve lesions.** Patients with multivalve disease requiring intervention, such as concurrent aortic stenosis

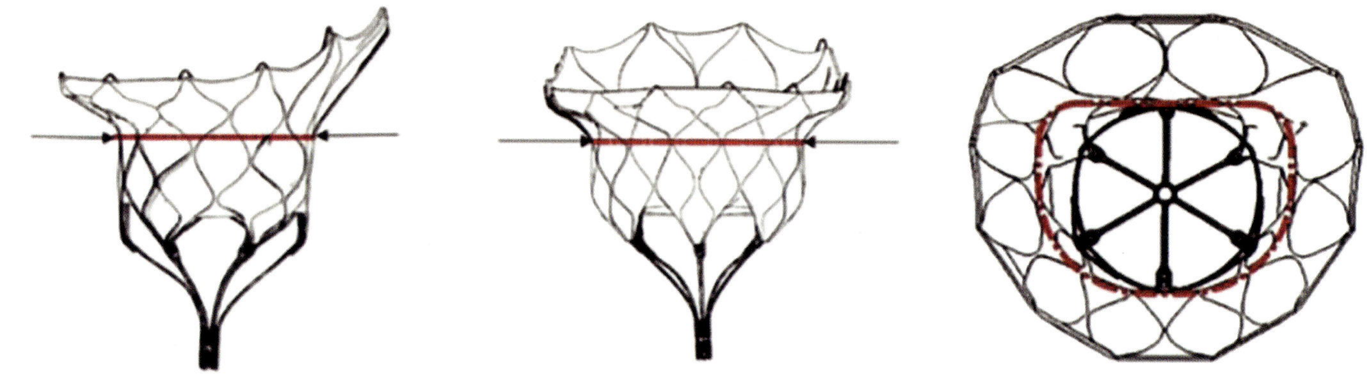

Fig. 24.4 Transcatheter mitral valve replacement. Valve size must incorporate (A) anterior-posterior (AP), (B) intercommissural (IC), and (C) perimeter (PER) dimensions. All three dimensions of the annulus must be considered in selecting the proper valve size. The more dynamic, irregular shape of the mitral valve in comparison to the aortic necessitates evaluating the annulus in all dimensions.

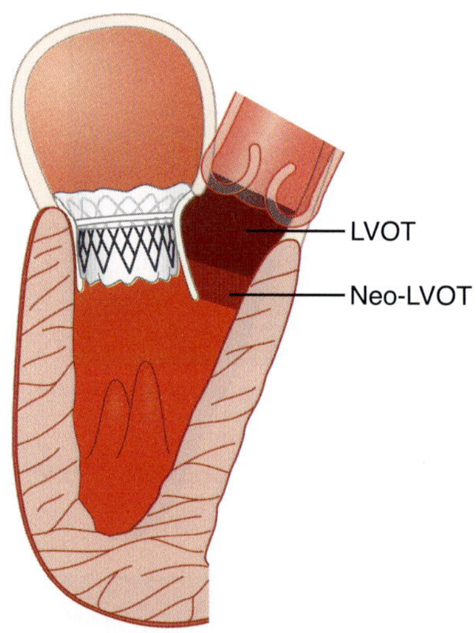

Fig. 24.5 Neo–left ventricular outflow tract (LVOT). The transcatheter valve can impinge upon the native LVOT, through both the valve apparatus itself and from pushing the anterior mitral valve leaflet forward, creating a "Neo-LVOT" that can compromise outflow.

or tricuspid regurgitation, will generally require surgical approaches. However, multiple transcatheter valve interventions, either staged or in a single session, appear to be a promising future option in select patients. Further investigation in this area is required.

Transcatheter Mitral Valve Replacement for Existing Bioprosthetic MVR

Currently, the most common indication for TMVR is for a failed bioprosthetic mitral valve. Prosthetic valve degeneration with stenosis or regurgitation requires re-intervention either by surgical re-do or a valve-in-valve TMVR, typically using an Edwards SAPIEN 3 TAVR valve. A transthoracic echocardiogram is generally performed first to confirm the pathology. If there is a doubt of vegetation or paravalvular mitral regurgitation, TEE is required. TMVR is not suitable for patients with significant paravalvular leak and requires either surgical replacement or a transcatheter plug. Valve sizing is based on the inner diameter of the existing bioprosthesis, which can be obtained from prior surgical reports, cardiac CT, or 3D TEE. Neo-LVOT should also be assessed by CT for valve-in-valve TMVR.

TRANSCATHETER APPROACHES FOR MITRAL VALVE REPLACEMENT

Transcatheter valve replacement may be done either via a transseptal or a transapical approach. While the techniques can vary for each individual valve, the following is a generic description of the valve placement procedures.

TRANSSEPTAL APPROACH PROCEDURE

Patient prep for TMVR is similar to TAVR. The procedure should ideally be performed in a hybrid operating room (OR). Femoral venous access should be obtained bilaterally, and arterial access obtained for invasive pressure monitoring. The transseptal sheath should be advanced into the left atrium under constant transesophageal echocardiogram guidance. Transseptal puncture is usually performed in a superior and posterior position to allow for best orientation once in the left atrium. An exchange wire is then advanced into the left atrium before exchanging the transseptal sheath for a steerable introducer sheath.

The atrial septum should then be further dilated. A 12-mm balloon dilation is usually sufficient. The catheter balloon should be advanced along the stiff wire and under TEE guidance, positioned across the atrial septum, and inflated. A larger balloon size may be needed depending on the valve delivery

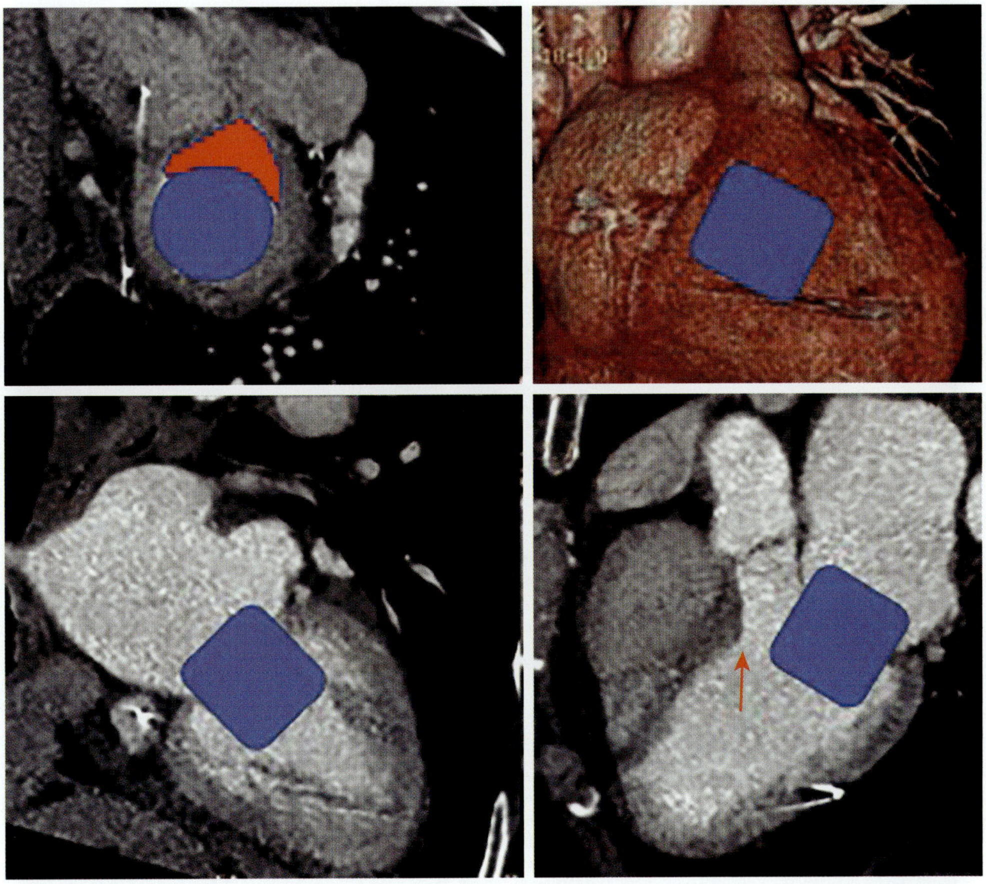

Fig. 24.6 CT-based simulation of neo–left ventricular outflow tract (LVOT). Prior to valve implantation, the post-implantation neo-LVOT should be predicted using MDCT and a simulated valve based on the size being implanted in the patient. This is of particular importance in patients with small cavity sizes or narrow native LVOTs. In this patient, a narrow predicted neo LVOT due to prominent basal septum and simulated valve placement can be seen *(red arrow)*.

system. The transcatheter heart valve (THV) delivery system is then carefully advanced over the stiff wire. Sheath alignment should be checked and adjusted before advancement into the right atrium. Under fluoroscopy and TEE guidance, the THV sheath should be advanced, and the septum slowly crossed. If difficulty arises crossing the septum, the THV sheath should be removed, and further balloon dilatation should be performed before re-attempting. Once into the left atrium, the THV catheter is oriented towards the mitral valve annulus and advanced. The THV should be positioned across the mitral orifice with 80% of the device into the left ventricle. Once the adequate position and orientation have been obtained, rapid ventricular pacing should be initiated and the valve deployed.[8]

TRANSAPICAL APPROACH PROCEDURE

Transapical access, as performed with the Tendyne valve, involves a small left anterior thoracotomy. The site for LV apical access is selected based on pre-procedural CT and intraprocedural TEE (Fig. 24.7). The access site selected must give good orientation to the mitral valve upon entry to the ventricle both in the commissural and septal-lateral planes. Once selected, the access site is punctured with a multipurpose needle, and a 7 Fr sheath advanced into the left ventricle. Under TEE guidance, a balloon tip catheter is advanced carefully to avoid chordal disruption into the left atrium. A 0.035″ guidewire is inserted, followed by a 36 Fr delivery sheath. The atrial aspect of the Tendyne prosthesis is advanced into the left atrium and oriented under TEE guidance to fit the shape of the native mitral valve. The prosthesis is then pulled back towards the apex of the heart until it is properly oriented in the mitral annulus and the valve is deployed. The deployed valve is fastened to the apex of the heart with an epicardial pad. The length of the attachment from the valve to the apex is adjusted to optimize position and left ventricular hemodynamics.

POST-PLACEMENT EVALUATION

Once the valve has been deployed, a complete TEE should be performed to confirm a satisfactory position. The valve should be assessed for a gradient or paravalvular leak. For transseptal valves, the atrial septum should be evaluated for the degree and direction of shunting. Very importantly, the LVOT should be evaluated for the presence of LVOT obstruction. Post-deployment heart block is rarely seen and much less common than what is observed with transcatheter aortic valve replacement.

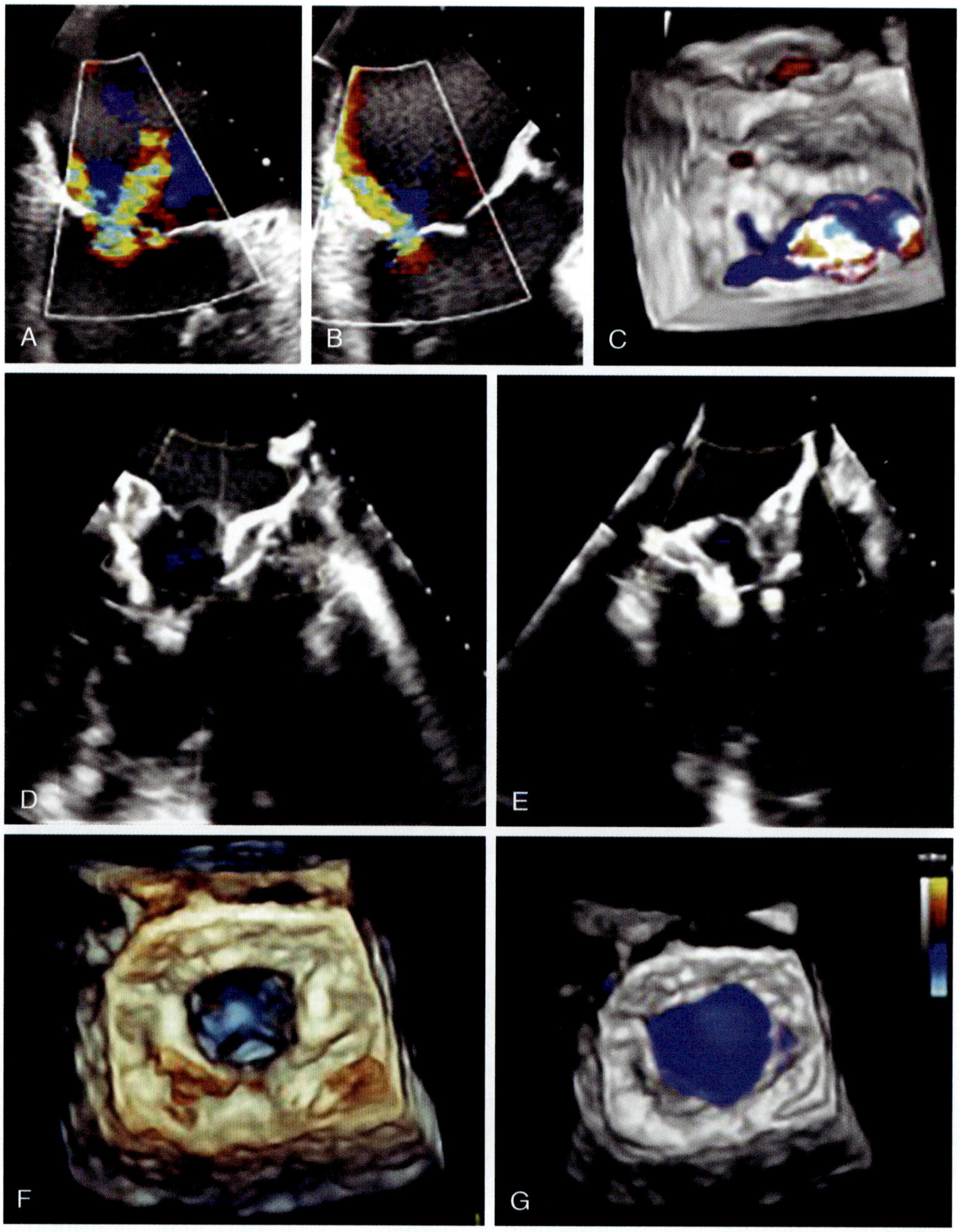

Fig. 24.7 Pre- and post-Tendyne case. (A) TEE, color Doppler, commissural view, demonstrating severe mitral regurgitation. (B) TEE, color Doppler, LV outflow view, demonstrating severe, eccentric posteriorly directed jet. (C) TEE, 3D reconstruction, surgeon's view, demonstrating poor coaptation of anterior and posterior leaflets. (D and E) TEE, color Doppler, post-Tendyne valve demonstrating no residual regurgitation. (F) TEE, 3D reconstruction, demonstrating Tendyne valve post-deployment. (G) TEE, 3D reconstruction color Doppler, no residual mitral regurgitation.

Improper position, with the valve either too far into the atrium or ventricle, carries a high risk of embolization for valve-in-valve TMVR. If noted acutely following deployment, a second transseptal valve may be deployed in order to secure it. The Tendyne valve can be repositioned by adjusting the apical tethering strain.

The degree of paravalvular or central regurgitation must be immediately assessed post-deployment. If large central regurgitation exists, manipulation of the stiff wire to a different position should be first performed to assess its effect on MR. If the central MR is still present, the wire should be withdrawn into the left atrium to reassess the MR. A second valve may be needed if there is still significant central MR, indicative of a defective implanted valve.

For valve-in-valve TMVR, no more than trace paravalvular MR post-implantation is expected. If a significant paravalvular leak is seen and the valve is positioned properly, post-dilatation with more volume to further expand the valve may be needed.

If the valve is positioned improperly, a second valve is usually needed. For native valve TMVR, some degree of paravalvular MR can be seen depending on the type of TMVR given the asymmetrical nature of the mitral valve. If severe paravalvular leak persists even after adjustments and repositioning, the attempt at TMVR should be considered failed, and a surgical valve may need to be implanted.

Given the degree of septal dilation needed for transseptal TMVR, atrial septal shunting post-procedure is common. A small degree of left-to-right shunting is generally well tolerated, with no need for intervention. Significant right-to-left shunting, which can be seen post-procedure in patients with pulmonary hypertension or RV dysfunction with high RA pressure, can result in hypoxia. A septal closure device can be deployed before the case is completed if deemed necessary.

Despite careful pre-operative assessment and precluding patients with a high risk of LVOT obstruction, LVOT obstruction can still occur after deployment of TMVR. The degree of LVOT obstruction and the contributing factors to the obstruction should be carefully assessed. Long or redundant anterior mitral leaflets, prominent basal interventricular septal hypertrophy, and/or small LV cavity can cause or worsen LVOT obstruction after implantation. Volume load, alcohol septal ablation, or laceration of anterior mitral leaflet technique have been used post-deployment to relieve LVOT obstruction. In severe cases with hemodynamic instability due to LVOT obstruction, urgent surgical intervention may be required as salvage.

POST-TRANSCATHETER MITRAL VALVE REPLACEMENT FOLLOW-UP

Given the relative infancy of TMVR, long-term follow-up data is lacking. Patients should be maintained on anticoagulation for 3 months following valve deployment. A transthoracic or transesophageal echocardiogram should be performed at this time to assess for elevated gradients or other signs of valve thrombosis. If normal function is noted, anticoagulation can typically then be stopped. A new paravalvular leak is rare and may suggest valve migration and warrants further workup. Recommendations regarding long-term surveillance with these valves are likely to significantly change over the next few years as more data is accrued.

! TIPS AND TRICKS

- Patient selection is very important with TMVR. An experienced surgeon with an experienced cardiac imager should evaluate the patient and deem them ineligible for repair prior to proceeding with TMVR, as surgical repair is often associated with better outcomes.
- Patients with native valves and patients with failing prior bioprosthetic valves or rings should be evaluated and treated as two separate clinical entities. Different valves are indicated depending on if this is a de novo valve or a valve-in-valve.
- In TMVR, there is a relatively long stent to host the valve, and the patient's native leaflets are not removed. The native anterior mitral leaflet may be pushed by the TMVR into the LVOT together with the TMVR stent, creating a narrowed neo-LVOT. Therefore, cardiac CT assessment of the predicted neo-LVOT is mandatory for selecting patients for TMVR. The anterior leaflet can be lacerated prior to valve deployment in order to help prevent this obstruction. High-risk patients with prominent basal septal hypertrophy or redundant anterior mitral leaflet may benefit from alcohol septal ablation or anterior leaflet laceration prior to valve implantation to maximize their LVOT diameter.

SUMMARY

TMVR is a technically challenging procedure that will continue to mature in both valve design and implantation technique before widespread adoption. The ideal valve in the future would likely offer transseptal delivery and be fully repositionable, with limited interruption of the LVOT. Given the complexity of pathology that leads to mitral regurgitation, patients in most circumstances historically have been best served with mitral repair or clip. Patients with severe primary mitral regurgitation that are not amenable to repair or surgical replacement, or patients with severe secondary mitral regurgitation that are not candidates for edge-to-edge repair, may be well served with transcatheter valve replacement techniques in the future.

ASSESSMENT QUESTIONS

1. Which of the following is a contraindication to receiving TMVR for severe mitral regurgitation?
   A. Moderate to severe mitral annular calcification
   B. Ejection fraction less than 35%
   C. A calculated neo-LVOT area of 140 mm^2
   D. Mitral stenosis
2. A patient is referred to you for TMVR. She is a relatively healthy 45-year-old female who has noticed exercise-limiting dyspnea over the past few months. She has been told she has had a heart murmur for the past 10 years. Echocardiography reveals a flail P2 scallop with severe eccentric regurgitation. What should be your next step in management?
   A. Proceed with TMVR
   B. Proceed with mitral clip
   C. Surgical consultation for mitral valve repair
   D. Medical management
3. Which of the following indications for TMVR has gained FDA approval?
   A. Severe native valve regurgitation
   B. Severe prosthetic valve regurgitation
   C. Severe native valve stenosis
   D. Severe functional mitral regurgitation

See page 318 for the answers.

REFERENCES

1. Testa L, Rubbio AP, Casenghi M, et al. Transcatheter mitral valve replacement in the transcatheter aortic valve replacement era. *J Am Heart Assoc.* 2019;8(22):e013352. doi:10.1161/JAHA.119.013352.
2. Niikura H, Gossl M, Sorajja P. Transcatheter mitral valve replacement with Tendyne. *Interv Cardiol Clin.* 2019;8(3):295–300.
3. Whisenant B, Kapadia SR, Eleid MF, et al. One-year outcomes of mitral valve-in-valve using the SAPIEN 3 transcatheter heart valve. *JAMA Cardiol.* 2020;5(11):1245–1252. doi:10.1001/jamacardio.2020.2974. PMID: 32745164; PMCID: PMC7391176.
4. Guerrero M, Urena M, Himbert D, et al. 1-year outcomes of transcatheter mitral valve replacement in patients with severe mitral annular calcification. *J Am Coll Cardiol.* 2018;71(17):1841–1853. doi:10.1016/j.jacc.2018.02.054. PMID: 29699609.
5. Suri R, Schaff H, Enriquez-Sarano M. Mitral valve repair in asymptomatic patients with severe mitral regurgitation: pushing past the tipping point. *Sem Thorac Cardiovasc Surg.* 2014;26(2):95–101.
6. Reid A, Zekry SB, Turaga M, et al. Neo-LVOT and transcatheter mitral valve replacement. *JACC: Cardiovasc Imaging.* 2021;14(4):854–866.
7. Lindman BR, Maniar HS, Jaber WA, et al. Effect of tricuspid regurgitation and the tight heart on survival after transcatheter aortic valve replacement: insights from the PARTNER II Inoperable Cohort. *Circ Cardiovasc Interv.* 2015;8(4):e002073.
8. Urena M, Himbert D, Brochet E, et al. Transseptal transcatheter mitral valve replacement using balloon-expandable transcatheter heart valves: a step-by-step approach. *JACC Cardiovasc Interv.* 2017;10(19):1905–1919. doi:10.1016/j.jcin.2017.06.069. PMID: 28982555.
9. Del Val D, Ferreira-Neto AN, Wintzer-Wehekind J, et al. Early experience with transcatheter mitral valve replacement: a systematic review. *J Am Heart Assoc.* 2019;8(17):e013332.
10. Pulerwitz T, Khalique O, Leb J, et al. Optimizing cardiac CT protocols for comprehensive acquisition prior to percutaneous MV and TV repair/replacement. *JACC: Cardiovasc Imaging.* 2020;13(3):836–850.
11. Hensey M, Brown R, Lal S, et al. Transcatheter mitral valve replacement: an update on current techniques, technologies and future directions. *JACC: Cardiovasc Interv.* 2021;14(5):489–500.

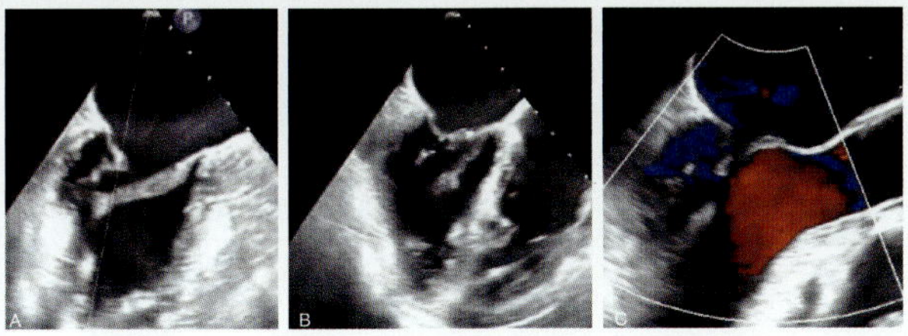

25

Percutaneous Mitral Valve Interventions: Evaluation, Pitfalls, and Complications

Rim Halaby, Howard C. Herrmann

CHAPTER OUTLINE

LEARNING OBJECTIVES

1. Review the indications for transcatheter mitral valve therapies according to American Heart Association/American College of Cardiology and European Society of Cardiology guidelines.
2. Review scoring systems for the assessment of favorable anatomy for mitral valve balloon valvuloplasty.
3. Review favorable and unsuitable anatomy for transcatheter mitral valve edge-to-edge repair for primary and secondary mitral regurgitation.
4. Discuss the importance of multidisciplinary heart team approach and optimization of medical therapy prior to mitral valve procedures.
5. Review common complications for transcatheter mitral valve procedures with emphasis on device-specific complications, in particular edge-to-edge repair and transcatheter mitral valve replacement.

INTRODUCTION

The field of transcatheter mitral valve interventions began with percutaneous mitral balloon valvuloplasty (PMBV) for mitral stenosis in the early 1980s. Since then, there has been a technological revolution that has permitted the treatment of regurgitant lesions. Transcatheter edge-to-edge repair (TEER) of the mitral valve with MitraClip (Abbott Vascular; Abbott Park, IL, USA) was first performed in 2003 and is now approved by the U.S. Food and Drug Administration (FDA) for the treatment of mitral regurgitation (MR) in selected patients. In addition, the success of transcatheter aortic valve replacement (TAVR) sparked interest in transcatheter mitral valve replacement (TMVR), which is now undergoing investigational assessment with a variety of devices. The major lesson learned throughout the journey of percutaneous mitral valve interventions is that appropriate patient selection is key for procedural success, especially given the complexity of the mitral valve apparatus and the heterogeneity of mitral valve diseases. Patient selection not only requires a global assessment of mitral valve anatomy, the underlying mechanism of mitral valve disease, the structure and function of the left ventricle, and patient comorbidities, particularly in the elderly and frail patients, but also the unique safety, efficacy, and results of specific devices and approaches.

PATIENT SELECTION AND EVALUATION

Percutaneous Mitral Balloon Valvuloplasty

According to the American Heart Association (AHA)/American College of Cardiology (ACC) and the European Society of Cardiology (ESC) guidelines, PMBV is indicated for the treatment of symptomatic severe mitral stenosis (mitral valve

TABLE 25.1 Summary of Recommendations for Transcatheter Mitral Valve Therapies According to the 2020 ACC/AHA Guidelines for the Management of Valvular Diseases

Percutaneous Mitral Valve Interventions	ACC/AHA Class, Level of Evidence
Percutaneous Mitral Balloon Valvuloplasty	
Symptomatic severe mitral stenosis (MVA<1.5 cm²), favorable anatomy, and absence of contraindications	I, A
Asymptomatic severe mitral stenosis (MVA<1.5 cm²), favorable anatomy, absence of contraindications, and elevated pulmonary pressures (PASP >50 mm Hg)	IIa, B-NR
Symptomatic severe mitral stenosis (MVA<1.5 cm²), suboptimal anatomy, and absence of contraindications	IIb, B-NR
Transcatheter Mitral Valve Repair for Primary Mitral Regurgitation	
Symptomatic chronic severe primary mitral regurgitation, favorable anatomy, life expectancy >1 year, and prohibitive surgical risk	IIa, B-NR
Transcatheter Mitral Valve Repair for Secondary Mitral Regurgitation	
Chronic severe secondary mitral regurgitation, persistent symptoms despite optimal GDMT, and approrpriate anatomy	IIa, B-R

ACC, American College of Cardiology; *AHA*, American Heart Association; *GDMT*, Guideline directed medical therapy; *MVA*, mitral valve area.

area <1.5 cm²) with favorable mitral valve anatomy and in the absence of any contraindications (AHA/ACC Class Ia, ESC Class Ib).[1,2] PMBV can be considered for asymptomatic patients with severe mitral stenosis and an aortic valve area of less than 1 cm² (Table 25.1). PMBV treats mitral stenosis through separation of the fused commissures with subsequent increase in the mitral valve orifice area. Transesophageal echocardiography (TEE) is necessary to evaluate the anatomy of the mitral valve and the presence of contraindications (Fig. 25.1). Contraindications include the presence of left atrial thrombus, massive or bicommissural calcification, more than mild MR, and concomitant other valvular diseases or severe coronary artery disease requiring surgical intervention. Multiple scoring systems exist for the assessment of the suitability of mitral valve morphology for PMBV, the most commonly used one is the original Wilkins score.[3] The Wilkins system assigns a score of 1 to 4 for each leaflet's mobility, thickening, calcification, and subvalvular thickening based on the transthoracic echocardiogram. A stenotic mitral valve with a Wilkins score of more than 8 is considered to have an unfavorable anatomy for PMBV due to advanced leaflet deformity, and a mobile mitral valve with limited thickening is more suitable for the procedure.[3] Among patients with unsuitable anatomical features and high surgical risk, a multidisciplinary approach is recommended, as some of these patients may be suitable for PMBV if the surgical risk is high or prohibitive.[4,5]

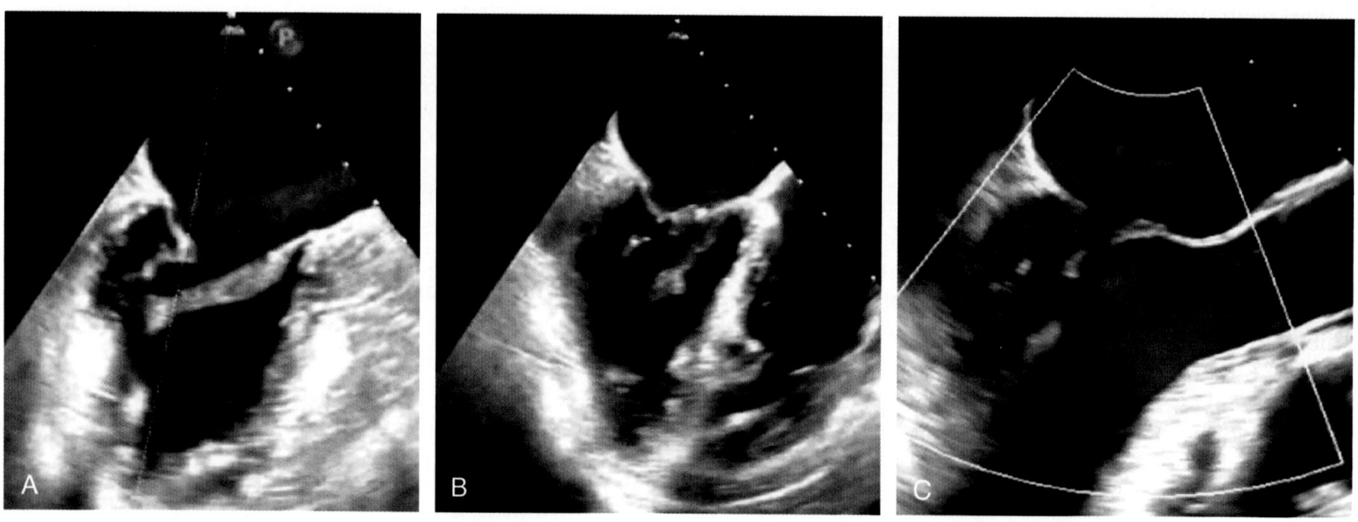

Fig. 25.1 Transesophageal echocardiography images of a patient with severe mitral stenosis undergoing evaluation for percutaneous mitral balloon valvuloplasty. (A) Transesophageal echocardiography 2-chambers view shows mitral valve leaflets and subvalvular thickening without evidence of significant leaflets calcification. (B) 4-chamber view demonstrates again the leaflets and subvalvular thickening. (C) There is absence of mitral regurgitation and left atrial thrombus that would preclude eligibility for mitral balloon valvuloplasty.

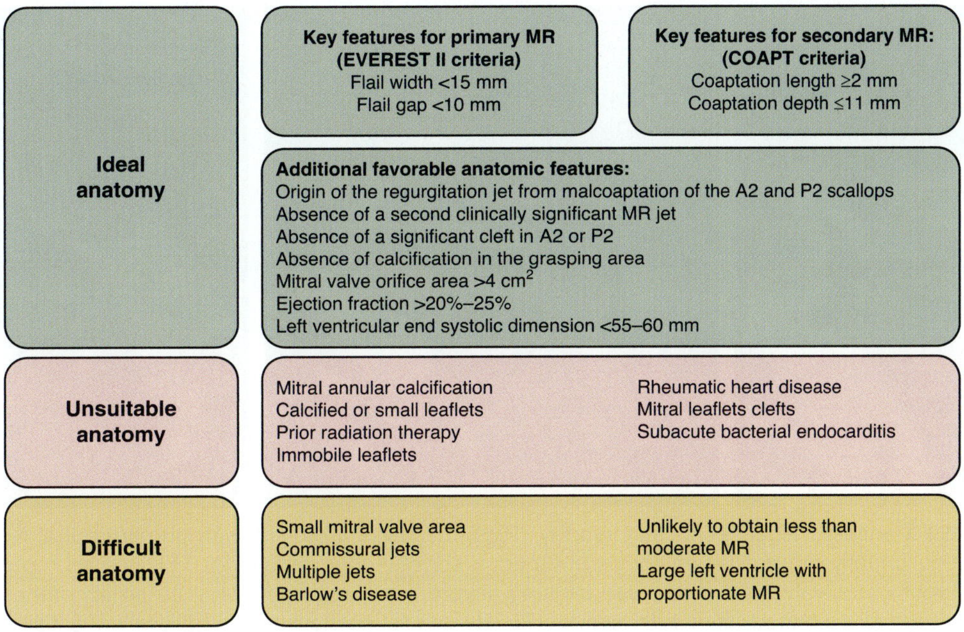

Fig. 25.2 Ideal, unsuitable, and difficult anatomy features for transcatheter mitral valve edge-to-edge repair. The assessment of mitral valve anatomy for adequate optimal clip positioning and implantation is required for patient selection. Ideal and unsuitable anatomy features reflect the inclusion and exclusion criteria of the EVEREST II (for primary mitral regurgitation) and COAPT (for secondary mitral regurgitation) trials. *MR,* mitral regurgitation.

Transcatheter Edge-to-Edge Repair

TEER with MitraClip (Abbott Laboratories, Abbott Park, IL, USA) is approved for the treatment of MR in selected patients. Primary MR is caused by an abnormality in the mitral valve leaflets or chords. On the other hand, mitral valve leaflets and chords are intact in secondary MR, and valvular regurgitation results from inadequate leaflet coaptation due to papillary muscle displacement and leaflet tethering in the setting of a distorted left ventricle. Given the different pathophysiology of primary and secondary MR, patient selection takes into account some different morphological features during the assessment for TEER eligibility. TEE plays a paramount role in the assessment of mitral valve anatomy for adequate optimal clip positioning and implantation (Fig. 25.2).

In primary MR, surgical mitral valve repair or replacement should be the first line therapy for most patients. TEER is a therapeutic option for chronic primary MR among symptomatic patients despite optimal medical therapy in the setting of favorable anatomy for TEER, reasonable life expectancy, and prohibitive surgical risk (ACC/AHA Class IIa, Level B-NR; ESC Class IIb, Level B) (see Table 25.1).[1,2] Ideal echocardiographic features for TEER for primary MR reflect the inclusion and exclusion criteria in the EVERST II trial, although current practice often extends the anatomic boundaries beyond the trial criteria.[6] As TEER replicates the Alfieri stitch of the middle scallops A2 and P2, favorable mitral valve features for edge-to-edge repair include origin of the regurgitation jet from malcoaptation of the A2 and P2 scallops, absence of a significant cleft in A2 or P2, lack of calcification in the grasping area, and absence of a second clinically significant MR jet (Fig. 25.3). In addition, key features for suitable anatomy in the presence of a flail leaflet are flail width smaller than 15 mm, flail gap smaller than 10 mm, and mitral valve area greater than 4.0 cm^2.[7,8] Bileaflet flail and severe bileaflet prolapse, multiple jets, and small mitral valve area all can preclude adequate clip positioning and implantation. Notably, patients enrolled in the EVEREST II trial had an ejection fraction greater than 20%, left ventricular end-systolic dimension 55 mm or smaller, and mitral valve orifice area greater than 4 cm^2.[7]

TEER has received approval for the treatment of moderate and severe secondary MR in heart failure patients who remain symptomatic despite optimal medical therapy based on the results of the COAPT trial.[9] In COAPT, enrolled patients had an ejection fraction more than 20%, left ventricular end-systolic dimension 60 mm or smaller, and mitral valve orifice area greater than 4 cm^2. When leaflet tethering is present, vertical coaptation length should ideally be 2 mm or larger and coaptation depth 11 mm or less (Figs. 25.2 and 25.4). Similar to primary MR, calcification in the grasping area of A2 and P2, cleft of A2 or P2, and lack of chordal support are unfavorable anatomic features for mitral valve clip implantation.[9]

Ideal candidates for edge-to-edge repair are patients who meet the inclusion and exclusion criteria of EVERST II (for primary MR) and COAPT (for secondary MR).[6,9] Additional unsuitable anatomy features include presence of mitral annular calcification, calcified leaflets, immobile leaflets, prior radiation therapy, and rheumatic heart disease. Patients who have been excluded from the edge-to-edge repair trials and who have difficult anatomy are those with a small mitral valve area, putting them at risk for severe mitral stenosis after TEER, commissural jets which add technical challenges to the procedure, and multiple MR jets. Clinical conundrums are cases with low likelihood

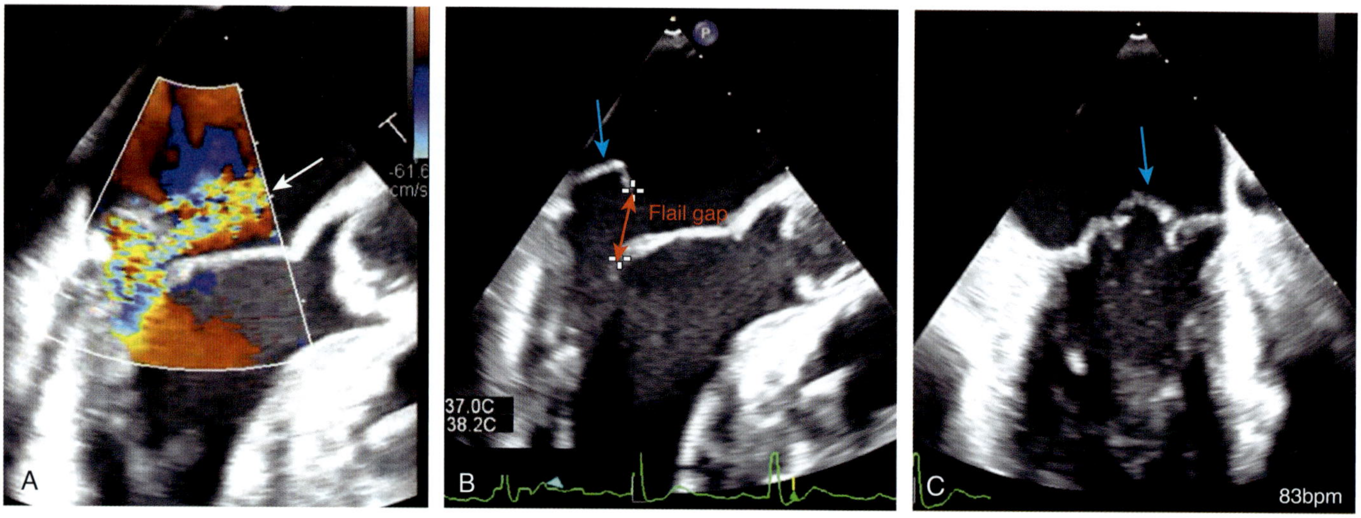

Fig. 25.3 Transesophageal echocardiography (TEE) images of a patient with primary mitral regurgitation undergoing evaluation for percutaneous edge-to-edge repair. (A) TEE shows ruptured posterior mitral valve leaflet chordae causing severe mitral regurgitation with an eccentric and anterolaterally directed jet *(white arrow)*. (B) The medial portion of the P2 scallop is flail with visible ruptured chordae *(blue arrow)*. One of the key features for suitable anatomy is flail gap <10 mm *(red arrow)*. (C) Commissural view shows medial portion of the P2 scallop is flail due to ruptured chordae *(blue arrow)*.

to obtain less than moderate residual MR, life expectancy less than 1 year, and large left ventricle size with proportionate MR that can be better treated with a left ventricular assist device or heart transplant.

Transcatheter Mitral Valve Annuloplasty

Transcatheter annuloplasty for the treatment of MR associated with dilated mitral valve annulus is under investigation and aims to reduce annular dimension by either direct or indirect mitral valve annuloplasty.[10] Some annuloplasty devices are delivered percutaneously into the coronary sinus, thus the anatomic relationship of the coronary sinus to the mitral valve annulus plays an important role in predicting procedural success. Ideally, the coronary sinus should be at the same level of the mitral valve annulus; however, in a proportion of patients the coronary sinus lies superiorly to the plane of the mitral valve

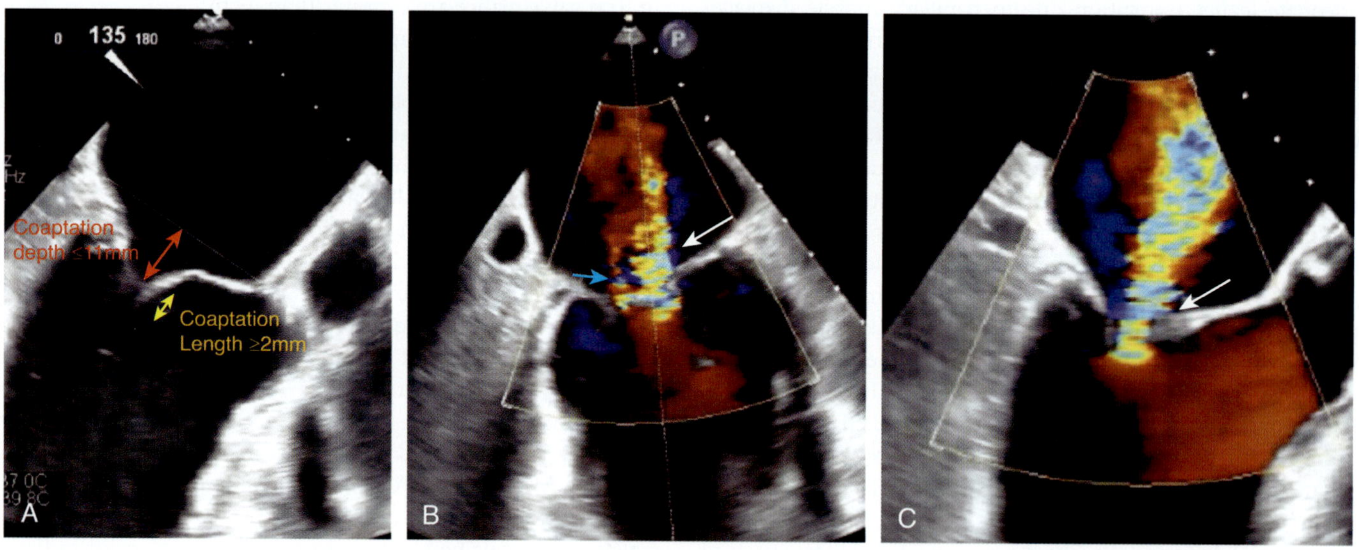

Fig. 25.4 Transesophageal echocardiography images of a patient with secondary mitral regurgitation (MR) undergoing evaluation for percutaneous edge-to-edge repair. (A) The ideal anatomic features for percutaneous edge-to-edge repair in secondary MR include vertical coaptation length ≥2 mm and coaptation depth ≤11 mm. The posterior leaflet is tethered and both leaflets are not calcified. (B) There is one predominant central mitral regurgitation jet arising between A2 and P2 *(white arrow)* and a small secondary jet *(blue arrow)*. (C) Long-axis view shows the predominant central regurgitation jet *(white arrow)*.

annulus, preventing adequate reduction of the mitral annular size. In addition, the course of the coronary arteries should be identified, particularly the left circumflex artery, which courses along the coronary sinus, raising the risk of intraprocedural coronary obstruction and myocardial ischemia.[11] The experience with percutaneous annuloplasty is in its early stages, and further studies are needed to better identify optimal anatomical features for this procedure.[12]

Transcatheter Mitral Valve Replacement

TMVR for treatment of severe mitral stenosis and severe MR is nascent compared to PMBV and TEER, and its use remains mostly investigational. TMVR began with the realization that TAVR devices can be placed in prior surgical rings or degenerated bioprostheses, and the Sapien balloon-expandable valve (Edwards Lifesciences, Irvine, CA, USA) is approved for placement in a prior surgical bioprosthesis who are high-risk for redo surgery. TMVR can also be performed in surgical rings and patients with severe mitral valve annular calcification. Challenges of TMVR in these settings include the complex anatomy of the mitral valve, large size of the mitral valve annulus, lack of annulus support, and difficulty of annulus sizing given its D-shape and asymmetrical configuration, which all increase the risk of device migration and paravalvular leak.[13] In addition, the proximity of the mitral valve to the left ventricular outflow tract (LVOT) is associated with LVOT obstruction following TMVR. Three-dimensional computed tomography is the imaging modality of choice for the assessment of TMVR patient eligibility, as it allows mitral annulus sizing, assessment of the predicted neo-LVOT size, and evaluation of annular calcification.[14] Finally, there are now multiple dedicated TMVR systems under development and investigation for placement, both transseptally and transapically in the native mitral valve.[15] The ideal patient, anatomy, and device for TMVR remain poorly defined, and further research is needed to improve patient selection and procedure planning.

PITFALLS AND COMPLICATIONS

General Principles

Prior to consideration of percutaneous mitral valve therapies, guideline-directed medical therapy should be optimized in patients with mitral valve diseases. Among patients with mitral stenosis, heart rate should be controlled to allow enough diastolic filling time for blood flow through the narrowed mitral valve. In patients with MR, preload reduction, afterload reduction, beta-blockade, and other evidence-based heart failure therapies, including cardiac resynchronization therapy, aldosterone antagonists, and SGLT2 inhibitors should be optimized. A heart team approach involving a dedicated multidisciplinary team of interventional cardiologists, cardiac imagers, heart failure specialists, and cardiac surgeons should be incorporated in the evaluation and management decisions of complex cases with unfavorable anatomy for percutaneous interventions and/or high surgical risks.

Percutaneous Mitral Balloon Valvuloplasty Complications

PMBV complications are related to vascular access, transseptal puncture, and equipment manipulation in the heart chambers (Table 25.2). Pericardial perforation and hemopericardium was previously reported to occur in up to 7% of patients, but more recent data suggest a lower rate of less than 1%, likely due to improvement in operators' technical skills and increased experience with this procedure.[16,17] The incidence of intraprocedural stroke is 1% to 3%.[16,17] Severe MR occurs in up to 15% of patients, and is usually the result of chordae rupture or leaflet tearing.[16] An echocardiographic score has been

TABLE 25.2 Summary of Complications of Percutaneous Mitral Valve Interventions

Complications of Percutaneous Mitral Valve Interventions
Percutaneous Mitral Balloon Valvuloplasty
Access related vascular complications and bleeding
Pericardial perforation and hemopericardium (<1%)
Intraprocedural stroke (1%–3%)
Severe mitral regurgitation (15%)
Transcatheter Edge-to-Edge Mitral Valve Repair
Access related vascular complications and bleeding (3.5%)
Air embolism or stroke (1.4%)
Tamponade (0.3%–1.4%)
Device implantation failure (4.2%)
Single leaflet device attachment (1%–1.5%)
Device embolization (0.1%–0.3%)
Cardiac perforation (1%)
Myocardial infarction (0.1%)
Iatrogenic mitral stenosis
Conversion to open-heart surgery due to intraprocedural complications (rare)
Transcatheter Mitral Valve Replacement
Access related vascular complications and bleeding
Left ventricular outflow tract obstruction with hemodynamic compromise (11.2%)
Valve embolization (4.3%)
Left ventricle perforation (1.7%)
Conversion to open heart surgery due to intra-procedural complications (3%–4%)
Transcatheter Mitral Valve Annuloplasty
Access related vascular complications and bleeding
Pericardial effusion and tamponade
High-degree atrioventricular block
Extrinsic obstruction of the left circumflex artery
Device dislodgement and fracture
Device failure
Periprocedural stroke

developed to predict the occurrence of severe MR, and it takes into account commissural calcification and the degree of thickness and calcification in each leaflet.[18,19] Patients who develop severe MR following PMBV most likely require subsequent mitral valve surgery.

Transcatheter Mitral Valve Repair Complications

Intra- and periprocedural TEER complications include access-related vascular complications, major bleeding, air or thrombus embolism, and pericardial effusion, as well as device-specific complications (see Table 25.2). In the EVEREST II, MITRA-FR, and COAPT trials, urgent conversion to heart surgery during the edge-to-edge repair procedure was extremely rare.[6,9,20] However, in MITRA-FR, device-implantation failure occurred in 4.2%, vascular complication requiring surgical intervention or bleeding in 3.5%, air embolism and stroke in 1.4%, and tamponade in 1.4% of patients.[20] In COAPT, the incidence of device-related complications at 12 months follow-up was 3.4% and included single leaflet device attachment (0.7%), device embolization (0.3%), and postprocedural pericardial effusion and tamponade (0.3%).[9]

Observational studies from real life experience with edge-to-edge repair with MitraClip showed a lower rate of complications with the learning curve of the procedure and improved institutional expertise. For instance, single clip detachment occurred in 9% of patients in EVERST I pilot study,[21] with an incidence of approximately 5% during the early experience after MitraClip approval in Europe,[14] and decreased to 1% to 1.5% in a recent analysis from the Society of Thoracic Surgeons/ACC Transcatheter Valve Therapy Registry.[22,23] Complete device embolization is rare, occurring in 0.1% of cases. Major or life-threatening bleeding happens in approximately 3.9%, and cardiac perforation in 1%. Less common periprocedural complications include myocardial infarction (0.1%) and stroke (0.4%).[23]

While transcatheter mitral valve repair reduces the severity of MR, it can lead to a decrease in the mitral valve orifice area and iatrogenic mitral stenosis, especially when more than one clip is implanted. These changes were first described in the EVEREST trials with a reduction of the mean mitral valve orifice area from 6.0 to 3.6 cm^2 and an increase in the mean mitral valve gradient from 1.7 to 4.1 mm Hg after MitraClip implantation.[24,25] The data on the effect of an elevated post-MitraClip mitral valve gradient is conflicting.[26,27] While one study suggests a mitral valve gradient greater than 5 mm Hg is associated with an increased rate of the combined endpoint of all-cause mortality, unsuccessful implantation, mitral valve surgery, left ventricular assist device implantation, and repeat procedures compared to patients with lower gradients,[26] another study suggests that the deleterious effects of an elevated post-MitraClip gradient are present in primary MR and not secondary MR.[27] A recent subanalysis of the COAPT trial showed lack of an association between an elevated mitral valve gradient following MitraClip and worse outcomes of mortality, heart failure hospitalization, and measures of functional status, suggesting that the reduction of MR severity with additional clips outweighs the negative effects of an elevated mitral valve gradient in secondary MR patients.[28]

Percutaneous Annuloplasty Complications

Percutaneous direct and indirect mitral valve annuloplasty devices are investigational for the treatment of mitral valve diseases. Device-specific complications reported in the literature are due to the spatial relationship of the coronary sinus and cardiac veins with surrounding structures, including pericardial effusion and tamponade, high-degree atrioventricular block, and extrinsic obstruction of the left circumflex artery (see Table 25.2).[29,30] Adequate procedural imaging guidance should theoretically decrease the risk of these complications. Device dislodgement and fracture, device failure, periprocedural stroke, and bleeding have also been described.[31]

Transcatheter Mitral Valve Replacement Complications

Early investigational experience with TMVR proved the feasibility of this procedure at the expense of an elevated risk of complications (see Table 25.2). Similar to transcatheter repair, procedural complications include access-related vascular complications and bleeding. Device-specific TMVR complications include inadequate valve positioning, device migration or embolization, LVOT obstruction, and valve thrombosis. A multicenter retrospective review of 116 extreme surgical risk patients with severe mitral annular calcification who underwent TMVR reported LVOT obstruction with hemodynamic compromise in 11.2% patients, valve embolization in 4.3%, and left ventricle perforation in 1.7%.[32] A second valve was implanted in 14.7% of patients due to either MR or valve migration.[32] Conversion to open-heart surgery has been reported in approximately 3% to 4% of TMVR cases due to intraprocedural complications.[32,33] A systematic review of existing TMVR studies reported long-term complications of device thrombosis (3%), endocarditis (4%), and stroke (4.5%) during a variable follow-up period ranging from 3 to 24 months.[33]

SUMMARY

Appropriate patient selection and detailed preprocedural assessment of the mitral valve apparatus are necessary to ensure the safety and efficacy of transcatheter mitral valve therapies. While multiple percutaneous mitral valve devices are still under development or investigation, the two procedures approved for the treatment of mitral diseases in the United States are PMBV and TEER with MitraClip. PMBV is indicated for the treatment of symptomatic severe mitral stenosis (mitral valve area less than 1.5 cm^2) with favorable mitral valve anatomy and in the absence of any contraindications (AHA/ACC Class Ia). MitraClip is approved for chronic primary MR among symptomatic patients despite optimal medical therapy in the setting of favorable anatomy for TEER, reasonable life expectancy, and prohibitive surgical risk (ACC/AHA Class IIa, Level B-NR). MitraClip is also FDA-approved for moderate and severe secondary MR in heart failure patients who remain symptomatic despite optimal medical therapy. (ACC/AHA Class IIa, Level B-R). Favorable anatomy and clinical features for edge-to-edge repair are those that meet the inclusion and exclusion criteria of EVERST II (for primary MR) and COAPT (for secondary MR). Procedural complications include vascular access and bleeding as well as device-specific complications.

CASE-BASED ASSESSMENT

An 88-year-old male with history of dyslipidemia presented to the hospital with acute shortness of breath and was found to have hypoxia in the setting of pulmonary edema. Transthoracic echocardiography showed new severe MR with preserved ejection fraction at 75% with no regional wall abnormalities. His respiratory failure progressed, requiring intubation, and he developed worsening cardiogenic shock with acute kidney injury and transaminitis, with subsequent placement of intraaortic balloon pump.

1. What is the next step in the management of this patient?
   - A. Optimize medical therapy with afterload reduction and diuresis
   - B. Obtain TEE
   - C. Urgent cardiac surgery and mitral valve repair
   - D. Urgent coronary angiography
2. TEE is performed (Videos 25.1 and 25.2). What is the diagnosis?
   - A. Acute primary MR
   - B. Secondary MR
   - C. Acute myocardial infarction
   - D. Cardiac tamponade
3. The patient is temporarily stabilized with the intraaortic balloon pump and remains intubated due to hypoxemic respiratory failure. What is the next best step in the management?
   - A. Urgent cardiac surgery and repair of the mitral valve
   - B. Urgent cardiac surgery and replacement of the mitral valve
   - C. Transcatheter edge-to-edge repair
   - D. Heart team evaluation
4. The heart team evaluated the patient. Cardiac surgery was thought to be high-risk given patient's age and comorbidities. The heart team's decision was to proceed with percutaneous edge-to-edge repair with MitraClip under real-time 2D and 3D TEE guidance (Videos 25.3, 25.4, and 25.5). A total of two MitraClips were implanted. Which of the following is NOT a favorable anatomy feature for MitraClip?
   - A. Flail gap 1.4 cm
   - B. Flail width 1.9 cm
   - C. Origin of the regurgitation jet from malcoaptation of the A2 and P2 scallops
   - D. Mitral valve orifice area 5 cm^2

See page 318 for the answers.

REFERENCES

1. Otto CM, Nishimura RA, Bonow RO, et al. Guidelines2020 ACC/AHA Guideline for the Management of Patients With Valvular Heart Disease: Executive Summary: A Report of the American College of Cardiology/American Heart Association Joint Committee on Clinical Practice Guidelines. *Circulation*. 2021;143(5). doi:10.1161/CIR.0000000000000932.
2. Vahanian A, Beyersdorf F, Praz F, et al. 2021 ESC/EACTS Guidelines for the management of valvular heart disease: Developed by the Task Force for the management of valvular heart disease of the European Society of Cardiology (ESC) and the European Association for Cardio-Thoracic Surgery (EACTS). *Eur Heart J*. 2021; doi:10.1093/eurheartj/ehab395
3. Wilkins GT, Weyman AE, Abascal VM, et al. Percutaneous balloon dilatation of the mitral valve: an analysis of echocardiographic variables related to outcome and the mechanism of dilatation. *Br Heart J*. 1988;60(4):299–308. doi:10.1136/hrt.60.4.299.
4. Herrmann HC, Wilkins GT, Abascal VM, et al. Percutaneous balloon mitral valvotomy for patients with mitral stenosis. Analysis of factors influencing early results. *J Thorac Cardiovasc Surg*. 1988;96(1):33–38.
5. Post JR, Feldman T, Isner J, et al. Inoue balloon mitral valvotomy in patients with severe valvular and subvalvular deformity. *J Am Coll Cardiol*. 1995;25(5):1129–1136. doi:10.1016/0735-1097(94)00063-v.
6. Feldman T, Foster E, Glower DD, et al. Percutaneous repair or surgery for mitral regurgitation. *N Engl J Med*. 2011;364(15):1395–1406. doi:10.1056/NEJMoa1009355.
7. Mauri L, Garg P, Massaro JM, et al. The EVEREST II trial: design and rationale for a randomized study of the evalve mitraclip system compared with mitral valve surgery for mitral regurgitation. *Am Heart J*. 2010;160(1):23–29. doi:10.1016/j.ahj.2010.04.009.
8. Hahn RT. Transcathether valve replacement and valve repair: review of procedures and intraprocedural echocardiographic imaging. *Circ Res*. 2016;119(2):341–356. doi:10.1161/CIRCRESAHA.116.307972.
9. Stone GW, Lindenfeld J, Abraham WT, et al. Transcatheter mitral-valve repair in patients with heart failure. *N Engl J Med*. 2018;379(24):2307–2318. doi:10.1056/NEJMoa1806640.
10. Feldman T, Guerrero M, Salinger MH. Emerging technologies for direct and indirect percutaneous mitral annuloplasty. *EuroIntervention*. 2016;12(Y):Y84–Y89. doi:10.4244/EIJV12SYA23.
11. Patterson T, Adams H, Allen C, et al. Indirect annuloplasty to treat functional mitral regurgitation: current results and future perspectives. *Front Cardiovasc Med*. 2019;6:60. doi:10.3389/fcvm.2019.00060.
12. Herrmann HC, Mack MJ, et al. Transcatheter therapies for valvular heart disease. In: Zipes DL et al, ed. *Braunwald's Heart Disease*. 11th ed: Philadelphia Elsevier; 2019.
13. Wyler von Ballmoos MC, Kalra A, Reardon MJ. Complexities of transcatheter mitral valve replacement (TMVR) and why it is not transcatheter aortic valve replacement (TAVR). *Ann Cardiothorac Surg*. 2018;7(6):724–730. doi:10.21037/acs.2018.10.06.
14. Taramasso M, Gavazzoni M, Nickenig G, et al. Transcatheter mitral repair and replacement: which procedure for which patient?. *EuroIntervention*. 2019;15(10):867–874. doi:10.4244/EIJ-D-19-00743.
15. Fiorilli PN, Herrmann HC. Transcatheter mitral valve replacement: rationale and current status. *Annu Rev Med*. 2020;71:249–261. doi:10.1146/annurev-med-051418-060028.
16. Herrmann HC, Lima JA, Feldman T, et al. Mechanisms and outcome of severe mitral regurgitation after Inoue balloon valvuloplasty. North American Inoue Balloon Investigators. *J Am Coll Cardiol*. 1993;22(3):783–789. doi:10.1016/0735-1097(93)90191-3.
17. Desnos C, Iung B, Himbert D, et al. Temporal trends on percutaneous mitral commissurotomy: 30 years of experience. *J Am Heart Assoc*. 2019;8(13):e012031. doi:10.1161/JAHA.119.012031.
18. Padial LR, Abascal VM, Moreno PR, et al. Echocardiography can predict the development of severe mitral regurgitation after percutaneous mitral valvuloplasty by the Inoue technique. *Am J Cardiol*. 1999;83(8):1210–1213. doi:10.1016/s0002-9149(99)00061-2.

19. Padial LR, Freitas N, Sagie A, et al. Echocardiography can predict which patients will develop severe mitral regurgitation after percutaneous mitral valvulotomy. *J Am Coll Cardiol.* 1996;27(5):1225–1231. doi:10.1016/0735-1097(95)00594-3.
20. Obadia J-F, Messika-Zeitoun D, Leurent G, et al. Percutaneous repair or medical treatment for secondary mitral regurgitation. *N Engl J Med.* 2018;379(24):2297–2306. doi:10.1056/NEJMoa1805374.
21. Feldman T, Kar S, Rinaldi M, et al. Percutaneous mitral repair with the MitraClip system: safety and midterm durability in the initial EVEREST (Endovascular Valve Edge-to-Edge REpair Study) cohort. *J Am Coll Cardiol.* 2009;54(8):686–694. doi:10.1016/j.jacc.2009.03.077.
22. Chhatriwalla AK, Vemulapalli S, Holmes DRJ, et al. Institutional experience with transcatheter mitral valve repair and clinical outcomes: insights from the TVT registry. *JACC Cardiovasc Interv.* 2019;12(14):1342–1352. doi:10.1016/j.jcin.2019.02.039.
23. Sorajja P, Vemulapalli S, Feldman T, et al. Outcomes with transcatheter mitral valve repair in the United States: an STS/ACC TVT registry report. *J Am Coll Cardiol.* 2017;70(19):2315–2327. doi:10.1016/j.jacc.2017.09.015.
24. Herrmann HC, Rohatgi S, Wasserman HS, et al. Mitral valve hemodynamic effects of percutaneous edge-to-edge repair with the MitraClip device for mitral regurgitation. *Catheter Cardiovasc Interv.* 2006;68(6):821–828. doi:10.1002/ccd.20917.
25. Herrmann HC, Kar S, Siegel R, et al. Effect of percutaneous mitral repair with the MitraClip device on mitral valve area and gradient. *EuroIntervention.* 2009;4(4):437–442. doi:10.4244/eijv4i4a76.
26. Neuss M, Schau T, Isotani A, et al. Elevated mitral valve pressure gradient after MitraClip implantation deteriorates long-term outcome in patients with severe mitral regurgitation and severe heart failure. *JACC Cardiovasc Interv.* 2017;10(9):931–939. doi:10.1016/j.jcin.2016.12.280.
27. Patzelt J, Zhang W, Sauter R, et al. Elevated mitral valve pressure gradient is predictive of long-term outcome after percutaneous edge-to-edge mitral valve repair in patients with degenerative mitral regurgitation (MR), but not in functional MR. *J Am Heart Assoc.* 2019;8(13):e011366. doi:10.1161/JAHA.118.011366.
28. Halaby R, Herrmann H, Lim S, et al. Lack of association of mitral valve gradient after mitraclip with outcomes in functional mitral regurgitation: results from the coapt trial. *J Am Coll Cardiol.* 2020;75(11 Suppl 1):1309. doi:10.1016/S0735-1097(20)31936-7.
29. Kim J-H, Kocaturk O, Ozturk C, et al. Mitral cerclage annuloplasty, a novel transcatheter treatment for secondary mitral valve regurgitation: initial results in swine. *J Am Coll Cardiol.* 2009;54(7):638–651. doi:10.1016/j.jacc.2009.03.071.
30. Sack S, Kahlert P, Bilodeau L, et al. Percutaneous transvenous mitral annuloplasty: initial human experience with a novel coronary sinus implant device. *Circ Cardiovasc Interv.* 2009;2(4):277–284. doi:10.1161/CIRCINTERVENTIONS.109.855205.
31. Gheorghe L, Ielasi A, Rensing BJWM, et al. Complications following percutaneous mitral valve repair. *Front Cardiovasc Med.* 2019;6:146. doi:10.3389/fcvm.2019.00146.
32. Guerrero M, Urena M, Himbert D, et al. 1-year outcomes of transcatheter mitral valve replacement in patients with severe mitral annular calcification. *J Am Coll Cardiol.* 2018;71(17):1841–1853. doi:10.1016/j.jacc.2018.02.054.
33. Del Val D, Ferreira-Neto AN, Wintzer-Wehekind J, et al. Early experience with transcatheter mitral valve replacement: a systematic review. *J Am Heart Assoc.* 2019;8(17):e013332. doi:10.1161/JAHA.119.013332.

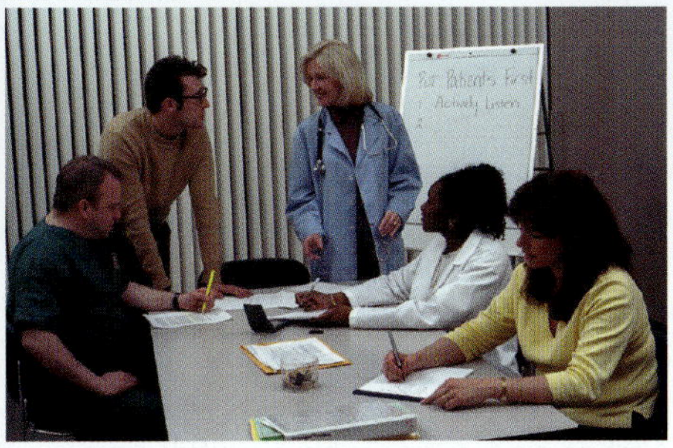

26

Developing Successful Structural Heart Programs

Carrie Redick, Lisa Hathaway Stella

CHAPTER OUTLINE

LEARNING OBJECTIVES

After reading this chapter, one should be able to:
- Identify the multidisciplinary team members.
- Define the steps for integrating mitral therapy into an established structural heart program.
- Describe efficient and effective patient care pathways for patients with mitral valve disease.

INTRODUCTION

Establishing the appropriate infrastructure is fundamental to optimizing outcomes in the delivery of care for patients undergoing treatment for mitral valve disease. Successful structural heart programs have considered the numerous factors which impact patient throughput from the first phone call through treatment to the follow-up care appointment. As additional structural heart programs begin to expand their treatment options to include mitral valve patients, the focus needs to be on the development of a well-defined care pathway that addresses all phases of care for this patient population. Adopting a multidisciplinary approach is central to ensuring appropriate coordination of care.

Conducting a thorough assessment of staffing, space, patient access, and definition of job roles must be considered in the early development of the program. This will allow for the provision of consistent processes resulting in the best possible care for patients. Best practice begins with a review of the existing structural heart program and the patient pathways previously established for the transcatheter aortic valve replacement (TAVR) patient as mitral valve patients follow similar care pathways. An ongoing careful review of outcome data, performance metrics, and the financial impact of the program should be diligently analyzed for process improvement opportunities.

THE MULTIDISCIPLINARY TEAM

Historically, the structural heart multidisciplinary team has been defined as the subspecialists on the team that traditionally has included an interventional cardiologist, a surgeon, an echocardiographer, an anesthesiologist, and other clinicians collaborating on the care of the patient. More recently, structural heart programs have begun to recognize the team is broader than physicians alone and has evolved to include administrators, advanced practice providers (APPs), schedulers, coordinators, and referring physicians as each of these members of the team has an impact on the patient experience and outcome. It is therefore essential for the first steps to include definitions of roles before expanding the program.

Role Definition

Without role clarity, workflows tend to be inefficient, with the focus shifting to the request or the immediate need demanding the staff member's attention. Often, this results in frequent distractions, forgotten details, and high levels of staff frustration. In addition, undefined responsibilities may lead to duplication of work thus reducing productivity. It is critical to the success of any program to take time to identify essential tasks and assign them to the appropriate job role.

Primary planning to assess skill task alignment and establish position responsibilities and functions begin with the entire team mapping out workflows. It is critical to have a concrete understanding of what is presently being performed before making changes that will ultimately impact patient care. Accordingly, frontline staff are critical to this discussion as they have first-hand knowledge of the workday roadmap. Engaging the team to outline future states will provide authentication of new workflows, elicit concordance, improve the likelihood of adherence, and consequently increase efficiency.

The process should start with categorizing tasks into buckets: preprocedural, peri-procedural, and post-procedure care. Scribing the patient throughput on a whiteboard or a visual display where all team members can see and contribute will accelerate and enhance the exercise. Decision points should be identified and tied into defined workflows. Once completed, a thorough review of the current state should be discussed, eliminating redundant and unnecessary steps.

The next phase includes a comprehensive review of job categories that may consist of the following roles: administrative support, APP, registered nurses (RN), certified medical assistants (CMA), and physicians. Other positions to consider depending on the size and scope of the program include research coordinators and analysts responsible for data abstraction and quality.

Although staffing models and job titles vary from institution to institution there are basic functions that are required for programs to run efficiently and successfully. One foundational role usually established at the onset is the valve coordinator (VC). This role is typically filled by an APP—either a physician assistant (PA) or a nurse practitioner (NP)—as clinical insights are essential to establishing appropriate patient pathways. Navigation through the pre-screening process to post-procedural care is complex and multifaceted so patients and their families rely heavily on the VC for support.

Depending on program volume, additional APPs may be required to support the valve clinic as well as assist with the educational and clinical needs of patients and their families. Program leadership may struggle with the decision to utilize an APN versus RN in this role. Factors contributing to the decision should include whether the hire is functioning to the top of his or her license. In addition, economic value should be considered when staffing valve clinics and assigning tasks, as having a licensed provider answering phones and scheduling testing may not be the most cost-effective use of personnel. Adequate administrative support is advised to facilitate timely referral to treatment times, support the clinical team, and increase patient and referring provider satisfaction. An alternative staffing model presents efficiencies through having an APN oversee RN team members, assisting in answering clinical questions, entering orders, and facilitating patient throughput. This blended example provides the advanced capabilities of having APN coverage while offering a less costly choice for organizations.

CMAs play an integral role in valve clinic triaging patients, scheduling any additional testing, and helping patients to navigate through their evaluation. The CMA also obtains historical medical records and test results prior to the first appointment. Additionally, CMAs room the patient, take vital signs, and enter pertinent information into the patient's record.

Another essential support role is that of the administrative coordinator who schedules clinical appointments and all associated testing and performs front-end duties including triaging phone calls. While some programs have APPs serve in this function, most programs find a clinical background is not necessary and that an administrative hire is less costly. Perhaps one of the most essential tasks for the administrative role is the interactions with the patients and families. The patient experience begins with the first phone call, which underscores the importance of hiring staff members who are professional and demonstrate both patience and compassion. Structural heart patients tend to be older and are likely to have a multigenerational family involved in their care requiring several points of contact that can be time-consuming and labor intensive, which should be factored into staffing ratios.

Time studies are an effective way to determine appropriate staffing ratios. These studies can validate daily responsibilities by tracking the number of minutes required to perform each task. Fig. 26.1 is an example of a time study for an APP. Although only a time study can definitively reveal how long it takes to complete each task, on average, structural heart programs have found that new team members should be added when the patient volume increases by a maximum of 100 procedures.

After all staff roles have been clearly defined by the planning team, attention should be directed to maintaining efficiency and ensuring accountability. A daily huddle, at a defined time each day, allows for the sharing of any pertinent patient information or concerns, allowing the team to remain focused and act upon issues in real time.

Structural heart remains a dynamic field with a continual pipeline of new innovations, medical devices, research, and best practices that need to be reviewed on a routine basis. It is therefore essential for the team to remain flexible when making decisions that are based on the current needs and latest reported evidence-based practice guidelines. Program leadership should meet regularly to examine and consider any necessary changes to the definition of roles and assigned workflows and make revisions accordingly.

Program Logistics

A thorough capacity assessment should be completed prior to adding a new procedure to a structural heart program. This can be accomplished internally or through an outside consultant but should be an initiative the program administrative director has the capability of completing.

Space in the valve clinic is a good starting point for a capacity assessment. The following questions should be explored:

Is there adequate space for the additional volume generated by adding mitral valve patients? How many exam rooms are available? How often does the clinic take place? Do clinic hours need to expand? What volumes do you envision over the next 5 years? What realistic options are available to the program?

Consideration must be also given to departments outside of the valve clinic as the decision to add mitral valve therapy will add volume to their programs as well and have ramifications on patient access. Resources in radiology, the cardiac catheterization lab (Cath Lab), the operating room (OR), non-invasive cardiology, anesthesia, and recovery units are among some of the areas that will be impacted. Considering resources are finite, it is important to remember that for every one mitral valve patient there will be multiple echocardiograms required over the course of care and treatment. Non-invasive cardiology will need to plan for the equipment and personnel necessary to deliver the required testing. The radiology department will be asked to make time for additional computed tomography (CT) scans and will be faced with increased staffing needs and growth in addition to cardiac procedures such as coronary computed tomography angiography (CCTA). These demands should not be the rate-limiting factor inhibiting growth and providing treatment for this patient population. Partnering with other services early on is critical to understanding their needs and the barriers they face providing care for the mitral valve patient.

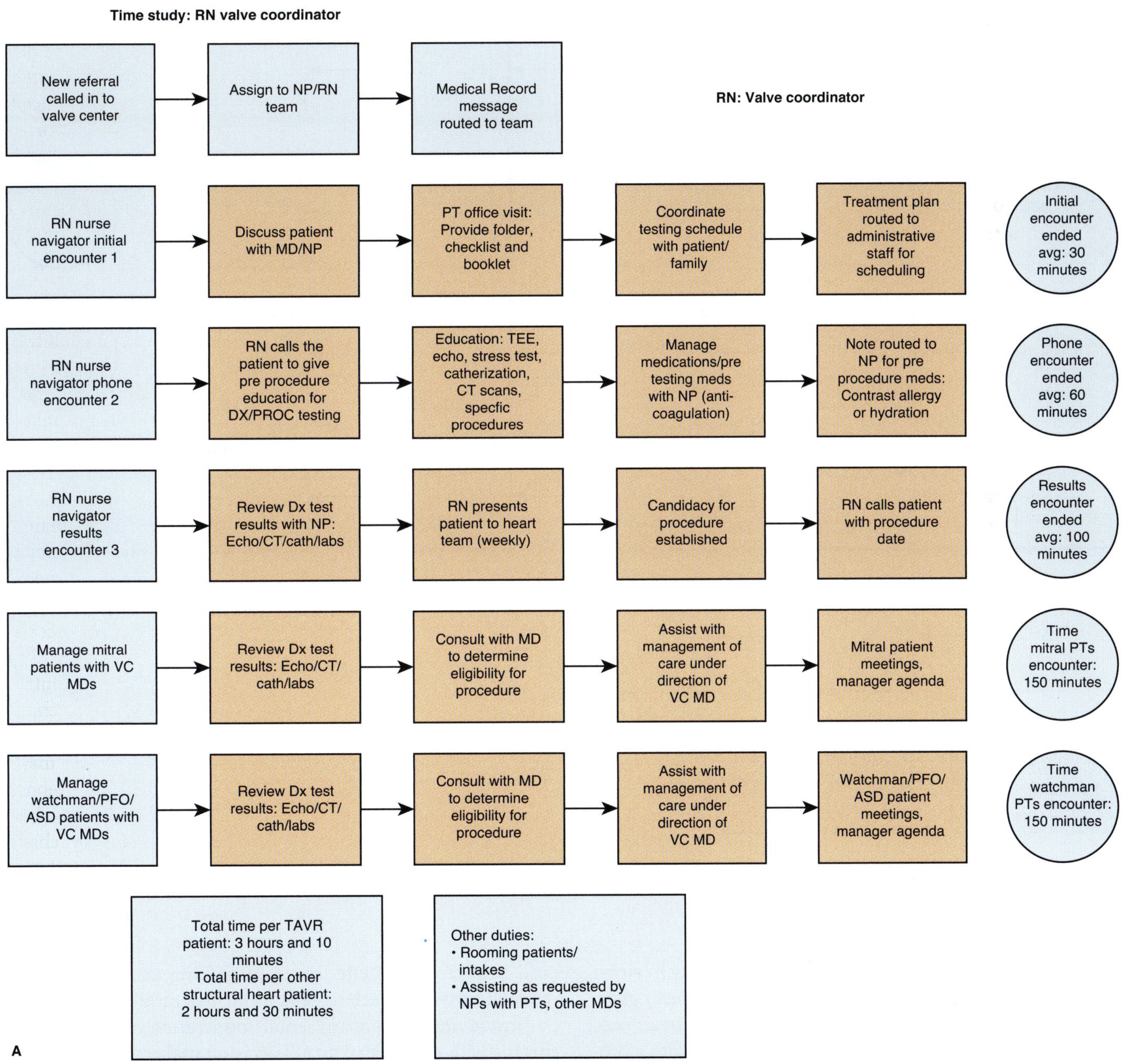

Fig. 26.1 (A) Time Study: RN Valve Coordinator. (B) Time Study Tool Worksheet. *ASD*, Atrial septal defect; *Dx*, diagnostic; *NP*, nurse practitioner; *PFO*, patent foramen ovale; *PROC*, procedure; *PTs*, patients; *RN*, registered nurse; *TAVR*, transcatheter aortic valve replacement; *TEE*, transesophageal echocardiogram; *VC*, valve coordinator.

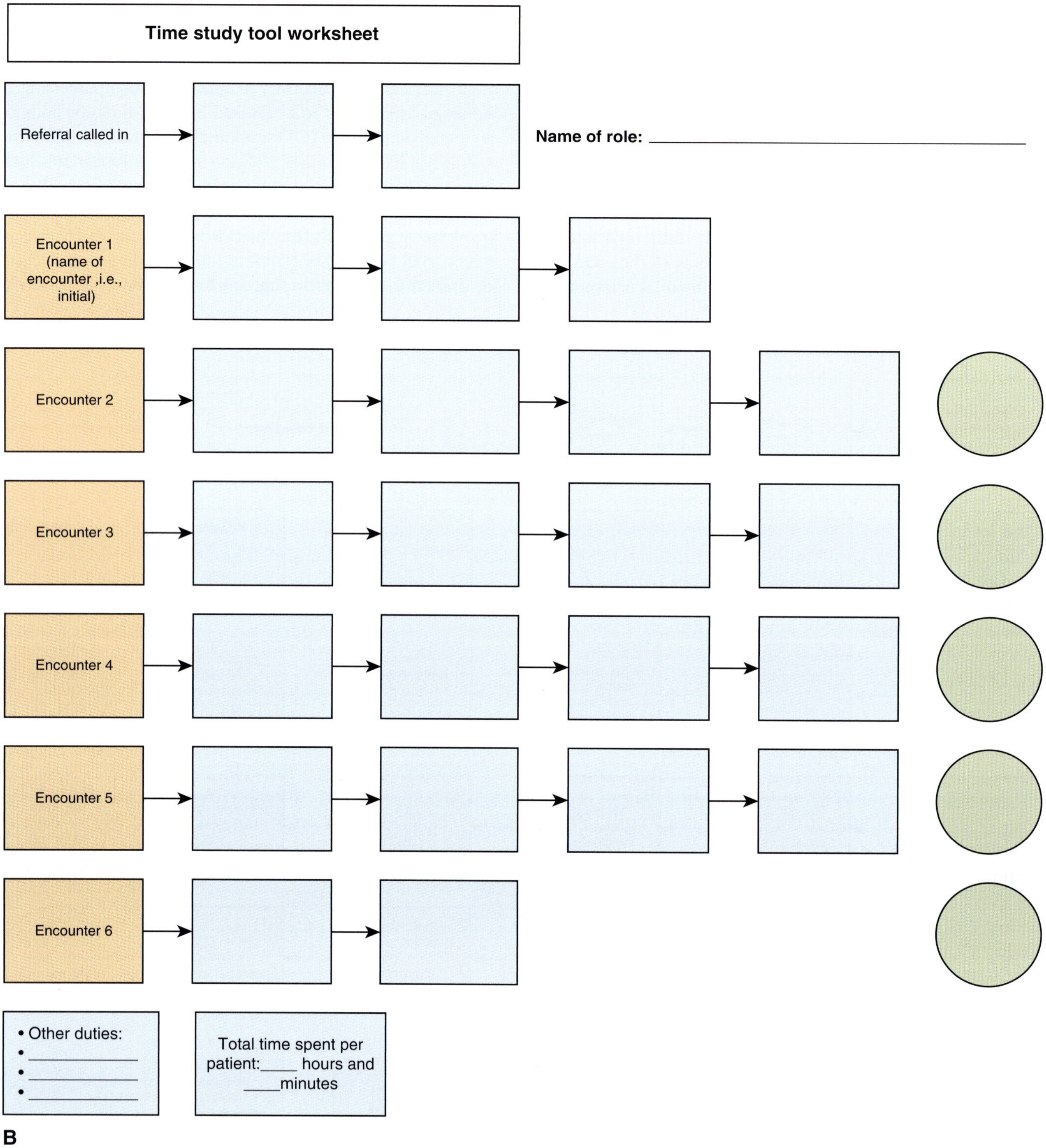

Fig. 26.1 Cont'd

Some programs are limited by case time availability in either the Cath Lab or the Operating Room, as they have been given assigned days and hours to perform their structural heart procedures. Meeting with the administrative leadership with a proposed new procedure and projected volumes is critical to growing the program. Being armed with an understanding of the impact the additional patients will bring to these departments will help facilitate better decision making and ensure a more collaborative approach to expanding programmatic services.

Improving interdepartmental cooperation begins with partnering with each department's decision maker. Developing subcommittees that meet monthly can be effective in promoting improved patient throughput and data-driven decision making. Routine meetings lead to the identification of potential barriers of care, improved communication, and ultimately decreased frustration. Additionally, as departments discuss shared challenges and develop solutions together, a more positive working relationship is fostered, allowing for increased efficiencies and patient throughput.

Planning not only for the present but prospectively looking 5 years out is an exercise that should be conducted at a minimum on an annual basis. Many programs have faced staffing shortages as burgeoning volumes have impacted patient throughput and delayed referral to treatment times, resulting in staff, physician, patient, and family frustrations. Program leadership should be aware of the tipping point by proactively adding new staff instead of waiting until team resentment builds, resulting in resignations, turnover, or burnout.

Patient Pathways

Preprocedural Evaluation

A mitral patient evaluation mirrors a TAVR evaluation, prompting the recommendation for mitral patients to follow the same structural heart team process presently in place for aortic patients. Ideally, patients should be seen within 10 days of the initial appointment request, although critical patients should be seen sooner. Prior to a clinic visit, it is important to obtain historical clinical notes, diagnostic images, and clinical assessments from any prior evaluation appointments. Patients can be empowered to gather their own information; however, it often leads to receiving incomplete or inappropriate information. Developing strong relationships with referring providers' offices and educating them on the importance of providing prior clinical information are key to making the evaluation process seamless. The intake process is an integral component of the scheduling and coordination of care. Relevant medical and surgical history should be taken at this point of contact so patients can be instructed on what types of information to bring with them to their appointment. Fig. 26.2 outlines the questions that should be asked at intake. Insurance information should be collected, allowing ample time for pre-authorizations. Additionally, referring physicians contact details should be collected as it is extremely important to engage referring clinicians as partners on the care team. Communication is vital to cultivating a good relationship and firmly establishing referral patterns.

Most patients will have a transthoracic echocardiogram (TTE) on the day of their evaluation unless a quality TTE has been completed within 30 days. Ideally, this exam should be performed prior to the evaluation appointment to ensure the images are available for the structural heart team to review. A CCTA may be needed depending on the type of mitral valve disease and the complexity of the case. Coordinating the diagnostic testing on the same day as the evaluation appointment will improve the patient experience as well as increase efficiency. Patients should be advised to dress comfortably and bring something to keep them occupied between appointments as their evaluation may take several hours.

The initial evaluation appointment should include the following: a history of present illness, pertinent past medical and surgical history, medication reconciliation, an electrocardiogram (EKG), a physical examination, and a review of past diagnostics studies. These steps are normally completed by an CMA, an APP, and a physician. Although not always required, a formal assessment by a cardiothoracic surgeon is best practice if there is a possibility of a surgical intervention or the patient is a potential candidate for a clinical trial. A Kansas City Cardiomyopathy Questionnaire (KCCQ) and a 5-m walk must also be obtained as it is required for the Transcatheter Valve Therapy Registry (TVT Registry) documentation.

Patients may be asked to return for a second set of diagnostic studies if clinically indicated based on the complexity of the pathology or anatomy. This may include a transesophageal echocardiogram (TEE) that will be helpful in delineating the best treatment modality and to complete an anatomical analysis of the mitral valve. Additionally, a left and right heart catheterization may be required to determine the best approach and access for the procedure.

The foundation of the structural heart team is the multidisciplinary approach to care. The heart team should meet weekly to discuss each patient and identify any barriers to care, eligibility for the procedure, and assess for gaps in data. Once all pertinent information and exam results for a patient are available, the patient's case should be presented and reviewed by the entire team. A thoughtful treatment plan is then developed with input solicited from all key constituents.

Procedural Considerations and Checklists

Once the screening process and work-up for the mitral valve patient has been completed, the procedure should be scheduled, ideally, within 30 days of the clinic visit. Careful thought and planning must be considered to ensure a safe and high-quality procedure with excellent clinical outcomes. A procedural checklist developed by the clinical leadership can confirm critical elements in planning prior to taking the patient to the procedure room. Functioning as a safety net, the checklist ensures the procedural steps are well defined and the operative team is all fully aware of the care plan for the case. In addition, it gives any team member the opportunity to ask questions or clarify details which results in a cohesive, well-developed procedural plan of care. Components of the checklist include the type of medical device, anatomic approach, sedation plan, imaging plan, and other crucial case details (Fig. 26.3).

Procedure logistics may vary between organizations; however, highly successful structural heart programs have embedded patient safety as a top priority by implementing mechanisms that standardize care. Checklists ensure all factors relating to the procedure have been addressed and are known to all team members. Ensuring a safe, high-quality procedure is performed consistently every time a mitral repair or replacement patient is brought to the operating table is the benchmark for all organizations.

Post-Procedural Care

Patients should be discharged with clearly written instructions that provide detailed explanations on what to expect following discharge. Documentation should also include post-procedure findings and identification of problems or symptoms for concern

Structural heart patient intake form

Today's date: ______/______/______

Evaluation requested: ❑ aortic valve ❑ mitral valve ❑ tricuspid valve ❑ Other __________

Patient name ______________________ **Sex** ❑ Male ❑ Female

Hospital MRN ______________ **DOB** ____/____/____

Address ______________________ ______________ ________
(Street) (City) (State)

________ ______________ ______________ ______________
(Zip code) Phone (home) Phone (cell) Email

Emergency contact ______________ Relationship ______________

Emergency contact phone ______________________

Insurance information

Primary carrier ______________________

Member ID no. ______________ Group ID no. ______________

Secondary carrier ______________________

Member ID no. ______________ Group ID no. ______________

Referring physician information

Name ______________________

Address ______________________ ______________ ________
(Street) (City) (State)

________ ______________ ______________
(Zip code) Phone (office) (Fax)

Cardiologist (if different from referring):

Name ______________________

Address ______________________ ______________ ________
(Street) (City) (State)

________ ______________ ______________
(Zip code) Phone (office) (Fax)

Appointment scheduled for ______/______/______ Time __________ ❑ AM ❑ PM

Previous echo – TTE (reports/images)	❑ Yes ❑ No	Records received	❑ Yes	❑ No
Previous echo – TEE (reports/images)	❑ Yes ❑ No	Records received	❑ Yes	❑ No
Previous cardiac cath (reports and images)	❑ Yes ❑ No	Records received	❑ Yes	❑ No
Prior heart surgery	❑ Yes ❑ No	Records received	❑ Yes	❑ No
Pulmonary function test	❑ Yes ❑ No	Records received	❑ Yes	❑ No
Recent lab work	❑ Yes ❑ No	Records received	❑ Yes	❑ No
Summary office notes	❑ Yes ❑ No	Records received	❑ Yes	❑ No
CT scan	❑ Yes ❑ No	Records received	❑ Yes	❑ No

Comments:

Fig. 26.2 Structural Heart Patient Intake Form *MRN,* Medical record number; *TEE,* transesophageal echocardiogram; *TTE,* transthoracic echocardiogram.

that includes clear instructions on when and how to reach out to the valve team. All instructions should be reviewed verbally with the patients and families using the "teach-back" method prior to discharge. Patients should be instructed to follow up with their cardiologist within the designated time frame, usually 7 to 10 days following discharge. Many programs have implemented a transitional care management strategy that includes a phone call to patients by a nurse navigator or a CMA 2 days following discharge, as it can prevent unnecessary re-hospitalizations and more importantly identify clinical issues before they become concerning. Fig. 26.4 lists the questions that should be asked during this call.

A 30-day follow-up appointment is recommended for all patients, although patients enrolled in a clinical trial likely will have to return more often depending on the research protocol. Often, a TTE will be performed on the same day to ensure there are no major changes to the valve function since discharge. Depending on the type of intervention, a CCTA may be ordered to evaluate the placement of the new valve. Again, scheduling all diagnostic testing and the follow-up appointment on the same day will have a positive impact on the patient experience and should be coordinated when possible. Fig. 26.5 illustrates a flowchart of the patient pathway.

Structural heart procedural checklist

- ☐ CTA (TAVR) or TEE (TEER) performed within 30 days for anatomical analysis
- ☐ Large bore access site: ____________ Vessel diameters: Right femoral: _________Left femoral: _________
- ☐ Other access sites: Pigtail: ______________ Other: ___________
- ☐ TVP access sites (select all that apply)
    - ☐ Femoral: Left _____ Right _____
    - ☐ Neck
    - ☐ Tempo wire
    - ☐ LV wire
    - ☐ Pacemaker implanted: Model _________
- ☐ Annulus measurement: Area: _________ Perimeter: _________ Mean diameter: _________
- ☐ Valve/device choice: ________________ Size: ___________
- ☐ Case complexity level:
    - ☐ Level 1: No anatomical or clinical adverse features
    - ☐ Level 2: Some adverse features easily overcome (LVOT calcium, low coronaries)
    - ☐ Level 3: Complex case; may require 3rd senior operator
        - ☐ Alternative access (suprasternal, transapical, transcarotid, transcaval)
        - ☐ High acuity (low EF, severe RV dysfunction, excessive tortuosity, and/or any other feature representing a high degree of complexity)
        - ☐ Neuro protection
        - ☐ Valve-in-valve
        - ☐ Bicuspid
        - ☐ Selected research cases
        - ☐ Consider discussing level 3 case with anesthesia
- ☐ Intra-Op imaging technique
    - ☐ TEE with CoreLab required, i.e valve sizing on table, complex case
    - ☐ TEE with CoreLab preferable
    - ☐ TTE: Reason why: ________________________
- ☐ Clinical field representative notified, i.e., valve, neuro protection, tempo wire, pacemaker

Fig. 26.3 Structural Heart Procedural Checklist. *ADLs*, Activities of daily living; *BNP*, brain natriuretic peptide; *EF*, ejection fraction; *FEV1*, first forced expiratory volume; *HTN*, hypertension; *LV*, left ventricle; *LVOT*, left ventricle outflow tract; *RV*, residual volume; *TVP*, temporary transvenous pacing; *TAVR*, transcatheter aortic valve replacement; *TEE*, transesophageal echocardiogram; *TEER*, transcatether edge-to-edge repair; *TTE*, transthoracic echocardiogram. *TIA*, transient ischemic attack; *TVP*, temporary transvenous pacing.

Structural heart procedural checklist

☐ **Conversion to open heart surgery** ☐ YES ☐ NO

☐ Health care proxy form in chart

Risk assessment:

Cardiac surgeon's assessment: ____________________ per __________________

Interventional cardiologist's assessment: ______________ per ______________

Frailty (5MG average): ________ Grip _______ ADLs _____

STS risk _______% for ___________________ (Procedure)

List of incremental and pertinent clinical findings, i.e. porcelain aorta, hostile mediastinum, frailty etc.

- **BNP 550 pg/mL, pro BNP 3200 pg/mL** = 3% ___
- **Prohibitive chest wall (deformity)** 5% ____
- **Severe LV diastolic dysfunction (grade 3 or 4)** = 4% ____
- **Prior stroke/TIA** = 3% _____
- **Hostile mediastinum** = 15% ____
- **FEV1 < 750 cc** = 20% ____ **FEV1 750–1000 cc** = 5% ____ **Home (supplemental) oxygen** = 5% ____
- **Nocturnal Bipap** = 2%____
- **Pulmonary systolic HTN**: 60–80 mm Hg = 5 %___ 80 mm Hg 15%____
- **Liver disease/ Childs A** = 5% ___**Childs B** = 7% ____**Childs C** = 25%_____
- **Aortic calcification: Porcelain** = 20%____ **Severe** = 3% ____
- **BMI < 21: < 80 y.o** = 4% ___ **80–90 y.o** = 5% ___ **>90 y.o** = 6 %___
- **Albumin < 3.3: < 80 y.o** = 4% ___ **80–90 y.o** = 5% ___ **>90 y.o** = 7%___
- **Wheelchair bound: < 80 y.o** = 7% ___ **80–90 y.o** = 8% ___ **>90 y.o** = 10%___
- **Does not live independently: < 80 y.o** = 5% ___ **80–90 y.o** = 6% ___ **>90 y.o** = 9%___
- ____
- **TOTAL SCORE** _________ **+ STS =** ______________

New York Heart Association (NYHA) Functional Classification

I ____ II ____ III ____ IV ____

Based on the above risk assessment and chart review, it is our clinical judgement that this patient is:

Low ____ **Intermediate**____ **High**_____ **Extreme**_____

Form completed by: ________________________________ Title: ________

Date: _____/_____/_______

Fig. 26.3 Cont'd on the top

TECHNOLOGY

Telehealth

Telehealth was not a major consideration prior to the COVID-19 pandemic, and most programs did not understand its potential until it was impossible to see patients in person. As we emerge from the pandemic, it is clear there remains a place for this important, virtual clinical tool. New patient evaluations are challenging when testing is required; however, telehealth can be an excellent option for a second opinion appointment when all testing has been completed. Additionally, it can be utilized for follow-up visits and post-procedural care. Telehealth has achieved pay parity and has allowed many programs to expand their reach in a clinically appropriate way. It is unclear whether some of the federal pandemic policies will remain intact, but what is unquestionable is that telehealth is here to stay and that structural heart programs should invest in defining a telehealth strategy for the future.

Artificial Intelligence

Many programs have benefited from investing in artificial intelligence (AI) platforms designed to scan images of patients who have had a recent echocardiogram. The software, based on defined

Post-procedural wellness call questions

1. **In the past 2 days (or since you left the hospital), have you experienced any of the following symptoms?**
   - Shortness of breath
   - Palpitations
   - Lightheadedness
   - Dizziness
   - Feeling like you are going to pass out
   - Weakness in the upper/lower extremities
   - Difficult speaking/swallowing
   - Chest pain
2. **In the past 2 days (or since you left the hospital), have you noticed any of the following with respect to your groin/leg:**
   - Bleeding
   - Pain
   - Swelling
   - Coolness
   - Discoloration of your toes

If a patient answers yes to any of the above, depending on the severity of the issue, patients should either be set up for a follow-up appointment, call their primary cardiologist, or be sent to the ER.

3. **Have you made your 10-day post-procedure follow-up appointment with your cardiologist?**

Fig. 26.4 Post-Procedural Wellness Call Questions. *ER*, Emergency room.

parameters, finds patients who have signs of valve disease but have not yet been referred for an evaluation appointment. Many of these AI products have the ability to push notifications to the ordering physicians through the electronic medical record (EMR) system to encourage them to refer their patients into valve programs for an evaluation appointment. A cost-benefit analysis should be done as these systems can be costly; however, they can yield a significant number of patients in need of mitral valve therapy and beyond.

FINANCIAL CONSIDERATIONS

The health of a structural heart program relies on many factors; however, both administrative and clinical leadership have an obligation to understand the financial impact of the mitral valve procedures. In an environment of declining reimbursements, health-care is under intense scrutiny to deliver the highest quality of care at the lowest cost. Structural heart programs must remain vigilant and fiscally responsible to allow for programmatic expansion including new procedures and personnel. Contribution margins, the amount of dollars the organization makes after variable expenses, should be scrutinized on a regular basis.

As transcatheter mitral valve technology continues to advance and treatment options expand, it is critical to the viability of the program to review the financial impact of the procedures. The

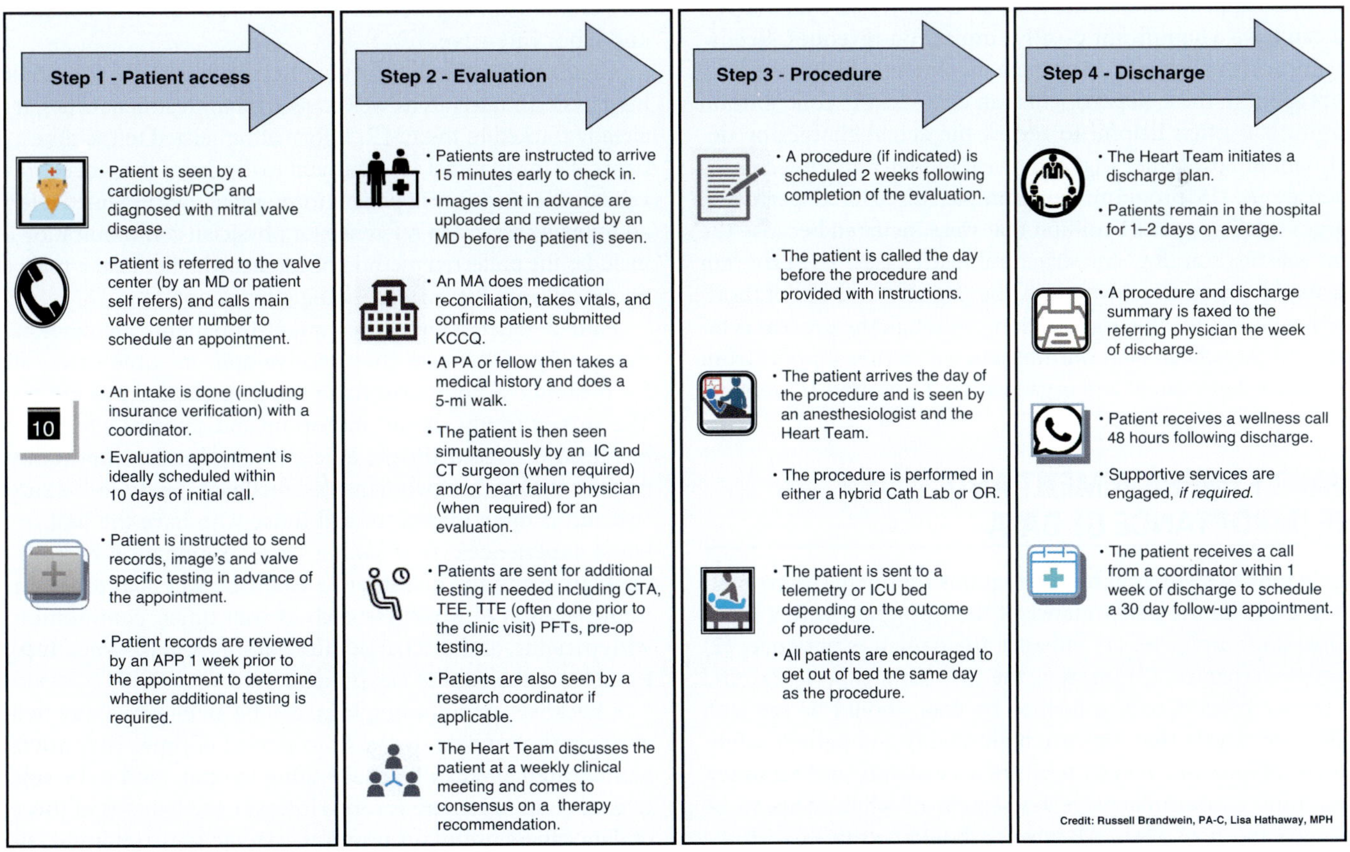

Fig. 26.5 Patient Pathway: Transcatheter Mitral Valve Therapy. *APP*, Advanced practice providers; *IC*, interventional cardiologist; *KCCQ*, Kansas City Cardiomyopathy Questionnaire; *OR*, operating room; *PA*, physician assistant; *PCP*, primary care provider; *PFT*, pulmonary function test; *TEE*, transesophageal echocardiogram; *TEE*, transesophageal echocardiogram.

operational budget should be reviewed, at minimum, monthly with variances investigated and reviewed for the potential to correct any identified concerns. In addition, financial programmatic analytics should be shared with the governing body of the program. Physicians should be aware that their decisions can have financial consequences for the organization. For example, bringing the patient in the night before a procedure increases the overall length of stay (LOS) or discharging a patient too quickly who requires a higher level of care can generate a penalty, thus lowering reimbursement.

Volume projections should be agreed upon by the team and presented to the executive finance committee for approval. Approved volumes should then be shared with other departments such as radiology and non-invasive cardiology to ensure all departments have the needed staff, equipment, and resources to support the program. Annual budgeting provides a financial infrastructure and should be as close to actual revenue and expenses as possible. If the pre-budget planning is thoughtfully completed with the input from both medical and administrative leadership, examining future device timelines, projected volumes, and reimbursement data, the program will have a solid financial foundation to begin the year.

Many administrators strategize cost savings through expense reduction rather than increasing efficiencies. Although opportunities for cost savings should be explored, leadership should not focus solely on supply cost reduction. Increasing efficiencies such as decreasing LOS or recovering a patient in a step down unit, when appropriate, rather than an intensive care unit (ICU) bed can have a significant positive impact on revenues. Recovery units often charge in 15-minute increments, so unnecessary hours spent in these departments can decrease the contribution margin. It is often helpful to review the actual charges by department or cost center that can reveal hidden and unnecessary expenses. A US program, for example, discovered perfusion charges totaling over $1 million that were incurred because the team was on "standby" for structural heart cases. The program was able to negotiate a lower rate, shaving off hundreds of thousands of dollars for the organization. Although the process is tedious, the payoff can be rewarding and will garner support from the finance department and organizational executive leadership.

QUALITY IMPROVEMENT AND THE IMPORTANCE OF DATA

Highly ranked structural heart programs routinely review metrics to evaluate the performance of their program with a focus on the "four aims" to: (1) enhance the patient experience, (2) improve outcomes, (3) improve the care team experience, and (4) reduce costs. Goals, informed by data, should be set with achievable targets that improve both quality and patient safety. Sources of data can vary in terms of accessibility and accuracy, warranting a comprehensive assessment of what needs to be reviewed and how often. All metrics should be shared with the entire team on a regular basis.

Data sources include the Society of Thoracic Surgery (STS) and the American College of Cardiology (ACC) TVT Registry, EMR and dashboards, clinical checklists, referral logs, patient satisfaction scores, and real-time monitoring. Reviewing the diverse sources of data can be a daunting task, so it is essential to choose the data sets that are most meaningful. Each source has its benefits and disadvantages, emphasizing the need to evaluate the relevance of the data to your program.

The TVT Registry is a surveillance database that reviews patient characteristics, treatments, and outcomes on a national level. Participation is tied to reimbursement, so it is required for all valve programs to comply if they wish to be paid. The TVT Registry, in return, provides national benchmarks that can be utilized to assess an individual program's performance. However, as the data are extracted retrospectively, it is usually not readily available until months later, so it may not be the best tool for real-time decision-making. However, the information provided is extremely valuable as it allows programs to see how they measure against their peers.

EMRs such as EPIC have the capability of extracting data in real time. EPIC dashboards can be built to display performance metrics as designated by the leadership team. Metrics can be pulled from any data field entered into the EMR including procedural volumes, procedural length times, LOS, pacemaker rates, mortality, stroke, and other defined data points. Data pulled into a dashboard should be validated through source reports. The downside to data mining an EMR is that anything entered into the system in a narrative format such as device type or procedure access site can only be obtained through chart review, which is time-consuming and labor intensive.

Creation of a referral tracking log can be helpful for monitoring physician referrals as well as referral to treatment times, if not already tracked in the EMR. Information related to the time a patient calls for an initial appointment to the day of the procedure can validate the efficiency of patient throughput. Documented referrals additionally serve as a reference for physician communication as it includes the preferred method of contact whether text, e-mail, or a phone call with the corresponding information.

Patient satisfaction scores quantify patients' perceptions of the quality of the care they receive and, in some cases, allow for meaningful comparisons to other institutions or programs. The survey results are an important indicator of whether care has been delivered timely, efficiently, and most importantly is patient centered. Obviously, the feedback tends to be subjective and is often biased toward those who have the best or the worst experiences. That said, a close examination of both the qualitative and the quantitative feedback will help programs to improve areas of weakness such as wait times, communication with patients, and discharge information, and inform strategies to improve the patient experience.

Checklists, or rounding logs, can be an effective way to look at a snapshot of data over a short period of time. They are often handwritten and can be challenging to read, tend to be subjective, or contain human errors. However, the benefits of this type of data can be useful for trending specific statistics in real time.

A peer review process, such as a morbidity and mortality (M&M) conference should be implemented for clinicians to review cases to evaluate and validate current practices. Any complications should be discussed to determine any needed changes in process or practice.

As additional mitral valve repair and replacement technologies become available it will be imperative for structural heart programs to review data relevant to the process and care delivery to meet this patient population's unique needs. Identifying areas for improvement as a group and developing action plans to alleviate issues, decrease complications, or improve performance metrics is essential to creating a quality program.

RESEARCH

A robust clinical trial portfolio allows a program to offer expanded treatment options to patients. Currently, there is only one approved minimally invasive way to treat mitral valve disease, the transcatheter edge-to-edge procedure. However, many promising transcatheter mitral valve replacement (TMVR) and transcatheter mitral valve repair (TMVr) devices and therapeutic techniques are currently in the investigational phase. Clinical trial work requires the addition of research coordinators to help identify, educate, and consent prospective patients and their families. Additionally, they are responsible for educating the heart team on the trial protocols including inclusion and exclusion criteria. Patients and their families must understand the benefit of research to existing and future patients as well as have a thorough understanding of the risks associated with being involved in a clinical trial. All clinical trials must also be submitted for Institutional Review Board (IRB) approval which can be a rigorous process, so a research coordinator, at minimum, is needed to interface with the IRB. Finally, most research protocols require several years of follow up with patients as well as associated testing that requires the proper scheduling support.

As valve programs look toward the future, there are also many clinical trials focused on tricuspid valve therapy that will require similar staffing appropriately embedded into the established valve program.

CONCLUSION

Developing a quality mitral valve program is a complex and multifaceted process. The foundational steps include building an appropriate infrastructure, clearly defining patient pathways, and, finally, frequently evaluating volumes to better understand the impact not just to the program but to the institution. Capitalizing on the lessons learned from existing TAVR programs, it is essential to focus on the following: (1) ensure that all members of the team are working to the top of their license, (2) regularly assess staffing ratios and resources to prevent patient access barriers, (3) communicate frequently to all stakeholders on projected growth so there is time to plan and prepare, and, (4) finally, set achievable program goals and make data-driven decisions based on financial performance and metrics.

SELF-ASSESSMENT QUESTIONS

1. What does "working" to the top of one's license mean?
   A. Practicing to the full extent of one's education and training
   B. Performing tasks as delegated by one's supervisor
   C. Assuming a leadership role because one is licensed
   D. Meeting the expectations of patients
2. Choose the forms of data a mitral valve program should review on a regular basis.
   A. Patient outcomes
   B. Financial data
   C. Length of stay
   D. Patient satisfaction scores
   E. All of the above
3. A mitral valve evaluation mirrors patients who receive the following therapy:
   A. PCI
   B. CTO
   C. TAVR
   D. Mechanical circulatory support
4. The success of a mitral valve program depends on:
   A. A team approach to care
   B. Thoroughly defined patient pathways
   C. Developing an appropriate infrastructure
   D. Communicating with all stakeholders on a regular basis
   E. Regularly reviewing performance metrics and adjusting, when necessary
   F. All of the above

See page 318 for the answers.

27

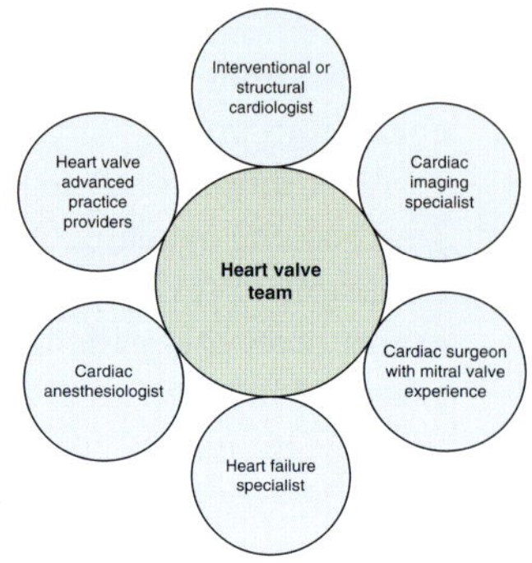

Quality Improvement and Outcomes

Wally Omar, Duane Pinto

CHAPTER OUTLINE

LEARNING OBJECTIVES

- Understand the principles of quality in care delivery and how they relate to mitral valve interventions.
- Recognize the need for a successful heart team, and each actor's specific contribution of a growing mitral valve program.
- Ensure that best practices are employed to improve patient outcomes, both by objective and self-reported measures.

ASSESSING QUALITY IN MITRAL VALVE INTERVENTION

Ensuring success in the delivery of mitral valve care necessitates answering the critical questions, "What is quality?" and "Who decides?" Active physician participation in developing the tools to measure and report quality outcomes is essential; otherwise, control over the process will be lost to those who do not possess an in-depth comprehension of interventional for valvular heart disease.

When defining "what is quality," one must recognize that quality measurement in the procedure suite goes beyond simply self-reporting excellent procedural outcomes, and there are several principles to guide this effort. While many models of quality can be employed, the well-established Donabedian model provides a simple, validated framework.[1] Quality in this model comprises three tenets: structure, process, and outcomes. Structure provides the physical and resource foundation for the procedure, and includes the hospital, staff, equipment, procedural volume, and so on. Process is the roadmap followed to deliver the care in question, and outcome assesses the effects of the procedure on the patient and the broader population.[2] Standardization of these tenets and their components has allowed for national standards of quality in percutaneous coronary intervention and surgical valve therapies through the American College of Cardiology and Society of Thoracic Surgeons (STS).[3]

Given the novelty of transcatheter valve interventions and how rapidly these technologies were adopted, a full consensus on standard policies has not been created. While the techniques may be novel, ensuring quality is not. This chapter will focus on the various components of building a quality mitral valve program by applying new data to the already-established frameworks, covering operator volumes, patient-centered team approach, procedural success rates, appropriate use, and outcomes. Adherence to these various components allows for the optimization and seamless operation of a transcatheter mitral valve program.

STRUCTURE

Building a Heart Team

Mitral valve therapies require a longitudinal, multidisciplinary approach for success. For an effective heart team approach, an institution should include the following members in its team (Fig. 27.1):

- Cardiac surgeon with experience in mitral valve surgery
- Interventional/structural cardiologist

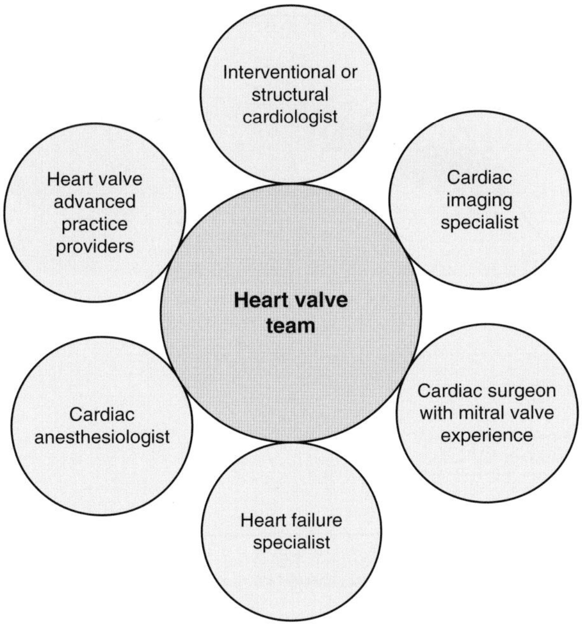

Fig. 27.1 The key members of a quality valve team as part of a valve center of excellence.

- Advanced heart failure cardiologist
- Cardiac imaging specialist
- Cardiac anesthesiologist
- Outpatient and inpatient team of advanced practice provider(s) and registered nurses

Each member of the team plays a key role in defining and ensuring implementation of the optimal mitral valve interventional process.

The cardiac surgeon has the greatest historical experience with mitral valve repair and replacement and is best equipped to properly risk stratify patients for surgery, ensuring both appropriate use and procedural success. Furthermore, current and future transcatheter techniques may still require surgical expertise, especially when alternative and/or transapical access are required. The Society for Thoracic Surgeons already has national benchmarks for surgeons to follow, some of which are described later in this chapter. These benchmarks can be used to determine their suitability for heart team involvement.

The interventional and/or structural cardiologist is most knowledgeable in catheter-based interventions and works alongside the cardiac surgeon to deliver the required therapy. They should be proficient in interpretation of intracardiac hemodynamics and shunts, obtaining large-bore access, performing transseptal puncture, and closing iatrogenic atrial septal defects in addition to the core skills required of an interventionalist. Their expertise is required for diagnostic hemodynamic assessment, procedural success, preprocedural optimization with percutaneous coronary intervention or ethanol septal ablations, as well as complication bailout including atrial septal defect (ASD) closure, device retrieval with snare catheters, and pericardiocentesis. Minimal procedure requirements for the structural cardiologist have started to emerge and are discussed later in the chapter.

An advanced heart failure specialist is not only an important member of the heart valve team but often the gatekeeper for referrals. In addition to establishing a longitudinal relationship with the patient's valve journey, the heart failure specialist assists in risk stratification and optimization of medical management prior the procedure. This component of care is crucial, especially when determining appropriate use for secondary mitral regurgitation in light of findings of both the cardiovascular outcomes assessment of the MitraClip percutaneous therapy for heart failure patients with functional mitral regurgitation (COAPT)[4] and percutaneous repair with the MitraClip device for severe functional/secondary mitral regurgitation (MITRA-FR)[5] trials where the differences in outcomes are in part related to differences in optimization of goal-directed medical therapy. Post-procedurally, the heart failure specialist will assist in left atrial or ventricular unloading and further optimize filling pressures and biventricular function.

Mitral valve therapies require cardiac imaging during evaluation and treatment. By extension, an expert cardiac imager is integral for success. This role can be filled by either a cardiologist or cardiac anesthesiologist with interest and knowledge of mitral valve anatomy and catheter based structural heart procedures. Prior to some procedures, cardiac CT is performed to define the mitral valve anatomy as it relates to the heart, and to determine risk for complications such as left ventricular outflow tract obstruction. Calling upon this expertise is of paramount importance to avoid complications. During the procedure, the operator relies on the cardiac imager to guide several portions of the procedure. As such, the imager must be facile with specific training in the various procedures and specifics such as delineating the interatrial septum for optimal septal puncture as well as the ability to rapidly shift between views, such as what is required during evaluation of the mitral valve leaflets during transcatheter edge-to-edge repair (TEER) clip deployment. The cardiac imager should be facile in obtaining and interpreting three-dimensional (3D) views of the mitral valve and characterizing mitral gradients in real-time.

The cardiac anesthesiologist, in addition to performing transesophageal echocardiography, ensures adequate hemodynamic support before, during, and after the case. Because these procedures are often performed in high-risk patients with reduced cardiac reserve, their role in maintaining patient stability before and after the procedure is emphasized. In addition, cardiac anesthesiologists play an important role when assessing procedural outcomes by employing blood conservation strategies, early extubation protocols, and pain management particularly in patients with reduced pulmonary reserve.

Advanced practice providers play a variety of roles in procedural planning, execution, and follow-up, working both in the inpatient and outpatient setting. They are integral in performing pre- and postprocedural visits (often 30-day and 1-year follow-ups), updating registry data as required, communicating with patient families to address their concerns, overseeing the completion of diagnostic testing, tending to inpatient consults, and triage urgent cases and more. One or more advanced practice provider (APP) is often required to fill these roles and are recommended for best practice in optimizing structural heart programs.[6]

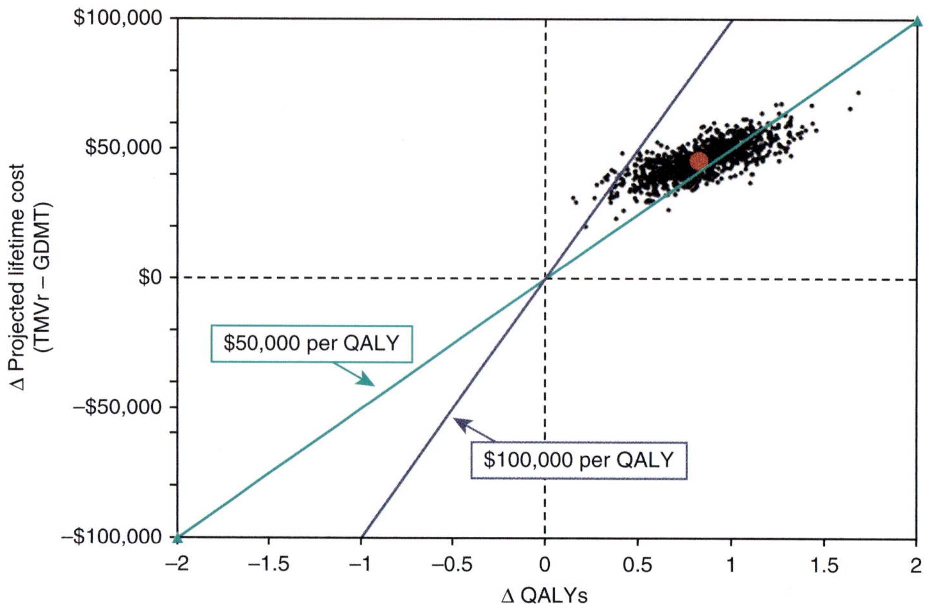

Fig. 27.2 Joint distribution of lifetime incremental cost and quality-adjusted life-years (QALYs) for transcatheter mitral valve repair (TMVr) versus guideline-directed medical therapy (GDMT). Incremental lifetime costs and benefits with TEER versus GDMT plotted on the cost-effectiveness plane with benefits expressed as QALYs. Solid red circle represents base case estimates; the surrounding small circles represent individual results for 1000 replicates of the study using bootstrap resampling; the solid green line represents a willingness-to-pay threshold of $50,000 per QALY gained; and the solid blue line represents a willingness-to-pay threshold of $100,000 per QALY gained. The base case results demonstrated a gain of 0.82 QALYs at an incremental cost of $45,648 per patient (after discounting), resulting in an incremental cost-effectiveness ratio of $55,600 per QALY gained. *TEER,* transcatheter edge-to-edge repair. (From Baron SJ, Wang K, Arnold SV, et al. Cost-effectiveness of transcatheter mitral valve repair versus medical therapy in patients with heart failure and secondary mitral regurgitation. *Circulation.* 2019;140:1881–1891.)

PROCESS

Once the necessary components of a valve center of excellence are established, a standardized operating process should be employed to ensure the delivery of quality care. While no single process has become standard in the United States, there are several key components to consider the appropriate procedure for a given patient, backed by the American College of Cardiology:

1. Understanding the U.S. Food and Drug Administration's indications for TEER in patients with (a) primary mitral regurgitation *and* high or prohibitive surgical risk and (b) selected patients with heart failure and secondary mitral regurgitation.
2. Recognition that surgical mitral valve repair for primary mitral regurgitation is associated with better outcomes than TEER when surgery is feasible.
3. A proper treatment algorithm for those undergoing TEER for secondary mitral regurgitation (MR), including documentation of the following:
   a. Clear establishment of the etiology of MR (primary vs secondary vs mixed)
   b. Persistent symptoms
   c. The use of adjunctive testing for patients with indeterminate MR severity, including but not limited to, right heart catheterization and exercise stress echocardiogram
   d. Maximally tolerated contemporary guideline-directed medical therapy (GDMT) in accordance with degree of heart failure for those with secondary MR
   e. Consideration of the associated hemodynamic consequences of TEER versus medical therapy
4. Determination of the decision to proceed with TEER made by multiple consultants, including one cardiac surgeon.

Adherence to the above not only ensures that the valve program is following established national guidelines, but that optimal multidisciplinary consideration was made for each procedural decision. Documentation from multiple consultants demonstrates that conservative measures were trialed for each patient, and that once the decision to intervene was made, all appropriate options were discussed. The process further promotes the heart team model, which remains at the core of a valve center of excellence.

OUTCOMES

Cost

Value-based care requires not only the delivery of high-quality care but doing so at a cost low enough to justify the care. In such a model, value is indirectly proportional to cost. Given the high cost associated with newer mitral valve interventions,

TABLE 27.1 Proposed Integration of Value Into Clinical Guideline Recommendations

High value: Better outcomes at lower cost of ICER <$50,000 per QALY gained
Intermediate value: $50,000 to <$150,000 per QALY gained
Low value: $150,000 or more per QALY gained
Uncertain value: Value examined but data are insufficient to draw conclusion because of no studies, low-quality studies, conflicting studies, or prior studies that are no longer relevant
Not assessed: Value not assessed by the writing committee

ICER, Incremental cost-effectiveness ratio; *QALY,* quality-adjusted life-year.

(Adapted from Anderson JL, Heidenreich PA, Barnett PG, et al. ACC/AHA statement on cost/value methodology in clinical practice guidelines and performance measures: a report of the American College of Cardiology/American Heart Association Task Force on Performance Measures and Task Force on Practice Guidelines. *J Am Coll Cardiol.* 2014;63(21):2304–2322.)

continuous efforts must be made to ensure value. Several studies have already investigated the costs and effects of TEER with the MitraClip for secondary mitral regurgitation and found the procedure to hold value over time. A 2-year retrospective analysis of the procedure demonstrated that postprocedural follow-up costs were lower with TEER than with GDMT alone ($26,645 vs $38,345), but cumulative 2-year costs were higher with TEER due to the upfront cost of the procedure ($73,416 vs $38,345). With the estimated increase in life span of greater than a year, the adjusted quality, adjusted life-years of 0.82 years yielded a cost effectiveness ratio of $40,361 per life year gained and $55,600 per quality-adjusted life-year gained, The conclusion is that 2-year follow-up costs were decreased by $11,000 per patient in TEER compared with GDMT (Fig. 27.2).[7] This result was found to be well below the threshold to be considered valuable for cardiac therapies in the United States, which is less than $50,000 per quality-adjusted life-year (QALY) gained (Table 27.1).[8] The above values are calculated for patients that met COAPT criteria, as follows: ischemic or nonischemic cardiomyopathy with left ventricular ejection fraction of 20% to 50%, grade 3+ or grade 4+ (moderate to severe) mitral regurgitation, symptoms consistent with New York Heart Association Class II–IV heart failure despite concurrent optimal medical therapies and/or cardiac resynchronization therapy.[9]

These findings have been replicated outside of the United States as well. A subanalysis of EVEREST and secondary MR patients in Canada found an incremental cost effectiveness ratio (ICER) of $32,300 per QALY gained over 10 years ($35,000), once again less than the $50,000 threshold of a valuable intervention. In the United Kingdom, the National Health Service Perspective found TEER to be reasonably cost effective with an ICER of $13,664 per QALY ($20,800).

While these data confirm mitral interventions to be of very high cost, the monetary value of the procedure is realized in follow-up and gained quality life-years over subsequent years.

Procedural Outcomes

Surgical Mitral Valve Replacement: Hospital Volume to Outcome Relationship

As mentioned, mitral valve surgery is not performed by every cardiac surgeon as it requires a yearly volume target to maintain proficiency. A 2020 study of the STS Mitral Valve Surgery Registry demonstrated a significant difference in outcomes after mitral valve repair and replacement according to hospital and operator volumes. Data from 2011 to 2016 found that the median annual isolated mitral valve surgery was 34 per hospital and 17 per surgeon. Surgeons and hospitals who fell into the lowest quartile were associated with not only a higher risk-adjusted composite outcome of morbidity (stroke, reoperation, prolonged ventilation, renal failure, and deep sternal wound infection) but higher risk-adjusted mortality at 30 days and 1 year as well when compared to those in the highest quartile. Furthermore, surgeons and hospitals in the lowest quartile were less likely to successfully attempt mitral valve repair. Authors of this trial concluded that mitral valve surgery should be considered at a regional level, as opposed to a hospital level, to optimize outcomes for patients.[10] It is important to note that the same volume-based variability was not demonstrated for heart failure hospitalizations and/or readmissions.

Similar metrics are used to determine the quality of an institution's mitral valve surgical program. As of 2015, the society of thoracic surgeons (STS) placed forth recommendations for public reporting on mitral valve replacement and repair. Using data from 2011 to 2014 and over 61,000 surgeries across 867 centers in the United States, mortality was 2.9% and morbidity was 17%. Based on the data, centers were awarded star values in accordance with event rates, such that those with one star had the highest rates of adverse events, and those with three stars the lowest. Out of the 867 centers, 32 centers had mortality rates of 5% or more, earning them a one-star rating, and 68 centers had mortality rates of 0.6% or less, earning them a three-star rating. There was fidelity in the morbidity rates such that they followed mortality.[11] Annual reporting at a hospital or group practice level on the three-star scale is now publicly available via the STS website to allow for transparency and accountability.[12,13]

MitraClip: Volume Outcomes

A study of pre- and post-FDA approval of MitraClip (Abbott Laboratories, Abbott Park, IL, USA) found similar trend when assessing hospital volumes and outcomes. When selecting for approximately 2000 patients undergoing MitraClip from the National Readmission Database, the authors found that performance of 10 or less procedures per year were associated with higher readmission at 30 days (OR 1.08) and higher mortality (OR 1.54).[14] A retrospective assessment of MitraClip procedures over the course of 5 years showed a similar trend in institutional volume and outcomes. The analysis found an inflection point at approximately 50 cases, after which procedural time and composite complication significantly decreased, and degree of MR reduction significantly increased (Fig. 27.3).[15] While not significant, specific adverse outcomes, including death, conversion to open-heart surgery, single leaflet device attachment, and

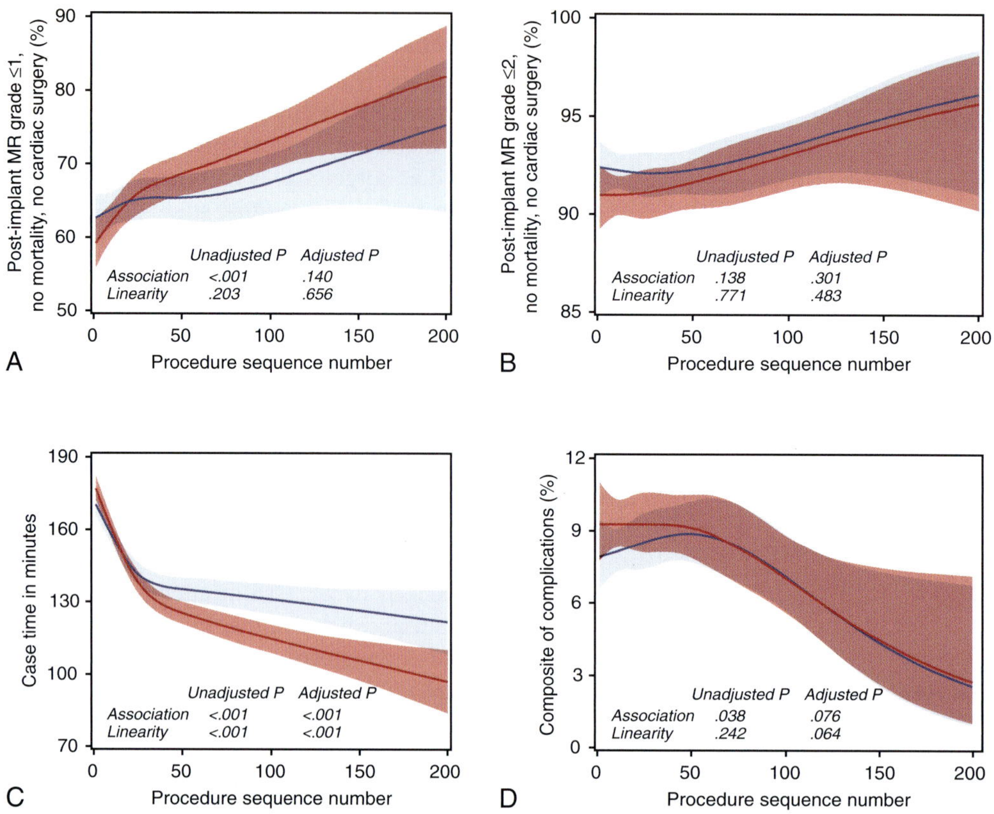

Fig. 27.3 (A) Learning curve for optimal procedure success. (B) Acceptable procedure success. (C) Procedure time. (D) Procedure complications. (From Chhatriwalla AK, Vemulapalli S, Szerlip M, et al. Operator experience and outcomes of transcatheter mitral valve repair in the United States. *J Am Coll Cardiol*. 2019;74:2955–2965.)

the need for blood transfusion were inversely related to institutional experience as defined by number of procedures.

These findings have motivated the American College of Cardiology to recommend minimum intervention targets for both operators and institutions. For new transcatheter mitral valve (MV) programs, the interventionalist should document 50 lifetime structural heart procedures, have prior transcatheter mitral valve repair experience with at least 20 lifetime transseptal punctures, 10 of which were performed as the primary operator, demonstrate board eligibility in interventional cardiology or cardiac surgery and complete certification in device-specific training.[16]

For institutions, broader recommendations have been set forth, suggesting the following: the presence of a surgeon who has performed 20 MV surgeries in the preceding year or 40 MV surgeries in the preceding 2 years, at least 50% of which should be a repair; minimum site mitral surgical volume of 40 cases in the previous year or 80 in the previous 2 years, 50% of which should be repair; an STS star rating of two or more for at least two consecutive reporting periods per year for both mitral valve replacement (MVR) and MVR + coronary artery bypass graft surgery (CABG). These recommendations carry forward when attempting to maintain a MV program, in addition to the following: a percutaneous coronary intervention volume of 300 or more per year, participation in the National Cardiovascular Data Registry (NCDR) Cath/PCI (percutaneous coronary intervention) or equivalent registry, and an in-hospital risk adjusted mortality rate above the lowest 25th percentile for the most recent four quarters.[16] Adherence to these standards may inform performance metrics set forth by the STS and transcatheter valve therapies (TVT) in the near future.

Should transcatheter TEER and future catheter-based valve interventions follow the pattern of transcatheter aortic valve replacement (TAVR), mortality and morbidity associated with the procedure is expected to decrease: TAVR had threefold higher mortality in 2014 than it did in 2019 (7.2% vs 2.5%), likely due not only to expansion of the procedure to lower risk populations but to operator experience as well.[17]

Procedural Outcome Requirements

Given a paucity of data to employ risk prediction models, such as what is available for surgical mitral valve intervention through the STS risk calculator, several procedural outcome benchmarks have been suggested to gauge the quality of an institution's mitral valve program. The initial outcomes of interest mimic those that determine procedurally success in surgical mitral valve interventions, seen in Table 27.2. They include mortality, stroke, bleeding, vascular complications,

TABLE 27.2 Proposed 30-Day Performance Requirement for MitraClip Operators

In-Hospital and 30-Day Outcome Metrics	Performance Requirement
In hospital + 30-day all-cause mortality	"As expected" or "better than expected" based on national benchmark data with 95% confidence intervals (CIs)
30-day stroke, transient ischemic attack	Performance falls within 95% outlier and/or 90% warning boundaries on funnel plot
30-day major vascular complication	Performance falls within 95% outlier and /or 90% warning boundaries on funnel plot
30-day major bleeding	Performance falls within 95% outlier and/or 90% warning boundaries on funnel plot
30-day moderate-to-severe or severe MR	Performance falls within 95% outlier and/or 90% warning boundaries on funnel plot
30-day significant mitral stenosis (MS) (mean gradient 8 mm Hg or more, valve area <1.5 cm^2)	Performance falls within 95% outlier and/or 90% warning boundaries on funnel plot

TABLE 27.3 Proposed 1-Year Outcome Metric Variables

- 1 year all-cause mortality
- Change in patient reported health status (KCCQ) at 1 year versus baseline
- 1 year rehospitalization for heart failure
- 1 year repeat MV intervention (transcatheter or surgical)
- 1 year moderate-to-severe or severe MR
- 1 year significant mitral stenosis (mean gradient 8 mm Hg or more, valve area <1.5 cm^2)

KCCQ, Kansas City Cardiomyopathy Questionnaire.

and reduction of mitral regurgitation to name a few. One-year outcomes are yet to be developed but will tend to focus not only on immediate procedural success, but effects on quality of life and heart failure readmissions as well (Table 27.3).[16]

As national benchmarks continue to develop, current data demonstrate low overall complication rates. A 5-year 2019 TVT analysis querying all participating TEER sites found that in over 12,000 cases performed, overall death rate was 2.1%. Complication rates for the remaining aforementioned variables, including single leaflet detachment, transient ischemic attack, stroke, and need for cardiac surgery were all 1% or less.[15]

Patient-Centered Outcomes

As shared decision-making is integrated into the valvular heart disease guidelines, patients are expected to not only have a say in the decision to proceed with a mitral valve procedure but confirm whether there was value in the intervention in the first place. Valve programs that participate in registries, including those that report to the TVT registry, are required to at least assess a KCCQ (Kansas City Cardiomyopathy Questionnaire) score and document the number of heart failure hospitalizations at 30 days and 1 year after the intervention. These metrics have shown improvement in past trials of mitral intervention:

a. In COAPT, quality of life was measured by the KCCQ. Patients who received the device had an improvement in their score by 12 points on average, and those who were in the medical group had a decrease in score by −3.6 points on average. The threshold for a significant change in KCCQ was 5 points.[9]
b. In MITRA-FR those who received MitraClip had an EQ5D (European Quality of Life Scale) score 50 points lower 1 year after the procedure, from 143 to 93.[18]
c. An analysis of 4226 patients from the Society of Thoracic Surgeons/American College of Cardiology Transcatheter Valve Therapy Registry found an overall improvement in patient-reported quality of life at 30 days and 1 year after the procedure (41.9 pre-TEER, 66.7 30 days post-TEER, without change at 12 months).
d. A trial of patients undergoing randomized surgical mitral valve replacement or mitral valve repair for severe ischemic mitral regurgitation demonstrated similar improvement in patient-reported quality of life at 1 year from the surgery: an average decrease of 22 points on the Minnesota Living with Heart Failure Questionnaire for the repair group and 30 points for the replacement group.[19]
e. Three-year outcome data from COAPT showed a maintenance of the favorable KCCQ changes seen in the initial study, as well as 6-minutes walk time/distance.[20]

While these metrics are a start, they do not encompass all of the factors that affect one's quality of life with mitral valve disease. Patient-centered outcomes, those that truly matter to the ones receiving the therapy, have become a means of assessing quality in oncology and are starting to be adopted in the heart failure population. Patients will play a growing role in understanding gaps in transition from hospital to home care, barriers to rehabilitation, and expected versus actual results as it pertains to their daily lives. These psychosocial effects of mitral valve interventions are to be understood and are part of a larger call to action by the National Heart, Lung and Blood Institute to be prioritized and studied in the years to come.[21]

The effectiveness of quality improvement in mitral valve therapies continues to evolve as new technologies are tried and tested. Given the rapid pace of change and implementation of new technology in the field, adherence to the core principles of quality becomes even more important. The structural elements of a multidisciplinary valve team with significant experience lay the foundation for quality work, while constant scrutiny and process improvement pave the way for optimal outcomes and delivery of high value care.

CASE-BASED ASSESSMENT

1. Which of the following is not an essential member of an institution's heart team as it pertains to mitral valve therapies?
   A. Cardiac surgeon
   B. Industry representative
   C. Heart failure specialist
   D. Advanced practice provider
2. Why is it recommended that a mitral valve interventions site should include a surgeon that performs at least 20 mitral valve surgeries per year?
   A. To make up for the cost incurred by performing transcatheter edge-to-edge repairs
   B. To ensure an adequate experience for patient satisfaction questionnaires and self-reported outcomes
   C. Surgical operator volumes correlate inversely with heart failure hospitalizations and readmissions
   D. Surgical operator volumes correlate inversely with morbidity and mortality
3. To ensure continued delivery of quality care in the face of a rapidly evolving field, mitral valve intervention centers should do which of the following?
   A. Participate in national registries like the ACC Transcatheter Valve Therapies (TVT) registry
   B. Independently assess patient-centered and self-reported outcomes on a regular basis
   C. Refer to the core tenets of structure, process, and outcomes when deciding to build or change the program
   D. All of the above

See page 318 for the answers.

REFERENCES

1. Donabedian A. The quality of care. How can it be assessed? *JAMA*. 1988;260:1743–1748.
2. Inohara T, Vemulapalli S. Transcatheter aortic valve replacement in the era of quality assessment. *Circ Cardiovasc Qual Outcomes*. 2018;11:e005233.
3. Krumholz HM, Keenan PS, Brush JE, et al. Standards for measures used for public reporting of efficiency in health care. *Circulation*. 2008;118:1885–1893.
4. Stone GW, Lindenfeld J, Abraham WT, et al. Transcatheter mitral-valve repair in patients with heart failure. *New Engl J Med*. 2018;379:2307–2318.
5. Obadia J-F, Messika-Zeitoun D, Leurent G, et al. Percutaneous repair or medical treatment for secondary mitral regurgitation. *New Engl J Med*. 2018;379:2297–2306.
6. Perpetua EM, Guibone KA, Keegan PA, et al. Best practice recommendations for optimizing care in structural heart programs: planning efficient and resource leveraging systems (PEARLS). *Struct Heart*. 2021;5:168–179.
7. Baron SJ, Wang K, Arnold SV, et al. Cost-effectiveness of transcatheter mitral valve repair versus medical therapy in patients with heart failure and secondary mitral regurgitation. *Circulation*. 2019;140:1881–1891.
8. Anderson JL, Heidenreich PA, Barnett PG, et al. ACC/AHA statement on cost/value methodology in clinical practice guidelines and performance measures. *Circulation*. 2014;129:2329–2345.
9. Stone GW, Lindenfeld J, Abraham WT, et al. Transcatheter mitral-valve repair in patients with heart failure. *New Engl J Med*. 2018;379:2307–2318.
10. Badhwar V, Vemulapalli S, Mack MA, et al. Volume-outcome association of mitral valve surgery in the United States. *JAMA Cardiol*. 2020;5:1092–1101.
11. Badhwar V, Rankin JS, He X, et al. The Society of Thoracic Surgeons Mitral Repair/Replacement Composite Score: A Report of the Society of Thoracic Surgeons Quality Measurement Task Force. *Ann Thorac Surg*. 2016;101:2265–2271.
12. The Society of Thoracic Surgeons. STS Public Reporting: Adult Cardiac Surgery Database Public Reporting; 2020.
13. Fernandez FG, Shahian DM, Kormos R, et al. The Society of Thoracic Surgeons National Database 2019 Annual Report. *Ann Thorac Surg*. 2019;108:1625–1632.
14. Panaich SS, Arora S, Badheka A, et al. Procedural trends, outcomes, and readmission rates pre-and post-FDA approval for MitraClip from the National Readmission Database (2013–14). *Catheter Cardiovasc Interv*. 2018;91:1171–1181.
15. Chhatriwalla AK, Vemulapalli S, Holmes Jr DR, et al. Institutional experience with transcatheter mitral valve repair and clinical outcomes: insights from the TVT Registry. *JACC Cardiovasc Interv*. 2019;12:1342–1352.
16. Bonow RO, O'Gara PT, Adams DH, et al. Multisociety expert consensus systems of care document 2019 AATS/ACC/SCAI/STS expert consensus systems of care document: operator and institutional recommendations and requirements for transcatheter mitral valve intervention: A Joint Report of the American Association for Thoracic Surgery, the American College of Cardiology, the Society for Cardiovascular Angiography and Interventions, and the Society of Thoracic Surgeons. *Catheter Cardiovasc Interv*. 2020;95:866–884.
17. Carroll JD, Mack MJ, Vemulapalli S, et al. STS-ACC TVT registry of transcatheter aortic valve replacement. *Ann Thorac Surg*. 2020;111(2):701–722.
18. Obadia JF, Messika-Zeitoun D, Leurent G, et al. Percutaneous repair or medical treatment for secondary mitral regurgitation. *New Engl J Med*. 2018;379:2297–2306.
19. Acker MA, Parides MK, Perrault LP, et al. Mitral-valve repair versus replacement for severe ischemic mitral regurgitation. *New Engl J Med*. 2013;370:23–32.
20. Mack MJ, Lindenfeld J, Abraham WT, et al. 3-Year outcomes of transcatheter mitral valve repair in patients with heart failure. *J Am Coll Cardiol*. 2021;77:1029–1040.
21. Lindman BR, Arnold SV, Bagur R, et al. Priorities for patient-centered research in valvular heart disease: a report from the national heart, lung, and blood institute working group. *J Am Heart Assoc*. 2020;9:e015975.

28

Establishing a Comprehensive Mitral Valve Program: Educating Patients and Referring Physicians

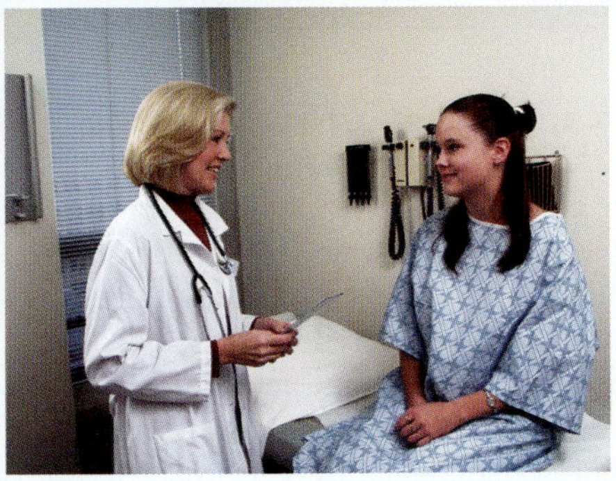

Roxanne DeStefano, Saif Anwaruddin

CHAPTER OUTLINE

LEARNING OBJECTIVES

1. Establish the key components necessary to market your program as a comprehensive mitral valve program
2. Learn to build a focused outreach plan to optimize internal and external outreach efforts
3. Learn to improve access to care through collaboration with the referral community

INTRODUCTION

In the past decade, structural heart programs have proven to be one of the largest areas of growth in the cardiovascular service line. This demand is due to both an aging population requiring complex treatment and technology enabling such patients to be treated. Mitral regurgitation (MR) is the most common form of heart valve disease in the United States, with a 10-fold increase in prevalence once patients reach 75 years of age.[1,2] Almost half of the patients who need and are eligible for a mitral valve intervention are not being identified and referred to a structural heart program; this potentially represents a large, unmet need.[3,4]

There are an increasing number of treatment options available for patients with mitral valve disease. In 2013, the first and only transcatheter mitral valve repair (TMVr) technology, the MitraClip (Abbott, Santa Clara, CA), received US Food and Drug Administration (FDA) approval and has pioneered the way forward for transcatheter mitral repair. The landscape for transcatheter edge-to-edge repair (TEER) widened following the FDA approval of the COAPT trial in 2018, as the indication was extended to include functional MR. COAPT demonstrated that TEER with MitraClip, in conjunction with guideline directed medical therapy, versus guideline directed medical therapy alone, in select heart failure patients with secondary MR improved survival, reduced heart failure related hospitalizations, reduced severity of MR, and provided symptomatic relief for this patient population.[5]

Advanced surgical techniques, especially those related to mitral valve repair, in conjunction with ongoing transcatheter clinical trials for both mitral valve repair and replacement, require formal, multidisciplinary collaboration to determine appropriate care on a patient-by-patient basis. One of the challenges that programs face is the challenge of developing a growth strategy for their mitral valve program. The introduction of the first (TEER) therapy into many structural heart programs was often incorporated as a new "procedure" and not adopted and marketed as a part of a comprehensive valve "program." Marketing a comprehensive mitral valve program may allow for the growth of all services offered by your team of experts to treat mitral valve disease.[6,7]

This chapter reviews the key components needed to create a comprehensive mitral valve program, how to build your plan prior to marketing your program, and strategies to execute hospital in-reach and community outreach initiatives. We provide examples on how to differentiate your program and create innovative ways to collaborate with referring physicians. Finally, we summarize the fundamental elements necessary to educate and engage patients in a program of this nature.

KEY COMPONENTS OF A COMPREHENSIVE MITRAL VALVE PROGRAM

The key components to building a comprehensive mitral valve program include: a cohesive team of key individuals with clearly defined roles, a multidisciplinary mitral valve clinic, and a mandatory, weekly, mitral valve team meeting. The first step is to ensure that you have a dedicated multidisciplinary team in place. A cornerstone of this endeavor is based on a collegial and collaborative partnership between the cardiac surgeon and the interventional cardiologist. Additional specialists on this team include a dedicated echocardiographer who specializes in structural imaging, a heart failure specialist with expertise in the treatment of heart failure and mitral valve disease, a dedicated structural heart valve coordinator (SHVC), and a dedicated cardiac anesthesia team.

The development of a multidisciplinary mitral valve clinic is essential for a comprehensive mitral valve program. A centralized evaluation location optimizes the patient process for thorough evaluation, proper diagnosis, and delivery of appropriate care by a team of experts.[8] The goal of the comprehensive mitral valve clinic is to provide patient-centric care based on evidence-based medicine and advanced treatment options provided by the institution. The clinic team should consist of cardiac surgeons, interventional cardiologists, echocardiographers and imaging specialists, heart failure specialists, and other clinicians such as the SHVC, advanced practice providers, and patient educators.

A member of the physician team of experts should work with hospital administrators to lead, coordinate, and optimize the patient pathway through the valve clinic. For patients who have not had an initial screening transthoracic echocardiogram (TTE), a certain number of reserved slots, staffed with sonographers and imaging experts, should be available for initial evaluation and quantification of MR. The multidisciplinary mitral valve clinic should focus on shared decision-making best practices throughout the patient evaluation continuum, the appropriate intervention pathway, and follow up care.

It is important to institute a mandatory, weekly, multidisciplinary mitral valve meeting. All MR patients should be presented at this meeting to ensure a collaborative approach towards the appropriate mitral valve treatment pathway. This meeting is a case planning meeting, and all specifics needs related to pre-, intra-, and post-procedural patient care should be discussed. At the conclusion of the meeting, all equipment needed for the mitral valve intervention, as well as specific members of the multidisciplinary team and vendor availability, must be confirmed.

The Multidisciplinary Team

The Cardiac Surgeon

The role of the cardiac surgeon is imperative to the growth of the comprehensive mitral valve program. Offering complementary therapies to treat patients with mitral valve disease may provide growth to existing therapies offered at the institution.[9] It is imperative for the surgeon to have a strong relationship with the interventional cardiologist in order to refer a patient for a transcatheter procedure and vice-versa. A hybrid team approach also creates new opportunities for the cardiac surgeon to acquire specific skillsets necessary to perform transcatheter procedures.

The Interventional Cardiologist

The role of the interventional cardiologist is to work with the multidisciplinary team to evaluate patients who are not surgical candidates for transcatheter options where the benefits outweigh the risks in certain patient candidates. The interventional cardiologist should be experienced in the treatment of mitral valve disease and have significant experience with the trans-septal technique. It is very important to develop a strong collaboration with the cardiac surgeon as it relates to patient evaluation, procedure planning, and intra-procedural success. A collaboration with the cardiac surgeon promotes dedication, motivation, and engagement in the team approach to treating mitral valve disease.

Structural Heart Valve Coordinator

The role of the SHVC is critical to the success and growth of any program. Many roles are included in the title of SHVC, such as (1) initial patient evaluation, (2) coordination of the patient pathway through the joint valve clinic, (3) arranging necessary testing for evaluation based on the type of procedure being considered, (4) guiding communication between patients and their family members, and (5) maintaining a constant mode of communication with the referring physician team. The SHVC presents the patient data at the multidisciplinary mitral meetings, collaborates within the industry for scheduling patient treatment, and collects required data for mandatory registry participation. Programmatic and outcome data are also captured, assessed, and reviewed by the SHVC to optimize efficiencies of the program. The data collected is utilized for demand planning that will determine additional headcount and additional resources necessary to optimize the overall efficiencies the program. Programmatic metrics should include patient volume, the number of days needed per month to treat patients coming into the valve center, appropriate utilization of staff and the delegation of responsibilities, and patient outcomes. This data can also be utilized to focus on the health economic impact to the institution with administration when looking at heart failure related admissions and length of stay.

Dedicated Structural Imaging

The cornerstone to any successful program is having dedicated structural imaging specialists. These imaging experts will develop and define a consistent algorithm and systematic approach to the patient screening and selection process within the institution. A well-defined investigation of the mitral valve will lead to appropriate acquisition of the images and measurements necessary to determine anatomic suitability for the specific treatment option for the patient. Having dedicated screening days built into the schedule will ensure optimization of capacity and reduce the time to treatment for patients. The individuals chosen to lead this charge are those that express interest in interventional echocardiography. They have a profound knowledge and skillset that incorporates three-dimensional echocardiography and multimodality imaging into planning and guiding structural heart disease interventions.

Heart Failure Specialist

The incorporation of a heart failure specialist as a part of the multidisciplinary team is essential to ensure that patients with heart failure and functional MR are appropriately managed on guideline directed medical therapy. The primary goal is to minimize late diagnosis and encourage early referrals to treat the heart failure population that suffers from functional MR. Another focus of the heart failure physician is to ensure that a frequent line of communication to referring physicians is instituted to standardize the adherence to guideline directed medical therapy and to evaluate all potential options available for advanced therapies for the patient with heart failure.

Building Your Business Plan

Common barriers to treatment of mitral valve disease include: (1) reluctance to refer frail or elderly patients, (2) patient reluctance to undergo mitral valve treatment, (3) uncertainty about the timing of intervention for functional disease, (4) limited local access to transcatheter mitral valve proceduralists, (5) limited local access to a skilled mitral valve surgeon, (6) inadequate quality of echocardiograms performed at the referring institution, and (7) difficulty interpreting reported imaging findings.[10] Addressing barriers to treatment should be approached with a careful strategy in mind–consistent and frequent education to the referral community.

MARKETING STRATEGY

A marketing strategy should coincide with a plan for outreach–a comprehensive mitral valve program that offers comprehensive outreach (Fig. 28.1). It is important to approach the referring providers by showcasing multiple members from the multidisciplinary team for all outreach events to effectively market your comprehensive mitral valve program. Prior to engaging the referring community, a strategic business plan should be built by the team, along with the coordinated efforts of administration, the marketing department, and physician liaisons. The team should develop a talk track summarizing why you are approaching the referring physician, how you can help them, and assuring them of what they can expect from your multidisciplinary team. It is important to highlight the differentiating factors of your mitral program, including outcomes, range of services,

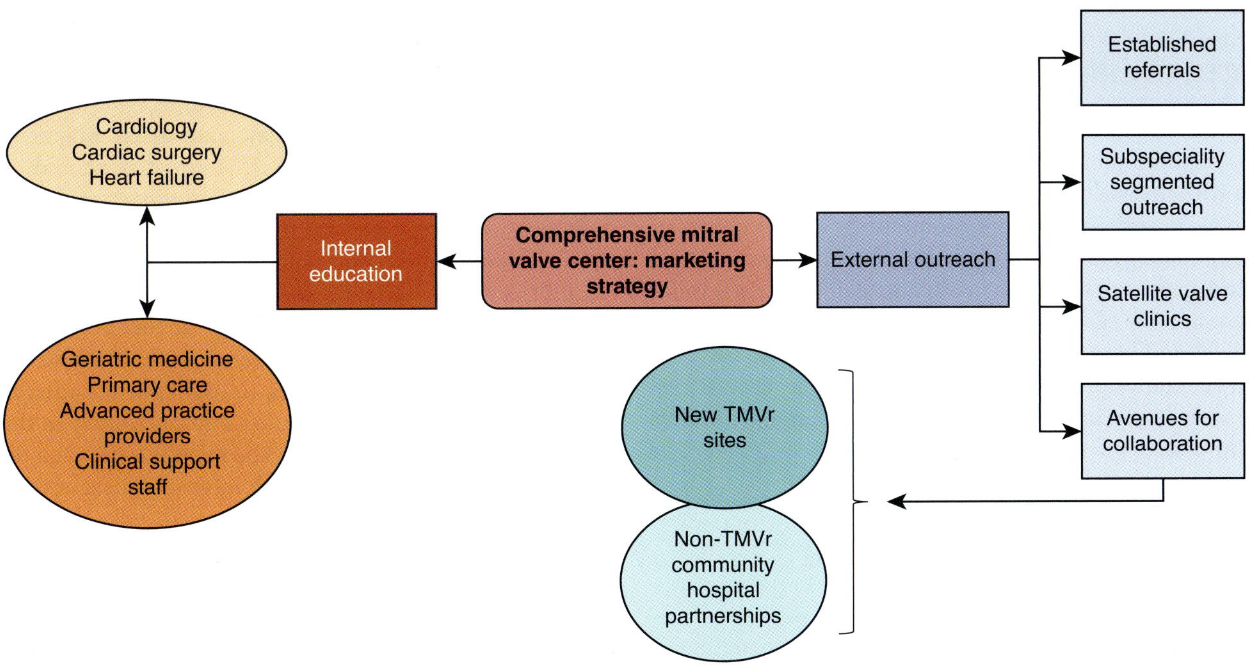

Fig. 28.1 A marketing strategy should coincide with a plan for outreach: a comprehensive mitral valve program that offers comprehensive outreach. *TMVr,* transcatheter mitral valve repair.

patient experience, efficiency, and referring physician customer service. Another part of your strategy should be to make the referral process seamless for the referring physician community.

Work with your marketing department to develop a customized comprehensive mitral valve program brochure and marketing packet containing the following information:

1. A picture of the multidisciplinary mitral valve team
2. A list of treatment options that are offered at your institution for mitral valve repair and replacement and insurance accepted
   a. Include pictures of the different treatment options that are available—both surgical and transcatheter
3. Map of the location of the valve center and the hospital
4. Biography on each member of the multidisciplinary team
5. Contact number and email address for the valve center
6. Business card for the valve program coordinator
7. Include a link to view a procedure that you have on your valve center website
8. Referral template to streamline the process for the referral into the valve center

OUTREACH

Prior to beginning your outreach strategy, it is important to designate an individual who will be responsible for tracking all referrals. This will be important so that you can plan the frequency of outreach with each physician. Current programmatic data can also be utilized to market outcome and efficiency data of the overall mitral valve program. The hospital/health system marketing department should assist in coordinating the marketing of the comprehensive mitral valve program through social media marketing, TV commercials, newspaper ads, social media platforms, billboards, and the hospital and valve center website.

STRUCTURAL HEART PHYSICIAN LIAISONS

It is very impactful to have dedicated structural heart physician liaisons. The overarching goal is for the physician liaisons to collaborate with the multidisciplinary team to create a specific plan of action for hospital in-reach and community outreach. Initiate a standing meeting once a month with the physician liaisons, the multidisciplinary team, the marketing team, and the administrative team. The agenda of each meeting should be to set goals to build referral base targets, collect data on referral patterns, and initiate follow up. The main strategy of dedicating physician liaisons to the structural heart program is to maintain, develop, and grow based on outcomes of the overall comprehensive mitral valve program.

COMMUNICATION WITH REFERRING PHYSICIANS

It is essential to develop a formalized and coordinated communication plan to share with the referring physicians as it relates to the patient's journey into the valve center, treatment provided, and plan for follow up. Follow up is a critical step that is essential to form long standing relationships and trust with the referring physician. The following templates should be created and utilized throughout each step of the patient journey:

1. Letter following initial visit stating the outcome of the valve center visit with next appointment date specified
2. Letter to referring physician following multidisciplinary mitral valve team meeting to describe treatment plan for patient and procedure date
3. Post-procedure follow up letter on your hospital letterhead that is mailed out to the referring physician after the procedure with next steps specified for follow up testing

Prior to any procedure, ensure that you have the referring physician's cell phone number. Commit to call the referring physician immediately after the mitral valve intervention takes place.

Create a de-identified video clip of pre-and post-images and text it to the referring physician immediately after the procedure. This offers a personal touch and showcases new and existing treatment options utilized.

If your team is dedicated to the execution of these best practices for all mitral valve interventions, your reputation as a comprehensive mitral valve program will flourish within the referral community.

EXECUTING YOUR PLAN: HOSPITAL IN-REACH, THE FIRST STEP TO OUTREACH

Internal Education

The multidisciplinary mitral team should initiate an aggressive hospital in-reach strategy prior to going out into the referring community. To drive patients into the valve clinic, you need to capture and reach a broad audience within your own institution. The goal should be to educate all faculty and staff on the comprehensive treatment options offered at the institution to increase mitral valve disease awareness. Be sure to include the departments of cardiology, cardiac surgery, geriatric medicine, heart failure, and primary care, advanced practice providers, and clinical support staff. This initiative should be driven and delivered by the entire multidisciplinary mitral team and should be coordinated by the SHVC and/ or physician liaisons at the hospital. The agenda should include peer reviewed data; changes to patient screening and selection protocols; and on-going education for the nurses and staff who provide pre- and post-procedural care for the patients. It is also important for the multidisciplinary team to highlight the metrics of the mitral program, such as volumes and outcomes, as they relate to specific treatment options. The overall goal is for the multidisciplinary team to partner with internal colleagues to network with their largest referral sources.

Streamlined Patient Screening and Selection Protocol and Process

Education surrounding the identification of patients with MR is essential to expanding the landscape for patients who may be eligible for treatment. Structural imagers can assist with the implementation of an echo alert system within the institution and throughout the health system. This can be constructed to ensure improved recognition of cardiac conditions utilizing 'triggers' identified by key words and critical values associated with MR. An echo alert system can be built into the system wide PACS system, and training and education should be implemented at each hospital within the health system.

Dedicated days should be established to screen for MR patients. The multidisciplinary team should implement a streamlined transesophageal echo (TEE) screening protocol for all MR patients. Any patient who receives a TEE for MR should receive the same thorough, systematic interrogation of the mitral valve. This should capture all data necessary to incorporate screening protocols for commercially available technologies and clinical trial protocols. When the team meets for the weekly multidisciplinary mitral meeting, they will have the images and anatomical information necessary to make the best treatment decision for each patient. This will also help to expand the screening process to all echocardiographers who perform TEEs at the institution to increase capacity and help decrease the need for a patient to receive a repeat TEE. The team should also identify a few dedicated sonographers who are super users on the streamlined TEE screening protocol. These super users will help to ensure that all necessary images are acquired to ensure all relevant data is captured.

Outreach

Begin your outreach strategy by focusing on established referrals first since there are existing relationships already in place. Make it a point to engage referring physicians who have referred a limited number of patients to educate them on a procedure that they referred a patient for. Invite your referring physicians to come to observe a procedure. Educate them on streamlined screening protocols to minimize the need for repeat imaging studies from the referring centers, while increasing overall awareness and early identification of patients. Host journal clubs with case presentations. Collaborate with industry to network with physicians outside of your network.

The next segment of your strategy should focus on subspecialty segmentation through education. The focus should be on:

1. peer-to-peer surgeon training for new surgical approaches to treating mitral valve disease
2. peer-to-peer interventional cardiologist training to optimize patient screening and selection
3. peer-to-peer training between the echocardiographer, the interventional cardiologist and the cardiac surgeon to establish consistent nomenclature to optimize the efficiencies within the procedure and to optimize strategic planning for cases
4. peer-to-peer training between the interventional cardiologist and the cardiac surgeon to teach the cardiac surgeon the trans-septal technique
5. peer-to-peer training for valve coordinators to optimize process efficiencies within the patient pathway and the programmatic pathway
6. peer-to-peer case reviews and presentations.

Also consider formal educational options, such as delivering a mitral valve symposium offering CME credits for internal faculty and referring physicians. A sample agenda should include expert leaders and scientific sessions on the services provided at the institution. This is an excellent opportunity to build awareness around new technologies and ongoing clinical trials.

AVENUES FOR COLLABORATION

Community Hospital Partnerships

The chance to partner with smaller community hospitals who do not offer advanced surgical mitral techniques or do not have the necessary infrastructure to offer transcatheter mitral valve procedures is an important consideration. The opportunity to become a referral center for patients who qualify for more advanced surgical therapies offered by your team is an opportunity to grow a referral network. The smaller community hospital can collaborate with the multidisciplinary team to develop a streamlined patient pathway for advanced management and treatment for their MR patients.

The option to partner with a structural heart program that does not have a transcatheter mitral valve program is also important to consider. A partnership with the team should include providing them privileges at your institution so they can refer and treat their patients at your center with the experience of your multidisciplinary team of experts. Focus on educating the referring structural heart program on the patient screening and selection process and testing required prior to TMVr. The opportunity for the referring center is to maintain the profitable open mitral surgical business and maximize the value of other structural heart offerings. This partnership will still provide the referring site access to care for their patients through a partnership with your multidisciplinary team. The referring site can promote TMVr as an offering for mitral valve patients. For the patients, this structure can help ensure optimal quality and outcomes given the collaborative nature within a large comprehensive program.

Partner With a Structural Heart Program Who Does Not Meet the National Coverage Decision Requirements to Offer Transcatheter Mitral Valve Repair

An additional opportunity would be to partner with a structural heart program who does not meet the TMVr National Coverage Decision (NCD) requirements. Provide education to their team on patient screening and selection to identify appropriate candidates for transcatheter mitral valve repair, TMVr. This will require identifying a program champion to act as the liaison between the centers.

Partner With a New Site Just Starting a Transcatheter Mitral Valve Repair Program

The goal of this arrangement with the new site would focus on identifying challenging cases to refer to your experienced team of experts for treatment. This will allow the referring center to focus on a successful TMVr rollout while they are overcoming the learning curve associated with new transcatheter procedures. The referring site can learn how to tackle challenging cases from your experienced multidisciplinary team while they focus on achieving optimal patient outcomes in their early learning process.

Mitral Valve Comprehensive Collaboration HUB

Offering comprehensive options to treat mitral valve disease, along with data that supports good clinical outcomes, will help your program towards a mitral valve center of excellence status. Partner with local, regional, and national structural heart centers to serve as a mentorship and training center of excellence. Foster collaboration by serving as a role model for other centers to learn how to run an efficient and successful comprehensive mitral valve program. Work with industry to provide a forum for others to learn how to grow and develop their programs. Mentor other programs on best practices and teach others how to tackle complex cases or improve in areas where they need help. Establish your site as a referral center for cutting-edge therapies that are only offered by your team of experts. This will ensure the formation of long- standing relationships with your peers.

Satellite Valve Clinics

Establish satellite valve clinics at hospitals within the health system and out of network. Partnering with hospitals who don't meet the requirements to have a comprehensive mitral valve program at their institution can be beneficial to increase programmatic visibility and patient access to comprehensive care. These clinics should be held regularly and in a joint and multidisciplinary fashion with the appropriate branding.

PATIENT EDUCATION

Providing patients with print materials that showcase illustrations and images to complement text descriptions can keep them engaged and will help them remember important details about their condition. Patient educators can refer patients and their family members to videos or animations that explain the anatomy, condition the patient is being treated for, and the procedure that will be performed on the patient. Building this relationship with the patient will help inform them and build trust with their valve team. It is also important to provide patients with online resources to allow them to explore on their own.

Coordinating patient level MR awareness groups or community screening events for patients is very valuable. Having multidisciplinary team presence will provide the patients with a forum to ask questions and help to alleviate misconceptions and concerns. Working with the marketing team and physician liaisons is important for engaging patients.

Finally, showcasing your team and your program in the media, such as the local evening news, will help to create awareness throughout the community on the services being offered within your comprehensive mitral valve program.

CONCLUSIONS

A tremendous amount of multidisciplinary commitment is needed to grow, build, and market a comprehensive structural heart program. The opportunity to create access to care for patients with previously limited treatment options is extremely rewarding to all members of the Team.

Marketing efforts should be focused on a programmatic approach to offering patient-centric care that spans across multiple disciplines and services, all within the breadth of services offered for the treatment of mitral valve disease. A concentrated focus should be placed on patient outcomes and the optimization of the patient pathway to create a boutique experience for the patients and their providers. Collaboration, coordinated teamwork, and direct communication are essential elements to building a sustainable program.

SUMMARY

A comprehensive mitral valve program must be created in order to extend outreach to patients and the referring community. Marketing a procedure is not enough to warrant a holistic approach to patient care. Marketing a program that offers patient-centric care and advanced treatment options, a multidisciplinary approach to shared decision-making, and services that extend across the continuum are essential to achieving optimal patient outcomes.

CASE-BASED ASSESSMENT

1. What are the three key components needed to build a comprehensive mitral valve program?
   - A. A cohesive team of key individuals with clearly defined roles, a multidisciplinary mitral valve clinic and a mandatory, weekly, mitral valve team meeting.
   - B. A collegial relationship between cardiac surgeons and interventional cardiologists only.
   - C. A hybrid OR, a defined treatment day, and a dedicated structural heart valve coordinator (SHVC).
2. How should you market your mitral valve program to referring physicians?
   - A. Market your program as a comprehensive mitral valve program that offers comprehensive outreach.
   - B. Build your marketing strategy around the new mitral valve procedure that is offered at your hospital.
   - C. Develop a marketing plan to target existing referring physicians with the interventional cardiologist and the cardiac surgeon only.

3. How can you collaborate with other centers to increase access to care for patients? Chose all answers that apply:
   A. Community hospital partnerships
   B. Partner with a Structural Heart Program who does not meet the National Coverage Decision (NCD) requirements to offer TMVr
   C. Partner with a new site just starting a transcatheter mitral valve repair program
   D. Mitral Valve Comprehensive Collaboration HUB
   E. Satellite Valve Clinics
   F. All of the above

See page 318 for the answer.

REFERENCES

1. Jones DL, Adams RJ, Brown TM, et al. Heart disease and stroke statistics 2010 update: a report from the American Heart Association. *Circulation*. 2010;121(7):e46–e215.
2. Nkomo VT, Gardin JM, Skelton TN, et al. Burden of valvular heart diseases: a population-based study. *Lancet*. 2006;368(16):1005–1011.
3. Mirabel M, Iung B, Baron G, et al. What are the characteristics of patients with severe, symptomatic, mitral regurgitation who are denied surgery? *Eur Heart J*. 2007;28(11):1358–1365.
4. Bach DS, Awais M, Gurm HS, et al. Failure of guideline adherence for intervention in patients with severe mitral regurgitation. *J Am Coll Cardiol*. 2009;54:860–865.
5. Stone GW, Lindenfeld J, Abraham WT, et al. Transcatheter mitral-valve repair in patients with heart failure. *N Engl J Med*. 2018;379(24):2307–2318.
6. Downs E, Lim S, Ragosta M, et al. The influence of a percutaneous mitral repair program on surgical mitral valve volume. *J Thorac Cardiovasc Surg*. 2015;150(5):1093–1097.
7. Conradi L, Lubos E, Treede H, et al. Evolution of mitral valve procedural volumes in the advent of endovascular treatment options: experience at an early-adopting center in Germany. *Catheter Cardiovasc Interv*. 2015;86(6):1114–1119.
8. Messika-Zeitoun D, Burwash ID, Mesana T. Educational series on the specialist valve clinic: challenges in the diagnosis and management of valve disease; the case for the specialist valve clinic. *Echo Res Pract*. 2019;6(4):T1–T6.
9. Niikura H, Gössl M, Bae R, et al. Impact of the commercial introduction of the transcatheter mitral valve repair of mitral surgical practice. *J Am Heart Assoc*. 2020;9(7):e014874.
10. Addressing mitral regurgitation: insights from CardioSurve. *Cardiol Mag*. Nov 16, 2018.

29

Ten Elements for a Successful Mitral Program

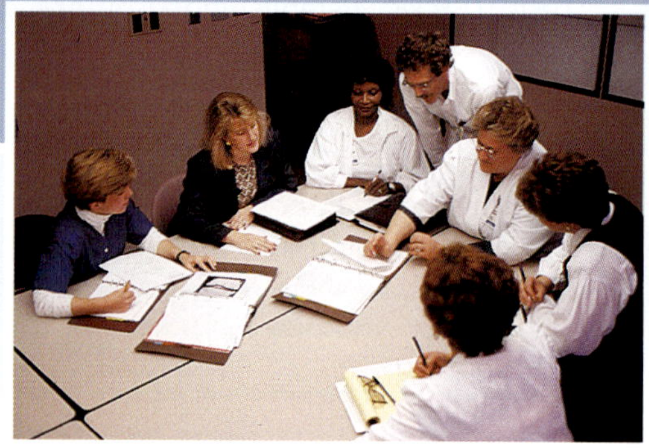

William A. Gray, Scott M. Goldman

CHAPTER OUTLINE

LEARNING OBJECTIVES

- Identify and understand the essential elements of establishing and nurturing a successful mitral valve program.
- Understand the importance of the skilled mitral surgeon to the success of an effective mitral valve program.
- Understand and evaluate advanced imaging techniques that are critical to a high-quality, expert mitral programs: transthoracic and transesophageal echocardiography, computerized tomography (CT), and cardiac magnetic resonance imaging (CMR).

This chapter endeavors to identify the essential elements of establishing/maintaining a successful mitral valve program based on at least two decades of personal experience and observation in this environment. Many readers will recognize that these will be largely the same elements inherent in a successful structural heart program and, to be fair, there is little light between the two.

As in most recipes, the best cooks will have a deep understanding of the fundamental ingredients but decide that certain modifications lead to a better meal—the same is true with this list, which is meant to be a starting point but is by no means exhaustive or exclusive.

CARDIAC SURGERY EXPERTISE

Many referrals for mitral valve disease to any institution by other cardiac specialists will be to surgeons for definitive therapy. This flow of patients will be the bedrock on which other diagnostic and therapeutic modalities—and resultant program expansion—will be built. Therefore, an experienced mitral surgeon skilled in all forms of repair, in minimally invasive access, and in the office and peri-operative management of mitral disease will be critical to a successful program. Mitral valve surgeons have a unique understanding of valve anatomy that can add valuable insight to whatever procedure is planned for.

Although there have been and will be fantastic innovations in the percutaneous treatment of mitral valve disease, at its core—historically and practically—it is a surgical domain. In the current environment, there are still many patients who will not qualify for percutaneous therapies by virtue of anatomical or access restrictions, durability of results, etc., and will require expert surgical care.

Last, although non-surgical specialists and cardiac surgeons may be well-versed in mitral disease (from multiple viewpoints), there is still much to learn from each other that will not only enrich our individual perspectives but also promote better patient outcomes.

ADVANCED IMAGING

Imaging is the keystone of a successful program and imagers need to progress for diagnostic imaging to interventional imaging, which does require a different mindset. They must become the eyes of the interventional cardiologists and surgeons performing the transcather based procedures. Three facets of cardiac imaging are each necessary for a high-quality, expert mitral program. First, transthoracic and transesophageal echocardiography expertise (physician and technician) in not only quantification of mitral disease, especially regurgitation, but also the mechanism of stenosis or regurgitation, location of principle pathology, and associated assessments of leaflet length, calcification, chordal location, fossa access suitability, etc. This will need to be married to interventional echo capability, which has almost become its own subspecialty within cardiology, to guide proceduralists and optimize outcomes.

Second, a quality computerized tomography (CT) program will allow for preoperative and preprocedural assessment of access points for bypass pump cannulation as well as the occasional inferior vena cava (IVC) filter for venous/transseptal procedures; and also, for evaluating mitral annular dimensions, sub valvar structures, and left ventricular outflow tract considerations. 4D CT is key for evaluating post procedural valve function.

Finally, especially for regurgitant lesions, cardiac magnetic resonance imaging (CMR) can be an invaluable adjunct to discordant or confounded findings echocardiographic imaging since CMR provides excellent regurgitant volume determinations.

INTERVENTIONAL CARDIOLOGIST WITH IMAGE INTERPRETATION SKILLS

With the advent of the structural heart field, this breed of interventional cardiologist is becoming more common than in the past. But there is a distinction to be made between a transcatheter aortic valve replacement (TAVR)-specialized physician who is used to working on a guidance system (the guidewire) and a mitral-specialized physician who will largely work untethered and need to understand his or her place in the heart in three dimensions and, further, know where specific maneuvers will take them relationally. Other skills including transseptal experience, paravalvular leak repair, valve-in-valve implantation, iatrogenic atrial septal defect repair, etc., will also be important in this space and all require a strong foundation in imaging. Add to this the lead interventionalist (surgeon or cardiologist) really should be the "captain" of the procedure and direct the imaging as they see the need; they cannot lead from behind. Therefore, they need a particularly good understanding not only of the echo imaging interpretation but also how those images relate to their tools, and what options they have for alternative views to best serve their needs.

ADVANCED PRACTICE PROVIDERS AND NURSE NAVIGATOR(S)

The outpatient mitral patient can be complex and, depending on the stage of the valvular disease, may have significant elements of heart failure that require active medication management. Two further, somewhat interrelated, factors can complicate their care: first, many of these patients will be involved with complex percutaneous therapies (approved or investigational) that require extensive test scheduling (non-invasive and invasive) with resultant needs for anticoagulation management and results tracking, and many of these patients will be elderly and require family to help them with information gathering, understanding of their condition and options, decision-making, and general communication through the process of evaluation. On the inpatient side, the pre- and postoperative or procedural management of these patient requires continuous "eyes-on" to assess for any change in status requiring an urgent response. It is obvious, then, given these complexities and need for multiple "touches" that advanced practice providers (APPs) will be an essential constituent in the care of the mitral patient.

Beyond these clinical needs, a nurse navigator is an invaluable role necessary to serve as a coordinator for all mitral-related activities: OR/cath lab scheduling; physician availability; coordination with research, with marketing, with quality assurance, with inventory/purchasing, and with billing compliance just to name a few. A program can run without such a person at the start but will be quickly hamstrung and limit its potential, so better to launch with than without. As a program achieves a critical mass of activity, a director will have fewer responsibilities involved with the day-to-day management and be more active in a broad, overarching capacity (referral outreach, data analysis of practice activity and outcomes, etc.) will further enhance program growth.

RESEARCH

The ability to offer patients the most advanced mitral care options available rests squarely on the capacity to conduct research at a high level, meaning appropriate patient selection, protocol adherence, reliable and complete data collection, and follow-up at pre-specified intervals, etc., which will usually attract sponsors. In addition, the relatively recent creation of the Food and Drug Administration's (FDA) Early Feasibility Study pathway further challenges research programs to create rapid turnaround on both Institutional Review Board protocol approvals and contract completion, as well as introducing generally more complex patient populations and earlier device iterations. Lastly, publication of both site outcomes and being part of larger national/sponsored research outcomes lends credibility to the program and usually leads to more research opportunities—an important byproduct of research. Therefore, strong institutional support and physician leadership in this realm is critical.

A FUNCTIONAL HEART TEAM

After the first five elements detailed above, the concept of a heart team might appear self-evident, and therefore redundant to separately list heart team as a critical component of success. But while the surgeon, cardiologist, imagers, APPs, and research coordinators are the heart team, they have to function as one entity and not a group of incongruent constituents with disparate goals. This ultimately boils down to the working relationship between the surgeons and cardiologists who should not compete for individual operative and procedural volumes but rather collaborate on each patient's management with all the tools that can be brought to bear, regardless of who brings them. This approach requires a cultural shift from the way many of us have grown up in our specialty silos and can be enabled by the incentive structures present in the background.

But a functional heart team is more than just about eliminating competition for volumes, it can also mean sharing office space and appointment times; carrying out weekly clinical and imaging reviews of all mitral patients being evaluated to the team for commentary and planning purposes; meeting with referring physicians and otherwise cooperating in marketing campaigns; carrying out data and quality assurance reviews; etc. Having a nonjudgmental colleague opine on difficult clinical decisions can only accrue to the patients' benefit.

MARKETING

Of course, marketing is an important element enabling and extending the growth of cardiac programs. This includes patient education, engaging with referring cardiologists, and primary care providers. Developing strong relationships with referring provider's offices and educating them on the importance of providing prior clinical information is key to making the evaluation process seamless. Communication is vital to cultivating a good relationship and firmly establishing referral patterns. This must also occur as part of the patient follow up process. Informing the referring cardiologist, the plan for medical therapy and expectations of a successful procedure. The tendency is to wait until new programs mature rather than integrating marketing activities into the program planning from the outset and then evolving the messaging as the program progresses.

QUALITY OVERSIGHT

Inherent in quality oversite (mortality and morbidity conferences, process improvement initiatives, etc.) is the ability to reliably collect data, collate, and analyze it so these mechanisms must be in place at the start of, and inclusive of, any mitral effort. The tenor of the quality meetings should be to identify opportunities for improvement in practice and in the system rather than to be punitive, which tends to inhibit discussion, self-reporting, and reflection. This is how improvement is fostered, especially in a new program with many novel experiences. At some point in the future, it is anticipated that public reporting of surgical and procedural outcomes will be public, so there are multiple incentives to foster continuous improvement.

INSTITUTIONAL SUPPORT

Regardless of whether the physicians integral to the mitral program are in private practice or hospital-employed, institutional support will be essential to program success. As can be seen in the aforementioned, hospital-based elements such as APPs, marketing, research, and quality oversight will require not only financial support, but also items not mentioned such as space, IT support, billing and coding optimization, inventory management, etc., will help grow the program and optimize both the clinical and financial mitral outcomes for the institution.

LUCK

With any early clinical experience, having a good string of initial outcomes will help build confidence and support of the program. But while this kind of "luck" can be created by excellent training, attention to procedural detail, and pre- and post-procedural care coordination, the most important element is patient selection, which requires an understanding of the patient's mitral anatomy and what available therapeutics best matches, and the patient's clinical condition including expected outcomes, risk of surgical repair or replacement, etc. Therefore, planning is key. Planning should occur at least three times for each patient centered procedure. The first should be when the patient is evaluated with the pertinent studies available. Next the patient should be presented to the multidisciplinary team where a detailed plan is formulated. Finally the team should meet just prior to the procedure, review the studies, and reiterate the procedural steps. Operating or intervening with the utmost skill on the wrong patient is the best way to ensure bad luck.

SELF-ASSESSMENT QUESTIONS

1. Identify the essential elements of a successful mitral valve program.
2. What areas, if any, will you need to address at your institution as you undertake to build a successful program?

See page 318 for the answers.

ANSWERS TO THE ASSESSMENT QUESTIONS:

Chapter 1:

1) E
2) C
3) A

Chapter 2:

- Ruptured papillary muscle—Carpentier Type II
- Restricted posterior leaflet—Carpentier Type IIIb

Chapter 3:

1) E. Class 1 indications (see Fig. 3.1) according to the ACC/AHA guidelines for treatment of primary mitral regurgitation include symptoms and LV dysfunction (defined as ejection fraction (EF) ≤60% or left ventricular end systolic diameter (LVESD) ≥40 mm) to prevent further deterioration. In asymptomatic patients, intervention may be considered if a successful repair is likely (<5% failure expectancy) with very low mortality risk (recommendation Class 2a, Level of evidence B-NR), when there is progressive increase in LV size or a decrease in EF (recommendation Class 2 b, Level of evidence C-LD).
2) F. TEER is recommended for patients with severe secondary MR and persistent symptoms on optimal guidelines-directed medical therapy in case LV EF is 20% to 49%, left ventricular end-systolic dimension (LVESD) ≤70 mm or/and pulmonary artery systolic pressure (SPAP) ≤70 mm Hg (recommendation Class 2a, Level of evidence B-R). Surgery is recommended with severe secondary MR and LV EF of 20% to 49% unsuitable for TEER (recommendation Class 2b, Level of evidence B-R), for "atrial MR" (recommendation Class 2b, Level of evidence B-NR; Fig. 3.2), or when CABG is indicated (recommendation Class 2a, Level of evidence B-R).
3) B. The minimal requirements for post-procedural echo are at 1 to 3 months post-procedure, and annually thereafter for transcatheter mitral valve repair and replacement, after 1 year and then every 2 to 3 years for surgical mitral valve repair, at 5 and 10 years with a surgical bioprosthesis but then annually, and only at an early postoperative time-point for a mechanical valve.
4) C. Percutaneous mitral balloon commissurotomy is Class 1 recommendation for severe symptomatic rheumatic mitral stenosis and Class 2a for patients with asymptomatic disease and elevated pulmonary artery pressure or Class 2b for patients with asymptomatic disease and new-onset atrial fibrillation.
5) D. In patients with severe symptomatic rheumatic mitral stenosis surgery is indicated as Class 1 in case of NYHA Class III-IV and contraindications to percutaneous mitral balloon commissurotomy, including a non-pliable valve, left atrial/appendage thrombus, and mitral regurgitation ≥+2.

Chapter 4:

1) C. Primary chordae tendinae are attached to ventricular surface of leaflets.
2) B. S1 is accentuated in early mitral stenosis disease and soften late in disease process
3) D. Standing increases end-diastolic volume and click murmur occurs later in systole

Chapter 5:

1) C. This study demonstrates severe functional MR due to an ischemic cardiomyopathy. In the parasternal long view, you can see failure of the leaflets to coapt in systole due to LV remodeling from a recent myocardial infarction. There is no evidence of a primary valvular abnormality.
2) C. Four specific signs for severe MR are present. Considering the PISA radius of 1.0, vena contracta width of 0.9 cm, the systolic reversal of pulmonary vein flow, and regurgitant color-flow jet greater than 50% of the left atrium, the severity of mitral regurgitation is severe. For confirmation, regurgitant volume, regurgitant fraction and EROA-PISA can be calculated.
3) A. Due to the increased stroke volume resulting from chronic, severe mitral regurgitation, the left ventricular cavity dilates in response. MR is a volume overloaded state which causes LV dilatation, rather than hypertrophy. Frequently, chronic, severe MR is accompanied by dilatation of other chambers but should always be accompanied by an enlarged left ventricular cavity.
4) C. Increased E wave on mitral inflow reflects increased stroke volume due to severe MR. It is a quick and easy variable to assess, but it is sensitive, not specific as other pathology may cause an elevated E wave such as mitral stenosis, diastolic dysfunction, atrial fibrillation, and high cardiac output states.
5) A. Patients with functional MR should be medically optimized regarding blood pressure, volume, heart rate, and heart rhythm, prior to final determination of MR. This patient should be treated with guideline-directed medical therapy for heart failure and then repeat a TTE.

Chapter 6:

1) D. All of the above.
2) B. Reversal of systolic pulmonary venous inflow is an important qualitative parameter suggestive of severe MR but is not a parameter used to assess anatomic feasibility. Multiple parameters may be used to determine anatomic feasibility for TEER devices. These include: location of the primary MR jet or leaflet abnormality, coaptation depth, coaptation length, coaptation (or flail) gap, and malcoaptation width.

In addition, the presence of clefts or deep folds, multiple prolapsing segments or MR jets, very large coaptation gaps or widths, calcification or marked restriction of leaflet mobility, and small mitral orifice areas may all reduce the chances of an optimal TEER result. Leaflet lengths will also determine the feasibility of TEER device stability and depending on the device, greater than 7 to 10 mm of leaflet length may be required.

Chapter 7:

1) C. Mid-esophageal mitral commissural view is the best view to assess the entire coaptation line and individual MR jets along the coaptation. All other views on the list represent a single cut across the coaptation.
2) C. Short posterior leaflets (<7 mm), rheumatic valves, large flail gaps (loss of secondary support), and small mitral valve area are examples of unfavorable features for TEER.
3) E. Iatrogenic mitral stenosis is one of the serious potential complications of TEER. After successful grasp, adequacy of the residual mitral inflow should be carefully assessed—before deploying the device—to exclude pathologic stenosis. In addition to Doppler interrogation, 3D multiplanar reconstruction and planimetry allow a relatively flow-independent assessment of the residual mitral valve area. Successful TEER reduces MR to ≤2+; therefore, there is no need to reposition or place additional devices in this case given only trace residual MR.

Chapter 8:

1) E
2) A
3) A and C

Chapter 9:

1) E
2) A

Chapter 10:

1) C
2) C
3) C

Chapter 11:

1) B. Transthoracic echocardiography. The patient has a physical exam which is concerning for volume overload and complains of dyspnea on exertion. She has a history of moderate mitral regurgitation with no previous echo documented in the vignette. Therefore, it would be best to start with a noninvasive test like a transthoracic echocardiography to assess LV function and valvular disease, such as mitral regurgitation suggested by the murmur documented on exam. A transesophageal echocardiography is too invasive as the first test and can be performed after transthoracic echocardiography to further define the etiology of mitral regurgitation if needed. Right heart catheterization is also too invasive as the first step and there is nothing on exam to suggest cardiogenic shock. A CT pulmonary embolism is not the next best step as patient has a low Wells score and the more likely diagnosis is cardiac in etiology. Left heart catheterization is also too invasive of a first test given patient is not having active chest pain, ECG shows no changes, and troponin is not significantly elevated.
2) B. Lasix. She has a new reduced ejection fraction and severe mitral regurgitation with poor coaptation of the leaflets. The physical exam and echocardiogram are also consistent with volume overload and patient is complaining of dyspnea on exertion. We should therefore start diuretics for initial relief to see the patient's response and potentially improve the severity of MR. By decreasing volume, we could decrease the left ventricular end-diastolic volume thus having better approximation of the mitral valve leaflets. Afterload reduction with enalapril and nitroglycerine is not the best first step given the need to reduce volume first, but certainly afterload reduction will be an important step. She does not have evidence of cardiogenic shock therefore milrinone is not indicated. Norepinephrine also not needed given patient is hemodynamically stable.
3) D. Switch enalapril to sacubitril-valsartan. This patient is currently being treated with diuretics and improved. She has adequate heart rate control with metoprolol succinate which like carvedilol is an evidence-based beta-blocker for reduced ejection fraction. Secondary mitral regurgitation can respond to afterload reduction and evidence-based therapies for reduced ejection fraction. Sacubitril-valsartan had superior outcomes to enalapril in the PARADIGM-HF trial and reduced mitral regurgitation more than valsartan alone as described earlier. Ivabradine is not indicated as first line therapy, nor indicated with her current heart rate of 68 beats per minute as well as only indicated for patients in sinus rhythm. Although she certainly may need mitral valve intervention, it is not the best next step.
4) A. Add empagliflozin. Although she is improved, she is not back to baseline and not necessarily full optimized from a medication standpoint either. Spironolactone could be a reasonable next step were it not for her elevated potassium. Resynchronization therapy is not clearly indicated for a QRS duration of 124 ms and right bundle branch block, nor has she had 3 months of maximal medical therapy. Therefore, it is also premature to check an echocardiogram which ultimately will help us know if a defibrillator or mitral valve surgical intervention is indicated.
5) B. Repeat echocardiogram. Digoxin has not shown a survival benefit for heart failure with reduced ejection fraction, and her heart rate is well controlled on metoprolol. Although she still has functional limitations, she does not have New York Heart Association Class IV symptoms to warrant home inotropes. At this point, the most reasonable next step is an echocardiogram for which mitral valve intervention would be warranted if mitral valve regurgitation is still sufficiently severe.

Chapter 12:

1) B. The ECG shows atrial standstill with a junctional escape at 55 bpm. This patient is otherwise stable and not requiring

hemodynamic support. There is no way to tell from this ECG if AV conduction is compromised. The use of dobutamine may increase junctional automaticity and therefore increase the rate, but may not speed up the sinus node, which is currently suppressed. If we pace the atrium at a slightly faster rate, we can assess AV conduction and if present, can increase the heart rate without the added wall stress and potential pro-arrhythmia of IV chronotropic agents. Temporary RV or permanent dual-chamber pacing are not indicated at this point.

2) C. This patient has long-standing persistent atrial fibrillation that is associated with suppression of sinus node function. The sinus node dysfunction is likely exacerbated by amiodarone and beta blockade. While stopping the medications may improve the sinus node function, it also markedly increases the chances of early return to atrial fibrillation, which would defeat the purpose of the ablation. Dobutamine may have a similar effect. By gradually decreasing the rate of pacing over a period of 5 minutes or more, the sinus node will be given more of a chance to recover and may be able to take over as the dominant pacemaker.

3) B. The entity of malignant mitral valve prolapse is not well understood and recommendations regarding ICD implant do not exist. While it is likely that surgical repair decreases the risk of sudden cardiac arrest, this theory has not been validated with any large trial. This patient survived VF arrest and has an indication for an ICD. The wearable vest defibrillator would not be appropriate in this case. This patient is suitable for either a subcutaneous ICD or an intravascular ICD, however he does not have an indication for an atrial lead, so dual-chamber ICD is not the best answer.

Chapter 13:

1) Sternotomy: Opening of the left pleura to allow the apex of the heart to drop into the left pleural space and retracting pericardial sutures placed at the level of the SVC, IVC, and PV.
2) The Cor-Knot device decreases cardiopulmonary bypass and total operative time, and the MICS instruments facilitate mitral repair or replacement for all approaches.
3) Aortic Insufficiency

Chapter 14:

1) D
2) D

Chapter 15:

1) B
2) A
3) C

Chapter 16:

1) C. Cardiac MRI is not required as part of the standard work-up for right thoracotomy mitral valve surgery.

2) B. Moderate obstructive lung disease is not prohibitive to right thoracotomy mitral valve surgery as the period of required single-lung ventilation is relatively short and can be accomplished with intervening periods of dual-lung ventilation. These patients are, however, at greater risk of requiring sternotomy should single-lung ventilation result in significant or persistent hypoxia or hypercarbia.

3) D. Ultrasonic debridement of a calcified mitral annulus is possible through a right thoracotomy approach. SITRAL mitral valve replacement is also possible.

4) C. In cases of small or severely diseased femoral arterial disease, right axillary arterial cannulation is possible. In instances where femoral arterial access is not utilized, percutaneous femoral venous cannulation is possible and avoids an additional incision. Although single venous cannulation can be performed, our preference is double venous cannulation to mimic cannulation strategies in open surgery.

5) A. Closure of the root vent after initiation of antegrade cardioplegia allows for de-airing of the aortic root and avoids air embolism to the coronary arteries.

Chapter 17:

1) A
2) B
3) A and B

Chapter 18:

A) Incorrect. Although a preoperative TEE can be very helpful in planning a repair strategy, it rarely demonstrates a valve pathology that would be a contraindication for a robotic approach. A stress test can be helpful in determining the presence of myocardial ischemia but does not rule in or out the need for concomitant coronary revascularization, which may contraindicate a robotic approach.

B) Incorrect. A right heart catheterization can determine the cardiac output and the volume status of the patient. It can be useful for a strategy of preoperative optimization. This is key to successful outcomes in all mitral valve procedures but is not unique to robotic mitral valve surgery. Pulmonary function testing in a patient without a history of significant lung disease is unlikely to change the planned approach to mitral valve surgery.

C) Correct. Coronary angiography can determine the need for coronary artery bypass in addition to the planned mitral valve repair. The requirement for concomitant revascularization is a contraindication for the robotic approach. CT angiography of the chest, abdomen, and pelvis is necessary for the planning of any approach that involves peripheral institution of cardiopulmonary bypass, including the robotic surgery. The presence of significant aortoiliac, peripheral arterial, or ascending aortic pathology is a contraindication to robotic mitral valve surgery.

D) Incorrect. Cardiac MRI can determine ventricular volumes and degree of regurgitation in patients with left ventricular dilation and severe mitral regurgitation demonstrated on transthoracic echo. It is unlikely that the additional information obtained from a cardiac MRI will change the planned surgery. Long-term cardiac monitoring may reveal the presence of episodes of atrial fibrillation. That finding may be an indication for an addition of an atrial ablation procedure. The need for this additional procedure is not a contraindication to robotic mitral valve surgery.

Chapter 19:

1) D
2) A
3) E
4) C
5) B

Chapter 20:

1) C
2) A
3) G
4) A

Chapter 21:

1) C. Does the patient have medical insurance?
2) A. Isolated mitral valve regurgitation with pathology limited to the posterior leaflet.
3) D. Primary mitral regurgitation due to posterior leaflet prolapse.

Chapter 22:

1) B
2) A
3) D
4) True
5) A

Chapter 23:

1) A
2) C
3) C
4) A
5) A

Chapter 24:

1) C. In TMVR, the native mitral leaflets are not removed. The anterior leaflet along with the valve strut/stent can protrude into the LVOT resulting in a smaller "neo" LVOT after valve implantation. Thus, TMVR is generally contraindicated in patients with small LV cavity or LVOT obstruction at baseline. A calculated neo LVOT of less than 150 mm^2 is generally considered not feasible.
2) C. This patient likely has history of mitral valve prolapse and is now presenting with a flail leaflet. Patients with simple posterior flail or prolapse should be considered for surgical repair as success rate is over 95%.
3) B. While expected to grow, the only current FDA approved indication for TMVR is valve in valve for a failing prosthetic valve.

Chapter 25:

1) B. Urgent TEE needs to be performed to evaluate the etiology of severe MR and the anatomy of the mitral valve.
2) A. TEE showed severe primary MR due to ruptured posterior mitral valve leaflet chordae. The jet is eccentric and is anterolaterally directed. The medial portion of the P2 scallop is flail with visible ruptured chordae. This extends to P3. The flail gap is large (approximately 1.5 cm), with a large flail width (approximately 1.9 cm).
3) D. A heart team approach involving a dedicated multidisciplinary team of interventional cardiologists, cardiac imagers, heart failure specialists, and cardiac surgeons should be incorporated in the evaluation and management decisions of complex cases with unfavorable anatomy for percutaneous interventions and/or high surgical risks.
4) B. Key features for suitable anatomy for TEER in the presence of a flail leaflet are flail width less than 15 mm, flail gap less than 10 mm, and mitral valve area greater than 4.0 cm^2. Flail width of 1.9 cm is large and considered unfavorable.

Chapter 26:

1) A
2) F
3) C
4) F

Chapter 27:

1) B
2) D
3) D

Chapter 28:

1) A
2) A
3) F

Chapter 29:

1) Answers should include surgical expertise, transthoracic and transesophageal echocardiography, computerized tomography (CT), and cardiac magnetic resonance imaging (CMR); interventional cardiologists; advanced practice providers and nurse navigator(s); research; functional heart team; marketing; quality oversight; institutional support.
2) Answer is an open-ended response.

INDEX

Page numbers followed by '*f*' indicate figures, '*t*' indicate tables, '*b*' indicate boxes, and 'e' indicate online content.